DIAGNOSIS OF SPEECH
AND LANGUAGE DISORDERS

DIAGNOSIS OF SPEECH AND LANGUAGE DISORDERS

James E. Nation, Ph.D.

Department of Speech Communication,
Case Western Reserve University,
Cleveland, Ohio

Dorothy M. Aram, Ph.D.

Department of Speech Communication,
Case Western Reserve University,
Cleveland, Ohio

Illustrated

THE C. V. MOSBY COMPANY

Saint Louis   1977

Library of Congress Cataloging in Publication Data

Nation, James E   1933-
    Diagnosis of speech and language disorders.

    Bibliography: p.
    Includes index.
    1. Communicative disorders—Diagnosis. I. Aram,
Dorothy M., 1942-   joint author. II. Title.
RC423.N25   616.8'55'075   76-28212
ISBN 0-8016-3631-0

GW/CB/B 9 8 7 6 5 4 3 2 1

To
students everywhere—for they are
the teachers of teachers

For
Brian and Bethany

Preface

Diagnosis of speech and language disorders is a professional skill. The basic goals of the diagnostician are to discover the client's speech or language problem, understand the potential causes of the problem, and propose appropriate management recommendations. To accomplish these goals the speech pathologist must have a basic fund of knowledge concerning normal and disordered speech and language, organize this information into a conceptual framework for easy retrieval, and understand the methodology necessary for solving the speech and language problem. Therefore diagnosis is a far different skill than just learning a series of testing procedures applicable to specific speech and language disorders, that is, tests for articulation disorders, voice disorders, stuttering, language disorders, and so forth.

The study of speech and language disorders is a field of inquiry within the realm of the behavioral sciences. As a behavioral science, a logical approach to diagnosis is available—the method of science. Scientific method as adapted to the clinical process should be the diagnostician's major tool. This approach can demonstrate a more unified ordering of information to students. They can acquire knowledge within a conceptual framework, behavior can be studied within this framework, advances in knowledge can be made, and arbitrary distinctions such as scientist and clinician can be broken down. The scientific orientation to diagnosis allows students to pursue diagnosis as a problem-solving process with the goal of understanding the nature, extent, and consequences of speech and language disorders.

The fundamental purpose of this text is to demonstrate how the method of science can be applied to the diagnostic process. What we feel students need is an organized framework for learning, recalling, and using information vital to the diagnostic process. Therefore the intent of this book is to present a conceptual framework for organizing the information needed by the diagnostician and a scientific methodology that demonstrates how this framework can be applied to the individual diagnosis.

The book is designed to teach an approach to diagnosis, not specific content about speech and language disorders or tests used in the diagnostic process. The emphasis is placed on how knowledge is acquired and used and how we must continue to expand on the information we need rather than on the learning of specific content. Throughout the text many projects and study questions are developed to assist students in thinking through their approach to diagnosis or problem solving.

Part I of the book presents the viewpoint that diagnosis is a professional skill requiring the acquisition of a fund of knowledge. To this end we define and delimit the problem area by ordering our fund of knowledge into an overall frame of reference about speech and language disorders within the context of normal human communication and its development. This framework is made up of a composite of what is known and what is theorized. We develop the diagnostician's funds of knowledge around a model called the speech and language processing model. The model emphasizes both speech and language behavior as well as the underlying physical processes by which language is received, comprehended, formulated, and produced. The components of the model are developed in some detail to demonstrate how information can be organized for retrieval and use.

Part II of the book contains a series of chapters that demonstrate specifically and systematically how the steps of the scientific method can be applied to the diagnostic process. Specific assignments that apply to each of the steps of the scientific method as related to diagnostic problems are designed. We demonstrate how students can retrieve information from their fund of knowledge and expand on it when attempting to define and delimit the clinical problem under consideration. We discuss how diagnostic hypotheses can be formulated, and we follow this with a discussion on the selection of tools to test these hypotheses. We then go on to discuss general and specific procedures for administering testing tools, how to analyze and synthesize the information obtained in order to make decisions as to whether a problem exists, and what should be done about it. We also consider report writing as a means of communicating the information obtained in the diagnosis, emphasizing that reports can also reflect the scientific method.

We believe the orientation considered in this book allows speech pathologists to approach diagnosis as an ongoing process of hypothesis formulation and testing, utilizing and expanding on the knowledge and theories we have about human communication and its disorders. This orientation should allow speech pathologists to feel more comfortable in approaching any diagnostic problem that may be presented. It should allow for flexibility and change rather than a static testing procedure approach, since the primary emphasis is placed on problem solving rather than on a series of tests for specific disorders.

Diagnosis of Speech and Language Disorders can serve as a textbook in courses at both the graduate and undergraduate levels. The student using this book should possess fundamental information in the areas of the normal human communication process, language acquisition and usage, child growth and development, and various speech and language disorders and their causes.

Many people are involved in preparing a textbook. To each person who has assisted we offer our thanks. Special acknowledgment and appreciation is expressed to Amy Lipkowitz, Robert Oberstar, Janet Whitney, and Ellen Wicker. Also, we are grateful to Dr. Genevieve Arnold, Professor of Speech Pathology at the University of Houston, for her helpful review of the final manuscript.

In the interest of simplicity and clarity, the diagnostician is referred to as "he" throughout the text. Since no singular pronoun aptly includes both sexes, this can be subtly downgrading to female diagnosticians. We wish to assure them that this was not our intent.

James E. Nation

Dorothy M. Aram

CONTENTS

Part I

A FRAME OF REFERENCE

Diagnosis as a professional activity

CHARACTERISTICS OF THE PROFESSIONAL

Diagnosis of speech and language disorders is a major professional activity of the speech pathologist. The speech pathologist applies his knowledge and diagnostic expertise to the speech and language problems presented by his clients. As a diagnostician, the speech pathologist is a professional who (1) possesses a fund of knowledge relevant to speech and language disorders, (2) is skilled in applying this knowledge to solving clinical problems, and (3) has an overriding concern in helping a person, his client, understand and manage his speech or language problem. These three characteristics—a fund of knowledge, a problem-solving skill, and client concern—are fundamental to the diagnostician's professional service.

Fund of knowledge

A profession is generally defined as a vocation based on specialized knowledge in some area of learning or science. To diagnose disordered speech and language the diagnostician requires specialized knowledge of the following:

1. Normal speech and language development and use
2. Variations and disorders of speech and language
3. Causal factors that disrupt normal speech and language
4. Various management alternatives

While relevant information comes from our study of the communication sciences, other important information comes from diverse areas, including, among others, the biological and physical sciences, linguistics, psychology, sociology, medicine, and education. Because the study of disordered speech and language is so multidisciplinary, one of the chief problems facing the diagnostician is drawing together all this information into an organizational framework that is readily usable for addressing clinical problems. Learning to become a diagnostician, therefore, is not simply a matter of learning a body of knowledge or course content. Developing a frame of reference for his fund of knowledge and making it readily applicable to clinical problems are equally, if not more, important to the diagnostician. Two notable implications follow from this orientation.

First, an organizational framework for funds of knowledge should not be directed to specific "problem types." The professional diagnostician is not a preprogrammed technician with certain information for certain conditions. Rather the professional's approach toward organizing knowledge should be integrative and not simply segmented or departmentalized into knowledge about voice disorders, stuttering, aphasia, autism, etc. The diagnostician must arrive at a framework that is equally appropriate to whatever speech and language behavior his client may present. Before he sees his new client, the diagnostician often does not know what "problem type" to expect. Even when he anticipates a certain pattern of behavior, the diagnostician is often surprised to find that what he expected did not turn out to be the primary disorder. For example, a child with a cleft palate may not experience significant difficulty in the peripheral production of speech, but he may experience difficulty in language formulation or perhaps he may even stutter. Therefore the diagnostician needs a superordinate view of speech and language processing and its disorders that allows him to flexibly shift gears and relate his fund of knowledge to whatever behavior occurs.

Second, our orientation implies that diagnoses are arrived at through application of this broad base of acquired knowledge. The diagnostic process stems from a culmination and integration of past experience and learning and may be viewed as the pinnacle of professional activity.

Although a diagnostician may have his current information organized for application, it should be understood that his frame of reference must allow for continued acquisition of knowledge. The diagnostician must realize that his present knowledge does not necessarily represent reality accurately. Instead, it only represents his understanding of his experiences and the available information at any given time.

The diagnostician keeps in mind that much of what is "known" may be theoretical. Additional knowledge not only will be forthcoming and acquired, but current information may change over time. The professional is committed to developing broad, solid funds of knowledge, while at the same time realizing the incompleteness and tentativeness of the knowledge he uses at any given time. It is vital that the diagnostician maintains an inquisitive, searching attitude toward knowledge acquisition that leads to a revitalization and a reevaluation of acquired information. He must keep current in his profession.

We have now stated that one characteristic of the diagnostician as a professional is his area of expertise, a fund of knowledge pertaining to normal and disordered speech and language that is organized into a frame of reference for clinical utility and professional expansion. We now turn to a consideration of the second characteristic of the diagnostician: a problem-solving skill.

Problem-solving skill

The diagnostician's primary professional activity is his problem-solving skill. He not only has an organized data base from which to work, but, equally important, he is skilled in a scientific method of using this knowledge to answer clinical questions. The professional diagnostician does not arrive at clinical solutions purely by intuition; rather, he approaches clinical problems through a systematic, explicit methodology based on his reasoning and training as a behavioral scientist. As a behavioral scientist, the diagnostician states cause-effect hypotheses pertaining to each client that he sees; he develops procedures for testing his clinical hypotheses; and he collects, analyzes, interprets, and generalizes from his clinical data.

The chief point to be made here is that diagnosis is something other than just testing or learning specified test procedures for a specific disorder. The diagnostician is a problem solver, a decision maker, not a technician or a "prescription filler." He carries with him a scientific methodology that allows him to systematically utilize his fund of knowledge in addressing the clinical problems presented to him. His scientific method organizes and guides his clinical work. While he may artfully employ procedures and relate to his clients, he has little use for "cookbook" approaches to diagnosis in which one routinely and invariably administers a set battery of tests for a given disorder. Rather, he approaches each diagnosis as a creative problem-solving activity that follows positively from a scientific methodology. Therefore, if confronted with symptomatology that does not fit a particular condition, he has a rational approach for studying the presented behavior. Similarly, he can readily assimilate new tests and testing procedures into his overall approach to diagnosis.

With the problem-solving methodology provided by his scientific orientation, the diagnostician is able to employ his professional judgment, discretion, and knowledge in tailor making each diagnosis. He is better able to efficiently and competently evaluate each client's unique speech and language disorder. As he continues to solve clinical questions with the scientific method, he learns more, he adds more information to his fund of knowledge, and his problem-solving abilities become more finely tuned.

Basic then to the development of a professional diagnostician is his utilization of a problem-solving methodology. A speech pathologist with a high level of knowledge but no approach to problem solving is not a diagnostician. Occasionally, we encounter very knowledgeable speech pathologists who have little ability to relate their knowledge to clients' problems. Because their knowledge is not available for clinical problem solving, these individuals, in our minds, are not diagnosticians.

We now turn to the third and final characteristic of the professional diagnostician: client concern.

Client concern

The diagnostician's ultimate professional concern is with the client he serves. Whatever we do as diagnosticians, we must acknowledge the wants and needs of the person who comes to us. Unless the diagnostic process benefits the client and addresses his needs, the activity becomes a sterile, academic exercise with little professional involvement. However, benefit to the client does not necessarily imply direct speech therapy. The diagnostician should be accountable for helping his client understand his speech and language disorder, its possible causes, and its prognosis as well as plan for appropriate future management of the problem when needed. Even if therapy or referral is not indicated, the diagnostician has added to his client's understanding of and future orientation to his problem.

The diagnostician must also know how and why the client was motivated to seek help. Does he come on his own volition, in agreement with the recommendation of another, or is he brought passively or actively against his will by a dutiful parent or spouse? The reality is that diagnosticians sometimes see people who do not want to be seen; for example, the preadolescent stutterer who does not take responsibility for his stuttering or cannot admit to having a problem or the aphasic who is so depressed about his total physical condition that he cannot accept the proddings of his spouse. These nonvoluntary clients should make us evaluate client concern carefully. To whom are we responsible? Is it always the client, or in some instances is it to an interested relative or professional?

Above all, the professional diagnostician must consider the client as a person with feelings, needs, and abilities beyond just the speech and language problem. It is the client who has the problem, not the problem that has the client. The diagnostician is the client's consultant in understanding that problem. His orientation should therefore be toward diagnosing a human being with a speech and language problem, not merely adding to his own sophistication and experience in recognizing and understanding disordered speech and language. If he has merely treated the client as a "problem type" to which he administers x number of tests, the diagnostician has failed to see the client as an individual and thereby neglects to meet an essential characteristic of his professional responsibility. Diagnosticians have not fulfilled their ethical contract with their client if they have not addressed *his* questions and provided as best they can for *his* needs.

THE DIAGNOSTICIAN'S JOB

We have presented an orientation to the organized fund of knowledge, the problem-solving skill, and the client concern that characterize the diagnostician as a professional. But what constitutes a diagnosis? We turn now to a discussion of the meaning and goals of diagnosis. We will first present our viewpoint and then relate our use of the term "diagnosis" to how others have viewed it and related terms.

A viewpoint

As viewed here, the diagnostician's job is to fulfill three purposes or goals. Incorporating his fund of knowledge with the method of science, the diagnostician addresses these three goals.

First, he focuses on the presented speech and language behavior to determine if the speech and language characteristics are disordered. Second, he wants to understand how that behavior came to be, that is, to understand what causal factors may be related to the behavior. Third, he utilizes the information gathered to decide what, if anything, to do with the client—client management.

Determining the speech and language variation/disorder

The first goal of diagnosis is to describe the client's speech and language behavior with particular emphasis on areas of greatest variation. This phase can be relatively objective, the primary interest being in gaining a detailed description of the variations of speech and language behavior presented. For example, if Amy is thought to have a generalized language disorder, a thorough specification of her language behavior would be in order. In addition, the diagnostician might note other aspects of Amy's speech such as voice and rhythm, although a detailed description of these may not be indicated.

After the speech and language variation has been described, the diagnostician's task is to judge if the observed variation is normal or disordered. He allows that speech and language behavior exhibits a range of acceptable variability. What he needs to determine is whether the given variation falls within or outside of this normal range. If the specific behavior departs far enough from what is accepted as normal, he then has identified a speech or language disorder. The diagnostician arrives at his determination that a disorder exists by comparing the observed speech and language behavior to normative data and acceptability criteria—all a part of the diagnostician's fund of knowledge. For example, 5-year-old Janet who only speaks in single-word utterances is clearly outside the range of normal syntactic expectancies.

Finally, through a comparison of the obtained behavioral variation with the diagnostician's known standard, a statement regarding the severity of the disorder may also be achieved. Thus, all other factors being equal, 2-year-old Ellen, demonstrating a total spoken vocabulary of 10 words, would not be judged to have as severe a language disorder as 4-year-old Sandra demonstrating the same behavior. While it is recognized that there is a considerable range in the ages at which children acquire certain features of their language, the competent diagnostician can arrive at a judgment of severity (1) by comparing the obtained behavior to normative data, (2) by noting the pattern of deviation, and (3) by referring to his own knowledge of the sequence of normal acquisition and usage when specific normative data is not available.

In determining the nature and extent of the speech and language disorder then, the diagnostician does three things. He describes the particular speech and language variation, he evaluates if the variation constitutes a disorder, and he judges the severity of the disorder.

Understanding causal factors

The second goal of diagnosis is to arrive at an understanding of causal factors that account for the presenting speech and language disorder. What does gaining such an understanding do for the diagnostician? Identifying causal factors allows him to have a better understanding of the nature of the speech and language disorder, its severity, and the prognosis. It also raises considerations for client management and serves as a guide to therapeutic intervention. For example, Robert's sibilant distortions may be caused by a malocclusion, an inability to hear or discriminate the appropriate sounds, a deviant model presented by his father, or a variety of other reasons. The approach to changing the distorted sounds would vary depending on the identified causal factors. The fact that Mr. Weiss' profound language problem resulted from a cerebrovascular accident (CVA) 5 years earlier has quite clear implications for prognosis. Learning that Margaret's hypernasality is due to lack of velopharyngeal closure raises the consideration of referral for surgical procedures. Innumerable examples can demonstrate that subsequent decisions and actions taken by the diagnostician rest on an understanding of causal factors.

When investigating causal factors, the diagnostician should not expect to identify a single cause for a given effect. Even in the physical sciences, one-to-one cause-effect relationships are difficult to demonstrate. When dealing with human behavior, the one-to-one relationship between a cause and an effect is even more tenuous. Rather, the diagnostician looks at multiple causation and interaction among numerous potential causal factors. He is not attempting to identify *the cause* but rather to suggest *probable causal relationships*. In approaching his search for causal factors, the diagnostician views causation in two ways.

First, he may search for *historical causal factors*, that is, past events that may have contributed to the current disorder. In this case he studies information about the client's past history.

Second, he investigates *contemporary causal factors*, that is, events that are currently operating to account for, perpetuate, or maintain the speech and language disorder.

Contemporary factors may include *extrinsic* situations that presently contribute to the disorder, for example, limited language stimulation from the immediate environment. In addition, contemporary causal factors may be viewed as internal processing deviations that are *intrinsic* to the client. For example, an auditory discrimination problem that is a processing deviation can be viewed as a contemporary causal factor contributing to or maintaining a client's disordered speech. Conditions that originally occurred in the past but are currently operating, sometimes referred to as maintaining causes, may be viewed as both historical and contemporary. While it is desirable to have an understanding of both historical and contemporary causation, many times historical causation is unknown or speculative. The more immediate contemporary disruptions in processing are more available for evaluation, more readily understood, and often serve as the basis for remediation.

Although at times the diagnostician may not be able to arrive at definitive causal factors, it is our contention that an attempt toward understanding causation is an indispensable goal of a complete diagnosis. Thus understanding causal factors, that is, searching for historical, contemporary, and multicausal factors that potentially contributed to and currently maintain the speech and language disorder, is the second major goal of the diagnostician.

Proposing client management

The final goal of diagnosis is to determine client management. As previously discussed, a fundamental characteristic of the diagnostician is client concern. The major reason for delineating speech and language disorders and understanding causal factors is to arrive at a plan of action for the client.

Before the diagnostician can proceed in making plans for client management, he must assess whether or not the speech and language variation/disorder constitutes *a problem for the client*. Here the diagnostician must use his professional judgment in evaluating the client and his speech and language behavior within the client's interpersonal, multisensory, and sociocultural contexts—his *multidimensional environmental context*. For example, Jim claims he is a stutterer; however, his speech does not evidence a deviant fluency pattern to the diagnostician. What appears "normal" from an observable viewpoint is not normal to the client. Thus, even if Jim's speech behavior is not considered variant to the diagnostician, Jim may still have a "speech" problem because of his own perceptions and feelings about his speech. Similarly, 4-year-old Philip's sound variations may be judged as a normal developmental variation by the diagnostician. If this evaluation is accepted by Philip's parents and significant others in his environment, the normal sound variation probably will not present a problem. However, if the parents or others do not regard the behavior as normal, a problem may exist. On the other hand, a foreign-born speaker of English may talk with a foreign accent, which, while at variance with standard English, may not present a problem for the speaker or his listeners. Similarly, a person judged by his listeners as having a strident voice quality may not consider his voice quality a problem.

The diagnostician may rely heavily on the client's verbal report of his feelings and attitudes about his speech and language, but he also gains information from observing the effect of the speech and language variation on the client and his listeners. The client's verbal statement may or may not coincide with the diagnostician's observations, which again calls for professional judgment by the diagnostician in evaluating if a "real" speech and language problem exists. Essentially, what we are proposing is that on identification of a speech and language variation/disorder, the diagnostician has to integrate the behavior into a broader context if he is to determine whether a problem exists for his client.

After establishing that a disorder constitutes a problem for the client, the diagnostician then develops a plan of action for him

—client management. This goal incorporates any further steps that are to be taken, including recommendations for speech and language therapy, educational placement, medical referrals, and psychological evaluations, among others. At times, no further plans are indicated. A consideration of client management should include a statement of probable prognosis given that the various management alternatives are carried out. Prognostic statements will weigh the nature and severity of the disorder, the causal factors, and the personal characteristics of the client such as age, motivation, and intelligence.

Other views of diagnosis and related terms

We have now presented the particular viewpoint toward diagnosis that is used in this book and will be expanded on in subsequent chapters. We do not wish to imply that all persons in speech pathology use the term "diagnosis" in the same sense as we do. Many writers have chosen other words to refer to the total activity we call diagnosis. Rather than assuming that everyone means the same thing by these words we will discuss our understanding of these related terms.

A medical heritage

The term "diagnosis" has a medical orientation: to determine by physical examination and laboratory tests the nature of a disease condition. The medical model generally implied that the symptoms and observable signs were not the underlying cause. Rather than deal with symptomatology, the focus in medicine generally has been an attempt to identify and treat the cause of a given condition. A number of writers in speech pathology use the word "diagnosis" in the medical sense and suggest that diagnosis should remain within the domain of the physician. Perkins writes:

Where assessment is the province of the speech pathologist, diagnosis is accomplished by the physician. The speech pathologist seeks to understand the disabilities that produce and maintain the speech disorder. The physician seeks the etiology of these disabilities. He seeks diseases and lesions that disable functions of the apparatus required for speech. The speech pathologist can often aid in this task. . . . Because the speech pathologist is interested in the biologic correlates of these skills, he may study them anatomically and physiologically. He may, if asked, be able to venture an informed opinion about the neurologic, laryngeal, respiratory, or orofacial conditon of a speech-handicapped patient. But if he is not asked, he will be well advised to limit his contributions to diagnosis to a report of information about which he has special competence: speech behavior. To venture unsolicited observations about the physical status of a patient can be construed by a physician as a novice telling a professional about his own specialty.*

Since the medical use of diagnosis focuses on underlying causation, other behavioral scientists also suggest that the term "diagnosis" is not appropriate for those who primarily want to describe and understand behavior (Palmer, 1970).

Despite these views, the term "diagnosis" has a long tradition in speech pathology. The primary texts to date in this aspect of speech pathology use the term "diagnosis" and support the causal implications it implies (Darley, 1964; Emerick and Hatten, 1974; Johnson et al., 1963). The activity engaged in is called diagnosis or diagnostics. Furthermore, Barnhart and Stein (1957) give an alternative dictionary definition of diagnosis: "a scientific determination, a description which classifies precisely, any analogous examination or analysis."

Aside from the tradition of common usage, we consider the term "diagnosis" to hold significant professional implications for speech pathologists. As specialists trained in describing and understanding speech and language disorders, their causes, and management procedures, speech pathologists rightfully should be in the most knowledgeable position to diagnose speech and language disorders. While we do not presume to make *medical diagnoses,* it is our position that because of his professional knowledge the speech pathologist takes a major role in searching for

and identifying probable causal factors. He should not be merely a passive recipient of medical diagnoses.

There are numerous instances in which speech pathologists as diagnosticians and physicians as diagnosticians work hand in hand to arrive at a determination of causal factors. In many situations the boundaries between the speech pathologist and physician are blurred in determining causal factors—active cooperation rather than abrogation should be the role of each. For example, a speech pathologist observing a client with a nasal voice quality, who fails to produce stops and fricatives and whose velum does not appear to make contact with the pharyngeal walls, may suggest that palatal insufficiency could be a primary cause of the observed speech variations. Depending on his work setting, the speech pathologist may refer the client to a physician for further evaluation that employs the use of more sophisticated cineradiographic techniques. Or the speech pathologist may be in a position to both perform and evaluate the cineradiographic studies as they relate to his client's speech and language disorder.

Knowing how certain medical conditions affect speech and language keeps the diagnostician aware that underlying the speech and language disorder being diagnosed there may be an undiagnosed medical condition requiring attention. Therefore referrals are made to physicians with clear statements as to the diagnostician's suspicions about medical conditions. For example, if he saw a client with a speech pattern characteristic of some form of dysarthria, he would certainly refer the client to a physician (neurologist), providing him with any information known about the relationship of the client's speech pattern to certain neurologic diseases. Or, in the case of a hypernasal client, if the examination of the velopharyngeal musculature along with the speech pattern led the diagnostician to suspect palatal paralysis or a submucous cleft of the palate, he would again refer to the appropriate physician

---

*From Perkins, W. H., *Speech Pathology: An Applied Behavioral Science*. St. Louis: The C. V. Mosby Co., 345-346 (1971).

with clear statements of his suspicions of the underlying physical condition.

It is the diagnostician's professional responsibility to communicate causal concerns to the physician; however, he must refrain from discussing them as if he had made a medical diagnosis. His job is to understand the onset and development of a speech and language disorder: How it came to be? What caused it? Some of the causal factors are medical, some are psychological, some are emotional, and some are unknown. In doing his job, the diagnostician must know his professional boundaries and how to relate to and work with other specialties that interact with his. Speech pathologists make speech and language diagnoses and not medical diagnoses, psychological diagnoses, psychiatric diagnoses, educational diagnoses, dental diagnoses, or neurologic diagnoses—nor should these other specialties make speech and language diagnoses. Each specialty uses information from other specialties to understand its own diagnostic concerns. Therefore to us there is a major difference between making a *medical diagnosis* (establishing the presence of and reasons for a condition, a disease, or other abnormality of structure and function in the individual) and making a *speech and language diagnosis* (analyzing, interpreting, and establishing causal relationships for observed speech and language disorders).

Comparison to similar terms

Numerous terms other than diagnosis have been used by writers in speech pathology to refer to the activity engaged in when determining the status of a given client. Words such as testing, examination, appraisal, evaluation, and assessment exist in the literature and are sometimes used interchangeably. While these words are often introduced within a textbook with little discussion as to their implication, we would like to point out some distinctions and make explicit our use of diagnosis as it relates to these terms.

Testing. While testing can refer to a form of data collection or one aspect of a more complete diagnosis, the term has come to suggest the routine administration of a test or battery of tests. Frequently the connotation is that few selective decisions have been made prior to testing and that this activity results in a test score with little or no interpretation of the test performance. Often testing has been used in a pejorative sense, as when a diagnostician denies being a "test giver."

Testing as a form of data collection is, in our view, both a part of determining the client's speech and language variation as well as understanding causal factors. Testing elicits data that allows the diagnostician to describe the presented speech and language variation and to some extent determine if it is disordered. Testing also aids in the understanding of causal factors, as when the results of audiometric testing reveal a hearing loss. Testing, to us, is the objective data-gathering level of diagnosis, allowing little role for the interpretive, evaluative aspects of a complete diagnosis. Thus we see testing as a limited part of diagnosis, contributing primarily to the goal of describing the speech and language variation and at times to the goal of understanding causal factors.

Examination. The term "examination" similarly has come to imply a systematic, although sometimes perfunctory, inventory of a client's behavior. As used by some writers, examination seems to carry a medical connotation and often is used to refer to physical inspection of the peripheral speech mechanism, or to determine auditory functioning. Examination, like testing, accounts for only a limited part of the total concept of diagnosis. While an examination may reveal information relevant to a description of the speech and language variation, most often examination implies inspection of the physical person rather than of his speech and language behavior per se. Such inspection provides information most directly pertinent to causal factors, particularly contemporary disruptions of speech and language processes. For example, an examination of tongue movement may reveal motor limitations contributing to faulty articulation.

Appraisal. As frequently used, appraisal also implies a certain routinization of activity. One author (Darley, 1964) sees appraisal as consisting of a series of steps that may be repeated over time to determine changes in the client's status. Appraisal is usually used to imply a description of particular behavior, frequently through noting strengths and weaknesses. The term seems to allow for some degree of interpretation by the diagnostician in determining what behaviors may be considered normal and disordered. Since appraisal encompasses interpretation, this term would be more inclusive than either testing or examination. Appraisal seems to parallel more completely our first goal of diagnosis, determining the speech and language variation/disorder. That is, appraisal provides not only a description of the variation but also interprets the gathered data to determine the presence of a speech and language disorder.

Evaluation. Evaluation as used by most writers incorporates both descriptive and interpretive functions. Behavior is described and then interpreted through reference to normative data and other client considerations. Although some writers (Palmer, 1970) suggest that evaluation carries a negative value judgment, for us this term again seems to refer most closely to our first goal of diagnosis, determining the characteristics of the speech and language variation/disorder.

Assessment. Assessment is the term chosen by several authors to imply a description of the nature, severity, and prognosis of the problem as well as a plan of remediation. We see assessment as including our goals of determining the speech and language disorder and proposing client management. What is lacking, usually through deliberate omission by some authors (Palmer, 1970; Perkins, 1977), is inclusion of probable causal factors. As stated, we feel all three goals should be addressed by speech pathologists during their diagnostic activity.

• • •

Thus we see testing, examination, appraisal, evaluation, and assessment as terms used to refer to only parts of the more total professional activity that we choose to term "diagnosis." Diagnosis not only represents the most complete meaning of the activity we intend to discuss but also carries the orientation to which we subscribe.

Setting, referral, and role modification

We have now discussed the professional characteristics of the diagnostician, presented the goals of the diagnostic process, and described various terms used to discuss the activities that make up diagnosis.

We have stated that the goals (purposes) of a complete diagnosis include evaluating the symptomatology, understanding causal factors, and determining client management. While we maintain that a professional diagnostician is capable of fulfilling all three goals of diagnosis, the three goals are not given equal attention or necessarily addressed in all practical diagnostic situations. We recognize that setting demands and referral requests require flexibility in the diagnostician's job focus.

Rather than promote different "types of diagnoses" such as the *survey, screening, appraisal,* and *etiologic* diagnoses as some authors do, we feel these "types of diagnoses" simply represent a *shift of focus* toward one of the three general goals of diagnosis. We do not believe that a change in the general orientation to diagnosis is needed but rather a shift of focus, adapting the diagnostic design to meet the specific purposes established by the setting or referral request.

As frequently happens, the referral statement can shift the focus of the diagnosis. For example, Mr. Kronenberg, an adult aphasic, is referred by a neurologist with the request that prognostic recommendations be given for language recovery. In this instance the primary speech and language disorder (aphasia) and causal factor (brain damage) are known. What is being requested is a determination of probable future language status of the client. While the diagnostician will have to further describe the nature and severity of the language disorder as well as look for other possible contributing causal considerations, as a consultant to the neurologist his major question to address, his diagnostic focus, would be client management. In other instances the diagnostician may focus primarily on a description of symptomatology or on underlying causal factors. Thus, while a diagnostician keeps in mind the three general goals of diagnosis, referral requests may focus his attention toward one primary goal of his diagnostic job.

Demands of a particular setting may also require a shift of diagnostic focus to one of the three stated goals of diagnosis. As discussed earlier, in some medical settings physicians and speech pathologists have joined forces to arrive at more exacting descriptions of the speech and language disorder, causal factors, and patient management. Darley (1973) has discussed the interdependent partnership between speech pathologists and neurologists in diagnosis and treatment of neurologic disorders. Settings such as Head Start and first-year education programs frequently wish to separate those children who have speech and language disorders from those who do not. Survey or screening procedures are frequently conducted in such settings to do this. The diagnostician's major focus is description of speech and language behavior for the purpose of locating problem cases.

Our profession also incorporates persons other than professional diagnosticians who may assume limited roles in the overall diagnosis of speech and language disorders. Students are trained to conduct all diagnostic functions; however, early in their training their main focus is to test for and describe speech and language behaviors or to administer certain tests that pertain to causal factors. While the student later in training tries out his interpretive and decision-making skills, the final responsibility for the diagnosis lies with the supervising professional.

In addition to the roles played by students, we often see nurses conducting hearing screening programs or administering other specific tests at the requests of physicians in a variety of health settings. Frequently, schools utilize parent volunteers to help administer routine tests. Paraprofessionals also perform designated tasks within speech and hearing agencies. In general these personnel are involved in administering a specific test for a specific reason. Their focus is generally on screening a large population or gaining specific, circumscribed information. Test interpretations are generally not part of their role. Rather, judgments and decisions are largely left to the speech pathologist, audiologist, or physician under whose direction they function. While these persons may be able to perform partial functions in the diagnosis, it is only the professional diagnostician who assumes full responsibility. It is the professional diagnostician who combines his knowledge and experience, his problem-solving skill, and his client concern for fulfilling all the diagnostic activities.

SUMMARY

Chapter 1 has presented the three goals that make up the diagnostician's job functions.

1. Determining the nature and severity of the speech and language disorder
2. Understanding historical and contemporary causal factors
3. Proposing appropriate client management

In order to perform his job functions the diagnostician must have three primary personal and professional characteristics.

1. An organized fund of knowledge and a frame of reference that are readily applied to the practicalities of diagnosis

2. A skilled problem-solving ability that stems from scientific methodology
3. Client concern as his ultimate professional responsibility

This chapter also considered the terminology used in our profession for describing the activities that go on during the diagnostic process as well as various shifts of focus required of the diagnostician because of work setting and referral considerations.

STUDY QUESTIONS

1. In this first chapter we described speech and language behavior in three ways: (1) as speech and language variations, (2) as speech and language disorders, and (3) as speech and language problems. The diagnostician's job is to view his client from these three perspectives. Compare other definitions of terms used to signify disordered speech and language with the three levels of description we discussed. See the contributions of Emerick and Hatten (1974), Leonard (1972), Ptacek (1970), and Van Riper (1972).
2. Schultz (1972, Chapter 1) considers the clinician as an information-processing system, making daily clinical decisions. What does he consider the primary sources of information available to the clinician for decision making?
3. Schultz (1972, Chapter 3) discusses the professional status sometimes accorded the diagnostician versus the therapist. React to Schultz's discussion.
4. Parents or children with speech and language disorders can be considered as part of the "client complex." Review Eisenstadt's (1972) points about weaknesses in client concern as evaluated by parents.
5. Schultz (1972, pp. 16-18) presents the complexities of decision making required of the clinician for performing screening procedures in a public school setting. Review these in relation to our concept of shifts of focus required of the diagnostician.
6. The student may be interested in pursuing the references in Chapter 1 to determine his reactions to our viewpoint regarding the meaning of diagnosis and the role of the diagnostician.

REFERENCES

Barnhart, G. L., and Stein, J. (Eds.), *The American College Dictionary*. New York: Random House, Inc. (1957).

Darley, F. L., *Diagnosis and Appraisal of Communication Disorders*. Englewood Cliffs, N.J.: Prentice-Hall, Inc. (1964).

Darley, F. L., Evaluation and management of neurogenic speech and language disorders: Interaction between neurology and speech pathology. Paper presented at the Annual Convention of the American Speech and Hearing Association, Detroit (1973).

Eisenstadt, A. A., Weakness in clinical procedures—A parental evaluation. *Asha*, **14,** 7-9 (1972).

Emerick, L. L., and Hatten, J. H., *Diagnosis and Evaluation in Speech Pathology*. Englewood Cliffs, N.J.: Prentice-Hall, Inc. (1974).

Johnson, W. J., Darley, F. L., and Spriestersbach, D. C., *Diagnostic Methods in Speech Pathology*. New York: Harper & Row, Publishers (1963).

Leonard, L. B., What is deviant language? *J. Speech Hearing Dis.,* **37,** 427-446 (1972).

Palmer, J. O., *The Psychological Assessment of Children*. New York: John Wiley & Sons, Inc. (1970).

Perkins, W. H., *Speech Pathology: An Applied Behavioral Science*. (2nd ed.) St. Louis: The C. V. Mosby Co. (1977).

Ptacek, P. H., The evaluative process in speech pathology. In J. Akin, A. Goldberg, G. Myer, and J. Stewart (Eds.), *Language Behavior: A Book of Readings in Communication*. The Hague: Mouton Publishers (1970).

Schultz, M. C., *An Analysis of Clinical Behavior in Speech and Hearing*. Englewood Cliffs, N.J.: Prentice-Hall, Inc. (1972).

Van Riper, C., *Speech Correction: Principles and Methods*. (5th ed.) Englewood Cliffs, N.J.: Prentice-Hall, Inc. (1972).

Chapter 2

Funds of knowledge: the diagnostician's data base

The diagnostician in practice and the student in training confront a wide range of speech and language disorders stemming from many possible causes and requiring countless management decisions. One day it may be a 4-year-old nonverbal child and the next an adult with a laryngectomy. The diagnostician must be prepared to work with many different types of clients. Only rarely will he work in a setting that specializes in a narrowly defined disorder, for example, in an aphasia rehabilitation unit. Also, the diagnostician is not likely to remain in the same professional setting throughout his career.

The first goal of this chapter is to outline the broad base of knowledge that the diagnostician must have to meet these circumstances, that is, to determine the speech and language disorder, understand causal factors, and recommend appropriate management plans for the wide range of clients he sees. The purpose is not to teach the content but to designate the funds of knowledge that must be acquired: the *diagnostician's data base*.

The second goal of this chapter is to help the diagnostician integrate this broad data base for clinical application. The data base is gained from a study of many areas related to the study of normal and disordered speech and language. It is not confined to *a discipline*, but draws from many disciplines—it is *interdisciplinary*. We will present the concept of theoretical models as a way of organizing and integrating the diagnostician's fund of knowledge: the *diagnostician's frame of reference*.

FUNDS OF KNOWLEDGE NEEDED BY THE DIAGNOSTICIAN

In order to accomplish his diagnostic goals the diagnostician must specifically study normal and disordered speech and language. The American Speech and Hearing Association *(Asha)* (1974) divides the academic information needed for professional certification into three broad areas.

1. Information that pertains to normal development and use of speech, language, and hearing
2. Information relative to communication disorders
3. Information and training in evaluation and management of speech, language, and hearing disorders

Asha explicitly has not stated specific course requirements; rather, it provides a description of the three areas of information needed.

While much of the information needed can be gained from study in our own discipline of speech pathology and speech and hearing sciences, for example, the work of Minifie et al. (1973) and Perkins (1977), the diagnostician also derives much information from other related disciplines. For example, *Asha* (1974) states that the required education in normal and disordered speech and language should be fulfilled within a larger general education framework with emphasis "in the areas of human psychology, sociology, psychological and physical development, the physical sciences (especially those that pertain to acoustic and biological phenomena) and human anatomy and physiology, including neuroanatomy and neurophysiology."

Thus the primary funds of knowledge needed by the diagnostician are about speech and language acquired within an interdisciplinary framework. We will now expand on the specific content needed. First, normal speech and language followed by a consideration of disordered speech and language will be discussed.

Normal speech and language

Knowledge of normal speech and language provides the diagnostician with a baseline needed for achieving the goals of diagnosis—for answering his clinical questions. (1) He determines if a speech and language disorder exists in reference to norms—knowledge of normal or expected behavior. (2) He identifies certain causal factors that may disrupt normal functioning from his knowledge of factors and determinants that contribute to normal speech and language development and use. (3) He develops a guide to client management from his knowledge of normalcy that establishes behavioral baselines toward which remedial efforts are directed. It is a truism that diagnosticians cannot understand or effectively work with disordered speech and language without firm roots in normal speech and language.

To look at normal speech and language, we have circumscribed four primary areas of needed information: language as a rule-based system, the normal speech and language user, speech and language development, and communicative interaction. Within each area we will briefly describe the needed information, the disciplines that provide the information, and the relevance of the information for the diagnostician.

Language as a rule-based system

Language, an ordered, predictable system for communication, can be abstracted from individual speakers and studied as an idealized system. Such study aims to describe language in and of itself and to present the rules that account for the creation of permissible language sequences. Students of language sometimes subdivide the language system into levels or parameters.

1. *Phonology,* which concerns the description of sounds in a language and the rules for ordering sound sequences
2. *Syntax,* which generally concerns word order and morphology
3. *Semantics,* which focuses on meaning
4. *Pragmatics,* which, as sometimes defined, attempts to understand the "rules" underlying the functional use of language

Linguistics has become the primary discipline devoted to the study of language as an idealized system. While writers have been intrigued with the study of language for hundreds of years, in the 1960's an outpouring of linguistic study and thought began with the advent of Chomsky's work (1957, 1965) in transformational-generative grammar. While differing approaches to the study of the language system have been presented such as descriptive linguistics (Francis, 1958; Gleason, 1961), stratificational grammar (Lamb, 1966), and case grammar (Fillmore, 1968), certainly Chomsky's influence has been a major force in accelerating the study of the structure of language.

With information for studying language as a rule-based system, the diagnostician is armed with an indispensable tool for clinical use. He may borrow the linguist's methods for describing, measuring, and understanding the language used by his clients (Compton, 1970; Menyuk, 1964; Morehead and Ingram, 1973). Linguistic description allows the diagnostician to capture on paper what his client is exhibiting.

How can the student diagnostician sort through the mass of information about language as a rule-based system that may be pertinent to his professional skill? Roberts (1964), Salus (1969), and Williams (1972) are helpful resources for organizing this information.

The normal speech and language user

The diagnostician needs knowledge about normal speech and language processes if he is to understand speech and language disorders. The focus here is on the normal person's ability to receive, comprehend, formulate, and produce speech and language—the human as a processing system.

The diagnostician needs knowledge of the biological, physiologic, and psychological requisites for speech and language. He needs information about human anatomy, especially concentrating on those structures involving hearing, understanding, and speaking. He also needs information about the psychological experience underlying and relating to speech and language. For example, when considering auditory reception, the diagnostician needs to know the anatomy and physiology of the hearing mechanism: its structure and function. He also has to understand the hearer's psychological response to sound and the role played by other psychological factors such as attention, motivation, and memory.

The biological sciences (including anatomy and physiology, neuroanatomy and neurophysiology, genetics, and embryology) have provided much information pertaining to the biological basis for speech and language. The speech and hearing sciences (speech perception, psychoacoustics, motor phonetics, etc.) have been central in accumulating and organizing pertinent anatomic and physiologic information as it relates to the study of speech reception and production. An understanding of the psychological dimensions of speech and language has been contributed to by a number of applied disciplines, including clinical neurology and psychology. In recent years the renewed vigor in the study of speech and language as a system has resulted in the emergence of new disciplines whose focal concern is with the normal speech and language user: psycholinguistics "wedded" the study of psychology and language; neuropsycholinguistics has come to refer to the interface between language behavior and its neuroanatomic basis.

Essentially the diagnostician's study of the normal speech and language user helps him understand why disorders do occur. For example, he may be able to relate an articulation disorder to a defective speech-producing mechanism as seen in a child with a cleft palate, or the language formulation disorder may be related to known left cerebral hemisphere damage. By understanding the relationship of anatomic, physiologic, and psychological factors to speech and language processing, the diagnostician can better determine the reasons for the speech and language symptoms presented by his client.

Several journals have come into being that emphasize this area: *Brain and Language, Cortex,* and the *Journal of Psycholinguistic Research.* In addition, Slobin (1971) and Williams (1972) provide readable introductions about the speech and language user.

Speech and language development

It is not enough for the diagnostician to acquire knowledge about speech and language as a fully developed system. Children begin the developmental process early in life, and the process continues throughout life. Speech and language disorders are seen at all ages, and diagnosticians must have an understanding of how the process develops and varies at different ages if they are to make appropriate comparisons of clients suspected of having speech and language disorders.

Knowledge related to child language development prior to the 1960's has been summarized by McCarthy (1954), including commentaries and criticisms. These earlier studies were primarily biographic and analytic, measuring quantitatively what a child did at a certain age in such areas as vocabulary development, sound development, sentence structure, and length of response.

Beginning in the late 1950's but with greater emphasis toward the late 1960's and early 1970's, a tremendous accumulation of language acquisition data resulted, corresponding to the outgrowth of theories regarding language as a rule-based system. New knowledge about speech and language development has come from many disciplines, including psycholinguistics, child psychology, education, and speech pathology.

From this outpouring of data new theories of speech and language acquisition are being proposed (Bloom, 1970; Clark, 1973; Schlesinger, 1971), and the developmental sequence of various parameters of language are being described in detail (Brown, 1973). Rather than striving for quantitative measures, the presumption is that each stage of development represents for the child his own rule-based system, which in some way reflects the adult system. In addition to the considerable attention now given to speech and language development per se, language acquisition is being more thoughtfully integrated with information about the child's physical, cognitive, and emotional development within his multidimensional environment.

Knowledge of normal speech and language development provides the diagnostician with a yardstick against which to judge the rate, sequence, and characteristics of the speech and language behavior presented by young clients, a yardstick that has great variability. Theories of acquisition provide insight into how and why the observed speech and language behavior may be disordered (Leonard, 1972; Menyuk, 1964; Morehead and Ingram, 1973; Sander, 1972), and descriptions of sequential development offer guides for remediation

(Lee, 1966, 1974; Miller and Yoder, 1974). Only by knowing what is expected in the way of speech and language during normal development can the diagnostician determine if a variation from normal constitutes a speech and language disorder.

The *Journal of Child Language* has been created expressly for the purpose of presenting information about child language. Additional references that summarize much of the work in language acquisition include Dale (1972), Hopper and Naremore (1973), Lee (1974), McNeill (1970), and Menyuk (1971).

Communicative interaction

Communicative interaction through creative speech and language use is unique to the human being. Speech and language as the primary means of human interaction can be considered as fulfilling the "human life-style." People talk to themselves and to one another to learn, impart information, control behavior, express anger, solve problems, fantasize, remember, reason, and persuade—the list is extensive and the categories are seldom mutually exclusive.

It is easy to see how the study of communicative interaction has become so multidimensional and interdisciplinary. Such diverse persons as business executives, psychologists, educators, philosophers, and health practitioners, among others, have all addressed communicative interaction, especially the problematic aspects. Academic areas such as speech communication, psycholinguistics, sociology, psychiatry, social psychology, and other "people-related" fields have all made contributions.

Because of this diversity of interest, we are often left with a fragmented framework. Mortensen (1972) has indicated that there may be as many definitions of communication as there are research interests about it. However, in his extensive work on communication as a study of human interaction, Mortensen (1972) provides us with a compelling organization. He sees human communication as made up of three interrelated systems: the *intrapersonal, inter-*

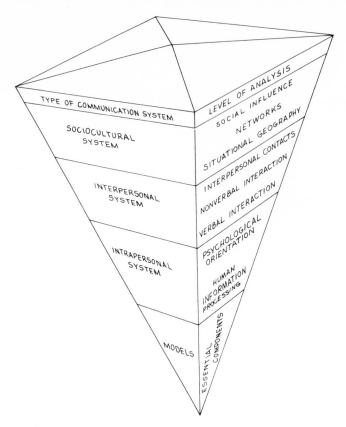

Fig. 2-1. Systems of human communication. The intrapersonal, interpersonal, and sociocultural systems of communication share certain essential components or common denominators. Each of the higher and successively more complex dimensions of behavior depends on the accumulative influence of the other systems and on their respective dimensions of activity. (From Mortensen, C. D., *Communication: The Study of Human Interaction.* New York: McGraw-Hill Book Co., [1972].)

personal, and *sociocultural.* Each of these systems shares essential components with the others within the overall human communication system (Fig. 2-1).

The use of speech and language in human communication forces the diagnostician to develop a broader perspective about speech and language. Apart from his focus on differentiating the disorders he hears, the diagnostician must evaluate how the disorder affects his client's overall communicative abilities (Siegel, 1967). For example, 42-year-old James who has an /s/ distortion may communicate effectively and be unconcerned about the distortion. If so, the diagnostician must question whether there is truly an interpersonal communication problem or if the speech disorder is merely an intrapersonal variation about which James has no concern.

Only when the diagnostician understands the effect any speech or language disorder has on communicative interaction will he have a true understanding of what constitutes a problem for the client and what needs to be done. We all know of people with "speech disorders" who feel no need to correct their disorder. Is it because they feel comfortable in interpersonal communication, or are they insensitive to their listeners, or do diagnosticians make too much out of some of the errors they hear?

For example, what is the difference between a speaker with a foreign dialect who is accepted readily by his listeners and considered to have a "charming" accent and the adult with an /r/ and /l/ distortion who may be spoken of as "that person who talks funny?"

In still broader perspective the diagnostician must understand how the speech and language disorder affects the overall psychological adjustment his clients make to their intrapersonal, interpersonal, and sociocultural worlds. Since speech and language are used for so many purposes, disorders frequently have significant effects on many areas of development and adjustment. For example, in the young child with a language disorder we may see significant subsequent effects on learning. The child who has no language because he is deaf also demonstrates this point clearly.

It is only when he understands the overall communication process as it relates to a specific language community with its personal, social, and cultural expectations that the diagnostician can place speech and language disorders into their appropriate contexts. His knowledge about communicative interaction gives him the broad perspective needed to interpret speech and language variations, disorders, and problems.

Summary

The diagnostician's funds of knowledge in normal speech and language behavior include four primary areas of information. (1) Understanding speech and language as a rule-based system offers a means of describing and ordering speech and language behavior. (2) Knowledge of the normal speech and language user allows understanding of speech and language processing within the normal individual. (3) Speech and language acquisition provides information for viewing normal changes in speech and language during growth and development. (4) Knowledge pertaining to communicative interaction places speech and language disorders within an intraper-

sonal, interpersonal, and sociocultural context to better appreciate the impact of the disorder on the person and his ability to communicate with others.

Disordered speech and language

While normal speech and language provide diagnosticians with a base for measuring and understanding disordered behavior, speech pathologists' unique area of expertise is their specific specialized knowledge about speech and language disorders. This knowledge equips them to fulfill the three purposes of diagnosis: determining the speech and language variation/disorder, understanding causal factors, and proposing client management. They therefore need detailed funds of knowledge related to each of these three goals of diagnosis.

Characteristics of speech and language disorders

To fulfill the first purpose of diagnosis, determining the speech and language variation/disorder, the diagnostician needs specific information about the symptoms and classifications used to describe speech and language disorders. When the behavior departs from normal expectations, the diagnostician has to know how to view, describe, and measure what he hears and sees. While, for example, his internalized normal standard may signal that a particular voice quality is not normal, he should have information that allows him to say more than "the voice quality is not normal." His detailed knowledge of voice disorders allows him to provide additional description and measurement of the behavior presented. He may study the client's voice range, listening for variations in quality as a function of pitch. He may have the client attempt different manners of voice production and note the effects on voice quality under each condition. The diagnostician's prior exposure to voice disorders allows him to descriptively classify the voice quality characteristics. In addition, he may wish to employ instrumental aids to provide objective study of the vocal tone. Thus what the diagnostician knows specifically about each speech and language disorder points the way for detailed analysis and description.

As specified by *Asha* (1974) certification requirements, speech pathologists must be trained in four primary disorder areas. These areas are disorders of *voice, fluency, articulation,* and *language.* Students are required to gain academic information and clinical practicum in each of these areas, usually through one or more courses, independent study, and clinical experience in each area.

Because of the emphasis placed on each disorder area, relating the disorders to each other has typically received less attention. The diagnostician is then left with a disjointed view of speech and language disorders. Often the student and professional diagnostician function as if they have mutually exclusive funds of knowledge for each disorder area rather than examining the relationships between, for example, articulation and language disorders. While it is essential to have information about specific speech and language disorders, it is equally essential to relate these areas to each other since the client may well present behaviors characteristic of more than a single disordered area.

Causal factors

To arrive at the second goal of diagnosis, understanding causal factors, the diagnos-tician must possess information pertinent to general and specific causes of speech and language disorders. He needs to gain knowledge about the intrinsic and extrinsic (biological-environmental) factors that may potentially affect the development and use of speech and language. He is interested in those physical, psychological, emotional, and environmental factors that may have a direct or indirect affect on the client's speech and language mechanisms and processes. For example, an amputated arm, although not directly needed for speech and language, may influence 2-year-old Bertheva's self-esteem, thus making her less outgoing and energized in attempting to communicate.

The diagnostician's fund of knowledge about causal factors should help him to:

1. Understand ways of categorizing causal factors that have a bearing on the speech and language disorder, information that helps him view and interpret various levels of causation
2. Gain a complete understanding of historical causal factors to assist in establishing how the present disorder came to be
3. Evaluate what interactions may have existed among multiple causal factors in the client's history to produce the disorder
4. Evaluate contemporary causal factors,

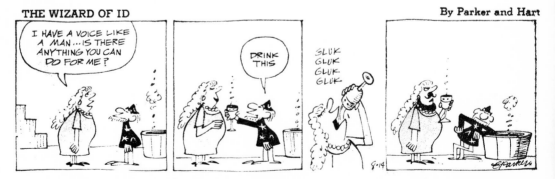

THE WIZARD OF ID By Parker and Hart

Fig. 2-2. Cause-effect relationship: a difference in judgment? (By permission of John Hart and Field Enterprises, Inc., August 14, 1974.)

as these are currently operating and may be more amenable to change

5. Identify probable cause-effect relationships in order to plan appropriate client management (Fig. 2-2)

In order to answer questions regarding causation, the diagnostician uses many sources. He considers his knowledge of normal speech and language development and use, emphasizing factors and determinants that could disrupt the process. Specific study of disordered speech and language provides considerable data about causation. As well, information that bears on questions of causation comes from disciplines outside speech pathology, including medicine, child growth and development, anatomy and physiology, psychology and psychiatry, and many others. With relevant information coming from many fields of study, cataloging potential causal factors has become significantly difficult for the diagnostician.

Client management

As previously discussed, the task of proposing client management includes determining if a disorder constitutes a problem for the client and, if so, recommending what to do about it. The diagnostician's data base in communicative interaction provides him with an intrapersonal, interpersonal, and sociocultural perspective from which to judge the importance of the disorder to both the client and others.

In addition the diagnostician must have specific knowledge regarding the range of management approaches needed for speech and language disorders. He must know when referrals are necessary to other professionals, what remedial programs (modes of therapy) are needed, and what effect the remedial program might have, that is, the skill of prognostication.

To make these decisions concerning client management, the diagnostician needs both theoretical and practical knowledge. He needs generalized information about what procedures and functions other professionals provide if he is to determine if a particular referral is indicated and appropriate. Practically, the diagnostician needs to know specific names of professionals and agencies that provide services in his community and how to go about obtaining that service. For example, on a theoretical level, a diagnostician may know that any one of a number of professionals can provide child guidance or psychotherapy; practically, however, the diagnostician has to know who is likely to accept the client within a reasonable period and at a manageable cost. In making recommendations for therapy programs, including speech therapy, the diagnostician must know the range of potential therapy alternatives and be aware of practical limitations in arranging for any of them.

Summary

The diagnostician's in-depth training comes from specialized study of the characteristics of speech and language disorders, causes of these disorders, and management considerations. The diagnostician must be able to relate all his areas of knowledge to specific clinical questions he may ask about a particular client. How can the speech and language disorder be described in detail? What may have caused the disorder? How did the disorder develop? What effects does the disorder have on the client's intrapersonal, interpersonal, and sociocultural life? What will be the best management of the disorder?

Once the diagnostician has gained a strong data base in both normal and disordered speech and language, he will be better equipped to answer these questions. He will be able to better understand that a speech and language variation, disorder, and problem are not one and the same.

The possession of this in-depth information helps the diagnostician meet the individual needs of the client, his ultimate concern. He is then able to make referral recommendations and to plan remedial programs, taking into account the symptoms, causes, and significance of the speech and language disorder.

ORGANIZATION OF THE DATA BASE

Having discussed the diagnostician's requisite funds of knowledge in normal and disordered speech and language, the task now is to organize this diverse information so that the diagnostician can use it. Not only has the relevant information come from multidisciplinary sources, but it also has arrived via different avenues. Research studies, clinical work, idiosyncratic observations, and "armchair philosophizing" all have been avenues for acquiring new information and developing new theories about normal and disordered speech and language. In short, the diagnostician has drawn from disparate disciplines and vantage points in his constant search for answers to problems presented by his clients.

Need for an organizing principle

Unless the data in the diagnostician's field of study is organized into a structured frame of reference, the information cannot be effectively applied to clinical problems. Bits of scattered data cannot be readily and selectively recalled. As a behavioral scientist and professional problem solver, the diagnostician must go beyond the "chunking," cataloging, and purely descriptive phases of scientific development. The diagnostician must organize and integrate the bits of knowledge into facts, inferences, hypotheses, theories, theoretical constructs, and conceptual frameworks in order to ask the most pertinent questions about speech and language disorders.

The problem facing the diagnostician is How can he organize and integrate the available information in such a way that is useful to him in pursuing the goals of diagnosis and allows him to assimilate, update, and discard information as he learns more about his discipline?

How has the field of speech pathology been organized and structured in the following major textbooks: Dickson (1974), Perkins (1977), and Van Riper (1972)? Is there a unifying theoretical position? A similar means of organization?

Models as organizing principles

Models offer a potentially useful organizing principle for the diagnostician's funds of knowledge. The use of models and schematic representations to portray and organize information has become prevalent in many disciplines. As well, speech pathology has been notable in using models to represent and relate various aspects of normal and disordered speech and language.

What follows now is a presentation of selected models to illustrate how they have been used to organize and integrate knowledge and to raise considerations for constructing a model for the diagnostician's purposes. Fig. 2-3 schematically represents our focus in the following discussion of models. We will start by looking at models of communication in their broadest sense, then restrict the scope somewhat to view models of human communication, and finally narrow our focus to models representing speech and language primarily as the auditory-oral system.

How have the terms communication, language, and speech been used? Can you accept any or all of the positions taken by various writers? Are the arguments purely semantic? Review the resources presented in this chapter. As well, consider the viewpoint presented by Cutting and Kavanagh (1975).

Communication models

Communication here is used in its most general sense to include all nonhuman and human means of transmitting and receiving messages. Models of communication in this broad scope take many forms, depending on whether they represent nonhuman communication systems, such as animal or computer communication, or human communication. Although many variations are in print, most communication models have four basic components in the complete process, as represented in Fig. 2-4: (1) a *sender,* presenter of a stimulus; (2) a *transmitting medium;* (3) a *receiver,* responder to the stimulus; and (4)

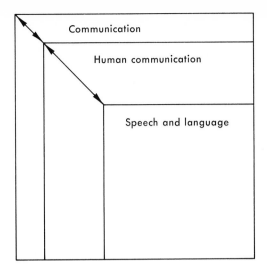

Fig. 2-3. Relationship between communication, human communication, and speech and language, focusing on speech and language.

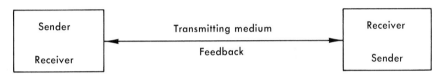

Fig. 2-4. The four basic components of the communication process.

a *feedback system* from receiver to sender, again through a transmitting medium. This model is general enough to represent virtually any communication system. For example, the model would be equally applicable to the Morse code, chimps' plastic token language, deaf sign language, or human speech. It is even applicable to computer communication, where computers are being designed to "talk" to one another and to "read human minds" (*Time Magazine,* July 1, 1974). The generalization of this model, however, is at the expense of explanatory power about the complexities occurring within any of the four components.

Human communication models

Models of human communication relate to all the means by which information is transmitted to and from one or more persons via various mediums. For example, people communicate with each other by sending telegrams, writing books and articles to be read, giving speeches, dancing, sending smoke signals, and gesturing with their hands and bodies. Numerous models have been developed to explain human communication.

Some human communication models *focus on communicative interaction.* An example of an interpersonal model of communication is one presented by Schein (1969) based on the Johari Window (Luft, 1961) (Fig. 2-5). The Johari Window hypothesizes that each person has several parts to himself. One part, represented by quadrant one, Open Self, includes those parts that the person is aware of and is willing to share with others. Quadrant two,

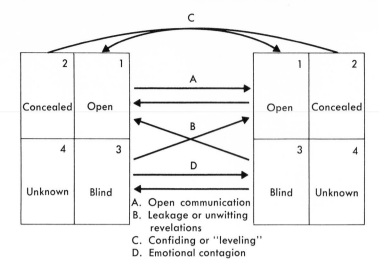

A. Open communication
B. Leakage or unwitting revelations
C. Confiding or "leveling"
D. Emotional contagion

Fig. 2-5. Types of messages in a two-person communication situation. (From Schein, E. H., *Process Consultation: Its Role in Organization Development.* Reading, Mass.: Addison-Wesley Publishing Co., Inc. [1969].)

Concealed Self, consists of aspects that the person is aware of but unwilling to share with others; therefore they are consciously concealed. Quadrant three, Blind Self, includes those aspects that the person is not aware of but that he communicates with others, for example, the mother who screams in a punctuated declaration, "I am *not* angry!" Quadrant four, Unknown Self, includes the aspects of the person that neither he nor others are aware of, for example, repressed feelings or undeveloped skills. Schein's (1969) model, then, illustrates the types of messages that occur when two people communicate, depending on the part of each involved in the communication.

How might a model like this be helpful in an interview with a client or his parents?

Other models emphasize the *multiple modalities through which people communicate*. Porch's model (1971) illustrates the multiple modalities of communication (Fig. 2-6). His model describes three input and output modalities of communication. Within the visual, auditory, and tactile input modalities, processes of reception, perception, and association occur, each process acting on the information in a specific way. The output modalities become functional when a decision has been made to respond, each process within the output modality performing a specific function on the message that is ultimately produced through the graphic, verbal, and gestural modalities.

Although Porch's model primarily reflects underlying speech and language processes, it highlights for the diagnostician the fact that human communication includes several modalities of "reception and expression" that can be integrated. Because of this process of modality integration, the diagnostician can present an auditory stimulus and ask for a written, oral, or gestural response. Each of the modalities of input can be related to each of the modalities of output, a concept of similar significance to the view of language processing held by Wepman et al. (1960).

Human communication models, therefore, are of interest to diagnosticians as they point up the various purposes and modes of human communication.

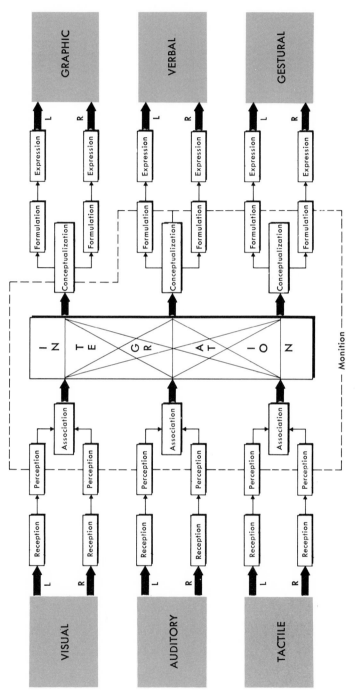

Fig. 2-6. A simple model of communication. (From Porch, B. E., *Porch Index of Communicative Ability: Administration, Scoring, and Interpretation.* [Vol. 2, Rev. ed.] Palo Alto, Calif.: Consulting Psychologist Press [1971].)

For further reading regarding human communication models see Mortensen (1972) and the delightful article by Harrison (1971) entitled "Other Ways of Packaging Information." Harrison demonstrates key points through interesting illustrations and models about the intrapersonal, interpersonal, and sociocultural aspects of human communication that would take thousands of words to say.

Speech and language models

Here we are treating language as an ordered system that associates sounds and meaning, with speech as the motoric production of language through the oral modality.

Speech and language models generally represent an idealized speech and language user, a person who sends and receives the spoken word. As such, these models have an intrapersonal focus; that is, they focus on the individual's processing of speech and language. Although reference to other language modalities frequently is made in many speech and language models (Fig. 2-6), our focus is on the auditory-oral (aural-oral) modalities. The following were selected as representative of several major approaches to modeling speech and language from the many models available. The models selected have been divided into those in which the primary focus is (1) the anatomic basis for speech and language, (2) the internal language processes, and (3) the interface between anatomy and language processing. A final model has been included for its importance in bringing to the diagnostician's awareness directly perceivable versus nondirectly perceivable speech events.

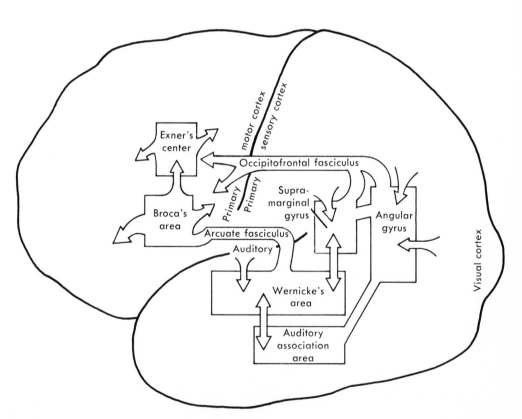

Fig. 2-7. Anatomic schematic and flow chart of central language mechanism. (Modified from Whitaker, H. A., Neurolinguistics. In W. O. Dingwall [Ed.], *A Survey of Linguistic Science*. College Park, Md.: Linguistic Program–University of Maryland [1971].)

Anatomic basis for speech and language. The anatomic basis for speech and language has been modeled in various degrees of specificity. For example, a rather specific model of the anatomic basis for speech and language has been presented by Whitaker (1971) (Fig. 2-7). His flow chart of the central language mechanisms suggests a number of central nervous system structures involved in language processing.

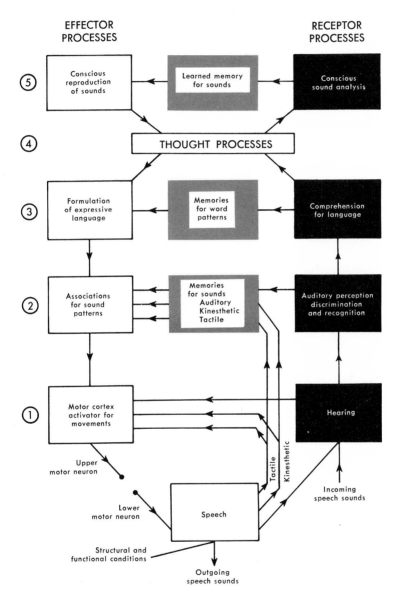

Fig. 2-8. Some processes involved in speech. Level 1: basic sensation and movements. Level 2: receptor-effector processes for articulate sounds. Basic articulation. Level 3: receptor-effector processes for integration of articulation with language. Level 4: mental processes associated with the reception and expression of thought through spoken language. Level 5: involves conscious sound analysis and synthesis. (From Morley, M. E., *The Development and Disorders of Speech in Childhood.* [3rd ed.] London: Churchill Livingstone [1972].)

Auditory information is received into this system at Wernicke's area, and oral information departs from Broca's area. These two major central nervous system structures separate for Whitaker the boundaries between the primary recognition and production systems and the central language system.

Anatomic models provide major assistance to the diagnostician for understanding the anatomic and processing basis for speech and language behavior, providing an essential foundation for the study of events that take place when a person uses language. They are particularly important for viewing and hypothesizing speech and language disorders resulting from damage or disruptions of the speech and language mechanisms at both the peripheral and central levels.

Internal speech and language processes. A number of writers have attempted to organize the internal language processes that operate between auditory input and oral output. Since these internal processes are generally inferred from observed behavior, they are basically hypothetical and are discussed differently depending on the writer's theoretical position.

A representative model of internal speech and language processes is that of Morley (1972) who presents five levels of processing (Fig. 2-8). She considers her diagram to be an illustration of the "receptive and expressive aspects of spoken language," deduced from her clinical experience with children demonstrating speech and language disorders. She discusses the processes that occur at each level of her diagram, from the basic sensation-movement processes to the mental processes for the reception and expression of speech through spoken language.

Some of the models we presented in earlier sections also incorporate internal processing concepts and can be viewed from this perspective as well as the focus in which they were presented. For the diagnostician, processing models along with anatomic models can be quite helpful for

inferring disrupted internal processes that might account for various types of speech and language disorders.

Anatomic and processing interface. For decades theorists and researchers have attempted to specify the speech and language processes that occur at various anatomic sites. For a period these "localizationists" were in disrepute, but the attempt to parallel language processes and anatomy has gained renewed respect. Models that attempt to explain this interface are among the more conceptual models of speech and language.

One such approach to modeling speech and language is that of Mysak (1966), whose central concern has been the development of a cybernetic analogue model for the "speech system." His two models presented here represent gross anatomic areas (Fig. 2-9) and the speech and language processing correlates for these areas (Fig. 2-10). His cybernetic analogue is made up of five units: the sensor, receptor, integrator, transmitter, and effector units. Each unit is discussed in terms of receiving, integrating, transmitting, or producing functions it performs while processing speech, emphasizing feedback and feedforward loops. Much of Mysak's emphasis in viewing speech within this servosystem framework is on the multiple channels, both internal and external, by which information is fed forward and backward in the system to provide control over speech and language processing. These feed-forward and feedback loops allow for monitoring, compensating, and correcting both the speech content and the speech product.

A schematic representation appearing in *Human Communication and Its Disorders: An Overview* (1969) conceptualizes the speech production process after the time the message has been formulated until it is realized as an acoustic response (Fig. 2-11). The diagram emphasizes the neuromuscular complexities of the speech production process as an interrelated yet sequential system requiring coordination of

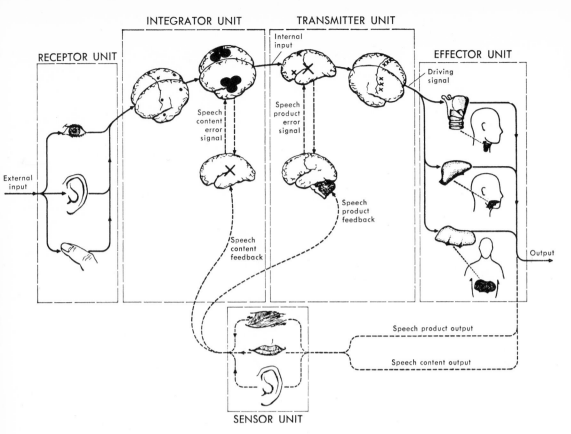

Fig. 2-9. Anatomic schema of the speech system. (From Mysak, E. D., *Speech Pathology and Feedback Theory.* Springfield, Ill.: Charles C Thomas, Publisher [1966].)

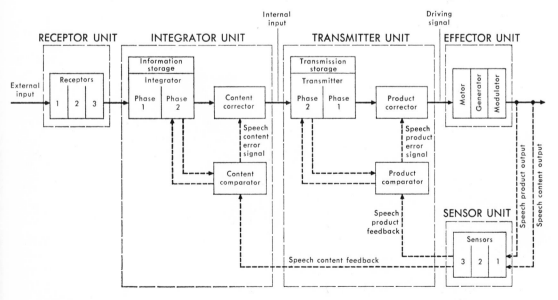

Fig. 2-10. Cybernetic analogue of the speech system. (From Mysak, E. D., *Speech Pathology and Feedback Theory.* Springfield, Ill.: Charles C Thomas, Publisher [1966].)

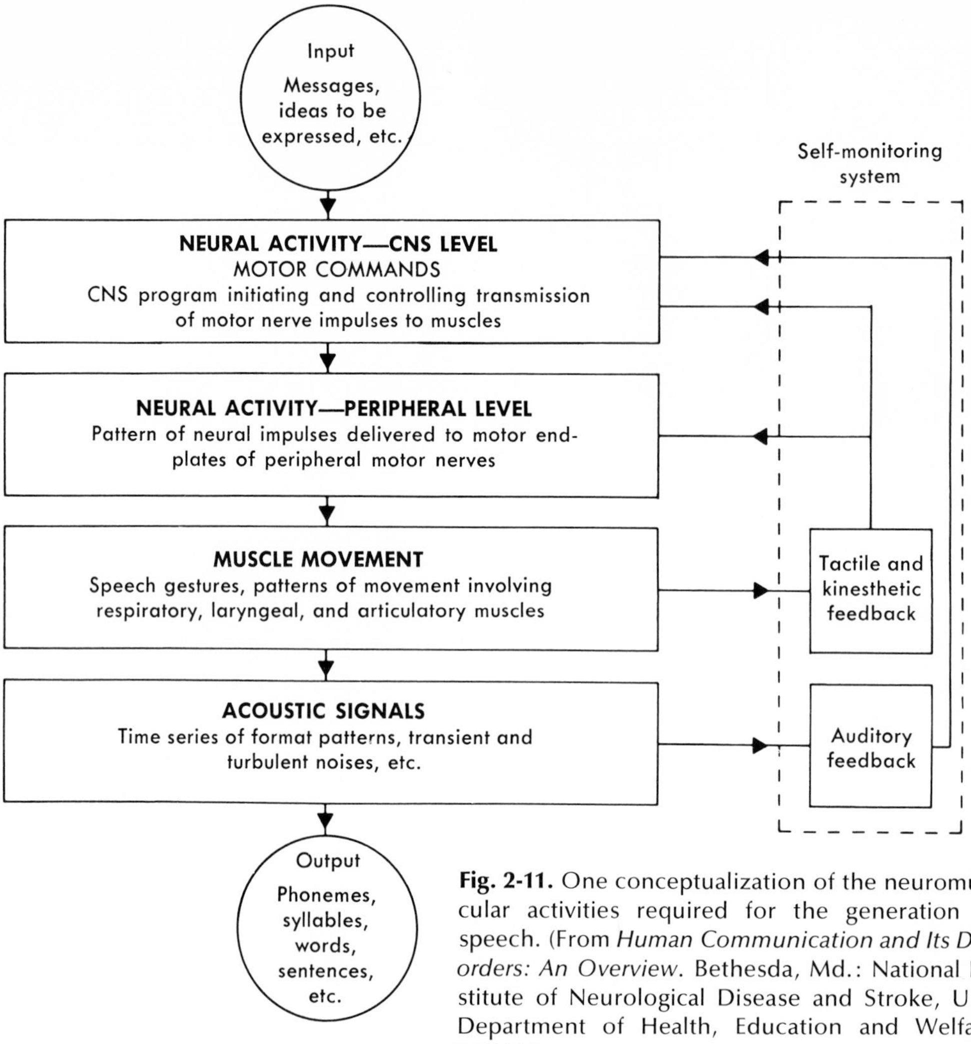

Fig. 2-11. One conceptualization of the neuromuscular activities required for the generation of speech. (From *Human Communication and Its Disorders: An Overview.* Bethesda, Md.: National Institute of Neurological Disease and Stroke, U.S. Department of Health, Education and Welfare [1969].)

all the levels. The diagram incorporates a self-monitoring system via auditory, tactile, and kinesthetic feedback loops that feed information back to the nervous system for monitoring and control of the physiologic events that take place in speech production.

Models attempting to specify the relationship between anatomy and physiology on the one hand and speech and language processing on the other offer the diagnostician a theoretical position for hypothesizing cause-effect relationships between physical causation, speech and language processing, and speech and language behavior.

We presented a schematic earlier by Whitaker (1971) as a representation of an anatomic model. This is only one of many developed by Whitaker (1970, 1971) in his comprehensive discussions of neurolinguistics. His articles are highly technical discussions of the relationship of speech and language to neural processing. We would suggest it for the reader who has a high level of interest in this subject matter.

Directly versus nondirectly perceivable speech events. Ptacek (1970) has presented a model focusing on what he calls stages

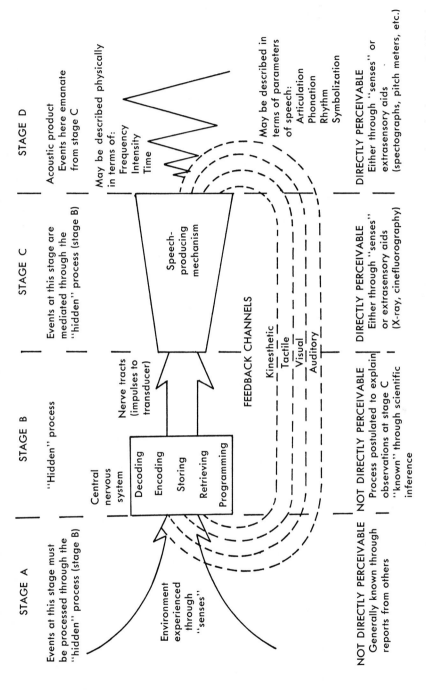

Fig. 2-12. Model of speech production. (From Ptacek, P. H., The evaluative process in speech pathology. In J. Akin, A. Goldberg, G. Myer, and J. Stewart [Eds.], *Language Behavior: A Book of Readings in Communication.* The Hague: Mouton Publishers [1970].)

in the speech production process (Fig. 2-12). At each stage of the process he considers how the diagnostician can obtain information about the processes and events involved, that is, how he comes to know the occurrences within each of the stages. Only at stages C and D does Ptacek feel the events are directly perceivable by an observer; whereas the events at stages A and B are not perceivable.

For the diagnostician the stages of the model express some of the important interrelationships and interactions between the environment and the human organism. The model assists the diagnostician in developing appropriate measurement strategies and techniques. At stage D he is given ways of directly measuring the acoustic product, either by measuring its physical components or by describing what Ptacek calls parameters of speech. At stage C he can take measures of the speech-producing mechanism either by direct observation and description or through the use of extrasensory aids. On the other hand, the model also helps the diagnostician focus on the inferences and hypotheses he develops about nonperceivable events on the basis of observable behavior. This is an extremely important concept for diagnosticians interested in determining cause-effect relationships in speech and language disorders.

As a project, compare and contrast the models presented here with any others you come across. Can you develop a comprehensive model of speech and language by abstracting from these models? Keep in mind that your model must be comprehensive yet simplified. Models as abstractions, by necessity, are simplifications of major concepts. Other suggested models are those of Adler (1964), Denes and Pinson (1963), Hardy cited in Hirsch (1966), McDonald (1964), Newman et al. (1973), and Wepman et al. (1960).

Models: cautions and considerations for the diagnostician

As we have pointed out, models of communication, human communication, and speech and language provide varying perspectives for the diagnostician in organizing his funds of knowledge. However, not all models are equally useful. What should the diagnostician keep in mind when he evaluates the usefulness of, or constructs models for diagnostic purposes?

The diagnostician must be cautious when attempting to apply models to diagnostic use. He must keep in mind that models are abstractions of complex behavior representing large chunks of data. The model maker assumes that the user brings knowledge to his model and therefore may have sacrificed one point in order to demonstrate what he thinks to be a more important point. The diagnostician must be aware that each model maker may feel his model best reflects reality, particularly since his model is based on his theoretical framework and conceptual organization. However, each model should be considered only as the "best thinking," the best representation of the model at the time the model maker presents it for view. Since models are abstractions of complex information, they should not be taken as either completely self-explanatory or as providing definitive answers to the theoretical issues in a given scientific field of inquiry. Just as in general semantics, "the map is not the territory," so also, the model is not the knowledge it represents.

Since not all models aid the diagnostician in the diagnostic process, we suggest seven considerations for critically evaluating a model's usefulness to the diagnostician for fulfilling the purposes of diagnosis.

1. *For a model to be maximally useful it should focus on speech and language.* While the broader context of communication, particularly human communication, is important, speech and language is the diagnostician's primary area of expertise. Because of this central interest, a model needs to allow for detailed specificity in organizing this most relevant fund of knowledge. If a model does not allow integration of considerable in-depth information related to speech and language, the

model may easily become superfluous, and the diagnostician will need to rely on alternate ways of integrating information. In other words, a diagnostician's model needs to organize as much of the most relevant knowledge he commands as possible or the model will not aid him.

2. *Since the auditory-oral modalities are the basic modalities of speech and language and the first to develop, these modalities may justifiably serve as the primary modalities explicated in a model.* This is not to say that a diagnostician does not need to maintain awareness of other modalities of input and output. Rather, it simply says that a detailed specification of information needs to be provided primarily for the auditory-oral modalities. While specifying the auditory-oral modalities will have the most specific application for the diagnostician, those working largely with special populations, such as the hearing impaired or adult aphasics, may also wish to have a general representation of other modalities in addition to the auditory-oral modality.

3. *A diagnostically useful model should carefully describe and delineate observable speech and language behavior.* The observed speech and language behavior needs to be dealt with in considerable specificity, not merely labeled output or speech and language behavior, which is the case in many models. The diagnostician in viewing the behavior presented to him needs a consistent framework that guides his observations and forces consideration of numerous observable parameters. A diagnostic model must provide for expansion of the observed speech and language characteristics.

4. *A model should allow for specification of the anatomy and "physiology" underlying language—the hypothesized internal language processes.* Much of a diagnostician's needed funds of knowledge concern the client's processing of speech and language; therefore a useful model must be able to expand on this crucial area.

5. *The diagnostic model should assist in developing the interface between the physical basis for language—anatomy and internal processing—and the observable speech and language behaviors.*

6. *The model should help the diagnostician understand causal factors and hypothesize cause-effect relationships.* Environmental input factors and the larger communication context need to be organized in addition to internal processing and observable speech and language parameters. Through representation of these three aspects the diagnostician can examine all potential causal factors and relationships. He can suggest relationships between input factors, internal processing, and observable speech and language. Such a model should aid the diagnostician in seeing, for example, that a client's observed pitch is related to laryngeal processes but may be related as well to input factors such as the pitch of another person who has a significant interpersonal relationship with the client.

7. *A diagnostician's model should help him develop ways of measuring speech and language disorders.* A model that contributes to maintaining an awareness of observable versus inferred behavior, factual versus theoretical information, helps the diagnostician in developing measurement strategies and in weighing the validity of the information obtained. For example, in diagnosing a stutterer's speech disorder, the diagnostician may decide to describe and measure the observed speech behavior or inferred processes. Measurement of observed behavior may give him data about the frequency, length, and contexts of repetitions and prolongations. The diagnostician might, however, hypothesize that the stutterer's nonfluencies are related to delayed auditory feedback processes and set out to measure and describe this inferred dimension. Given these two sets of information, one concerning observed behavior and the other inferred processes, the diagnostician must keep in mind the level of abstraction and inference in arriving at each.

Evaluate the models we have presented and any others in relationship to the seven critical considerations presented.

Summary of models as organizing principles for the diagnostician's data base

Models have served as a means of organizing and integrating information in many disciplines, including speech pathology. They provide a potentially useful frame of reference for the diagnostician's diverse data base. We have viewed illustrative models relating to communication, human communication, and speech and language. From these models we discussed seven considerations necessary for constructing and evaluating a model for diagnostic use.

REFERENCES

Adler, S., *The Non-verbal Child.* Springfield, Ill.: Charles C Thomas, Publisher (1964).

American Speech and Hearing Association, *1974 Directory.* Washington, D.C.: American Speech and Hearing Association (1974).

Bloom, L., *Language Development: Form and Function of Emerging Grammars.* Cambridge, Mass.: The M.I.T. Press (1970).

Brain and Language. New York: Academic Press, Inc.

Brown, R., *A First Language: The Early Stages.* Cambridge, Mass.: Harvard University Press (1973).

Chomsky, N., *Syntactic Structures.* The Hague: Mouton Publishers (1957).

Chomsky, N., *Aspects of the Theory of Syntax.* Cambridge, Mass.: The M.I.T. Press (1965).

Clark, E., What's in a word? On the child's acquisition of semantics in his first language. In T. E. Moore (Ed.), *Cognitive Development and the Acquisition of Language.* New York: Academic Press, Inc. (1973).

Compton, A. J., Generative studies of children's phonological disorders. *J. Speech Hearing Dis.,* **35,** 315-339 (1970).

Cortex. Varese, Italy: La Tipografica Varese.

Cutting, J. E., and Kavanagh, J. F., On the relationship of speech to language. *Asha,* **12,** 500-506 (1975).

Dale, P. S., *Language Development: Structure and Function.* Hinsdale, Ill.: Dryden Press (1972).

Denes, P., and Pinson, E., *The Speech Chain.* Murray Hill, N.J.: Bell Telephone Laboratories (1963).

Dickson, S. (Ed.), *Communication Disorders: Remedial Principles and Practices.* Glenview, Ill.: Scott, Foresman & Co. (1974).

Fillmore, C. J., The case for case. In E. Bach and R. J. Harms (Eds.), *Universals in Linguistic Theory.* New York: Holt, Rinehart & Winston, Inc. (1968).

Francis, W. N., *The Structure of American English.* New York: The Ronald Press Co. (1958).

Gleason, H. A., *An Introduction to Descriptive Linguistics.* (Rev. ed.) New York: Holt, Rinehart & Winston, Inc. (1961).

Harrison, R. P., Other ways of packaging information. In J. A. DeVito (Ed.), *Communication: Concepts and Processes.* Englewood Cliffs, N.J.: Prentice-Hall, Inc. (1971).

Hirsch, I. J., Audition in relation to perception of speech. In E. C. Carterette (Ed.), *Brain Function: Speech, Language, and Communication.* (Vol. 3) Berkeley, Calif.: University of California Press (1966).

Hopper, R., and Naremore, R., *Children's Speech: A Practical Introduction to Communication Development.* New York: Harper & Row, Publishers (1973).

Human Communication and Its Disorders: An Overview. Bethesda, Md.: National Institute of Neurological Disease and Stroke, U.S. Department of Health, Education and Welfare (1969).

J. Child Lang. London: Cambridge University Press.

J. Psycholing. Res. New York: Plenum Press.

Lamb, S. M., *Outline of Stratificational Grammar.* Washington, D.C.: Georgetown University Press (1966).

Lee, L. L., Developmental sentence types: A method for comparing normal and deviant syntactic development. *J. Speech Hearing Dis.,* **31,** 311-330 (1966).

Lee, L. L., *Developmental Sentence Analysis.* Evanston, Ill.: Northwestern University Press (1974).

Leonard, L. B., What is deviant language? *J. Speech Hearing Dis.,* **37,** 427-446 (1972).

Luft, J., The Johari window. *Hum. Rel. Trade News,* **5,** 6-7 (1961).

McCarthy, D., Language development in children. In L. Carmichael (Ed.), *Manual of Child Psychology.* New York: John Wiley & Sons, Inc. (1954).

McDonald, E. J., *Articulation Testing and Treatment: A Sensory-Motor Approach.* Pittsburgh: Stanwix House, Inc. (1964).

McNeill, D., *The Acquisition of Language: The Study of Developmental Psycholinguistics.* New York: Harper & Row, Publishers (1970).

Menyuk, P., Comparison of grammar of children with functionally deviant and normal speech. *J. Speech Hearing Res.,* **7,** 109-121 (1964).

Menyuk, P., *The Acquisition and Development of Language.* Englewood Cliffs, N.J.: Prentice-Hall, Inc. (1971).

Miller, J. F., and Yoder, D. E., An ontogenetic language teaching strategy for retarded children. In R. L. Schiefelbusch and L. L. Lloyd (Eds.), *Language Perspectives—Acquisition, Retardation, and Intervention.* Baltimore: University Park Press (1974).

Minifie, F., Hixon, T., and Williams, F., *Normal*

Aspects of Speech, Hearing, and Language. Englewood Cliffs, N.J.: Prentice-Hall, Inc. (1973).

Morehead, D. M., and Ingram, D., The development of base syntax in normal and linguistically deviant children. *J. Speech Hearing Res.,* **16,** 330-352 (1973).

Morley, M. E., *The Development and Disorders of Speech in Childhood.* (3rd ed.) London: Churchill Livingstone (1972).

Mortensen, C. D., *Communication: The Study of Human Interaction.* New York: McGraw-Hill Book Co. (1972).

Mysak, E. D., *Speech Pathology and Feedback Theory.* Springfield, Ill.: Charles C Thomas, Publisher (1966).

Newman, P. W., Low, G. M., Haws, R. J., and Bone, J. W., Communication, its disorders and professional implications. *Asha,* **15,** 290-292 (1973).

Perkins, W. H., *Speech Pathology: An Applied Behavioral Science.* (2nd ed.) St. Louis: The C. V. Mosby Co. (1977).

Porch, B. E., *Porch Index of Communicative Ability: Administration, Scoring and Interpretation.* (Vol. 2, Rev. ed.) Palo Alto, Calif.: Consulting Psychologists Press (1971).

Ptacek, P. H., The evaluative process in speech pathology. In J. Akin, A. Goldberg, G. Myer, and J. Stewart (Eds.), *Language Behavior: A Book of Readings in Communication.* The Hague: Mouton Publishers (1970).

Roberts, P., *English Syntax.* (Alternate edition) New York: Harcourt Brace Jovanovich, Inc. (1964).

Salus, P. H., *Linguistics.* Indianapolis: The Bobbs-Merrill Co., Inc. (1969).

Sander, E. K., When are sounds learned? *J. Speech Hearing Dis.,* **37,** 55-63 (1972).

Schein, E. H., *Process Consultation: Its Role in Organization Development.* Reading, Mass.: Addison-Wesley Publishing Co., Inc. (1969).

Schlesinger, I. M., Learning grammar: From pivot to realization rules. In R. Huxley and E. Ingram (Eds.), *Language Acquisition Models and Methods.* New York: Academic Press, Inc. (1971).

Siegel, G. M., Interpersonal approaches to the study of communication. *J. Speech Hearing Dis.,* **32,** 112-120 (1967).

Slobin, D. I., *Psycholinguistics.* Glenview, Ill.: Scott, Foresman & Co. (1971).

Time Magazine, Science: Mind reading computer (July 1, 1974).

Van Riper, C., *Speech Correction: Principles and Methods.* (5th ed.) Englewood Cliffs, N.J.: Prentice-Hall, Inc. (1972).

Wepman, J. M., Jones, L. V., Bock, R. D., and Van Pelt, D. V., Studies in aphasia: Background and theoretical formulations. *J. Speech Hearing Dis.,* **25,** 323-332 (1960).

Whitaker, H. A model for neurolinguistics. *Occasional papers 10,* Language Centre, Colchester, England: University of Essex (1970).

Whitaker, H. A., Neurolinguistics. In W. O. Dingwall (Ed.), *A Survey of Linguistic Science.* College Park, Md.: Linguistic program, University of Maryland (1971).

Williams, F., *Language and Speech: Introductory Perspectives.* Englewood Cliffs, N.J.: Prentice-Hall, Inc. (1972).

Chapter 3

The speech and language processing model: an introduction

In the behavioral sciences, theorizing and model making are tricky and hazardous endeavors. The determinants of human behavior, particularly species-specific language behavior, are extremely complex, poorly understood, and difficult or impossible to measure directly. In Chapter 2 we discussed seven important considerations for constructing a model as an organizing principle for use by the diagnostician. Focusing on these seven considerations the speech and language processing model (SLPM) was constructed specifically for application to the clinical process of diagnosis. It represents one way of conceptualizing the many different facets that make up the study of speech and language disorders, placing the client in a biological perspective. Our basic intent in this chapter is to introduce the reader to the concepts and terminology presented in the SLPM. Therefore we will not provide technical or detailed information now about the derivation of any specific component of the model. Instead, we want to first present an orientation to the SLPM as a framework for organizing normal and disordered speech and language and as a measurement framework for establishing cause-effect relationships.

FRAMEWORK FOR ORGANIZING NORMAL AND DISORDERED SPEECH AND LANGUAGE
Components of the speech and language processing model

The SLPM has been constructed with three major components that are schematically represented in Fig. 3-1.

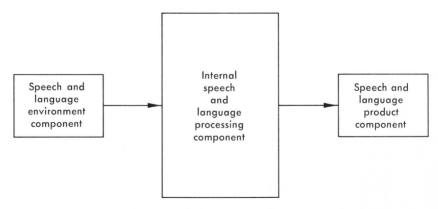

Fig. 3-1. Schematic of the three components of the speech and language processing model.

1. The *speech and language environment component* emphasizes those environmental events, either historical or immediate, that help explain the individual's current development and use of speech and language.
2. The *internal speech and language processing component* emphasizes a schema for understanding the underlying anatomy and processing events that occur when the individual uses speech and language.
3. The *speech and language product component* specifies the observable parameters of the speech and language behavior that result when an individual speaks.

Speech and language environment component

To learn and use speech and language the individual must be exposed to appropriate speech and language experiences over time, experiences gained within a broad environmental background. If the diagnostician is to understand speech and language disorders, he must consider his client as a biological being within this broad, complex environment. The SLPM assists in this task by viewing the environment in continued interaction with the individual speech and language user. The SLPM considers two major divisions of the speech and language environment component: the speech and language input and the multidimensional environmental context.

Speech and language input. The study of language acquisition has been central to understanding speech and language input. From his direct sensory experiences and interpersonal communicative interactions the child receives his primary speech and language stimulation (input) for processing. He, thereby, learns the language practices of those around him. To acquire a complete speech and language system the child must be exposed to all the parameters and levels of speech and language. He must have exposure to the *words, sentences, sounds,* *voice qualities, resonance patterns,* and *prosodic features* of those important people in his environment if he is to learn to communicate effectively. As well, he must learn the *communicative contexts* in which people use speech and language.

Evidence exists that demonstrates the dependency of the child's developing speech and language system on the speech and language input he receives. For example, one child may not have been exposed to much naming of objects and events in his environment, thus affecting his development of semantic categories. Another child, exposed primarily to dialectal speech, will be expected to deduce the rules of language based on this dialectal input; thus he too will speak with a dialectal pattern. Still, a third child may not be exposed to language as a form of information exchange and thus be limited in his pragmatic use of language.

Language acquisition is, of course, a major emphasis in the diagnostician's study of speech and language disorders; however, he must not lose sight of the relationship of input stimulation to language usage beyond the primary acquisition stage. After the primary speech and language system is learned, the language user continues to develop sophistication in speech and language use. Continued speech and language stimulation allows him to increase and change his vocabulary, develop greater command of syntax, learn to "speak" better, and develop the many "rules" of interpersonal communication.

Multidimensional environmental context. Besides the speech and language input that is available to the individual, there are other environmental factors to consider in language development and use. For example, factors such as family constellation, ethnic membership, birth order, etc. have been related to measures of children's speech and language. Perhaps every environmental variable is in some way relevant. Exactly how these environmental determinants should be discussed in relation to their influence on speech and language often is not clear. The literature cites numerous factors that at times have a high statistical correlation with certain measures of language; however, we generally do not know how these environmental factors influence the development or use of language. It is not easy to determine what relationship, if any, specified factors have to the onset, development, and use of speech and language. For example, how does a numerical figure reflecting socioeconomic status relate to an adult's restricted use of syntax or a child's limited vocabulary? As McCarthy (1954) indicated some time ago, we need explanatory concepts to assist in our interpretation of statistical correlations.

To understand disordered speech and language the diagnostician must bring order to the diversity of potential environmental determinants. To do this, we suggest that all environmental factors considered as determinants of speech and language learning and use be viewed in relationship to the parameters of speech and language input. The diagnostician must study how these multidimensional environmental factors might have affected the speech and language stimulation received by the client.

Measurement considerations. When the diagnostician attempts to discover information about the client's speech and language environment, he is primarily measuring information that is, at best, only *partially observable* to him. The speech and language stimulation the client received in the past cannot be observed directly by the diagnostician. Instead, measurements of this *historical speech and language environment* usually take the form of a report of past events. The diagnostician asks for information from various sources, be it from a parent, social worker, referring physician, or the client himself. The diagnostician must not confuse this information with direct observation of the environment, but rather he should take this information for what it is. It is partially observable information based on an informant's perception and recall of past events, not even necessarily the past as reality. The diagnostician can only assume that the informant has observed the historical speech and language environment. From the information he obtains about the historical speech and language environment the diagnostician can only draw inferences, that is, make interpretations about how the information obtained relates to the client's current speech and language disorder.

In addition to the historical speech and language environment the diagnostician himself creates an *immediate speech and language environment* through the tasks he presents and his own interpersonal characteristics. The diagnostician can *directly observe (control)* the immediate speech and language environment. That is, he can specify the speech and language stimulus, the sounds, words, and sentences he presents to the client to elicit certain responses. He also can control the context of the diagnostic setting, the room size, the clothes he wears, the objects and materials he uses, etc.

Through the use of the speech and language environment component of the SLPM, the diagnostician focuses on the speech and language input within the multidimensional environmental context. The diagnostician measures the partially observable historical environment and controls the observable immediate environment. From his observations he interprets the role the speech and language environment has played in the client's speech and language disorder. Chapter 4 will expand on the speech and language environment component of the SLPM.

Internal speech and language processing component

In Chapter 2 models were discussed exemplifying several perspectives on the anatomic and physiologic bases for speech and language, what we term the *physical basis* for speech and language. This physical basis for speech and language is highly complex (Berry, 1969) and little understood. However, to fulfill the purposes of diagnosis, the diagnostician must make an attempt to understand what intervenes between the speech and language input and output of his client. Environmental influences only account for some of the causal factors contributing to disordered speech and language. Disruptions of the physical basis for speech and language account for a large number, perhaps the largest number, of the speech and language disorders seen. Therefore, if the diagnostician is to understand disordered speech and language and its causes he must develop a schema that considers how the physical basis of speech and language relates to speech and language disorders. This schema must be open-ended, allowing for easy adaptation as knowledge accrues about the physical basis for speech and language.

The internal speech and language processing component of the SLPM presents a schema for viewing the physical basis for those events that occur within the human as he listens and speaks, a *schema for the auditory-verbal modality.*

Segments of the internal processing component. Our schema is based on the assumption that different internal processing events take place at different anatomic levels within the human being. As a primary example, we know that receptor organs are designed to respond to specific types of input stimulation; the ear receives auditory data, the eyes visual data, etc. We also know that certain structures are used to perform motor tasks; for example, the structures of the speech mechanism are used to speak. However, the motor systems do have greater flexibility than the sensory systems—the ears cannot see, but we can write with our feet, "talk" with our hands, and speak with a part of our digestive tract.

From this assumption we have divided the internal speech and language processing component into three segments. These three segments representing anatomic and processing boundaries are the *auditory re-*ception *segment, central language segment,* and *speech production segment.*

Anatomically, we are concerned with those primary structures by which speech and language are processed. Therefore, in general, the auditory reception segment is made up of the structures of the *auditory modality;* the central language segment is composed of those brain structures frequently called *central language mechanisms,* primarily located in the left cerebral hemisphere; the speech production segment is made up of those structures generally viewed as the *verbal modality,* the "motor" systems responsible for speech production.

Processing events occur within these anatomic boundaries. These *physical processes* receive and comprehend the speech and language input or formulate and produce speech and language responses. Different types of speech and language processes occur in the three segments.

The auditory reception and speech production segments are best considered as *modality specific*—the auditory input and the verbal output modalities by which language is received and produced. In this sense these two segments are differentiated from the processes within the central language segment, best considered as *nonmodality specific,* the segment where language is represented as a linguistic system.

Processing schema for the internal processing component. Having divided the internal speech and language processing component into three segments, we now further develop our schema for viewing the processes that take place within the segments. Our processing schema incorporates two major concepts.

First, our schema incorporates what we have termed *physical processes.* From our study of the anatomy and physiology of speech and language we have derived and named a series of physical processes within each segment of the internal processing component. These physical processes have been hypothesized to account for the events that take place internally when the individual uses speech and language. On the SLPM we have derived those processes that seem most reasonable based on our reading of the literature.

These physical processes for the most part are *not directly observable* to the diagnostician. They are processes that occur on an anatomic-physiologic basis; thus they are abstractions, conceptualizations from many ideas about the physical basis for speech and language. We have attempted to keep the specified processes clinically useful, those that we consider most helpful to the diagnostician in looking at underlying reasons for the speech and language disorders they observe. We are interested in a parsimonious, although theoretical, view of speech and language processing. Therefore on the SLPM we present a series of *nine primary physical processes*.

Second, our schema incorporates what we have termed *behavioral correlates*. Behavioral correlates are sets of behaviors *observable* to the diagnostician. From the client's behavioral responses to specified tasks the diagnostician gains information about the client's ability to process speech and language. Thus the behavioral corre-lates are viewed on the SLPM as the client's observable responses to tasks that are intended to "measure" the internal physical processes. It is the physical processes that give rise to the sets of behaviors measured as behavioral correlates. In our schema, behavioral correlates are considered as behavioral "stages" or "behavioral processes" reflective of the internal physical processes within each segment of the internal processing component. What we are calling behavioral correlates often have been called psychological processes. Each behavioral correlate presents different information to the diagnostician for observation. On the SLPM we present a series of *seven primary behavioral correlates*.

Table 1 demonstrates the relationship of the seven behavioral correlates to the nine physical processes within each segment of the internal speech and language processing component of the SLPM. The dotted lines represent the anatomic and processing overlap and exists among the segments.

A processing overview. In Chapter 5 we will expand on the meaning of each of the behavioral correlates and the physical processes. At this time, to demonstrate the re-

Table 1. Schema for internal speech and language processing component demonstrating how physical processes for speech and language give rise to a set of behavioral correlates within each segment of component

Segment	Physical processes	Behavioral correlates
Auditory reception segment	Auditory acceptance-transduction Auditory analysis-transmission Auditory reception-analysis	Sensation Perception
Central language segment	Auditory programming Language representation Speech programming	Comprehension Formulation Repetition
Speech production segment	Speech initiation Speech coordination-transmission Speech production	Sequencing Motor control

lationship between these two major concepts of the internal speech and language processing component, we will present a processing overview. Our intent in this processing overview is to provide a basic introduction to the terms and concepts presented. Table 1 should be followed in this discussion.

AUDITORY RECEPTION SEGMENT. The auditory reception segment is considered as a *primary recognition system*. The physical processes that take place here are referred to as *prelinguistic processes*, that is, analyses that take place before spoken messages can be understood.

When a speech stimulus enters the auditory reception segment (auditory modality), it undergoes a series of three auditory processes that perform prelinguistic analyses on the stimulus. These prelinguistic analyses occur as a result of the physical processes of (1) *auditory acceptance-transduction*, (2) *auditory analysis-transmission*, and (3) *auditory reception-analysis*. These processes give rise to the behavioral correlate of *sensation*. Diagnostic tasks performed here are generally concerned with the client's ability to hear, to detect the presence of sound, measured by many types of hearing tests.

Adding the physical process of (4) *auditory programming*, we would be able to measure a more complex behavioral correlate, that of *perception*. Perception refers to the ability to perceive, to auditorally realize, similarities and differences in the auditory stimulations. Again, the diagnostician uses tasks to measure aspects of the client's ability to "hear." Now, the tasks go beyond sensation and involve complex measurements of sound localization, discrimination, sound sequencing, auditory closure, etc.

CENTRAL LANGUAGE SEGMENT. The physical processes that take place within the central language segment are *linguistic processes*. They allow the individual to understand (decode) what he hears, to create (encode) messages to be spoken, and to repeat what he hears. Thus it is considered as the *linguistic system*.

In the central language segment the physical processes include (4) *auditory programming*, (5) *language representation*, and (6) *speech programming*. Note in Table 1 that auditory programming overlaps the auditory reception and the central language segments. The prelinguistic information processed within the auditory reception segment is first received in the central language segment. Once received, the three physical processes turn the data into representational, symbolic information. These linguistic processes act to program, integrate, retrieve, and store information in a representational form.

Language representation and auditory programming perform a series of linguistic analyses that finally allow the listener to derive meaning from the stimulus. These processes *decode* the words, sentences, and sounds that make up the received message. They give rise to the behavioral correlate of *comprehension*. Comprehension is here viewed as the listener's ability to make sense of the pragmatic, semantic, syntactic, and phonologic parameters of the message.

Disruption of any of these physical processes can have a direct effect on the client's ability to understand what has been said to him. The diagnostician uses many tasks to determine how well a client understands language. Most of the tasks focus on having the client follow spoken directions. Thus a client might be asked to point to a picture that has been named, follow a series of commands increasing in linguistic complexity, or select the syntactically correct sentence from two spoken by the examiner.

The physical processes of language representation, auditory programming, and speech programming are needed to *create and encode* a message. Each of these processes appears to have a somewhat different linguistic function; yet each is needed for the complete act of message creation. They account for the selection of the appropriate words, syntax, and phonology needed for the specific message within a communicative context. Thus they give rise to the behavioral correlate of *formulation*. Formulation can be defined as the ability of a person to create a message, either self-initiated or in response to something that he has comprehended. Disruption of any of these physical processes would be seen as disordered pragmatic, syntactic, semantic, and phonologic formulation. Again, the diagnostician uses many tasks to measure the client's ability to formulate messages —naming, defining words, spontaneous speech, etc.

Repetition is also seen as a behavioral correlate within the central language segment. Repetition is the *meaningful or non-meaningful* reproduction of a speech and language stimulus. If an auditory stimulus is repeated meaningfully, repetition would require the same physical processes as needed for language comprehension and formulation. However, a stimulus can be repeated nonmeaningfully, without comprehension. Whatever the listener hears he says. In this instance, processing presumably bypasses language representation, going from auditory programming to speech programming.

SPEECH PRODUCTION SEGMENT. The speech production segment is considered as a *primary production system*. The processes that take place in this segment are referred to as *postlinguistic processes,* that is, *motor events* that occur after a message has been formulated. These processes turn the message into spoken form.

To express a formulated message a series of interrelated physical processes occur within the speech production segment. The physical processes of (6) *speech programming,* (7) *speech initiation,* (8) *speech coordination-transmission,* and (9) *speech production** are responsible for the motoric actualization of the formulated message; that is, they allow for speech to occur. Note in Table 1 that speech programming overlaps the central language and speech production segments. Following from the more

------

*Note carefully that within the speech production *segment* there is also a speech production *process.*

central process of speech programming, a motor response is initiated by the physical process of speech initiation. The behavioral correlate to these two processes can be measured as *sequencing*. From speech initiation the motor response is then transmitted and coordinated, the speech coordination-transmission process; and finally, a motor response is actualized, the speech production process. The physical processes of speech initiation, speech coordination-transmission, and speech production can be observed in *motor control,* a behavioral correlate primarily related to these three processes. The speech production process is the final physical process for actualizing the message that has been formulated. Speech production involves the actual movements of the speech mechanism. *Breathing for speech, phonation, resonation, articulation,* and *prosodation* are subprocesses of the speech production process. Together all the physical processes of the speech production segment are responsible for initiating, transmitting, coordinating, and actualizing the motor activity required for producing a spoken response.

Within the speech production segment the diagnostician can take measures of the behavioral correlates of sequencing and motor control. Measurements of these behavioral correlates are concerned with speech production as a motor system—how well the speech production segment works in producing the various parameters of speech. Sequencing involves the appropriate ordering and timing of speech events. Motor control relates to the ability to move and control the speech musculature for speech production. The diagnostician can observe these correlates directly by listening to the parameters of the speech product (see discussion of speech and language product component) or by observing the muscular movement that occurs during speaking. For example, he can see if the tongue, lips, jaws, etc. move in the right direction and with appropriate tension for producing any specific sound of the lan-

Table 2. Summary of concepts presented in construction of internal speech and language processing component

	Auditory reception segment	Central language segment	Speech production segment
Anatomy	Structures of auditory modality	Central language (brain) mechanisms	Structures of "verbal" modality

Physical processing concepts	Primary recognition system
	Prelinguistic processes receive and analyze auditory input
	Auditory acceptance-transduction
	Auditory analysis-transmission
	Auditory reception-analysis
	(Auditory programming)
		Linguistic system
		Linguistic processes; language is represented
		
		Auditory programming
		Language representation
		Speech programming
			Primary production system
			Postlinguistic processes produce motor activity for speech
			(Speech programming)
			Speech initiation
			Speech coordination-transmission
			Speech production
			  Breathing for speech
			  Phonation
			  Resonation
			  Articulation
			  Prosodation

Behavioral correlates	Sensation Perception	Comprehension Formulation Repetition	Sequencing Motor control

guage; or he can listen for excess resonance, inappropriate pitch, etc.

Table 2 summarizes the concepts that underly the construction of the internal speech and language processing component.

Measurement considerations. The basic schema provided by the internal speech and language processing component directs the diagnostician's measurements and observations toward any physical bases for his client's speech and language disorder. The SLPM states that various behavioral correlates (reflective of speech and language use) occur as a result of a series of interrelated physical processes within rather well-defined anatomic boundaries. Therefore the diagnostician directs his measurements to the three aspects presented: *anatomy, physical processes,* and *behavioral correlates.*

For the most part, the physical bases for speech and language cannot be observed directly. There are some notable exceptions. The diagnostician can directly observe cer-

tain peripheral structures of the ear and the speech mechanism (the outer ear, the teeth, the tongue, etc.). Other structures are partially observable through the use of instrumental aids. Brain structures can be viewed via radiographic procedures such as the brain scan. In postmortem examination, brain structures can be observed directly to determine if lesions exist that could have accounted for the disorder present prior to death.

In the case of physical processes few of these can be observed directly or even with instrumental aids. Certain movements of the speech mechanism during speech can be observed, but this is a limited view of physical processing. Instead, the diagnostician infers disrupted physical processes based on behaviors he can observe. His source of information comes from behaviors that can be reported by the client or behaviors observed directly by the diagnostician. When a client speaks, the diagnostician is able to learn something about the client's ability to formulate and produce a message by observing the speech and language behavior. Similarly, when a client responds in some way to a language stimulus, the diagnostician can make observations of the response and then make a statement about the client's ability to receive and comprehend a language stimulus.

The diagnostician measures these *externalized behaviors*—correlates to the physical processes. The behavioral correlates represent different stages of physical processing where the diagnostician can "ask for" and then observe the response. Therefore each of the behavioral correlates can be defined by specifying tasks for its measurement.

The behavioral correlates of sensation, perception, and comprehension can be measured from either a verbal or nonverbal response. For example, if we asked a client, "Is your name Brenda Star?" and she responded correctly, "Yes, it is," we would be able to measure her spoken response and infer that comprehension of the stimulus was present. However, in diagnosis we often rely on *secondary* nonverbal responses to obtain information about the behavioral correlates of sensation, perception, and comprehension. If a spoken response is not wanted, not possible, or deviant, the diagnostician will use other avenues for obtaining a response such as pointing, finger raising, carrying out commands, etc.

The diagnostician interested in measuring sensation may ask the client to raise his finger when he hears a tone. Perception may be measured by asking the client to nod his head yes or no when asked if two sounds presented are alike or different. There are many tasks that have been devised to assist the diagnostician in measuring the behavioral correlates of sensation and perception, particularly the testing techniques devised by audiologists. These measures are taken by presenting stimuli to the client and asking him to report his auditory experience: "I hear the sound, I hear the differences between those sounds, I've heard that sound before, those are the same, etc."

Similarly, to measure comprehension the diagnostician observes a verbal or nonverbal response to the stimulus. What he measures is the appropriateness of the response in relationship to the stimulus. Comprehension may be measured by asking a client to physically carry out a command. For example, if we said to an aphasic client, "Go to the door" and he got up from his chair and opened the window, the diagnostician would judge the aphasic's comprehension as being less than adequate. But this particular response may well have shown some degree of comprehension as the behavior that occurred seems to relate tangentially to the command. Other tasks could be developed to allow the diagnostician to know if the client knows the difference between "Laura hit Arick" and "Arick hit Laura," a task for syntactic comprehension.

Diagnosticians need more sophisticated tasks that measure comprehension at the various linguistic levels to determine if the client's difficulty in understanding is because of phonologic, syntactic, semantic, or pragmatic elements of the message. And, in children's language disorders there is a significant need for measures that give an estimate of how well a child understands in comparison to how well he formulates language (Aram and Nation, 1975).

Measurement of comprehension is receiving greater attention. In the aphasia literature more emphasis is being placed on measuring comprehension at various linguistic levels (DeRenzi and Vignolo, 1962; Goodglass, 1968; Goodglass et al., 1966). In the literature on child language disorders more tasks are being developed for observing the emergence of comprehension abilities as they relate to formulation and production (Bloom, 1974; Ingram, 1974; Menyuk, 1974). Waryas and Ruder (1974) have been exploring various research strategies for measuring and interpreting responses that provide information about grammatical comprehension abilities.

The behavioral correlates of formulation, repetition, sequencing, and motor control generally require observation of a verbal response. There are exceptions. For example, when the diagnostician observes the diadochokinetic rate of the tongue in nonspeech activities, he is making an observation of motor control. However, keep in mind that this nonspeech activity is not a direct observation of motor control during the speech production process. The tasks the diagnostician designs for measuring these behavioral correlates should specify the type of verbal response to be observed. He may ask the client to name pictures, repeat sentences, talk about what is happening in a picture, prolong a vowel sound, produce a sequence of phonemes, sing the musical scale, etc.

Diagnosticians thus set up tasks that allow measurement of externalized behaviors reflecting physical processes. The SLPM attempts, throughout the internal processing component, to relate behavioral correlates to the anatomic and physical processing bases for that behavior. From his observations the diagnostician can seek the physical basis for the observed behavior.

Cautions. Objections are frequently raised about viewing processes in a way that makes them seem to be isolated events occurring only at a given anatomic level. These objections are justifiably raised. They help prevent oversimplified views of speech and language processing as discrete, discontinuous steps rather than a continuous interrelated processing system. Even though anatomic and processing boundaries are presented on the SLPM and processing is discussed this way, we caution the reader that the internal speech and language processing component is an interacting, continuous processing system; a disruption in one segment will have an effect on the processes in other segments.

Each of us will have to come to a decision about the theoretical position presented in the SLPM. The SLPM reflects the belief that there are underlying anatomic structures and processing events that can be delineated in relationship to different speech and language behaviors.

Different behaviors and disorders can be viewed in terms of anatomic and processing disruptions. Diagnosticians see speech and language disorders that are reflective of differential disruptions in the auditory reception, central language, and speech production segments. Disorders may sound similar but stem from different disrupted physical bases. We believe that the SLPM aids in sorting out the complicated physical basis for the disorders observed. Such a view assists in hypothesizing cause-effect relationships for clients whose speech and language is disordered.

Chapter 5 expands the details from which our schema for the internal speech and language processing component of the SLPM was derived.

Speech and language product component

When a speaker utters a message, the resulting product is an *acoustic waveform* made up of physical dimensions: frequency, intensity, spectrum, and duration. This end *acoustic product* can be viewed and structured differently depending on the purposes of the observer. For example, a speech scientist may be interested in using various types of instruments to study the frequency or intensity characteristics of the acoustic waveform. A voice teacher may be interested in listening to the pitch, loudness, and quality characteristics of the voice. A psycholinguist may be interested in describing the syntactic structure of the speaker's message. The diagnostician of speech and language disorders may be interested in any or all of the above observations of the acoustic product, along with many others to help define his client's speech and language disorder.

Acknowledging that many viewpoints exist about speech and language behavior, we have designed the speech and language product component of the SLPM for the diagnostician. It has been constructed to assist the diagnostician in ordering the many details of the speech and language behavior he may observe when a client speaks. To this end the speech and language product component has two divisions: the speech product and the language product.

Within each of these divisions, we developed a *basic set of speech and language parameters*. These parameters of the speech and language product were developed after considerable review of many systems of nomenclature presented in the literature. An attempt was made to provide a set of product terminology consistent with usage in the fields of speech and language disorders as well as normal development and use of speech and language. Knowledge from linguistics was carefully considered in the development of the terminology of the speech and language product component.

The speech product is seen as a direct reflection of the processes that occur in the speech production segment. The five basic parameters of the speech product are *vocal tone* and *resonance,* which in combination provide us with the third parameter, *voice.* The fourth parameter of the speech product is *phonetic structure.* Adding phonetic structure to voice provides the fifth parameter, *prosody.* The following diagram illustrates the relationships among these five parameters of the speech product division.

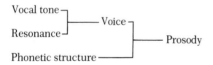

The language product is viewed as a direct reflection of the series of physical processes responsible for message formulation within the central language segment.

The language product includes four parameters or levels of language: *phonologic, syntactic, semantic,* and *pragmatic.*

Measurement considerations. The speech and language product is the diagnostician's *most accessible behavior for direct observation.* It is the client's spoken response. As a spoken response, the speech and language product can be observed by the diagnostician for two basic purposes. First, the product can be observed as an end result,

a set of parameters to be observed by the diagnostician to determine if the client's speech and language behavior is normal or disordered. Second, the product can be observed as behaviors that are reflective of internal speech and language processes. As stated previously, the speech product is most directly reflective of the physical processes within the speech production segment, and the language product is most directly reflective of the physical processes within the central language segment. Thus the diagnostician can observe the parameters of the speech and language product to provide information rather directly about the behavioral correlates of formulation, repetition, sequencing, and motor control (see discussion of internal processing component). At the same time the diagnostician should not lose sight of the fact that the client's spoken response, the speech and language product, can also provide information and insight into the client's ability to sense, perceive, and comprehend speech and language. Thus, the speech and language product component of the SLPM is perhaps the diagnostician's most powerful measurement tool. What the speech and language product does for the diagnostician is dependent on his *diagnostic intent*—what he wants to measure and why he is measuring it.

With this in mind the speech and language product component was designed to provide a specific set of parameters to which the diagnostician can direct his observations of normal and disordered speech and language behavior. He can direct his attention to all the parameters, the entire spoken response, or to a parameter of basic concern. For each parameter he can specify his detailed observations of the errors and variations he hears his clients produce.

The diagnostician could measure the physical characteristics of the acoustic product. Through instrumental analysis he can analyze the acoustic waveform, specifying the frequency, intensity, spectral, and durational characteristics of the acoustic product. This form of measurement is particularly useful where exact, specific physical data is wanted; for example, when the following diagnostic question is asked, "What are the format characteristics of Howard's hypernasality?" Because the measurements are typically made through refined instrumentation, human error and judgment are minimized. Use of physical measurement allows exactness of measurement that is readily quantifiable and gives high observer agreement.

Several difficulties, however, are associated with utilizing physical measurement in many clinical situations. Frequently the instrumentation required is expensive, bulky, and time-consuming, thus reducing the ease and flexibility with which it may be adapted to nonpredictable clinical situations. Furthermore, while instruments give data, they usually do not provide judgments. Yet most diagnostic problems require judgment; for example, does Howard's /s/ fall within the range of acceptable production of the English phoneme /s/ or is Mr. Hardee's voice quality excessively breathy?

Although measurement of the physical characteristics of the acoustic product are sometimes made by the diagnostician, his most frequent method of observation resides in his knowledge and skill as a "listener." His eyes and ears take in information that he uses to make auditory and visual analyses and comparisons to judge if speech and language are disordered.

The diagnostician designs diagnostic tasks to elicit speech and language responses, and his formal knowledge of the details of the speech and language products directs the specific observations he makes. His interest may be in listening to parameters of language to determine if his client has a disorder of syntax, semantics, or phonology. Or he may design tasks to address questions such as, "Is Amy's /r/ phoneme, voice quality, pitch, or rate essentially within normal limits?"

Since the diagnostician "carries" this method of observation with him, it provides maximum flexibility and efficiency in terms of cost, equipment, and ease of administration. However, considerable measurement error may be introduced into his observations, since they are dependent on the training and skill of the specific diagnostician. If the diagnostician has not learned to differentiate between phonetic variations, he may not "hear" or be able to record the difference between his client's lingual and lateral productions of the /s/ sound. If the diagnostician has not experienced hypernasality versus hyponasality, he is going to have difficulty identifying and specifically describing the distinctions he hears in the resonance product. Or two diagnosticians with different skill levels may not agree on the amount of hoarseness heard in the client's vocal tone.

Chapter 6 presents a more detailed discussion of the speech and language product component of the SLPM.

MEASUREMENT FRAMEWORK FOR ESTABLISHING CAUSE-EFFECT RELATIONSHIPS

As well as providing the diagnostician with a conceptual framework for viewing and measuring normal and disordered speech and language, the SLPM provides a measurement framework for establishing cause-effect relationships. The SLPM can guide and direct the measurement strategies the diagnostician utilizes for determining when speech and language are disordered and why they are disordered. He must discover potential cause-effect relationships if he is to provide appropriate management procedures. The diagnostician attempts to discover all types of information about his client.

To do this the diagnostician must learn how to *systematically elicit, observe,* and *interpret* the data needed to establish cause-effect relationships. He must attain these three major skills.

First, the diagnostician must learn how to direct his observations. He must separate what he can observe from what he can only partially observe, and from what is not directly observable by him.

Second, the diagnostician must learn what strategies he can use to elicit and measure the behaviors he wants to observe. He must become highly skilled at designing tasks—developing *measurement strategies*—that reveal relevant information about the client's ability to use speech and language. The behaviors he elicits and measures may be as simple as the raising of a finger in response to hearing a sound or as complex as the many verbal responses client's make to questions asked by the diagnostician. In some instances, as previously discussed, the diagnostician may choose instruments, *extrasensory aids,* to assist him in making his observations and measurements.

However, the diagnostician's major measurement tool is his own skill as a *systematic observer*. Through his knowledge, experience, and training, the diagnostician becomes a *"calibrated instrument."* He is his own best friend and worst enemy when it comes to making appropriate observations of the information needed to isolate his client's speech and language disorder. His observations will be only as good as his developed skill level.

How the SLPM assists the diagnostician in attaining these first two skills has been discussed in some detail. Measurement considerations were pointed out to the reader during our presentation of each of the components of the SLPM. Our intent there was to focus the diagnostician's attention on what could be observed in each component. Within each component of the SLPM, the formal knowledge, the major concepts to which the diagnostician directs his observations, was specified. Information and behavior that was observable was separated from information that was only partially observable, nonobservable, or only observable through the use of extrasensory aids.

Ptacek's model (1970) presented in Chapter 2 (Fig. 2-12) is extremely relevant to this concept of observable and nonobservable aspects of speech and language.

Third, the diagnostician must learn how to describe and interpret the information he has obtained. Beyond his powers of observation and measurement, he must develop his ability to *explain, infer,* and *predict*. Based on a limited amount of observable information, the diagnostician makes many inferences about his client's speech and language disorder. As a part of being a "calibrated instrument," the diagnostician must develop this complex inferential skill, keeping his errors of interpretation to a minimum.

This third skill has been discussed somewhat, primarily in our presentation of the internal processing component. It is the diagnostician's use of the SLPM for developing his inferential skill to establish cause-effect relationships that we want to expand on here. We have termed this skill the diagnostician's *inferential measurement strategy*.

Inferential measurement strategy

The diagnostician's behavioral observations do not always specify cause-effect relationships. More often the information needed by the diagnostician for interpretation of cause-effect relationships was only partially observable to him. Therefore he must interpret cause-effect relationships on the basis of inference, the inferential measurement strategy.

The essence of the inferential measurement strategy is to say something about an event that is not fully understood, based on whatever observations and theoretical understanding one has of the event. It is the *problem-solving level of measurement*. For the diagnostician involved in investigating the nature and causes of speech and language disorders it becomes one of his most crucial measurement strategies.

The SLPM assists the diagnostician in developing the use of the inferential measurement strategy by addressing the *interface*, the relationships and interactions, among the physical and behavioral aspects of speech and language. This interface is represented by the three components of the SLPM.

From the information he gathers and the observations he makes within each component of the SLPM, the diagnostician draws cause-effect relationships. Each client can be thought of as a *"mini-SLPM."* The client's environmental background can be studied; his anatomy and physical processing systems can be investigated; and the speech and language product can be observed. From the data he gathers the diagnostician can draw his inferences about what the disorder is, what has caused it, and what he might propose for remediation.

The diagnostician's use of the inferential measurement strategy can be represented by demonstrating the directional route the inference takes as seen in the following examples.

If the diagnostician saw a child with a significant disorder on the phonologic level of language, he might decide on the following directional route for his inferential strategy.

Language product → Physical process →

          Speech and language environment

This strategy represents his study of a cause-effect hypothesis.

Following the preceding inferential strategy, the diagnostician would first investigate information that might be indicative of a disrupted physical process for phonologic formulation. Then he would investigate the child's speech and language environment. In this example, if the diagnostician found nothing to signal a processing disruption but did discover that the child's mother spoke with a similar phonologic pattern, he would most likely conclude that the child's phonologic disorder (effect) was related to the speech and language stimulation (cause) provided by his mother's speech pattern.

Or, in another example, the diagnostician may observe that his client's responses to auditory tasks were faulty; the client could not hear the sounds; he could not discriminate between sounds. Depend-ing on the responses observed, the diagnostician may hypothesize impaired anatomy of the hearing mechanism and suggest that the client has an auditory processing disorder, disruption of the physical processes within the auditory reception segment. The inferential measurement strategy might look like this:

Behavioral correlates → Physical basis →
  (sensation, per-   (anatomy)
  ception)

                Physical basis
                (auditory processing)

Or, in still another example, if the diagnostician hears faulty vocal tone, he will want to know why and how it was produced. He knows that vocal tone is related to the speech production subprocess of phonation. Therefore his first level of investigation might be into the process of phonation, including an investigation of the condition and function of the laryngeal mechanisms. However, the nature of the vocal tone disorder could lead the diagnostician to infer other physical processing disorders from which he may hypothesize certain anatomic disruptions. This inferential strategy might look like this:

Speech product → Speech production process →
  (vocal tone)   (phonation)

           Other physical process → Anatomy
           (e.g., speech coordi-
           nation-transmission)

Relating the observed speech product to its physical basis allows the diagnostician to state and to test cause-effect relationships, thereby aiding in his understanding of causal factors and planning for client management.

Any number of these diagrams, singly or in combination, could be used to demonstrate how inferences are made among the components of the SLPM. Thus a most important aspect of the SLPM for the diagnostician is that it has been designed to help specify and measure cause-effect relationships. The SLPM helps the diagnostician to measure all aspects of speech and language, not only the product but also the underlying processes and the input stimulation that may help to explain the speech and language disorders heard. Is the speech and language product different for a child who is significantly hearing impaired (disrupted auditory reception segment), from the product of a child who has experienced reduced verbal stimulation (environmental input disruption), from the product of a child with a lesion of the left posterior temporal parietal lobe (central language segment disruption)? It is cause-effect questions such as these that the SLPM attempts to answer.

Chapters 7 and 8 expand on cause-effect relationships and measurement strategies employed by the diagnostician.

EXPANDED DIAGRAM OF THE SPEECH AND LANGUAGE PROCESSING MODEL

Now that we have provided an introduction of the SLPM and its use, we present the reader with a diagram representing the expanded version of the model. Fig. 3-2 presents the three components of the SLPM and incorporates the concepts and terminology we have presented to this point.

The figure demonstrates the relationship among the three components. The speech and language input parameters of the speech and language environment component are processed by the internal speech and language processing component. The physical processes within the internal processing component receive, comprehend, formulate, repeat, and produce messages. The messages produced are then broken down as the parameters of the speech and language product component.

The diagrammatic representation and nomenclature of the speech and language environment and speech and language product components are self-explanatory at this point. However, some additional comments about the diagrammatic representation of the internal processing component are needed for interpretation of Fig. 3-2.

First, the three segments of the component are notated at the bottom, demonstrating loosely the boundaries of the seg-ments but at the same time showing that the boundaries are not totally separated. Instead, the segments have a degree of anatomic and processing overlap.

Second, the internal physical processes are presented entirely within the large internal box; for example, auditory acceptance-transduction, language representation, etc. Inclusion within the box indicates that these are internal processes conceptualized as physical events that occur when speech and language are being processed. For the most part these physical processes are not observable to the diagnostician.

Third, the arrows within the component indicate the basic sequential flow of processing operations that take place; although as previously mentioned, they are in no way meant as an exact representation of processing events.

Fourth, the nomenclature for the behavioral correlates, for example, sensation, perception, etc., and with the exception of repetition, is written half-in and half-out of the large box representing internal processing. This demonstrates that the behavioral correlates relate to the physical processes but at the same time are external behaviors amenable to observation and measurement. The dotted lines indicate that the behavioral correlates are a result of the interaction of a series of physical processes rather than a direct one-to-one counterpart for a specific physical process.

It is suggested that the student return to the material in this chapter and restudy it in light of this figure of the expanded version of the SLPM. It is essential for understanding the later detailed discussion of the SLPM that the student have a good grasp of the components.

SUMMARY

As with all models of the speech and language process, the SLPM is only a reflection of its authors' viewpoint at the time it was constructed. It, too, has many missing pieces of information about the speech and language process, a process that is incompletely understood. However, as an organizing principle and a mea-

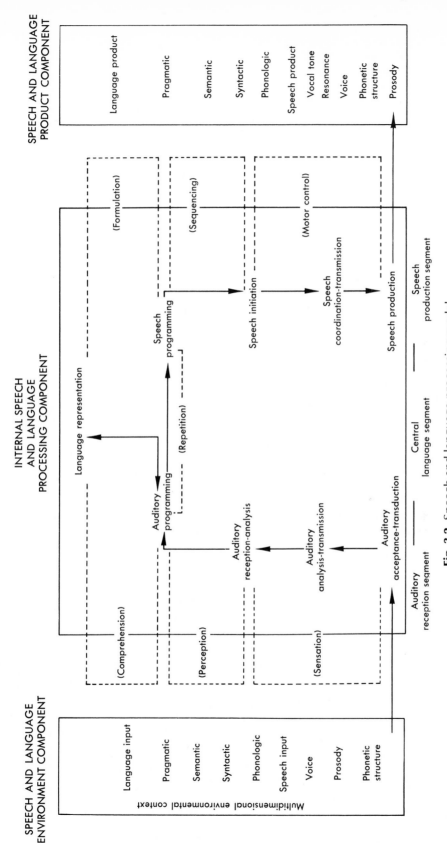

Fig. 3-2. Speech and language processing model.

surement framework for the diagnostician, the SLPM is structured to allow for continued modification and interpretation as information about speech and language accrues.

A speech and language interface is represented by the three components of the SLPM. By showing the relationship between the speech and language environment, the internal speech and language processing, and the speech and language product components, we feel the SLPM serves as an important conceptual framework in accomplishing the purposes of diagnosis.

The SLPM provides the diagnostician with:

1. A means for viewing the events that have taken place in the speech and language environment that may help explain the client's current speech and language functioning
2. A means for viewing any disruptions in the underlying physical basis for speech and language that may explain the observed disorder
3. A direct organization of speech and language behaviors that can be observed and used to isolate and define the speech and language disorder

The speech and language product component guides in delineating the speech and language disorder, while the linkage to the environment and internal processing components aids in understanding potential causal factors and in proposing client management.

As a project the student might evaluate the SLPM to determine how well it meets the seven considerations for construction of a diagnostic model discussed by the authors in Chapter 2. These considerations state that the model should:

1. Emphasize speech and language as the central concern of the diagnostician
2. Develop the auditory-verbal modalities as the primary speech and language channels
3. Specify in detail the observable parameters of speech and language behavior

4. Develop a schema for viewing the internal speech and language processing systems
5. Demonstrate the relationships (the interface) between anatomy, internal processing, and speech and language behavior
6. Aid in hypothesizing cause-effect relationships in speech and language disorders
7. Assist in developing diagnostic measurement strategies by differentiating observable behavior from that which is inferential

---

REFERENCES

Aram, D. M., and Nation, J. E., Patterns of language behavior in children with developmental language disorders. *J. Speech Hearing Res.,* **18,** 229-241 (1975).

Berry, M., *Language Disorders of Children: The Bases and Diagnoses.* New York: Appleton-Century-Crofts (1969).

Bloom, L., Talking, understanding, and thinking. In R. L. Schiefelbusch and L. L. Lloyd (Eds.), *Language Perspectives—Acquisition, Retardation, and Intervention.* Baltimore: University Park Press (1974).

DeRenzi, E., and Vignolo, L. A., The token test: A sensitive test to detect receptive disturbances in aphasia. *Brain,* **85,** 665-678 (1962).

Goodglass, H., Studies on the grammar of aphasics. In S. Rosenberg and J. H. Koplin (Eds.), *Developments in Applied Psycholinguistics Research.* New York: Macmillan Inc. (1968).

Goodglass, H., Klein, B., Carey, P., and Jones, K. J., Specific semantic word categories in aphasia. *Cortex,* **2,** 74-89 (1966).

Ingram, D., The relationship between comprehension and production. In R. L. Schiefelbusch and L. L. Lloyd (Eds.), *Language Perspectives—Acquisition, Retardation, and Intervention.* Baltimore: University Park Press (1974).

McCarthy, D., Language disorders and parent-child relationships. *J. Speech Hearing Dis.,* **19,** 514-523 (1954).

Menyuk, P., Early development of receptive language: From babbling to words. In R. L. Schiefelbusch and L. L. Lloyd (Eds.), *Language Perspectives—Acquisition, Retardation, and Intervention.* Baltimore: University Park Press (1974).

Ptacek, P. H., The evaluative process in speech pathology. In J. Akin, A. Goldberg, G. Myer, and J. Stewart (Eds.), *Language Behavior: A Book of Readings in Communication.* The Hague: Mouton Publishers (1970).

Waryas, C., and Ruder, K., On the limitations of language comprehension procedures and an alternative. *J. Speech Hearing Dis.,* **39,** 44-52 (1974).

Chapter 4

Speech and language environment component of the speech and language processing model

The speaker/first-language learner functions in a multidimensional environment filled with innumerable influences that can affect his speech and language learning and processing. Given the complexity of the speech and language environment, how can diagnosticians make sense out of all the potential environmental influences on a client's speech and language? Why is it important to organize information about the relationship of the environment to speech and language? As diagnosticians we want to understand how environmental factors affect speech and language since they have causal and remedial implications.

In Chapter 3 an orientation to the speech and language environment component was developed. Two major divisions of the environment component were presented: the multidimensional environmental context and the speech and language input. This component is now expanded and is represented in Fig. 4-1, which presents our schema for viewing the relationship between the multidimensional environmental context and the speech and language input received by the individual.

MULTIDIMENSIONAL ENVIRONMENTAL CONTEXT

While the complex contribution of various environmental influences defies clear understanding, the overall context in which language is learned and used includes at least three significant interacting contexts (Fig. 4-1): the interpersonal context, the multisensory context, and the sociocultural context.

First, we know that language originates and is used largely in an *interpersonal context*. In order for a child to develop and use speech and language appropriate to his environment, people in his interpersonal environment must talk to him; he must be exposed to the speech and language of his language community. To understand the interpersonal contribution to speech and language development and use the diagnostician relies on his broad knowledge in human communicative interaction (Chapter 2).

Second, the speech and language environment has a *multisensory context*. Multisensory influences include physical-technologic and experiential factors, that is, the environmental stimuli and sensory explorations that form the real world symbolized by language. For the young child this may mean the sensory information he discovers through his explorations that provide perceptual categories represented by his early words. In addition, multisensory experiences may initiate speech and language within a speaker; for example, an adult may see a cloud or a horse race that

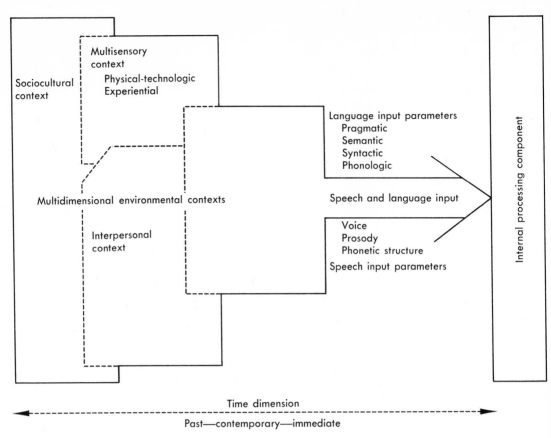

Fig. 4-1. Speech and language environment component of the SLPM.

prompts him to comment on these sensorily derived events. Thus the multisensory context may provide the perceptual-cognitive basis for language or may act as a stimulus to instigate speech and language within the speaker.

Third, the interpersonal and multisensory contexts are embedded into a broader *sociocultural context*. However, it is generally the continuous interpersonal environment that transmits sociocultural practices and values. The people in a child's environment provide him with the information that allows him to know the sociocultural practices involved in how, when, and where to use speech and language appropriately.

From this interacting multidimensional environmental context the speaker/first-language learner must abstract the pertinent speech and language data. However, speech and language stimulation is not always in the form of a clear, uncomplicated message. Language, as spoken, is frequently indistinct and fragmented. Rarely are the language rules made explicit; rather, the language learner and speaker must piece together the fragments to deduce the regularities of the system that he is to learn and use. To complicate matters further, the spoken message is only one of a number of competing auditory stimuli. From the noise of the television, street, children playing nearby, and whatever, the listener must bring to the foreground the speech and language directed toward him. The listener's task, then, is to abstract the relevant speech and language data from disjointed interpersonal, multisensory, and sociocultural contexts that make up his speech and language environment.

In examining his client's environmental contexts the diagnostician searches for factors that may have contributed to his client's speech and language disorder. He needs a framework for interpreting environmental determinants as potential causal factors. We turn now to the framework offered by the speech and language environment component for considering environmental influences on speech and language.

SPEECH AND LANGUAGE INPUT

In developing our framework for the environment component we wanted to keep the diagnostician's major concern paramount—speech and language. Although our clients exist in a complex environment, what they most directly need for speech and language development and use is speech and language stimulation (input). Therefore we can use the parameters of speech and language as a focal point around which to organize and scan the diverse, potential environmental influences and determinants.

This approach to considering the environment forces the diagnostician to carefully examine just what it is about a specific environmental factor or event that may have had an effect on speech and language. Often it is difficult to discern the relationship between an identified factor, for example, maternal deprivation, and its effect on speech and language. Frequently it appears that the specified factor is not the most direct influencing factor but rather serves as an umbrella term to cover a variety of experiences that may affect speech and language more directly. For example, Rutter (1972), in reexamining the concept of maternal deprivation, suggests that the restrictions in verbal development of maternally deprived children can be explained most directly by the linguistic deprivation rather than the maternal deprivation per se.

Speech and language parameters

The parameters of speech and language, then, would seem to provide a logical means for organizing environmental data. For our purposes, the primary task of a language learner is to learn to speak as others in his environment speak. This perspective suggests that for a person to use various features in his expressed speech and language he would have to be exposed to these same features in his speech and language environment.

The environment component of the SLPM incorporates the same set of speech and language parameters for input as it does for the speech and language product. Thus, paralleling the product component of the SLPM, speech and language input has been broken down into the *language input* and the *speech input.*

The language input has been subdivided into the *pragmatic, semantic, syntactic,* and *phonologic* levels. Pragmatics concerns how language is used in the environment, the effects various factors have on the use of language, what functions or purposes language serves, and how these uses are related to broader interpersonal and sociocultural variables. Semantics includes the meaning underlying words and the meaningful relationships between words. Here the concern is with both interpersonal and multisensory contributions to the development and use of meaning. Syntactics focuses on the grammar of language, including word order and morphology; while phonology deals with the sounds and rules for ordering sounds in a language.

Speech input has been subdivided to include the parameters of *voice, phonetic structure,* and *prosody.* While each of these parameters will be discussed more thoroughly later in the product discussion, briefly these parameters consist of the following. Voice includes loudness, pitch, and quality characteristics as well as resonance. Phonetic structure focuses on the specific instances, the actual occurrences of speech sounds heard, regardless of the phonemic categorization. Prosody includes the rate, fluency, intonation, and stress patterns that give spoken language a flow and rhythm.

Using these speech and language parameters, we can then order and interpret the diverse environmental information available to us. Much may be learned about a client's environment—the maternal grandmother is an alcoholic, the mother is a "working woman," the older brother is a delinquent, etc. Although helpful in understanding the client as a totality, unless these bits of information can be related to speech and language input, they are not helpful to the diagnostician's purpose of attempting to understand causal factors and may, in fact, be extraneous to his central concern.

For example, an alcoholic grandmother who sees Amy only on short, yearly visits probably has little if any direct effect on her delayed speech. However, an alcoholic grandmother who assumed primary care for Amy may indeed provide significantly inappropriate speech and language stimulation. If she is the primary caretaker, she may talk and read little to the child, thus restricting speech and language input on all levels. Depending on her state of stupor, the phonetic structure input she provides may be slurred and misarticulated or she may provide a pragmatic model that teaches Amy that language is primarily a tool for verbal abuse. In any event, the diagnostician cannot just "red flag" the information, "alcoholic grandmother," assuming an effect on speech and language, but rather he needs to show specifically how the grandmother's condition contributes directly or indirectly to the speech and language input per se.

While our example may be a little far-fetched, diagnosticians do encounter "red flags" and must be on guard. They must not assume an influence on speech and language when one may not be present.

Consider, for example, the isolated terms "divorced parents," "bilingualism," and "lower socioeconomic status," all terms that are frequently used to explain speech and language disorders and yet in themselves provide insufficient information for causal interpretation.

TIME DIMENSION

In addition to structuring environmental factors that may affect speech and language input, the environment component also incorporates a time dimension (Fig. 4-1). The time dimension is divided into the historical speech and language environment and the immediate speech and language environment.

This time dimension is seen as a continuum. It encompasses the client's cumulative past experiences ranging from day one, the *distant past,* to the *contemporary environment,* to those events that are *immediate,* that is, currently occurring in the diagnostic setting. Viewing the time dimension on this continuum allows the diagnostician to note changes in environmental circumstances and forces him to consider carefully what effect he and the tasks he uses have on the client's speech and language behavior. The historical continuum and the immediate diagnostic situation give the diagnostician a *time of occurrence* organization to events within the speech and language environment.

Historical speech and language environment

Our historical time dimension considers all the past interpersonal, sociocultural, and multisensory experiences that have contributed to an individual's speech and language history; it is an accumulation of experiences from the distant past to the present.

Yet, the importance of the environment to language acquisition is a point of disagreement among theorists. At one extreme are those who maintain that all aspects of speech and language are learned from environmental presentation and reinforcement, attributing little innate predisposition to the child. At the other extreme are those theorists who suggest that the environmental speech and language stimuli merely act as a trigger for a child's intrinsic mechanisms, which are highly specialized and predisposed to learn language.

While these positions represent the extremes, most viewers of child language fall somewhere between, crediting the child with some degree of innate specialization to handle language, while at the same time recognizing that the language stimulation from the child's environment provides information—a model from which the child learns language. This is the position represented by the SLPM; neither the environment nor the speaker/language learner alone accounts for all facets of speech and language development or use. Rather, the environment has a role in providing the data that allows the child to learn the special characteristics of speech and language as used by those around him. And the child's specialized biological self allows him to readily learn the language system available to him.

Some documentation is available on the kind of linguistic environment parents provide for their children. Some writers (Brown and Bellugi, 1964; Brown et al., 1969) have suggested modeling, expansion, and constituent-prompts as activities parents use during verbal interchanges with their children. Other writers are concerned with the roles that imitation, operant conditioning, and self-motivated practice play in learning language (Mowrer, 1960; Skinner, 1957; Staats, 1968). Some writers have suggested that children may use different learning strategies for different parameters of their language system. For example, Hopper and Naremore (1973) indicate rule induction and possibly modeling as primary strategies for early syntax learning, while they suggest rule induction and imitation as important for phonologic learning.

The type of speech and language stimulation varies with the age of the child, thus the importance of considering the time dimension. Broen (1972) and Ringler (1973) have studied the changes in parental speech in relation to age. Generally, these studies have indicated that the mother's speech with children just learning to speak is shorter, slower, and less complex semantically and syntactically than her speech with older children or adults.

While research has begun to accrue regarding the linguistic characteristics of the normal child's speech and language environment, the questions of quality, quantity, source, and timing of speech and language input remain largely untouched. How do competing environmental stimuli affect the language learner's ability to receive speech and language input? How direct must the stimulation be for the learner to profit from its information? Must the language learner be actively involved in receiving, manipulating, and reformulating the language input, or may he be a passive observer of the speech and language scene? A basic question yet unanswered is how much stimulation is enough and under what conditions. Is one-shot exposure sufficient for a child to have gained from the language experience, or is repeated presentation necessary? What do we know about the differential effects of various sources of language input? Is one source, possibly the mother, a more potent language provider than other sources? What contribution, if any, do the radio and television make to language learning? What is the appropriate timing of speech and language stimulation, and how do the requirements change over time? Is one form of stimulation more effective at one age than at another or more appropriate for providing data for one level of language than for another?

While we do not have conclusive answers to questions of quality, quantity, source, and timing of speech and language input, for the present we can operate with the assumption that the historical speech and language environment must provide some degree of stimulation pertaining to all parameters of speech and language.

The diagnostician will have to cull information from his funds of knowledge that supports the environment's historical role in the learning and disrupting of the various parameters of speech and language. For example, in viewing the environment's relation to voice input, the diagnostician must consider the evidence that children model to some degree their vocal tone and resonance characteristics on significant adults in their environment by imitation and identification. Lieberman (1967) found that the fundamental frequency of a 10-month-old boy and a 13-month-old girl during babbling tended to approach that of the speaker with whom they were in contact. The fundamental frequency of the 10-month-old boy when alone averaged 430 Hz, was 390 Hz with his mother, and 340 Hz with his father. The 13-month-old girl's average fundamental frequency was 390 Hz with her mother and 290 Hz with her father. Similarly, Murphy (1964) suggests that children may adopt deviant vocal tone or resonance through identification with someone with a deviant voice. Klinger (1962) did report a case study of a normal child whose resonance was an imitation of his cousin's hypernasality, which was secondary to a cleft palate.

The prosodic features of intonation, stress, rate, and fluency have been related only to a minimal degree to speech and language input. For example, children between 6 and 8 months of age have been reported to imitate contrasting intonation patterns, including changes in pitch and stress (Nakazima, 1962). Rate of the language stimulus has also been related to older children's ability to comprehend language (Berry and Erickson, 1973). Speech patterns characterized as foreign dialect in second-language learning provide evidence of the role played by intonation, stress, and timing of a speaker's native speech environment.

As well, a speaker's phonetic structure has been related to environmental models as seen in dialectal patterns or sound errors that are similar to parental and sibling speech errors.

Children learn the language system heard in their environment. Not only does a Chinese child learn the Chinese phonologic and syntactic system, but also a black inner-city child learns the phonologic and syntactic features of his community's black dialect. While the phonologic and syntactic parameters are most directly learned because of the language input a child hears, semantic and pragmatic parameters of language learning draw from a broader range of environmental experience.

In considering semantic input the diagnostician will need to account for not only how a lexicon is acquired but also the referential-meaningful relationship between the words and the concepts they represent. He will want to view both the meaning features underlying single words as well as the meaningful relations between words. Clark (1973) has suggested that the earliest semantic features underlying single words are derived from a child's early perceptual experience with the world. Later features are contributed by social or functional factors within the cultural context. Brown (1973a, b) has suggested that semantic relations expressed in early sentences are the terminal achievement of the child's learning the physical-perceptual characteristics of his world through sensorimotor exploration. Thus, in understanding the environment's contribution to semantic development and use, the diagnostician will want to carefully evaluate perceptual, social, and cultural experiences that may underly the semantic system.

The contribution of the environment to pragmatic development and use may draw from multiple aspects of the environment. In particular, three sources would appear to be basic for providing pragmatic information: interpersonal relationships, sensory and cognitive experiences, and sociocultural practices in the use of language.

Most forms of language usage occur in

an interpersonal setting; in fact, language could be said to rest on or be supported by interpersonal relations. Many writers have referenced the importance of the mother-child interaction in laying the groundwork for communicative interaction (Mowrer, 1952; Wyatt, 1962). The social context, particularly between the mother and child, has been implicated as important for further communication participation, even considerably before 1 year of age. Oral gratification, maternal bonding, and identification have all been cited as important in developing interpersonal interactions basic to verbal communication (Freud, 1965; Mowrer, 1952, 1960).

Sensory exploration and cognitive experience provide the subject matter for content and context-oriented speech. Through his sensory experiences the child learns that his environment may be segmented, named, and described (Sinclair-de-Zwart, 1971, 1973). Cognitive experience allows the speaker to displace thought from the present and to comment on content or the media itself, thus freeing him from the present experiential bounds of the context (Macnamara, 1972).

Sociocultural practices in the use of language provide models and expectations for the use of language. The bulk of the work in the field of sociolinguistics has been directed to understanding the relationship between a speaker's sociocultural context and his use of language. Bernstein (1970), among others, has described the relationship between social class, roles, and the language codes of its speakers. A major tenet of his position is that learning a given linguistic code is a primary means by which social structures perpetuate themselves in the children of parents who use those codes.

Whenever the diagnostician is considering any past or contemporary environmental influence on speech and language input, he is considering the historical speech and language environment, whether the event occurred 10 years or 10 minutes earlier. The historical continuum, then,

allows examination of these environmental factors within a time-related frame. When a historical factor occurs that may restrict any parameter of speech and language input, this factor becomes causally suspect. The more extreme the limitation or deviation of speech and language input created by the factor, the more probable an effect on speech and language.

Immediate speech and language environment: the diagnostic setting

The immediate speech and language environment is concerned with the present diagnostic situation. The diagnostician becomes the central figure in the client's immediate environment. Too often the influences of immediate environmental variables on the client's speech and language behavior go unexamined by the diagnostician. Therefore the immediate speech and language environment time dimension directs attention to the specific speech and language tasks presented and to the interpersonal characteristics of the diagnostician.

Sensory experience is purposefully manipulated by the diagnostician's presentation of speech and language tasks. Diagnostic stimuli are generally presented through the auditory or visual modalities, although with young children or in special situations other modalities may be used. The diagnostician must examine the given stimulus items to determine what level or levels of speech and language input are included. For example, one phonemic discrimination test utilizing nonsense syllables does not provide semantic information, whereas a second phonemic discrimination test using single words introduces semantic information into the discrimination task. Typically, syntactic test items include phonologic, syntactic, and semantic information even though the level under test is said to be syntactic. In addition, the syntactic contrasts are frequently pictured, thus requiring processing of visual stimuli paralleling the auditory information. Implicit in all these test presentations are the pragmatic expectations of a diagnostic setting. Is the diagnostician's speech and language used for meaningful communicative interaction, or is the stimulus presented as a "test" of the client's abilities? For what purposes is the language used—to ask, direct, facilitate? Do the pragmatic conditions created by the diagnostician require the client to fill in the blank, spontaneously generate language, repeat the examiner's words, or elicit some other use of language?

The topic of conversation has been found to have an important bearing on the amount and complexity of verbal responsiveness. Personal involvement in the topic and novel and interesting topics of conversation have been shown to increase measures of verbal expression (Cazden, 1970). Children have been shown to talk more about toys and films than still photographs (Strandberg, 1969), and the variable effect of different pictures in eliciting verbal responses has also been demonstrated (Cowan et al., 1967).

What is required of the client has also been related to verbal responsivity. Pictures and other concrete stimuli have been found to limit the diversity of syntactic and vocabulary usage. Cazden (1970) has suggested that an absence of pictures seems to free children to work more with linguistic knowledge. Other research has shown that some subjects offer increased diversity of response when the examiner probes more frequently for additional information. Williams and Naremore (1969) have demonstrated that the type of question asked by the interviewer influences the complexity of the response offered by children, particularly lower-class children. Simple questions—for example, "Do you play baseball?"—tended to elicit yes/no or one word responses. Naming questions—for example, "What TV programs do you watch?" —tended to be followed by lists of names. Questions requiring explanation or elaboration—such as, "How do you play kick the can?"—tended to gain the most complex responses and evidenced less difference in output productivity between lower- and higher-class children than did the simple questions and naming questions.

The diagnostician also needs to be aware of extraneous sensory experiences within the diagnostic setting and their effect on the client. All too often our "quiet" examining room is invaded by hall or street noise. Or the light-colored clothing barely visible through the one-way observation mirror catches the discerning client's eye. While these random sensory variables may not be of much consequence for the diagnostician, they may become prominent for the client and therefore worthy of the diagnostician's attention.

Perhaps one of the most determining and yet least considered aspects of the diagnostic setting is the effect of the examiner on the client's speech and language behavior. Several studies have considered the influence of the examiner on children's verbal and intellectual performance (Cazden, 1970; Jensen, 1969; Katz, 1964), although speech pathologists are just beginning to examine such interactions (Shriberg, 1971). Writers have noted that testing situations combine a relationship of interpersonal formality and power with cognitive demands and thus are especially threatening to clients. Hopper and Naremore (1973) suggest that children are particularly sensitive to the physical and interpersonal context. Labov (1970) has been outspoken in implicating the silencing effect of a white adult examiner on the verbal performance of black inner-city children. He has demonstrated that black children's verbal expressiveness can be changed by altering the power relations in the testing situation, making the test procedures less formal, including a friend of the subject, and talking about topics of interest. Children from impoverished backgrounds improve their test performance after repeated opportunities to become familiar with the testing situation. Cazden (1970) has reported that children tend to converse more readily with a greater number of exchanges when the conversation is initiated by the child rather than the adult.

The diagnostician, then, considers the present diagnostic setting in terms of the speech and language variables inherent in the given tasks as well as the interpersonal characteristics that may influence the verbal output of his client.

SUMMARY

The speech and language environment component of the SLPM proposes that the multidimensional environmental variables in a client's background be considered in terms of their influence on the parameters of speech and language input. In addition, this component leads the diagnostician to consider environmental information within a time dimension continuum. The historical environmental continuum concerns the client's cumulative life experiences with speech and language, ranging from the distant past through contemporary events. The immediate environment focuses on the diagnostic setting, chiefly the tasks presented and the interpersonal interactions between the diagnostician and client.

REFERENCES

Bernstein, B., A sociolinguistic approach to socialization: With some reference to educability. In F. Williams (Ed.), *Language and Poverty: Perspectives on a Theme*. Chicago: Markham Publishing Co. (1970).

Berry, M. D., and Erickson, R. L., Speaking rate: Effects on children's comprehension of normal speech. *J. Speech Hearing Res.*, **16**, 367-374 (1973).

Broen, P. A., The verbal environment of the language-learning child. *Asha Monogr.*, No. 17 (1972).

Brown, R., *A First Language: The Early Stages*. Cambridge, Mass.: Harvard University Press (1973a).

Brown, R., Development of the first language in the human species. *Am. Psychol.*, **28**, 9-106 (1973b).

Brown, R., and Bellugi, U., Three processes in the child's acquisition of syntax. *Harvard educ. Rev.*, **34**, 133-151 (1964).

Brown, R., Cazden, C., and Bellugi, U., The child's grammar from I to III. In J. P. Hill (Ed.), *Minnesota Symposium on Child Psychology*. (Vol. 2) Minneapolis: University of Minnesota Press (1969).

Cazden, C., The neglected situation in child language research and education. In F. Williams (Ed.), *Language and Poverty: Perspectives on a Theme*. Chicago: Markham Publishing Co. (1970).

Clark, E., What's in a word? On the child's acquisition of semantics in his first language. In T. E. Moore (Ed.), *Cognitive Development and the Acquisition of Language*. New York: Academic Press, Inc. (1973).

Cowan, P. A., Weber, J., Hoddinott, B. A., and Klein, J., Mean length of spoken response as a function of stimulus, experimenter, and subject. *Child Develpm.*, **38**, 191-203 (1967).

Freud, A., *Normality and Pathology in Childhood: Assessments of Development*. New York: International Universities Press, Inc. (1965).

Hopper, R., and Naremore, R., *Children's Speech: A Practical Introduction to Communication Development*. New York: Harper & Row, Publishers (1973).

Jensen, A. R., How much can we boost IQ and scholastic achievement? *Harvard educ. Rev.*, **39**, 247-277 (1969).

Katz, I., Review of evidence relating to effects of desegregation on the intellectual performance of Negroes. *Am. Psychol.*, **19**, 381-399 (1964).

Klinger, H., Imitated English cleft palate speech in a normal Spanish speaking child. *J. Speech Hearing Dis.*, **27**, 379-381 (1962).

Labov, W., The logic of nonstandard English. In F. Williams (Ed.), *Language and Poverty: Perspectives on a Theme*. Chicago: Markham Publishing Co. (1970).

Lieberman, P., *Intonation, Perception and Language*. Cambridge, Mass.: The M.I.T. Press (1967).

Macnamara, J., Cognitive basis of language learning in infants. *Psychol. Rev.*, **79**, 1-13 (1972).

Mowrer, O. H., Speech development in the young child: I. The autism theory of speech development and some clinical applications. *J. Speech Hearing Dis.*, **17**, 263-268 (1952).

Mowrer, O. H., Hearing and speaking: An analysis of language learning. *J. Speech Hearing Dis.*, **23**, 143-153 (1960).

Murphy, A. T., *Functional Voice Disorders*. Englewood Cliffs, N.J.: Prentice-Hall, Inc. (1964).

Nakazima, S., A comparative study of the speech development of Japanese and American English in childhood. *Studia Phonologica*, **2**, 27-39 (1962).

Ringler, N., Mothers' language to their young children and to adults over time. Doctoral dissertation, Case Western Reserve University (1973).

Rutter, M., Maternal deprivation reconsidered. *J. psychosom. Res.*, **16**, 241-250 (1972).

Shriberg, L. D., The effect of examiner social behavior on children's articulation test performance. *J. Speech Hearing Res.*, **14**, 659-672 (1971).

Sinclair-de-Zwart, H., Sensorimotor action patterns as a condition for the acquisition of syntax. In R. Huxley and E. Ingram (Eds.), *Language Acquisition: Models and Methods*. New York: Academic Press, Inc. (1971).

Sinclair-de-Zwart, H., Language acquisition and cognitive development. In T. E. Moore (Ed.), *Cognitive Development and the Acquisition of Language*. New York: Academic Press, Inc. (1973).

Skinner, B. F., *Verbal Behavior*. New York: Appleton-Century-Crofts (1957).

Staats, A. W., *Learning, Language and Cognition*. New York: Holt, Rinehart & Winston, Inc. (1968).

Strandberg, T. E., An evaluation of three stimulus media for evoking verbalizations from preschool children. Master's thesis, Eastern Illinois University (1969).

Williams, F., and Naremore, R. C., On the functional analysis of social class differences in modes of speech. *Speech Monogr.*, **36,** 77-102 (1969).

Wyatt, G. L., and Herzan, H. M., Therapy with stuttering children and their mothers. *Am. J. Orthopsychiat.*, **32,** 645-660 (1962).

Internal speech and language processing component of the speech and language processing model

The diagnostician's interest goes beyond the speech and language behaviors he can observe. He must, as well, be concerned with the "hidden processes," that is, the internal physical events taking place that are generally not directly observable. The diagnostician must understand the relationship between the speech and language behaviors he observes and the physical basis for these behaviors.

Historically, the study of this relationship has interested scientists and clinicians for many years. Neurologists, speech pathologists, psychologists, psycholinguists, and others have presented theories as to how language is processed by the human being. They have attempted to delineate the anatomic structures and the physical (physiologic) processes underlying language behavior. We are all aware of such major contributions as those made by Broca (1861a, b) and Wernicke (1874) regarding the functions of the frontal and temporal lobes in language formulation and comprehension.

Many controversies have occurred concerning whether or not an anatomic and physiologic basis can be specified for given speech and language behaviors. Many specifics continue to be disputed, but some commonality can be seen. Unanimity of thought is greater in the peripheral than the central systems. Thus virtually all theorists viewing speech and language agree that reception of the auditory stimulus within the auditory modality and speech production through movement of the structures of the speech mechanism are indisputable aspects of speech and language processing. What goes on in the brain is much less clear and far from universally agreed on. Its representation may range from the "black box" approach to highly inferential, complex processing concepts.

Today there are still remnants of the controversy regarding localization of function within the central nervous system. However, as more data have accrued, particularly those studies relating speech and language disorders to anatomic and neurologic dysfunction, there is greater understanding of the relationship between speech and language behavior and the functional organization of the nervous system. As we learn to specify where damage occurred in the organism and measure the resultant behavior more precisely, we can develop more sophisticated hypotheses about the physical basis for speech and language; we can develop better conceptual and theoretical positions regarding speech and language processing systems.

Even though we must be cautious when attempting to delineate the interface between anatomy, physical processing, and

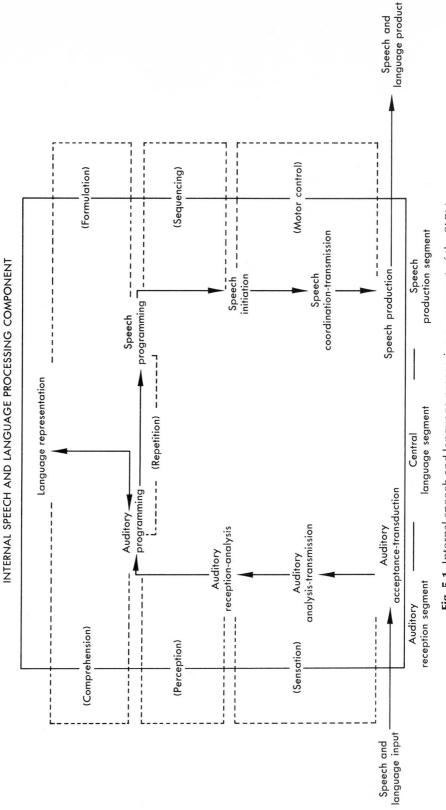

Fig. 5-1. Internal speech and language processing component of the SLPM.

behavior, the available data allow us to make some tentative statements about these relationships. The internal speech and language processing component of the SLPM, abstracted from a large body of information, is *our* statement of these relationships. Its intent is to help the diagnostician relate speech and language disorders to the physical basis for such disorders. The internal processing component viewed in relationship to the other two components of the SLPM allows the diagnostician to do two things:

1. Infer potential physical disruptions from observed behaviors.
2. Predict potential speech and language disorders from knowledge about physical disruptions.

For example, if the diagnostician has been provided with medical data that his client has a lesion of the posterior area of the left first temporal convolution, the diagnostician would likely predict that the client would be aphasic and that the client's language disorder would be characteristic of what is called fluent or Wernicke's aphasia. Therefore a model that can demonstrate, albeit abstractly, the interface between speech and language behavior and its physical basis affords the diagnostician with a tool for developing better hypotheses about cause-effect relationships.

An orientation to the internal speech and language processing component of the SLPM was presented in Chapter 3. The component is reproduced in Fig. 5-1. At this time we will present in greater detail some of the specific and technical information from which the internal processing component of the SLPM was derived. The detailed discussion of the three segments of the internal processing component will be approached by providing, first, a discussion of the physical basis of the segment (anatomic and processing considerations) and, second, a discussion of the behavioral correlates to the physical processing. The discussion centers more on behavioral correlates, since behavior is more primary and accessible to the diagnostician; it is the behavioral correlate that provides the diagnostician with his means of measuring speech and language processes.

AUDITORY RECEPTION SEGMENT

The *prelinguistic* physical processing that takes place in the auditory reception segment *(auditory modality)* allows the listener to derive *sensory* and *perceptual* information from the physical characteristics of the auditory stimulus. Within this segment the listener does not comprehend the message. This segment has been referred to as a *primary sensory system* or a *primary recognition system.*

Physical basis of auditory reception segment
Anatomy

The anatomy of the auditory reception segment is made up of the *bilateral structures of the auditory modality,* from the outer ear to Heschl's gyrus, the primary auditory cortex. Whitaker (1970) provides us with an anatomic schematic of the auditory modality, except he has not included the outer and middle ear structures (Fig. 5-2). As demonstrated in Whitaker's schematic, the SLPM would extend the auditory reception segment to include some interactions with Wernicke's area, auditory association cortex. This anatomic interaction is necessary when discussing processing events taking place within this segment; however, the internal processing component views Wernicke's area primarily as a structure of the central language segment.

Physical processes

Within the auditory reception segment a series of four prelinguistic processes that give rise to the two behavioral correlates of sensation and perception are hypothesized. These processes are auditory acceptance-transduction, auditory analysis-transmission, auditory reception-analysis, and auditory programming.

Auditory acceptance-transduction. The physical process, auditory acceptance-transduction, incorporates the activities

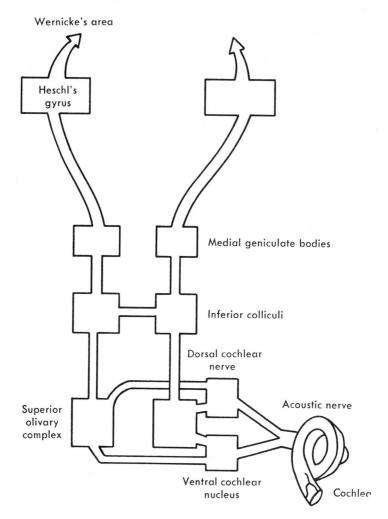

Fig. 5-2. Anatomic schematic of the auditory modality. (From Whitaker, H., A model for neurolinguistics. *Occasional Papers 10.* Language Centre, Colchester, England: University of Essex [1970].)

that occur from the time the auditory stimulus enters, is *accepted by,* the outer ear until it reaches and stimulates the hair cells of the organ of Corti in the inner ear (Chalfant and Scheffelin, 1969). In this process the auditory stimulation undergoes a series of *transductions,* changing the acoustic energy into mechanical, hydraulic, and electrochemical forms of energy. Auditory acceptance-transduction, then, is basically viewed as a process that allows the accepted auditory stimulus to be altered in such a way as to allow for further neurologic processing.

Auditory analysis-transmission. Once the hair cells of the organ of Corti have been stimulated, the physical process termed auditory analysis-transmission begins. The process begins at the level of the hair cells in the cochlea and "ends" at the level of the primary auditory cortex. Various "way stations," synaptic junctions, exist within the pathway (Fig. 5-2). Prelinguistic neural *"analysis"* (coding) takes place within the process of auditory analysis-transmission, a coding of the frequency, intensity, and durational characteristics of the auditory stimulus.

The cochlea first provides for primary coding of these physical characteristics. The eighth cranial nerve (auditory nerve) then *transmits* the coded auditory data from the cochlea to the cochlear nuclei in the medulla. From here, the data are *transmitted* to the primary auditory cortex via two auditory pathways: the direct lemniscal and the indirect reticular pathways (Rose, 1971). During the transmission along the auditory pathways some other *analyses* undoubtedly occur, for example, comparing the coded physical characteristics of the incoming auditory stimulus to previously established auditory patterns (*Human Communication and Its Disorders*, 1969).

Auditory analysis-transmission then is a prelinguistic coding of the frequency, intensity, and durational characteristics of the auditory stimulus, from the time the hair cells of the cochlea are stimulated until the coded data reach the primary auditory cortex.

Auditory reception-analysis. Auditory reception-analysis begins once the coded auditory information has arrived at (been *received* by) Heschl's gyrus, the primary auditory cortex.

The primary auditory cortex is not simply a passive receiver of the auditory information. Complex activities and pattern analyses take place here. The cortical divisions of the primary auditory cortex participate in selectively *receiving* and *analyzing* the coded frequency, intensity, and durational data through differential inhibition and facilitation of the arriving auditory data (Chalfant and Scheffelin, 1969).

According to Luria (1966), this part of the auditory cortex deals with precise differentiations and integration of the arriving auditory data. He views the primary auditory cortex as important for complex differential auditory analyses—for continued discrimination and comparisons of auditory patterns with previously established patterns.

Thus auditory reception-analysis is viewed as the prelinguistic physical process where the coded auditory data arriving at the primary auditory cortex are further analyzed and synthesized into *complex auditory patterns*. These complex auditory patterns are compared to previously established patterns.

Auditory programming. The auditory programming process is presented on the SLPM as part of *both* the auditory reception segment and the central language segment. Here, we will limit our discussion of the process to its prelinguistic functions. Later, when we discuss the physical processes of the central language segment, we will consider the linguistic functions of the auditory programming process. This prelinguistic-linguistic distinction draws attention to the sequential, interacting activities of the physical processes as represented in the internal processing component.

The *prelinguistic auditory programming process* begins when the auditory patterns analyzed and synthesized in the primary auditory cortex are sent to Wernicke's area, particularly the posterior aspect of the superior temporal convolution at the sylvian margin. The prelinguistic activities of auditory programming include at least *three major activities:*

1. Sorting speech from nonspeech auditory patterns
2. Changing auditory patterns into phonetic patterns (features)
3. Storing these phonetic features

First, to sort speech stimuli from other auditory stimuli, auditory programming must determine the auditory patterns inherent in speech stimuli that make them different from other auditory stimulations. The human probably has a built-in ability to discriminate and recognize speech data, as there is evidence that the cortical areas related to speech perception are innately organized. The left cerebral hemisphere functions for the temporal analysis and organization of the auditory patterns of speech, and therefore it plays the significant role in speech perception, whereas the right hemisphere seems more responsive to auditory information of a nonverbal nature (Kimura, 1973).

The second prelinguistic activity for which auditory programming is responsible is that of changing the analyzed auditory patterns into phonetic patterns. One way in which auditory programming organizes the information may involve a type of grouping process related to the temporal nature of auditory stimulation. Certain features of the auditory pattern may be clustered, while others retain their distinct characteristics. This grouping process of auditory programming requires the ability to select and abstract from the continuous stream of stimulation those features that are distinctive and those that are considered nondistinctive, thereby grouping the auditory data into appropriate phonetic notations. In this way, phonetic constancies are programmed into the system.

The third prelinguistic activity of auditory programming is the ability to store the phonetic patterns that have been abstracted and grouped. In this sense the auditory programming process includes a "memory" component for holding and comparing the information being processed.

Thus the prelinguistic activities of auditory programming within the auditory reception segment sort speech from nonspeech stimulation, change auditory patterns into phonetic patterns, and store this information for comparative purposes.

In summary, the four physical processes within the auditory reception segment are prelinguistic processes involved in receiving, coding, analyzing, transmitting, and programming the auditory stimulus. These processes code and analyze the incoming physical characteristics of the auditory stimulation, ultimately turning the data into phonetic feature patterns. These processes prepare the speech data for linguistic analysis, which takes place in the central language segment.

For an overall review of the auditory modality see Glattke (1973) and Whitfield (1967).

Behavioral correlates within auditory reception segment

As hypothesized on the SLPM, sensation and perception are the two behavioral correlates that result from the prelinguistic physical processes taking place within the auditory reception segment. These two correlates reveal the processing events prior to language comprehension, although the boundary between speech perception and language comprehension may be very narrow and perhaps quite arbitrary. These behavioral correlates reveal the listener's ability to become aware of and attach significance to the auditory stimulations he receives or, as Myklebust (1954) would say, to structure his auditory world. Thus measurement of the sets of behaviors that define sensation and perception allow the diagnostician to say something about his cleint's ability to process auditory information prior to language comprehension.

Sensation

On the SLPM, sensation is tied to the physical processes of auditory acceptance-transduction, auditory analysis-transmission, and auditory reception-analysis. Sensation is viewed as a low-level *behavioral response to the presence of sound*.

Sensation does not occur until cortical activation has taken place—auditory reception-analysis. As Luria (1966) would say, it occurs in the first stages of arrival at the primary auditory cortex. Sensation, in this view, is a "preliminary" behavioral response to the neural activation that occurs when the intensity, frequency, and durational characteristics of the stimulus are received by the primary auditory cortex. Sensation is associated with the primary selection, sorting out, and registration of the essential components of the auditory stimulus.

Theoretically, at this stage the auditory stimulus is not interpreted by the listener; he cannot give the stimulus meaning relative to other auditory stimuli. The listener can report if he is aware of the presence or absence of sound, but supposedly he cannot identify the sound (Chalfant and Scheffelin, 1969). Sensation is rather like an "on-off" registration process; the sound is or is not heard.

Thus, when the diagnostician measures sensation, he is particularly interested in his client's ability to hear. He searches for the client's threshold of hearing. He wants to know if the client can respond to the presence of a sound without regard for recognition of the characteristics of the sound. If the stimulus is presented at the threshold of hearing, the listener, most likely, would only say that he hears (senses) sound. Even if words were presented at the threshold of hearing, the listener probably would not recognize or interpret the phonemic and semantic features of the words presented; he would again only hear sound. Therefore, when diagnosticians are interested in discovering if there are disruptions in the auditory processing system that affect the ability to hear, they usually present nonlinguistic stimuli—pure tones and noise.

Perception

On the SLPM, perception as a behavioral correlate occurs when the prelinguistic auditory programming process has been added to the process of auditory reception-analysis.

Auditory perception is modality bound; it occurs as the end result of the activities taking place within the auditory modality. Thus perception is dependent on the sequencing, grouping, and storing of innumerable auditory patterns.

For most types of auditory stimulation an active listener would be able to report more information about its auditory characteristics than just hearing it. In everyday listening, reports of sensation probably seldom occur alone. Thus, as the next "highest" behavioral correlate after sensation, perception differs from sensation in that the listener can now recognize and sort the auditory information as well as compare and discriminate it in relation to previously stored information. In short, the listener

can *derive significance* from the characteristics of the auditory stimulation.

Many authors consider discriminatory activities as a major part of perception. Schuell et al. (1964), for example, view the process of perception as a discriminatory activity, scanning and sampling the incoming signals and matching them with previously stored signals. Luria (1966) views perception as a complex, active process that includes the identification of individual signals, integration of like signals into categorical groups, selection of their meaning from a series of alternatives, and discrimination of the components of the signal that are essential to the listener from those components that are considered unessential.

Certainly, discrimination is seen in the literature as a major aspect of perception. However, it is a process that requires more than a simple same-different comparison, since each incoming stimulation varies in its auditory features. For example, the phonetic features of incoming speech vary from speaker to speaker, and yet the listener is able to discriminate these variations into patterns that are considered the "same."

Liberman et al. (1967) ask the question "Why are speech sounds, alone among acoustic signals and in spite of the limitations of the ear, perceived so well?" What answers to their question do they arrive at in their extensive article?

Many other tasks go into perception, making a clear delineation of the nature of perception difficult. Operationally, perception has included *measuring a set of behavioral responses* to tasks defined as auditory attention, stimulus recognition, localization, auditory closure, categorization of auditory patterns, discrimination, temporal ordering, temporal judgment, and patterning the auditory stimulation into significant features.

Therefore diagnosticians study the perceptual abilities of their clients by selecting specific stimulus tasks that ask for specific response patterns, depending on what aspect of perception they wish to study.

Berry (1969), Chalfant and Scheffelin (1969), Hirsch (1966), Johnson and Myklebust (1967), and Mysak (1966) all present viewpoints about the nature of auditory perception. How do they define perception and what tasks do they use to measure it? What information do Eisenberg (1970) and Eisenson (1972) present about perception as a developmental phenomenon?

CENTRAL LANGUAGE SEGMENT

The physical processes that occur in the central language segment *decode and encode linguistic information,* allowing the individual to *derive meaning* from a message, to *repeat* a message, or to *formulate*

a message. This segment has been referred to as the central language system or primary linguistic system.

Physical basis of central language segment
Anatomy

The brain-language relationship has undergone extensive study since the excitement generated by Broca's presentation of the relationship between "articulated language" and the cortical area now known as Broca's area, the third frontal convolution. Today there is general concensus that language behavior is, in most instances, located in the left cerebral hemisphere. The internal processing component of the SLPM takes the view that the anatomic structures of the central language segment are located primarily in the left cerebral hemisphere.

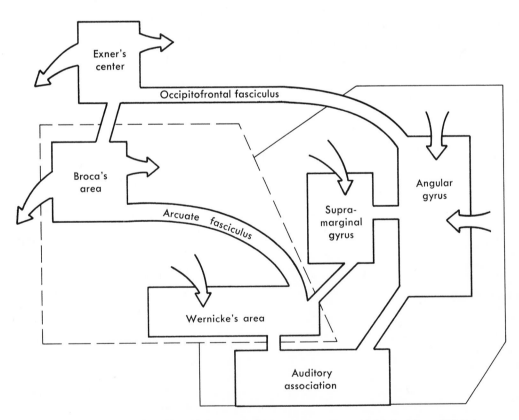

Fig. 5-3. Anatomic schematic of the central language system. (Adapted from Whitaker, H., A model for neurolinguistics. *Occasional Papers 10.* Language Centre, Colchester, England: University of Essex [1970].)

The following sources can be used as a review of cerebral localization of language functions: Berry (1969), Eisenson (1972), Lenneberg (1966), Penfield and Roberts (1959), and Russell and Espir (1961). Does cerebral localization differ between children and adults?

Many neuroanatomic models have been worked out to represent the anatomic structures for language. Whitaker (1970) provides an anatomic schematic compatible with the SLPM schema of the central language segment anatomy. Fig. 5-3 presents these structures as represented on the left cerebral hemisphere.

The anatomic areas of the central language segment viewed primarily as an *auditory-verbal* system are made up of:

1. Broca's area, the third frontal convolution
2. Wernicke's area, the first temporal convolution
3. Auditory association areas, the second and third temporal convolutions
4. Supramarginal gyrus
5. Angular gyrus

Note carefully the location of the supramarginal and angular gyri; the arrows feeding into these areas show their location relative to other important association areas for language. They lie adjacent to the auditory, visual, and somesthetic association areas.

Besides these anatomic areas, there are major pathways that connect these areas to one another. On the schematic these are shown by the use of arrows and connecting pathways for input and output of information among the structures. Of major importance is the long association pathway, the *arcuate fasciculus,* that connects Wernicke's area to Broca's area.

Physical processes

Even though the neuroanatomy of the central language segment is beginning to be worked out, there is still much speculation as to how these neurologic structures process linguistic information. Since language is organized in the left cerebral hemisphere, it seems logical that the anatomic structures may be "set" to interpret auditory patterns into a representational language form. These anatomic areas and physical processes could be considered *ideational* (symbolic) in nature; that is, the central language segment may interpret the auditory patterns by *deriving representational meanings* based on established linguistic rules. This process of building up representational forms within the central language segment is developmental; rules are learned over time, children responding differently than adults.

We are yet a long way from knowing how this process of representational activity takes place within the central language segment. A great step forward in our understanding of language processing was brought about by the work of Geschwind and his associates. Geschwind's two-part article "Disconnexion Syndromes in Animals and Man" (1965) was a landmark. It provided significant insight into the organization of language in the brain by studying behavioral syndromes of patients with different central nervous system pathologies.

Continual study is going on, and more theories about brain-language functions are being developed. A specialty is coming into existence called neurolinguistics, psychoneurolinguistics, or neurobehavior. The basic intent of this specialty is to discover the processes by which man represents language in his nervous system. However, Hughlings Jackson's caution of some time ago is still apt: it is one thing to locate a lesion that disrupts language and quite another to locate language processing in the central nervous system.

With this in mind the central language segment of the internal processing component of the SLPM (Fig. 5-1) hypothesizes three interacting linguistic physical processes that give rise to the three behavioral correlates of comprehension, formulation, and repetition. The processes are auditory programming, language representation, and speech programming.

Auditory programming. Auditory programming as a *prelinguistic process* contributing to auditory perception was discussed within the auditory reception segment. As a prelinguistic process, it turned the analyzed auditory patterns into phonetic features, readying them for further linguistic analysis.

Auditory programming as a *linguistic activity* of the central language segment is a function of Wernicke's area as well as its interactions with the remainder of the auditory association cortex, the second and third temporal convolutions (Fig. 5-3). Geschwind (1965) and Luria (1966), among others, assign a linguistic processing role to these anatomic areas. Various linguistic *decoding* and *encoding* activities have been ascribed to the auditory programming process, presumably based on established linguistic rules.

Auditory programming is responsible for *decoding phonologic information* from the phonetic features it receives. This process is apparently governed by linguistic rules that determine if the features received are made up of permissible phonemes and phonologic sequences.

Geschwind (1968) discusses this activity of the auditory association cortex as a "theory-making" activity, in that it must classify the auditory patterns (phonetic features) into phonemes, classifying the entire set of allophones that belong in a single phonemic class. Luria (1966) offers further support to this process. He considers that lesions in this area would result in difficulties analyzing complex auditory information. Disturbances of "phonemic hearing," where the individual has difficulty identifying isolated sounds from the sound complex, differentiating similar sounds, and maintaining proper "phonemic ordering," would be seen.

In addition to its phonologic processing role, Geschwind (1968) speculates that the auditory association areas are also operational in "syntactic comprehension." He feels that grammar is something that grows up within the auditory association area (our auditory programming process), and that perhaps a good part of *syntactic decoding* takes place within this area.

Thus auditory programming allows the listener to make his first linguistic interpretations, specifically phonologic and possibly some syntactic interpretations. These interpretations are made by comparing the incoming auditory information as it is decoded with previously programmed and stored linguistic information.

Abbs and Sussman (1971) have hypothesized a feature detector theory of "speech perception." They hypothesize neurosensory receptive fields that operate as feature detectors capable of decoding the phonologic features of speech from the physical parameters of the auditory stimulus. How does their concept of feature detectors correspond or differ from our hypotheses about the prelinguistic-linguistic divisions of the auditory programming process?

Auditory programming is also involved in *encoding phonologic and syntactic* aspects of the message to be expressed. Once a message has been created by the language representation process (see later discussion), it is thought to be sent back to the auditory programming area (Fig. 5-3). It is very likely that the *"auditory" phonologic patterns* are retrieved and applied here. As well, it has been speculated that certain *syntactic units may be inserted* into the message. Geschwind (1968) goes on to suggest that impulses arriving here from the angular gyrus arouse the "heard name" of words to be expressed.

In summary, the auditory programming process has been hypothesized as having *encoding* as well as *decoding linguistic functions.* It has been assigned the following linguistic tasks:

1. Decoding phonetic features into phonemes and phonologic sequences
2. Decoding some aspects of syntax
3. Encoding (applying) the auditory phonologic pattern of the message being expressed

4. Encoding (inserting) certain syntactic units into the message being expressed

Therefore the auditory programming process has been assigned linguistic functions that are related to all three behavioral correlates of the central language segment: comprehension, formulation, and repetition.

As mentioned, the auditory programming process is considered to have both prelinguistic and linguistic activities. Separating the auditory programming process into a prelinguistic and linguistic division may be a highly arbitrary distinction. The anatomic areas involved in this process are contiguous and interacting, and when damaged, more than a single activity is likely to be disrupted. However, there are theoretical advantages for making the separation. It assists the diagnostician in separating prelinguistic disorders such as phonetic discrimination from linguistic disorders such as phonologic decoding and encoding.

Language representation. Language representation as a physical process occurs when the activities of the angular and supramarginal gyri interact with the activities of the auditory association area (Fig. 5-3).

The anatomic sites of the angular and supramarginal gyri are located in the inferior parietal lobe. These areas lie at the junction of the classical visual, auditory, and somesthetic association areas (Geschwind, 1965), making them ideally suited for the establishment of associations between different types of sensory information (*cross-modal associations*). Therefore Geschwind calls this area the "association area of association areas."

The physical process of language representation then introduces the most complex form of *language decoding* and *encoding*. As a physical process, it is of tremendous significance for semantic and pragmatic integration to say nothing of its importance to reading, writing, and gestural modes of human communication.

Prior to the process of language representation, phonologic and some syntactic interpretations of the auditory message have taken place. However, it is the process of language representation that *completes message decoding*. Language as meaning is represented here based on the complex multiple stimulus analysis that occurs in this major association area.

Message encoding begins when the process of language representation retrieves information that has been integrated and stored within this area. The angular gyrus in particular has been suggested by Geschwind (1965) as having the function of naming. Luria (1966) concurs that the semantic aspects of language are handled in this area but also suggests that logical-grammatical operations occur as well.

Within this process, auditory, visual, and somesthetic information is related, integrated, stored, and retrieved. Relationships are formed among the various types of perceptual information. The human develops the capability of relating words to words and words heard to objects seen; he can label a visual event and visualize an auditory event; he can interpret and discuss his sensory world through language.

Language representation thus is seen as an additive synthesis of information from more than one modality. It is a meeting and exchange between auditory, visual, and somesthetic experience that is stored and becomes available for future interpretation and retrieval. *Semantic, pragmatic,* and *some syntactic decoding* and *encoding* are seen as activities of language representation.

Speech programming. Once the message is ideationally encoded by the language representation process, it is sent back to the auditory programming areas for phonologic and more syntactic encoding (see discussion of auditory programming process). The encoded message is then conducted across the arcuate fasciculus to Broca's area (Fig. 5-3), bringing the message to the final physical process within the central language segment, speech programming. The arcuate fasciculus provides the essential anatomic linkup between auditory programming and speech programming.

The basic activity of speech programming is to *change the auditory program received via the arcuate fasciculus into a motor program.* It turns the message into a *series of motor speech commands.* These programmed motor speech commands are then sent to the primary motor cortex, which initiates the postlinguistic production processes.

Geschwind (1965) describes Broca's area as a complex way station between the auditory association areas and the primary motor cortex. He considers Broca's area to function as an "auditory-motor transducer" and suggests that it contains the rules for turning the sounds of speech into motor acts. These rules are utilized to program phonologic sequences so that speech is sequential and there is a smooth transition from one phoneme to the next. Sequential programming is not meant to imply that a linear series of discrete phonemic units are being programmed, but rather sequential programming that would account for coarticulation, the sequential muscular movements seen in speech production (Daniloff and Moll, 1968). These rules also provide the speech program with the *prosodic features of speech* so that the melody of the speech pattern is present.

In a sense it could be said that the speech programming process *"reads" the phonologic representation* of the message that was applied by the auditory programming process and *transduces this into a series of motor speech representations.* These motor representations then tell the primary motor cortex what information to send to the muscles as sequential movement patterns. As stated by Kent (1973), this process "orchestrates the motor reactions." These motor commands determine the final sequence of events that would then be heard in the speech product, given that the speech production segment carries out these commands appropriately.

Developmentally, the speech program-

ming process has been considered by some to provide automaticity and efficiency to language. As the language learner gains more and more experience transducing auditory programs into speech programs, his speech programming process may assume some activities from the auditory programming process. Green (1970) has stated that Broca's area inserts functor words such as "the," "and," and "of" into the message. He feels that automaticity and efficiency of language would be greatly reduced if every functor word had to be inserted into the message before arriving at Broca's area. It is also possible that certain morphophonemic rules are implemented here providing for automatic insertion of such syntactic features as tense and pluralization.

Speech programming as the final physical process in the central language segment basically *programs the sequence of motor commands* to be used for phonemic and prosodic production. As well, in later life, the process may begin to automatically insert certain syntactic units into the message.

• • •

In summary, the three physical processes within the central language segment (auditory programming, language representation, and speech programming) are linguistic processes involved in decoding the message after its prelinguistic analysis and in encoding the message to be produced by the speech production segment.

The position we have taken regarding the anatomic and processing basis for language is that it is primarily cortical activity; Broca's area and the auditory association areas in interaction with the large temporoparieto-occipital complex. However, other views have been presented in the literature. Penfield and Roberts (1959) hypothesized a centrencephalic system for the "elaboration" of speech. The centrencephalic system is suggested by them as the means by which cross-modal integration takes place. They consider this system as including all the subcortical gray matter and connecting tracts that serve inter- and intrahemispheric integration. This system is primarily thalamic; nerve fibers from parts of the thalamus are projected to and from the cortical speech areas, and by means of these circuits, speech and language information is coded, organized, and synthesized. The speech areas are thus coordinated by this centrencephalic system. The January, 1975 (vol. 2), issue of *Brain and Language* is devoted to the topic of the role of the thalamus in language. These articles suggest that there is a thalamic role in language that is different from the cortical role. Among the views presented is the role of the thalamus in language as arousal, alerting, activation, and attention in interaction with memory mechanisms, timing mechanisms, etc. How, as speech pathologists, would you interpret these findings? As language? As linguistic operations? As prelinguistic operations? As nonlinguistic operations?

Behavioral correlates within central language segment

The physical processes within the central language segment give rise primarily to three measurable behavioral correlates. As measurable sets of behaviors, the correlates of comprehension, formulation, and repetition reveal the individual's ability to process linguistic information.

Comprehension

Comprehension is seen to occur on the SLPM as a result of interactions between the physical processes of auditory programming and language representation. These processes decode the auditory patterns into linguistic information, drawing information as well from other sensory modalities.

Comprehension implies that the listener has *made sense of the message* he has received. He not only has grasped the meaning of the words he has heard but also the relationships the words have to each other. Language is comprehended because the listener applies linguistic rules to his auditory perceptions and derives meaning from the message. Through these rules the listener can combine current language input with stored information, giving rise to new meaningfulness. He develops *representational abilities*—the ability to decode the phonologic, syntactic, and semantic parameters of the message as well as place them within a pragmatic context.

In order to do this the listener must be able to turn the prelinguistic phonetic features into phonologic, semantic, and syntactic representations for comparison with stored information. The data suggest that different processes are responsible for decoding different components of the message. Processing of linguistic information for comprehension is suggested to "begin" with phonologic comprehension that primarily occurs as a result of the auditory programming process followed by syntactic, semantic, and pragmatic comprehension, which result primarily from language representation.

Thus the diagnostician interested in measuring comprehension can develop tasks that isolate the linguistic levels of language comprehension. At the same time he can work toward separating comprehension problems that stem from prelinguistic disruptions versus those that stem from disruption of the linguistic processes.

Rees (1973), analyzing literature relating auditory processing to language disorders, developed the argument that "there is no basis for the assumption that the comprehension of heard speech depends on the fundamental ability to analyze the utterance into a string of phonemes—or larger segments—in the order produced." What alternate hypotheses does she offer?

Formulation

Formulation on the SLPM is a behavioral correlate resulting from the physical processes of language representation, auditory programming, and speech programming.

Formulation is considered to be the behavioral correlate that reveals the speaker's *active creation and planning of a message on all linguistic levels* prior to production of the message. Formulation is the representational creation and planning of a message. This linguistic creativity allows the speaker to formulate novel messages that convey different meanings to suit the purposes of the speaker and his listeners. Formulation implies that the speaker has a system by which he can plan the intent of the message and structure it according to the standards of his language community.

To formulate a message the speaker must first know his intent (pragmatic purpose), and from this intent he can plan the linguistic structure of the message. As Lenneberg (1967) indicates, the elements of the message cannot be ordered without the knowledge of the intent of the entire sentence or message. Formulation, therefore, implies that the speaker implements the linguistic rules by which messages are created and planned. By implementation of linguistic rules the speaker retrieves representational information and derives the pragmatic, semantic, syntactic, and phonologic features of the message he wants to produce. He selects the appropriate words (lexical selection), orders the words into appropriate syntactic patterns, and selects the appropriate phonologic sequences, which are then turned into speech programs.

As in comprehension, there is information suggesting that different underlying physical processes are responsible for encoding different components of the message during formulation. Thus processing of linguistic information for formulation is suggested to "begin" with pragmatic, semantic, and syntactic formulation as a result primarily of the language representation process, followed by more syntactic and phonologic formulation from auditory programming. Final phonologic formulation occurs when the speech programming process turns the phonologic program received from auditory programming into a motor speech program.

Therefore the diagnostician interested in measuring the behavioral correlate formu-

lation would observe the language product. He can design tasks to isolate the various levels of language and from his observations potentially determine the physical processes that may be disrupted.

Repetition

Repetition implies that a language stimulus presented is reproduced with no assumptions made regarding the meaningfulness or purposefulness of the response. The SLPM (Fig. 5-1) suggests that repetition may occur in one of two ways.

First, repetition may proceed through the usual comprehension-formulation sequence that would involve all central language processes. In this case, the language stimulus would be comprehended as well as purposefully reproduced—*meaningful repetition*.

Alternatively, repetition may result via a shortcut. Information can be *shunted* directly from auditory programming to speech programming, thus bypassing language representation—*nonmeaningful repetition*. But for repetition to be intact, the auditory programming process must arouse the appropriate sequence of sounds to be sent to the speech programming process for motoric representation. Anatomically, as we have already seen, Wernicke's area (auditory programming) possesses conduction links with Broca's area (speech programming) via the arcuate fasciculus. This route permits transmission of auditory-verbal sequences without reference to meaning. An individual shunting information across this route presents behavior observed essentially as a rote response, independent from meaningful comprehension or purposeful formulation.

Note how other model builders have also included this lower level shunting of information: Kirk et al. (1968), Morley (1972), Osgood and Miron (1963), and Wepman et al. (1960). This short circuiting of information also gains support from other investigators: Fay and Butler (1968), Fraser et al. (1963), Howes (1967), and Kent (1974).

SPEECH PRODUCTION SEGMENT

The speech production segment of the internal processing component of the SLPM has received extensive study in speech pathology. The *postlinguistic* physical processes that occur in this segment are responsible for turning the formulated message into an actualized speech event, the acoustic waveform. The speaker *initiates, transmits, coordinates,* and *produces* the motor activities necessary for speech production. This segment has been referred to as a *primary motor system, primary production system,* or *the verbal modality.*

Physical basis of speech production segment
Anatomy

The anatomy of the speech production segment is made up of the bilateral structures of the verbal modality—from the primary motor cortex to the muscles and structures of the speech mechanism. Again, Whitaker (1970) presents anatomic schematics basically in keeping with our definition of the speech production segment (Figs. 5-4 and 5-5).

The reader is referred to the following texts for detailed reviews of information about the speech production segment: Kaplan (1971), Minifie et al. (1973), Palmer (1972), and Zemlin (1968).

Physical processes

The complexity of speech production results from the incorporation of a seemingly infinite number of component acts and the combination of these component acts into appropriately timed, ordered, and executed sequences. The internal processing component of the SLPM (Fig. 5-1) hypothesizes a series of four interacting physical processes within the speech production segment. Following speech programming, they are speech initiation, speech coordination-transmission, and speech production. The speech production process itself incorporates five subprocesses: breathing for speech, phonation, resonation, articulation, and prosodation.

Speech programming. Since the formulated message is sent from Broca's area, the site of speech programming, this area could be considered as overlapping with the speech production segment. However, as we have discussed, Broca's area is considered primarily a part of the central language segment. Its speech programming role in formulation has been discussed. We will not discuss its role in the speech production segment until we consider the behavioral correlate of sequencing.

Speech initiation. Once the formulated message has been given its speech program, it is sent to the primary motor cortex, the primary anatomic site for speech initiation. The speech-producing musculature is neurologically represented at the base of the primary motor cortex, which is contiguous to Broca's area.

In order to produce speech the motor plan sent from speech programming must be turned into a series of neural impulses. Speech initiation, then, is the process of *initiating these neural impulses* in the primary motor cortex. Speech initiation "reads" the motor program and translates it into sequential neuromotor impulses to be sent to the speech mechanism. The physical process of speech initiation thereby guides the sequential motor movements of the speech production subprocesses of breathing for speech, phonation, resonation, articulation, and prosodation.

Speech initiation is far more complex than portrayed here. Other anatomic sites and processes are involved. What role does Luria (1966) ascribe to the secondary motor cortex (Brodmann's area 6) and the postcentral regions of the left cerebral hemisphere?

Speech coordination-transmission. The physical process of speech coordination-transmission is responsible, along with speech initiation, for the *smooth on-target movements* of the speech musculature.

The neural impulses initiated in the primary motor cortex are interactive with many interrelated motor and sensory systems. These systems have been studied ex-

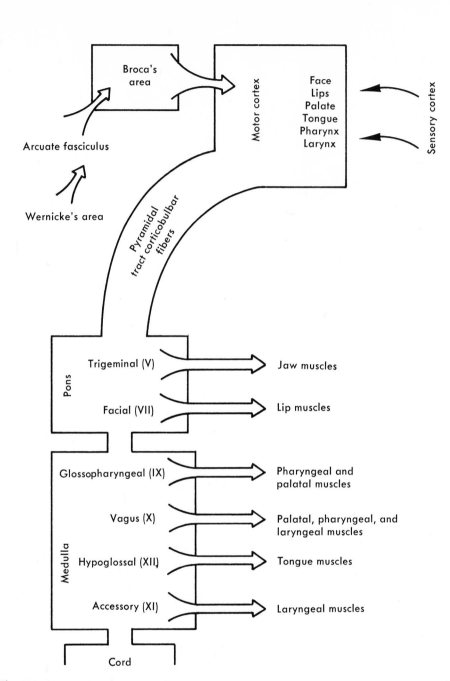

Fig. 5-4. Anatomic schematic of the verbal modality. (From Whitaker, H., A model for neurolinguistics. *Occasional Papers 10.* Language Centre, Colchester, England: University of Essex [1970].)

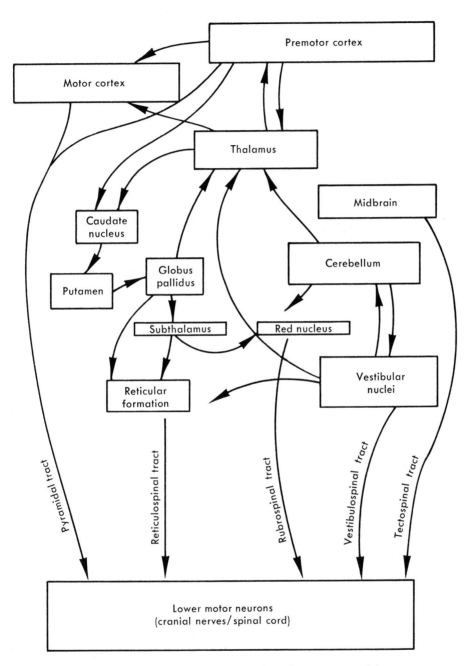

Fig. 5-5. Anatomic schematic of the pyramidal and extrapyramidal motor systems. (Adapted from Whitaker, H., A model for neurolinguistics. *Occasional Papers 10.* Language Centre, Colchester, England: University of Essex [1970].)

tensively. Gardner (1968) views them as levels of motor organization from the lowest (spinal) to the highest (cortical), and Darley et al. (1975) discuss hierarchies of motor organization. Others have viewed these systems from a more functional viewpoint. They have studied the interactions of the pyramidal, extrapyramidal, cerebellar, and reticular systems in terms of the roles they play in mediation, transmission, modulation, coordination, facilitation, and inhibition of motor activities. Whitaker's (1970) schematic only begins to spell out the complexities and interactions of those systems involved with all motor activities, including speech production (Fig. 5-5).

The speech coordination-transmission process is seen as the activity of all these neural structures, pathways, and interactions that have an effect on muscular activity. Therefore speech coordination-transmission concerns the *control* of the hundreds of muscular adjustments made very rapidly during each moment of speech production.

Berry (1969) provides extensive information about "tracking language in the nervous system" that relates to the concepts presented here about speech coordination-transmission.

Speech production. The speech production process is viewed on the SLPM as the organized, controlled, and coordinated neuromuscular activities of the breathing, laryngeal, pharyngeal, oral, nasal, and facial structures that make up the speech mechanism.

Breathing for speech, phonation, resonation, articulation, and *prosodation* as *subprocesses* of speech production interact continuously during the act of speaking. The sequential activities that occur as a result of the preceding neurologic processes must be accurate in terms of force of contraction, timing of contractions, speed of contractions, range of movement, direction of movement, sequence of movement, etc.—all controlled in relationship to all

other bodily activities taking place while an individual is talking.

The complexity of this muscular activity has been described by Lenneberg (1967). Lenneberg discussed some physiologic correlates to these activities. What hypotheses does he propose to account for the complexities of speech production?

The study of the structures and subprocesses of speech production has long been a part of the discipline of speech pathology. As a study and review guide the student might find it useful to develop a detailed table of the structure and functions of the speech-producing mechanism. Kaplan (1971), Palmer (1972), and Zemlin (1968) can serve as general resources as well as the table on p. 145 of *Human Communication and Its Disorders: An Overview* (1969). For more detailed information reflecting specific viewpoints, Dickson et al. (1974, 1975) could be consulted. The following are useful sources related to the specific subprocesses of the speech production process.

Breathing for speech (respiration)	Boone, 1971; Hixon, 1973; McDonald and Chance, 1964; Van Riper and Irwin, 1958
Phonation	Boone, 1971; Hollien, 1962; Moore, 1971; Sheets, 1973
Resonation	Boone, 1971; Dickson and Dickson, 1972
Articulation	Brown et al., 1973; Daniloff, 1973; Darley, 1964; Klatt, 1974; McDonald, 1964; Perkins, 1977
Prosodation	We have developed a somewhat artificial subprocess of speech production that we have termed prosodation. It is considered as a unified, integrated process incorporating aspects of the other subprocesses of speech production. This process is responsible for the speech product we later view as prosody. We know of no literature that specifically discusses a prosodation process. However, there is beginning to be more study of the underlying physiologic events that result in the product we call prosody. What does Netsell (1973) consider as the physical basis for prosody?

• • •

In summary, the physical processes that occur in the speech production segment are postlinguistic processes. They carry out the *motor activities* required for producing speech. Fig. 5-6 summarizes the activities of the speech production segment.

Behavioral correlates within speech production segment

The internal processing component of the SLPM (Fig. 5-1) specifies two be-havioral correlates reflective of the physi-cal processes within the speech production segment. The behavioral correlates of se-quencing and motor control assist the diag-nostician in determining how well the speaker can carry out the postlinguistic motor activities needed for speech produc-tion.

Sequencing

On the SLPM sequencing is tied to the physical processes of speech pro-

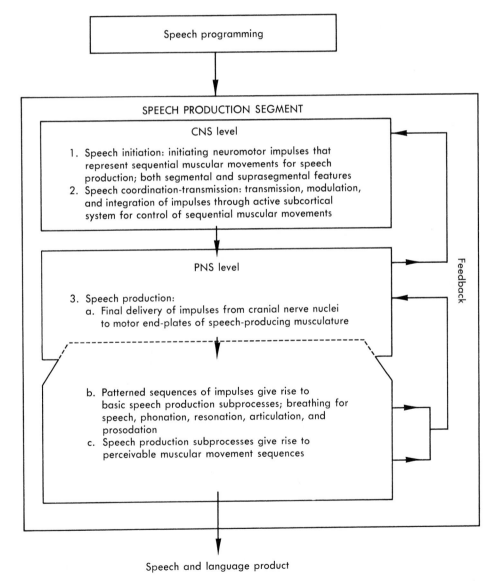

Fig. 5-6. Summary of the activities of the speech production segment of the SLPM.

gramming and speech initiation. Speech programming is responsible for planning the motor sequence for speech production, and speech initiation is responsible for translating the program into a sequential series of neuromotor impulses. This sequential order of neuromotor commands is sent to the speech mechanism to be actualized as a *sequence of muscular movements*.

Sequencing as a behavioral correlate then has to do with observing the *order of motor activities* that occur when speech is produced. The diagnostician can observe some of the muscular activities of the speech mechanism to determine if sequencing is disrupted, or he may listen to the production of speech sounds to gain cues about disruptions of sequencing.

Motor control

The final behavioral correlate of the speech production segment is motor control tied to the physical processes of speech initiation, speech coordination-transmission, and speech production. This behavioral correlate allows the diagnostician to observe if *on-target, precise movements* of the speech-producing structures have occurred. He can observe patterned movements, tension, position, manner of production, etc. to arrive at an estimate of muscular activity and control. There are also instrumental measures available for gaining information about motor control during speech production. Cinefluorography, electromyography, and laryngoscopy are among those extrasensory measures that provide rather direct instrumental analyses of the processes within the speech production segment.

Motor control along with sequencing gives the diagnostician information he needs regarding the *temporal coordination of muscular contractions* that take place during speech production. They allow him to view the timing, the serial ordering of muscular movements. When observing the behavioral correlates of motor control and sequencing, it must be kept in mind that they are reflections of physical processes that are carrying out a preprogrammed message. As Kent (1973) has indicated in his development of a preprogramming model for speech movements, the motor program inherently includes timing control. He adds that once the program is triggered (speech initiation in the SLPM) the serial movements of speech are produced in the planned sequence.

SUMMARY

The internal speech and language processing component of the SLPM presents speech and language processing as an interface between behavior and its physical basis. The point has been emphasized that the diagnostician can observe behavioral correlates that provide him with information about internal physical processes.

The internal processing component was constructed based on the following concepts. First, the component was broken into three segments representing anatomic and processing boundaries. Second, within each segment the model presents the hypothesized sequence of physical processes responsible for speech and language behavior. Nine physical processes were hypothesized. Third, the model presents a set of behavioral correlates within each segment. These behavioral correlates are presumed to arise from the activities of the physical processes; that is, they are sets of external behaviors that the diagnostician can observe. Seven behavioral correlates were presented.

Having traversed this more technical discussion of the internal processing component, the reader may wish to refer again to the *processing overview* presented in Chapter 3.

REFERENCES

Abbs, J. H., and Sussman, H. M., Neurophysiological feature detector and speech perception: A discussion of theoretical implications. *J. Speech Hearing Res.*, **14**, 23-36 (1971).

Berry, M., *Language Disorders of Children: The Bases and Diagnoses*. New York: Appleton-Century-Crofts (1969).

Boone, D. R., *The Voice and Voice Therapy.* Englewood Cliffs, N.J.: Prentice-Hall, Inc. (1971).

Broca, P., Nouvelle observation d'aphémie produite par une lésion de la mortié posterieure des deuxieme et troisième circonvolutions frontales. *Bull. Soc. Anat. Paris,* 398-407 (1861a).

Broca, P., Remarques sur le siège de la faculté du langage articulé, suivés d'une observation d'aphémie. *Bull Soc. Anat. Paris,* 330-357 (1861b).

Brown, W. S., McGlone, R. E., and Proffit, W. R., Relationship of lingual and intraoral air pressure during syllable production. *J. Speech Hearing Res.,* **16,** 141-151 (1973).

Chalfant, J., and Scheffelin, M., *Central Processing Dysfunctions in Children: A Review of Research.* NINDS Monogr. No. 9. Bethesda, Md.: U.S. Department of Health, Education and Welfare (1969).

Daniloff, R. G., Normal articulation processes. In F. D. Minifie, T. J. Hixon, and F. Williams (Eds.), *Normal Aspects of Speech, Hearing, and Language.* Englewood Cliffs, N.J.: Prentice-Hall, Inc. (1973).

Daniloff, R. G., and Moll, K., Coarticulation of lip rounding. *J. Speech Hearing Res.,* **11,** 707-721 (1968).

Darley, F. L., *Diagnosis and Appraisal of Communication Disorders.* Englewood Cliffs, N.J.: Prentice-Hall, Inc. (1964).

Darley, F. L., Aronson, A. E., and Brown, J. R., *Motor Speech Disorders.* Philadelphia: W. B. Saunders Co. (1975).

Dickson, D. R., and Dickson, W. M., Velopharyngeal anatomy. *J. Speech Hearing Res.,* **15,** 373-381 (1972).

Dickson, D. R., Grant, J. C. B., Sicher, H., Dubrul, E. L., and Paltan, J., Status of research in cleft palate: Anatomy and physiology. I. *Cleft Palate J.,* **11,** 471-492 (1974).

Dickson, D. R., Grant, J. C. B., Sicher, H., Dubrul, E. L., and Paltan, J., Status of research in cleft palate: Anatomy and physiology. II. *Cleft Palate J.,* **12,** 131-156 (1975).

Eisenberg, R. B., The organization of auditory behavior. *J. Speech Hearing Res.,* **13,** 453-471 (1970).

Eisenson, J., *Aphasia in Children.* New York: Harper & Row, Publishers (1972).

Fay, W., and Butler, B., Echolalia, I.Q. and the developmental dichotomy of speech and language systems. *J. Speech Hearing Res.,* **11,** 365-371 (1968).

Fraser, C., Bellugi, U., and Brown, R., Control of grammar in imitation, comprehension, and production. *J. verb. Learning verb. Behav.,* **2,** 121-135 (1963).

Gardner, E., *Fundamentals of Neurology.* (5th ed.) Philadelphia: W. B. Saunders Co. (1968).

Geschwind, N., Disconnexion syndromes in animals and man. I and II. *Brain,* **88,** 237-294; 585-643 (1965).

Geschwind, N., Neurological foundations of language. In H. R. Myklebust (Ed.), *Progress in Learning Disabilities.* New York: Grune & Stratton, Inc. (1968).

Glattke, T. J., Elements of auditory physiology. In F. D. Minifie, T. J. Hixon, and F. Williams (Eds.), *Normal Aspects of Speech, Hearing, and Language.* Englewood Cliffs, N.J.: Prentice-Hall, Inc. (1973).

Green, E., On the contribution of studies in aphasia to psycholinguistics. *Cortex,* **6,** 216-235 (1970).

Hirsch, I. J., Audition in relation to perception of speech. In E. C. Carterette (Ed.), *Brain Function: Speech, Language, and Communication.* (Vol. 3) Berkeley, Calif.: University of California Press (1966).

Hixon, T. F., Respiratory function in speech. In F. D. Minifie, T. J. Hixon, and F. Williams (Eds.), *Normal Aspects of Speech, Hearing, and Language.* Englewood Cliffs, N.J.: Prentice-Hall, Inc. (1973).

Hollien, H., Vocal fold thickness and fundamental frequency of phonation. *J. Speech Hearing Res.,* **5,** 237-243 (1962).

Howes, D., Hypotheses concerning the functions of the language mechanism. In K. Salzinger and S. Salzinger (Eds.), *Research in Verbal Behavior and Some Neurological Implications.* New York: Academic Press, Inc. (1967).

Human Communication and Its Disorders: An Overview. Bethesda, Md.: National Institute of Neurological Disease and Stroke, U.S. Department of Health, Education and Welfare (1969).

Johnson, D., and Myklebust, H., *Learning Disabilities: Educational Principles and Practices.* New York: Grune & Stratton, Inc. (1967).

Kaplan, H. M., *Anatomy and Physiology of Speech.* (2nd ed.) New York: McGraw-Hill Book Co. (1971).

Kent, R. D., Is the seriation of speech movements governed by motor programs or feedback? Paper presented at the Annual Convention of the American Speech and Hearing Association, Detroit (1973).

Kent, R. D., Auditory-motor formant tracking: A study of speech imitation. *J. Speech Hearing Res.,* **17,** 203-222 (1974).

Kimura, D., The asymmetry of the human brain. *Scient. Am.,* **228,** 70-78 (1973).

Kirk, S. A., McCarthy, J. J., and Kirk, W., *Examiner's Manual: Illinois Test of Psycholinguistic Abilities.* Urbana, Ill.: University of Illinois Press (1968).

Klatt, D., The duration of /s/ in English words. *J. Speech Hearing Res.,* **17,** 51-63 (1974).

Lenneberg, E. H., Speech development: Its anatomical and physiological concomitants. In E. C. Carterette (Ed.), *Brain Function: Speech, Language, and Communication.* (Vol. 3) Berkeley, Calif.: University of California Press (1966).

Lenneberg, E. H., *Biological Foundations of Language.* New York: John Wiley & Sons, Inc. (1967).

Liberman, A. M., Cooper, F. S., Shankweiler, D. P., and Studdert-Kennedy, M., Perception of the speech code. *Psychol. Rev.,* **74,** 431-461 (1967).

Luria, A. R., *Higher Cortical Functions in Man*. New York: Basic Books, Inc., Publishers (1966).

McDonald, E. T., *Articulation Testing and Treatment: A Sensory-Motor Approach*. Pittsburgh: Stanwix House, Inc. (1964).

McDonald, E. T., and Chance, B. C., *Cerebral Palsy*. Englewood Cliffs, N.J.: Prentice-Hall, Inc. (1964).

Minifie, F. D., Hixon, T. J., and Williams, F. (Eds.), *Normal Aspects of Speech, Hearing, and Language*. Englewood Cliffs, N.J.: Prentice-Hall, Inc. (1973).

Moore, P. G., *Organic Voice Disorders*. Englewood Cliffs, N.J.: Prentice-Hall, Inc. (1971).

Morley, M. E., *The Development and Disorders of Speech in Childhood*. (3rd ed.) London: Churchill Livingstone (1972).

Myklebust, H., *Auditory Disorders in Children*. New York: Grune & Stratton, Inc. (1954).

Mysak, E. D., *Speech Pathology and Feedback Theory*. Springfield, Ill.: Charles C Thomas, Publisher (1966).

Netsell, R., Speech physiology. In F. D. Minifie, T. J. Hixon, and F. Williams (Eds.), *Normal Aspects of Speech, Hearing, and Language*. Englewood Cliffs, N.J.: Prentice-Hall, Inc. (1973).

Osgood, C., and Miron, M., *Approaches to the Study of Aphasia*. Urbana, Ill.: University of Illinois Press (1963).

Palmer, J. M., *Anatomy for Speech and Hearing*. (2nd ed.) New York: Harper & Row, Publishers (1972).

Penfield, W., and Roberts, L., *Speech and Brain Mechanisms*. Princeton, N.J.: Princeton University Press (1959).

Perkins, W. H., *Speech Pathology: An Applied Behavioral Science*. (2nd ed.) St. Louis: The C. V. Mosby Co. (1977).

Rees, N. S., Auditory processing factors in language disorders: The view from Procrustes' bed. *J. Speech Hearing Dis.*, **38**, 304-315 (1973).

Rose, D. E. (Ed.), *Audiological Assessment*. Englewood Cliffs, N.J.: Prentice-Hall, Inc. (1971).

Russell, W. R., and Espir, M. L. E., *Traumatic Aphasia. Oxford Neurological Monographs*. London: Oxford University Press (1961).

Schuell, H., Jenkins, J. J., and Jimeniz-Pabon, E., *Aphasia in Adults: Diagnosis, Prognosis, and Treatment*. New York: Harper & Row, Publishers (1964).

Sheets, B. V., *Anatomy and Physiology of the Speech Mechanism*. New York: The Bobbs-Merrill Co., Inc. (1973).

Van Riper, C., and Irwin, J. V., *Voice and Articulation*. Englewood Cliffs, N.J.: Prentice-Hall, Inc. (1958).

Wepman, J. M., Jones, L. V., Bock, R. D., and Van Pelt, D. V., Studies in aphasia: Background and theoretical formulations. *J. Speech Hearing Dis.*, **25**, 323-332 (1960).

Wernicke, K., The symptom-complex of aphasia (1874). In A. Church (Ed.), *Diseases of the Nervous System*. New York: Appleton-Century-Crofts (1908).

Whitaker, H. A., A model for neurolinguistics. *Occasional Papers 10*. Language Centre, Colchester, England: University of Essex (1970).

Whitfield, I. C., *The Auditory Pathway*. Baltimore: The Williams & Wilkins Co. (1967).

Zemlin, W. R., *Speech and Hearing Science: Anatomy and Physiology*. Englewood Cliffs, N.J.: Prentice-Hall, Inc. (1968).

Speech and language product component of the speech and language processing model

This chapter focuses on the verbal response that comes out of the speaker's mouth—his speech and language product. An orientation to the speech and language product component can be reviewed in Chapter 3.

What is or is not heard in the client's speech and language product at any stage during his learning and use of speech and language usually forms the basis for identification of a speech and language disorder and likewise serves as the basis for a diagnostic referral. The parameters of the speech and language product are typically the diagnostician's initial concern. From what he hears and observes of the client's speech and language product, the diagnostician then considers the physical basis and environmental factors that may account for the disordered product. For example, observing 7-year-old LaVerne's distortion of the /s/, /z/, /ʃ/, and /ʒ/ phonemes could lead the diagnostician to investigate physical processing disruptions in the speech production segment that may account for LaVerne's phoneme distortions. Thus the diagnostician often first uses information from the speech and language product to identify, classify, and uncover the causal basis for speech and language disorders.

As discussed in Chapter 3, the speaker's verbal response is essentially an acoustic waveform. This acoustic waveform (prod-

uct) can be subjected to various forms of measurement, analyzed from diverse viewpoints, and segmented into various frameworks. A multitude of possible speech and language product frameworks are available in speech pathology. Here, we present one such framework: the speech and language product component of the SLPM. The details of this component are expanded in Fig. 6-1.

Although the component represents our current thinking, we in no way expect every diagnostician to adopt all aspects of this particular framework. But we do consider the speech and language product component to exemplify a number of strengths.

1. It is comprehensive and terminologically consistent.
2. It is theoretically consistent—it relates speech and language behavior to underlying speech and language processes.
3. It is adaptable to multiple measurement approaches.

First, we consider the nomenclature developed for the product component to be comprehensive and consistent with current terminology. As can be seen in Fig. 6-1, we have separated the product into two major product levels—the speech product and the language product. Within each product level, major behavioral parameters are specified. As well as incorporating

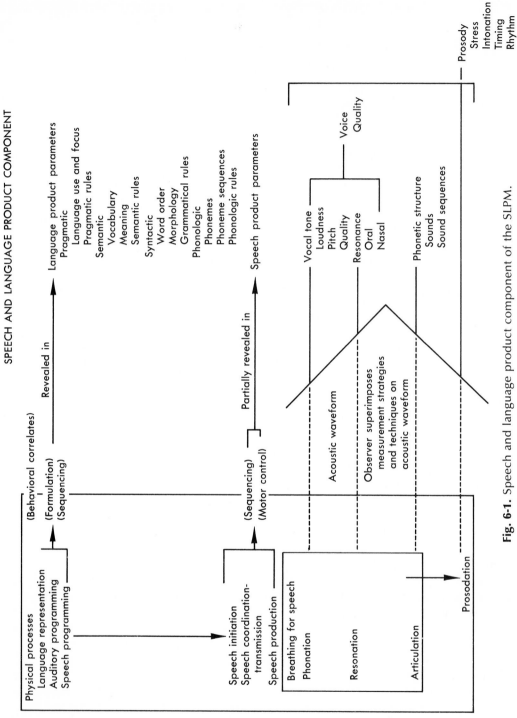

Fig. 6-1. Speech and language product component of the SLPM.

linguistic terminology, these parameters allow for easy adaptation to disorder classifications. The diagnostician can talk about speech disorders, language disorders, voice disorders, pitch disorders, phonetic structure disorders, etc.

As well, consistency was developed in the SLPM between the speech and language product terminology and the speech and language input terminology. The SLPM views the two as the same, another way of saying that the parameters of the spoken product are the parameters the listener receives as speech and language input.

Second, the product framework makes the relationship between the speech and language product and its physical basis explicit: it is theoretically consistent. Each level and parameter in the product component may be traced back to one or more physical processes and behavioral correlates from which it arises. This forces the diagnostician to recognize the fundamental connection between internal processing and speech and language behavior.

The speech product is considered a direct reflection of the activities of the speech production segment and more specifically of the subprocesses of speech production (Fig. 6-1). It is a "motoric" response. The language product, on the other hand, is not a reflection of motoric processes. Instead, it is considered a direct reflection of the physical processes of the central language segment as revealed by the behavioral correlate of formulation.

Third, the speech and language product component is adaptable to many different measurement strategies and techniques (Chapter 3). Since these strategies are dependent on choices made by the observer, no single approach to measurement inherently provides a "true" characterization of the speech and language response. Rather, the tasks are designed to elicit responses, and the measurement techniques chosen provide information to suit different purposes. Recognizing that there is no superior measurement strategy, the diagnostician can benefit from having diverse strategies available and selecting those techniques that best answer the questions he asks.

For example, a specific production of the [l] phone could be measured physically, perceptually, or linguistically, dependent on the question asked. If the diagnostician is interested in knowing if Bethany's [l] production in the word *l*amb is acceptable, he would probably choose a perceptual measure. The diagnostician would listen to Bethany's [l] production and perceptually compare her [l] with his internalized norm (acceptable limits) for the /l/ phoneme. In this way the diagnostician obtains the most direct answer to his question. If the diagnostician chose to describe the spectral characteristics in more exacting detail by instrumental measurement, he would gain physical data, but this measure would not tell him if the sound was acceptable. Or, if the diagnostician chose to consider all the allophonic variations of the /l/ phoneme, he would gain linguistic information; but again, this measure would not add considerably to his judgment of the acceptability of Bethany's [l] production.

It is vital that the diagnostician maintain a clear focus on what he is measuring and inferring when he uses the speech and language product component. At times he measures the product in order to describe speech and language behavior. At other times he measures the product to enable him to infer about the behavioral correlates and, from that, to infer about physical processes. And still, there are instances where the diagnostician can infer from observations of the speech and language product to the speech and language environment. Thus the speech and language product component serves as a framework for measuring and describing speech and language disorders as well as answering questions about cause-effect relationships.

With these three considerations in mind, the primary emphasis of this chapter will be a description of the speech and language product to which the diagnostician can direct his measurements. As well, certain major points about speech and language acquisition will be made. The diagnostician needs both an understanding of speech and language as a standard adult system and as a standard developing system. What follows, then, is an explication of the terms used in the speech and language product component of the SLPM. Fig. 6-1 should be consulted regularly throughout this discussion.

SPEECH PRODUCT

Just as the speech production subprocesses are truly inseparable so are the speech products that result. However, it is necessary for the observer to isolate convenient parameters of the speech product for his use in diagnosis. The diagnostician directs his observations to five primary speech products: vocal tone, resonance, voice, phonetic structure, and prosody.

Vocal tone

Produced by vocal fold movement, vocal tone relates most directly to the speech production subprocess of phonation (Fig. 6-1). While the subprocess of breathing for speech provides the underlying breath stream for phonation, sound is not produced until there is laryngeal participation. Thus breathing provides the power source for phonation, but phonation contributes most directly to vocal tone.

In analyzing vocal tone the diagnostician aims to describe three primary physical and perceptual parameters: *intensity,* or its perceptual correlate, *loudness; frequency,* perceived as *pitch;* and *spectral complexity,* perceived as *vocal quality.*

What are your speculations as to the "sound of the voice" as it comes directly from the larynx prior to the addition of any resonation? Can you find any literature that may support your speculations? How do people who study speech acoustics consider it (Minifie, 1973)?

To obtain physical measurements of the characteristics of the vocal tone would re-

quire instrumental analyses. Instruments such as the spectrograph, pitch meter, phonelograph, and sound level meter are some that give information about the intensity, frequency, and spectrum of the vocal tone.

Diagnosticians, however, generally measure the *perceptual correlates* of the physical characteristics. *Loudness* is typically judged as appropriate or inappropriate for a given situation. Judgments of too loud, too soft, or fading generally serve as rough indicators of the unacceptability of the loudness dimension of vocal tone.

Pitch, the perceptual correlate of vocal fold vibration, refers to the highness or lowness of vocal tone. Diagnosticians describing this aspect of vocal tone are generally concerned with the total possible pitch range, the optimum range (the range of most easily produced tones), the habitual range, and the modal pitch. Inappropriate pitch fluctuations and breaks in the tone as well as a monotone or stereotyped use of pitch may be noted if present (Boone, 1971).

Quality disorders introduced at the laryngeal level generally result from hyper- or hypotension of the laryngeal mechanism or aperiodic vibration of the vocal folds. Laryngeal hypertension may produce qualities described by some as harshness and glottal shock. Laryngeal hypotension frequently results in excessive loss of air, producing a breathy quality. Aperiodic vocal fold vibration introduces noise elements creating qualities such as hoarseness.

In addition to describing the loudness, pitch, and quality of the vocal tone, diagnosticians also encounter clients who produce no vocal tone. The two most common occurrences of absence of vocal tone are in hysterical aphonia, where the structural mechanism is intact, but the client does not phonate normally and in laryngectomized patients, where all or part of the laryngeal mechanism has been removed.

To augment information relating to a description of vocal tone, the following resources are suggested: Darley (1964), Emerick and Hatten (1974), Fisher (1966), Luchsinger and Arnold (1965), and Perkins (1977).

Resonance

Before the vocal tone exits from the speaker, it is modified by contributions of the pharyngeal, nasal, and oral cavities and their interactions—the resonation process. The primary functions of these cavities are to increase the loudness of the vocal tone and to add quality modifications, the sounding board and open cavity effects.

The study of resonance as a speech product has been emphasized primarily from an interest in the acoustic characteristics of the three normally nasal sounds of English, the /m/, /n/, and /ŋ/, and a significant concern for the resonance deviations in speakers with inadequate velopharyngeal closure, particularly the individual with a cleft palate. Resonance as a speech product, other than these two concerns, has primarily been studied as a feature of voice quality.

There are many instrumental measures that have been devised to study nasal air flow, air and sound pressure, and the acoustic spectrum of nasality as a product (Counihan, 1971a, b; Schwartz, 1971). While resonance contributions can be measured objectively through instrumentation, typically, clinical descriptions are qualitative and note too much or too little contribution of a particular resonating cavity. For example, nasal resonance may be described as appropriate, too great (hypernasality or simply nasality) or too little (hyponasality), or of a certain type (cul-de-sac).

Nasality as a product to be measured by the diagnostician resides primarily in his perceptual judgment. This perceptual judgment must be based on a knowledge of the effects of nasal coupling with the oral cavity. As with all attempts to separate a product for a perceptual analysis, the diagnostician must take into account how his perceptions may be accounted for by degrees of interactions. All that is heard as nasal resonance may not be a simple matter of nasal coupling, rather it may also stem from other characteristics of the vocal and nasal tracts. His judgments should consider how much is related to what.

Is "nasal twang," a dialectal variation, considered a resonance or a voice quality difference? How is this product considered from a production viewpoint? What contributes to the effect called "nasal twang"?

Voice

Often the voice problem presented cannot be referred easily to vocal tone or resonance alone, but rather as an interaction between these two products. Voice as a speech product and a disorder is clearly an ambiguous phenomenon. Our profession has gone "round the bush" many times in attempting to define voice in relationship to underlying production processes. Quality as an aspect of vocal tone has defied description by speech pathologists. Many types of voice quality disorders are described by terms that are seldom agreed on by those listening to the voice.

Perkins (1977) states, "Whereas glottal vibration rate stands in a direct (though not linear) relation to pitch, and intensity of glottal pulses to loudness, what production process stands in direct relation to perceived quality? None." What dimensions does Perkins suggest as basic to the production of the product we call voice quality? How can it be measured instrumentally?

We indicated earlier that voice quality is a component of vocal tone related to phonation; now we are indicating that voice is a product related as well to resonation. Of course, we could go on to add that voice is a reflection of articulation and prosodation; again, we feel we would be correct. For example, Boone (1971) discusses the oral cavity as a single or multiple resonator depending on the position of the tongue and other oral structures. Thus changes in articulatory structures can have an effect on oral resonance, resulting in changes in perceived voice quality during speech. However, we want to reserve our concept of the voice product to the perceptual quality of the sound we perceive as uncontaminated as possible by these other speech production subprocesses. For our purposes here, then, the voice product comprises the products of vocal tone and resonance in varying degrees of combination.

Perhaps our concept of voice would be best exemplified by the quality of the vocal sound produced when a speaker prolongs vowels at various pitch and loudness levels. The perceptions we make of these productions come closest, for us, to the meaning of voice as an interaction of phonation and resonation. In these productions the diagnostician is very likely to hear the many variations in voice quality that are produced by normal and deviant producers of the product, voice. For example, laryngeal hypertension may produce a harsh vocal tone quality, but this tone when coupled with insufficient pharyngeal resonation, resulting in damping of lower frequencies and amplification of high overtones, may yield an overall thin, relatively high and "tinny" voice quality termed by some as strident.

Emerick and Hatten (1974) concur that the "imprecision of labels" has been a basic ingredient in our difficulties studying voice. They list 10 factors that have contributed to imprecise definitions and consequent clinician insecurity.

Phonetic structure

Phonetic structure refers to the sounds that are produced during the speech production process. Phonetic structure is most directly referable to the subprocess of articulation, the process by which the voiced and voiceless airstream is modified by the

articulators to produce the characteristic acoustic spectrum for the sounds of our language. The utterances that we segment in phonetic structure are referred to as phones (speech sounds) and are classified in a number of ways.

1. *Production (physiologic) systems* are concerned with the place and manner of articulation.
2. *Acoustic systems* describe the physical characteristics associated with each speech sound.
3. *Perceptual systems* have their basis in an understanding of the sound system of a given language; the listener categorizes a sound produced in comparison to his knowledge of standard sounds.

When analyzing phonetic structure, it is important to distinguish between the phonetic product and the phonemic product. The former has its basis in a physiologic-acoustic analysis, the latter in an acoustic-perceptual analysis.

When describing the *phonetic product,* the diagnostician is interested in the way speech sounds are actually produced by the speaker, referred to frequently as motor (physiologic) phonetics. Observation of phones tells the diagnostician about the idiosyncratic production of particular sounds by a given speaker. These are phonetically transcribed using diacritics to aid in recording the actual specific productions of phones. Thus the diagnostician can note phonetic differences of length, nasalization, lip-rounding, tongue height, voicing, etc. The interest is in a refined description of how a given sound was produced during the articulation process. Fig. 6-2 presents a view of the articulators and places of articulation used to describe speech sounds from a production point of view.

Another branch of the study of phonetics, acoustic phonetics, provides the diagnostician with another form of description. He can, through instrumental analysis, study the acoustic properties of speech sounds, properties such as formant structure, fundamental frequency, dura-

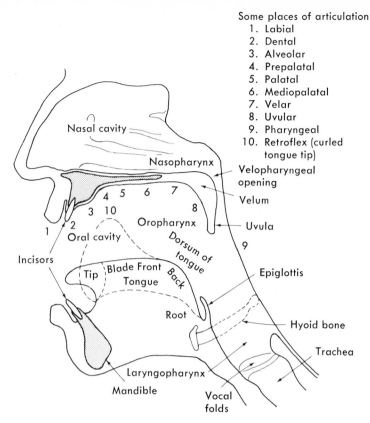

Some places of articulation
1. Labial
2. Dental
3. Alveolar
4. Prepalatal
5. Palatal
6. Mediopalatal
7. Velar
8. Uvular
9. Pharyngeal
10. Retroflex (curled tongue tip)

Fig. 6-2. Schematic view of the articulators, vocal tract cavities, and places of articulation. (From Daniloff, R. G., Normal articulation process. In F. D. Minifie, T. J. Hixon, and F. Williams [Eds.] *Normal Aspects of Speech, Hearing, and Language.* Englewood Cliffs, N.J.: Prentice-Hall, Inc. [1973].)

tion, and intensity. Minifie (1973) has constructed a table of the acoustic properties of English fricatives using several sources (Table 3). The table provides a physiologic description, a source spectrum, and an output spectrum. The source spectrum refers basically to the glottal spectrum, whereas the output spectrum refers to the characteristics of the sound after modifications have occurred along the vocal tract. Minifie's (1973) information gives acoustic data that are the basis for the diagnostician's perceptual judgments.

Minifie (1973) has developed his table for fricative sounds. Can this table be expanded for the /p, b, t, d, k, and g/ sounds? For other sounds?

The *phonemic product,* on the other hand, is more concerned with the diagnostician's perceptual judgment of speech sounds. He wants to know if a sound that is produced meets the standard for that sound in a given language. To do this he listens to the acoustic characteristics of the sound and determines perceptually if it fits a specific sound category. Thus the phonemic product is measured by the diagnostician's judgments and is dependent on his knowledge about normal speech sounds.

The phonemic product treats specific occurrences of phones as members of idealized sound categories (phonemes). Phonemic transcriptions ignore fine nonmeaningful distinctions between members of the same phoneme category and only

Table 3. Acoustic properties of English fricatives*

Physiologic description	Source spectrum	Output spectrum
Interdental		
/θ/ and /ð/ produced with tip of tongue close to, or touching, inner edge of upper incisors; air forced through narrow slit between bottom of upper teeth and top surface of tongue, broad width-to-height nature of orifice shape yielding low-intensity level, broad bandwidth of noise	Flat noise spectrum from about 1,000 to 10,000 Hz; energy may drop off at about 3 dB/octave	Strevens observes /θ/ has low-intensity noise with highest center of gravity in frequency domain of any English fricative; largest amplitudes of energy from 7,000 to 8,000 Hz; Heinz and Stevens found listeners identified wide band noises with resonances from 6,500 to 8,000 Hz as either /f/ or /θ/
Labiodental		
/f/ and /v/ produced with upper teeth close to inner surface of lower lip; airstream passing between teeth and lower lip and also through some interstices between upper teeth; broad width and low height to elliptical orifice offering large resistance to outward flow of air as well as causing low-intensity wide band noise to be produced; noise source relatively unmodified by vocal tract since noise source located near output of resonance tube	Low-intensity noise band from 800 to 10,000 Hz; amplitude of noise drops approximately 3 dB to 6 dB/octave	Low-intensity noise ranging from approximately 1,500 to 7,500 or 8,000 Hz; Strevens identified low-level resonances at 1,900, 4,000, and 5,000 Hz; Fant suggests major resonance occurring at 6,000 to 7,000 Hz and dependent on the resonance of air column in constriction and shallow cavity formed by lips in front of upper incisors; Fant suggests this high-frequency resonance very low in amplitude and /f/ sound perhaps better described by broad band noise with no observable resonances
Linguoalveolar		
/s/ and /z/ produced with tongue tip or tongue blade raised to approximate alveolar ridge; tongue grooved forming narrow air channel down center of tongue; closer approximation to circular orifice providing more efficient conversion of aerodynamic power to acoustic power than does wide but low elliptical orifice required for /f/ and /θ/; turbulence generated at constriction and also at cutting edge of upper incisor teeth	Sound source spectrum flat from 300 to 4,000 Hz followed by 6 dB/octave drop above 4,000 Hz	Due to an antiresonance around 3,500 Hz, very little energy observed in output spectrum below 4,000 Hz; no characteristic resonance pattern but usually major energy peak between 4,000 and 7,000 Hz
Linguopalatal		
/ʃ/ and /ʒ/ produced with blade of tongue or tip and blade approaching palate approximately where alveolar ridge joins hard palate; require tongue to be only slightly grooved, providing larger area for turbulence; airstream set into turbulence in constriction and possibly at teeth	Approximately flat-source spectrum (0 dB/octave) from 300 to 6,000 Hz	Lowest output energies around 1,600 to 2,500 Hz; very sharp cutoff of high-frequency energies around 7,000 Hz; most of fricative energy in lower frequencies; Strevens and Heinz and Stevens show first two resonances occurring at about 2,500 and 5,000 Hz, respectively

*From Minifie, F. D., Speech acoustics. In F. D. Minifie, T. J. Hixon, and F. Williams (Eds.), *Normal Aspects of Speech, Hearing, and Language.* Englewood Cliffs, N.J.: Prentice-Hall, Inc. (1973). Minifie developed this table from the following primary sources: Fant (1960), Heinz and Stevens (1961), and Strevens (1960).

Table 3. Acoustic properties of English fricatives—cont'd

Physiologic description	Source spectrum	Output spectrum
Glottal		
/h/ produced by increasing airflow through larynx and creating turbulence within partially constricted glottis	Broad-spectrum noise	Output spectrum ranging from about 400 to 6,500 Hz; several peaks in output spectrum for /h/, one around 1,000 Hz and another around 1,700 Hz; since whole vocal tract resonating during /h/, lower frequency energies resonated than for fricatives with more forward places of articulation; no physiologic constraints placed on tongue during /h/, providing maximal coarticulation with following vowel; hence, resonances for /h/ closely approximating those for following vowel

record sounds that function as linguistically different.

Minifie (1973) has indicated that the phonemic concept may have outlived its usefulness. His comments are based on what appears to be a lack of physiologic and perceptual reality to phonemes. Does it appear to you that the use of the phoneme as a concept may be irrelevant in our study of speech sounds?

While the phonetic and phonemic products may in fact be the same segmented behavior (a phone), it is how the behavior is viewed that gives rise to the phonetic/phonemic distinction. When the concern is the specific production of sounds as they are formed in the speech production process, the phonetic viewpoint is primary. When the production of sounds as representative of linguistic differences is the concern, the phonemic viewpoint is primary.

Diagnosticians studying phonetic structure use both viewpoints. The phonetic viewpoint is used particularly when sounds are heard in error. For example, when Jonathan utters the [θ], the diagnostician may say that his phonetic structure is an appropriately produced phoneme (perceptual), it has characteristic frequency components (acoustic), and it sounds as if it were produced with the tongue between the teeth (physiologic). Of course, if the diagnostician were watching as well as listening, he could have observed the place of articulation. All of these ways of analyzing phonetic structure by the diagnostician are built into his perceptual measurements. His perceptions will be as good as his knowledge of speech sound production, what he knows about the physiologic, acoustic, and phonemic aspects of speech sounds. When he uses these systems for observing the product phonetic structure, he is basically interested in what sounds were produced, how they were produced, and if they are on target. He is interested in the sounds as phonetic structure, not as meaningful linguistic units. Therefore notations of the phonetic product require a system for describing all the significant sounds for a given language, in English between 40 and 45 vowels and consonants.

Peterson and Shoup (1966a-c) have presented three articles discussing the physiologic and acoustic phonetic theories. They include an extensive discussion and description of a notational system for representing the phonetic product. Would their system be practical for a diagnostician?

Not only does the diagnostician segment out the vowels and consonants from the stream of speech when he views phonetic structure, but he also observes the sequential relationship of sounds. He is not concerned about meaningful sequences here so much as he is concerned about the influence of one sound on another. That is, he is interested in observing the effect of coarticulation—the phonetic context (Daniloff and Moll, 1968; Klatt, 1974). For example, Bertheva produces a nasalized vowel following an /n/, but she does not do this following an /m/. The diagnostician would be interested in discovering this phenomenon when he studies phonetic structure even though, in this example, the phonetic variation would not change the meaning of Bertheva's utterance.

Suprasegmental features could also be considered a part of phonetic structure. These are features that signal stress, intonation, and durational aspects of the utterance. However, suprasegmental features are generally viewed in relationship to speech segments larger than a phone. Therefore in the speech product we will view the suprasegmentals as a part of prosody, which is contributed to by phonetic structure.

Prosody

Prosody as a speech product is referable to the subprocess we have termed prosodation. It is an integrated process, incorporating aspects from the other four speech production subprocesses. Thus prosody is related to the other speech products: vocal tone, resonance, voice, and phonetic structure. Prosody is a fundamental aspect of speech behavior, but there is little general agreement as to the boundaries of the actual behavior observed. Sometimes it is called "the melody of speech" (Berry, 1969) or vocal variety. It is made up of both segmental and suprasegmental features.

As a perceptual correlate to the process we have called prosodation, there is little definitive information. Prosody as an acoustic phenomenon has sometimes been identified as fundamental voice frequency, voice intensity level, and acoustic phonetic duration. Netsell (1973) operationally defines three prosodic features: intonation, stress, and rhythm. To him, intonation is perceptually related to the fundamental frequency of vocal fold vibration. Stress relates to syllable emphasis, and rhythm is the perception of the phonetic events over time.

Most authors include the following in some combination as features of prosody: pitch, loudness, time, rhythm, fluency, stress, pauses, quality, juncture, duration, intonation, rate, and phrasing. Darley (1964) speaks of stress, rhythm, and pitch comprising the prosodic quality of speech. Fisher (1966) mentions rate, stress, phrasing, and intonation as components of prosody. Perkins (1977) in discussing the "speech flow processes" comments that rhythm, established by patterns of stress and rate, is identified in speech as prosody.

Drawing from these and other authors, then, prosody seems to include at least two major dimensions: one that focuses on *intonation and stress patterns* and a second that has to do with *timing-rhythm*. Timing-rhythm includes two factors: *rate* and *fluency*. Rate concerns the overall speed of message utterance, phrasing characteristics, pause length, syllable length, and hesitancies. Fluency addresses how smoothly phonemes, syllables, words, and phrases are joined together into longer utterances. Repetitions and prolongations of these features create disruptions in fluency, a prosody variation.

As has been stated, these prosody characteristics are a result of the entire set of speech production subprocesses, but as behaviors (products) they can be isolated to some extent and viewed as an independent parameter of the speech product. The dimensions that make up prosody can be observed in the same way that phones and phonemes are viewed (Francis, 1958). The diagnostician can notate how words are stressed, if a pause occurs between two words, if a sentence was said with a downward inflection, if a vowel was prolonged, if rate is fast, etc.

Prosody is typically viewed as extending over an utterance, suprasegmental, rather than specific instances, segmental. The overall stress patterns used, the overall intonation patterns, the overall timing-rhythm patterns, and the rate and fluency are noted rather than viewing a specific instance of stress, intonation, or time. This is primarily because a specific instance provides little information about the nature of the prosody product, nor would a specific instance of a prosody error, even if consistent, do much to the meaning intended by the speaker. Some speakers may even have an overall variation of prosodic features without interfering significantly with communication. We know of any number of people who speak with little change in intonation, stress, and timing; they sound boring, but we can understand their message.

Prosodic features, as well, serve to signal meaningful differences between utterances, for example, the rising pitch used when asking a question. They also signal semantic relationships in certain ambiguous sentences; for example, "He is a French teacher." They also serve in extralinguistic ways to express certain emotions and to give each speaker a distinct vocal quality; they do seem to add to the "beauty" of languages. Here the diagnostician would be looking at the use of prosody to convey subtleties of meaning, to express various emotional states, to ask questions versus making statements, to distinguish between words that are written alike, etc.

Thus prosody observations can be made strictly as a production phenomenon; or, on the other hand, they can be observed as a function of meaning.

Prosody as a parameter of the speech product important to the diagnostician is just coming into its own. True, many of its features have been embedded in discussions of speech disorders for some time, for example, voice and stuttering; however, the disorders were not considered primarily as prosodic variations. Prosody seemed to be reserved more for voice and

diction classes, a part of acting and public speaking. Prosody is receiving greater attention in speech pathology. Emphasis is being given to the prosodic disorders seen in patients with neurologic disorders (Darley et al., 1969, 1975). Moncur and Brackett (1974) devote an entire chapter to the treatment of prosody. And in this book we are considering stuttering and fluency disorders as having their primary basis in a prosody variation, the timing-rhythm component.

Does Moncur and Brackett's (1974) concept of prosody coincide with that used here? Pay particular attention to their discussion of pitch. How does their concept of prosody compare to that of Bronstein and Jacoby (1967)?

LANGUAGE PRODUCT

The framework for viewing language as a product evolves largely from theoretical schemata developed in linguistics and psycholinguistics, treating language as a rule-based system. Language behavior as a rule-based system has been segmented into the phonologic, syntactic, semantic, and pragmatic parameters (levels) of language structure (Fig. 6-1). However, it must be kept in mind that these levels of language co-occur and interinfluence each other.

Phonologic level

Whereas phonetic structure aims primarily to describe the actual production of instances of phones, the phonologic level treats specific phones as representative of phoneme categories, both segmental and suprasegmental phonemes. The concern shifts more to generalized characteristics and rules of the system that signal meaning rather than individual sound description. Segmental features include the sounds or phonemes of the language and their rules of permissible order. Suprasegmental features include juncture (the difference between giant's eyes and giant size), stress (the difference between cónduct and condúct), and intonation (the dif-

Table 4. Classification of sound "features"*

Phoneme	Keywords	Sound classification — Consonants	Vowels	Glides	Diphthongs	Manner — Nasal	Oral	Voiced	Voiceless	Continuant C₁	Continuant C₂	Interrupted I₁	Interrupted I₂	Bilabial	Labiodental	Interdental	Linguaalveolar	Linguaalveopalatal	Linguavelar	Glottal	High 1	High 2	Mid 1	Mid 2	Low	Front	Central	Back
p	*pipe*	+					+		+			+		+														
b	*baby*	+					+	+				+		+														
t	*tot*	+					+		+			+					+											
d	*dad*	+					+	+				+					+											
k	*kick*	+					+		+			+							+									
g	*gig*	+					+	+				+							+									
tʃ	*church*	+					+		+				+					+										
dʒ	*judge*	+					+	+					+					+										
f	*fife*	+					+		+	+					+													
v	*verve*	+					+	+		+					+													
θ	*ether*	+					+		+	+						+												
ð	*either*	+					+	+		+						+												
s	*sis*	+					+		+	+							+											
z	*buzz*	+					+	+		+							+											
ʃ	*ship*	+					+		+	+								+										
ʒ	*vision*	+					+	+		+								+										
h	*high*	+					+		+	+										+								
m	*mom*	+				+		+			+			+														
n	*nine*	+				+		+			+						+											
ŋ	*sing*	+				+		+			+								+									
l	*let*	+					+	+			+						+											
l̩	*table*	+		+			+	+			+						+											
w	*wet*	+		+			+	+			+			+					+									
j	*yet*	+		+			+	+			+							+										
r	*rye*	+		+			+	+			+						+	+										

i	me	+ + + + +			2	
ɪ	bid					
e	play					
ɛ	get					
æ	hat	+ + + + + + + + + + + + + + + +				
ʌ-ə	mud/about					
ɝ-ɚ	bird/another	+ + + + + + + + + + + + + + + +				
a	father	+ + + + + + + + + + + + + + + +				
ɔ	jaw					
o	tone	+ + + +				
ʊ	push	+ + + + + + + + + + + + + +				
u	pool					
aɪ	smile					
aʊ	ouch					
ɔɪ	toil					
ju	fuel					

+ = "Feature" present for that sound.

Table developed by J. E. Nation who is grateful for the contributions of Ellen Wehrle and Julie Mayerovitch.

ference between "Mary is going" said with a rising intonation pattern as a question or falling intonation as a statement; see previous discussion of prosody).

In describing the phonologic level of language, then, the diagnostician aims to make an inventory of the client's phonemic system and to identify the rules by which he selects and joins these phonemes together. He studies the phonologic level of language from the same data (phones) as he uses to study phonetic structure.

When studying the client's phonemic inventory, the diagnostician may choose to describe the client's own phonemic system or to note how the client's phonemic usage differs from mature standard English. If he chooses the former, he would have to identify all sound categories that signal a change in meaning in much the same manner that a linguist identifies phonemes in an exotic language. More commonly, in clinical situations the diagnostician surveys a client's phonemic inventory in comparison to standard English, keeping in mind the speech and language environment from which the client learned language.

For some time clinicians have been analyzing a client's phonologic system by charting the place and manner of his productions (Van Riper and Irwin, 1958) as would be done in an analysis of phonetic/phonemic structure. More recently, distinctive feature theory is being widely used (Schane, 1973). Diagnosticians have begun describing the distinctive features present in the phonologic system of their clients. Distinctive feature systems for analysis of phonology have been presented by Chomsky and Halle (1968), Jakobson et al. (1963), and Miller and Nicely (1955) and have been adopted for clinical use (Compton, 1975; McReynolds and Engmann, 1975; McReynolds and Huston, 1971; Pollack and Rees, 1972).

In 1973, because of concern about the difficulties of applying certain distinctive features to clinical work, a table of "sound features" that were felt to be more applicable to clinical analysis of the phonetic-phonemic-phonologic aspects of speech and language was developed (Table 4). The table was developed keeping in mind that the acoustic basis for what we hear as speech sounds is rooted in the subprocesses of speech production. Along with Walsh (1974), we feel that certain features presented in distinctive feature analysis systems are not perceptually realized; therefore this classification returns to a place and manner (physiologic) emphasis. The table classifies sounds into vowels and consonants, a time-honored differentiation. However, two other classes of sounds, the glides and the diphthongs, have also been incorporated. For example, the /w/ is given a + as being both a consonant and a glide to demonstrate that it is seen in its traditional classification as a consonant but also as representing a glide. A set of definitions for each of the categories of sound "features" used in Table 4 follows.

DEFINITION AND DESCRIPTION OF TERMS USED IN TABLE 4
Sound classification

Consonants: /p, b, t, d, k, g, tʃ, dʒ, f, v, θ, ð, s, z, ʃ, ʒ, h, m, n, ŋ, l, l̩, w, j, r/

Vowels: /i, ɪ, e, ɛ, æ, ʌ-ə, ɝ-ɚ, a, ɔ, o, ʊ, u, aɪ, aʊ, ɔɪ, ju/

Glides: Formed by first placing the articulators in the position for one consonant and then gliding to the position of the following vowel, as in /l, w, j, r/

Diphthongs: Formed by first placing the articulators in the position for one vowel (position 1) and then gliding to the position of a second vowel (position 2), as in /aɪ, aʊ, ɔɪ, ju/

Manner of articulation

Nasal: Sound characterized by nasal cavity resonance, as in /m, n, ŋ/

Oral: Air escaping primarily through the oral cavity, as in /p, b, t, d, k, g, tʃ, dʒ, f, v, θ, ð, s, z, ʃ, ʒ, h, l, l̩, w, j, r, i, ɪ, e, ɛ, æ, ʌ-ə, ɝ-ɚ, a, ɔ, o, ʊ, u, aɪ, aʊ, ɔɪ, ju/

Voiced: Vocal cords vibrating during production, as in /b, d, g, dʒ, v, ð, z, ʒ, m, n, ŋ, l, l̩, w, j, r, i, ɪ, e, ɛ, æ, ʌ-ə, ɝ-ɚ, a, ɔ, o, ʊ, u, aɪ, aʊ, ɔɪ, ju/

Voiceless: Vocal cords not vibrating during production, as in /p, t, k, tʃ, f, θ, s, ʃ, h/

Continuant: Primary constriction of vocal tract not narrowed to point where air flow past the constriction is blocked, as in /f, v, θ, ð, s, z, ʃ, ʒ, h, m, n, ŋ, l, l̩, w, j, r, i, ɪ, e, ɛ, æ, ʌ-ə, ɝ-ɚ, a, ɔ, o, ʊ, u, aɪ, aʊ, ɔɪ, ju/

Continuant 1: Sounds made by narrowing the opening of the mouth so that the flow of air is not entirely blocked but is obstructed, as in /f, v, θ, ð, s, z, ʃ, ʒ, h/

Continuant 2: Sounds where the flow of air is not blocked or obstructed, as in /m, n, ŋ, l, l̩, w, j, r, i, ɪ, e, ɛ, æ, ʌ-ə, ɝ-ɚ, a, ɔ, o, ʊ, u, aɪ, aʊ, ɔɪ, ju/

Interrupted: Sounds made by closing off the flow of air completely and then releasing it, as in /p, b, t, d, k, g, tʃ, dʒ/

Interrupted 1: Air released instantaneously (plosion), as in /p, b, t, d, k, g/

Interrupted 2: Air released gradually (affrication), as in /tʃ, dʒ/

Place of articulation

Consonants and glides

Bilabial: Made with lips, as in /p, b, m, w/

Labiodental: Contact between lower lip and upper teeth, as in /f, v/

Interdental: Tongue between teeth, as in /θ, ð/

Linguoalveolar: Made with tongue tip touching or approximating alveolar ridge, as in /t, d, s, z, n, l/

Linguoalveolopalatal: Made by raising tongue toward the palate, as in /tʃ, dʒ, ʃ, ʒ, l̩, j, r/

Linguovelar: Contact between back of tongue and velum, as in /k, g, ŋ/

Glottal: Vocal cords brought together sufficiently to obstruct passage of air but not to produce voice, as in /h/

Vowels: Place of articulation for vowels referring to position of the highest part of the tongue along a vertical and a horizontal axis (for both high and mid-vowels, position 1 higher than position 2)

High vowels 1: /i, u, ju/

High vowels 2: /ɪ, ʊ/

Mid-vowels 1: /e, ɝ-ɚ, o/

Mid-vowels 2: /ɛ, ʌ-ə, ɔ, ɔɪ/

Low vowels: /æ, a, aɪ, aʊ/

Front vowels: /i, ɪ, e, ɛ, æ, ju/

Central vowels: /ʌ-ə, ɝ-ɚ/

Back vowels: /a, ɔ, o, ʊ, u, aɪ, aʊ, ɔɪ/

Diphthongs: Listed on the chart as beginning (1) and ending (2) positions

---

Walsh (1974) has reacted to the indiscriminate use of distinctive feature systems for clinical use. Even though Table 4 was developed prior to the appearance of Walsh's article, much of what he says is relevant to this sound feature approach. It is important clinically that a student understand thoroughly the system he uses for analyzing a client's sound system. Compare Table 4 to Walsh's proposed system and to that of Chomsky and Halle (1968), Jakobson et al. (1963), McReynolds and Huston (1971), and Miller and Nicely (1955).

In addition to surveying the phonemes and sound features used by the client, the diagnostician also wants to describe the rule system for selecting and combining phonemes into sequential patterns. He may describe the client's phonologic rules and compare these rules to that of standard English. He would also draw from information pertaining to the influence of the phonemic context on a specific phoneme.

Thus the diagnostician is interested in ascertaining what rules apply when phonemes are used together. For example, why does Darrell employ consonants only prevocalically, producing no postvocalic consonants? Or why does Philip produce an appropriate [r] with lip-rounding in the context of lip-rounded vowels (*rope, ru*by) but inappropriately in the context of lip-spread vowels (*reed, ri*d). Although expli-

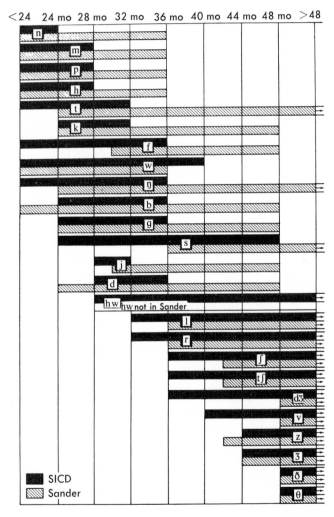

Fig. 6-3. Comparison of SICD with Sander's analysis (1972) of Templin (1957) and Wellman et al. (1931) data showing average age estimates (50%) and upper age limits (90%) of customary consonant production. When the percentage correct at 24 months exceeded 70%, the bar extends to the left <24. When the 90% level was not reached by 48 months, the bar extends to the right >48. (From Prather, E. M., Hedrick, D. L., and Kern, C. A., *J. Speech Hearing Dis.*, **40,** 186 [1975].)

cation of the development of phonologic rules is just beginning, Compton (1970, 1975), Ingram (1974), and Schane (1973) suggest some general rules that may aid the diagnostician in evaluating sequences of phonemes.

When studying the phonologic level of language, the diagnostician must understand how it is acquired. Many of his clients are young children that have, as yet, not completed the development of phonology. Therefore the diagnostician must understand the "standard" system at various ages during the developmental process.

Several early investigations of the age of acquisition for English phonemes are well known (Poole, 1934; Templin, 1957; Wellman et al., 1931), and both Templin (1957) and Winitz (1969) have provided comparative tables summarizing these findings. Although providing normative data relevant to sound acquisition, these studies have received considerable criticism as to the criteria for acceptance of a phoneme as learned as well as the methodology employed in the studies. Sander (1972) has reinterpreted several of these studies and has charted the variability in sound acquisition from the age when 50% to 90% of children produce a given sound in two out of three positions in a word.

More recently, phonologic development has focused on recognition and production of the distinctive features employed in the language. Jakobson (1960) was one of the first to suggest that children did not learn specific sounds but rather through development differentiated the contrasts between distinctive features. He suggested that these distinctive features, bundles of which represented specific phonemes, were universal to all languages. With Halle, Jakobson (1956) proposed a universal developmental hierarchy of distinctive feature contrasts. While Jakobson's theory has not always been supported by subsequent research findings, much of the evidence is consistent with his predictions (Ervin-Tripp, 1966). Possibly more important, his theory has shifted the focus of phonologic development from sound learning to differentiation of distinctive features. Menyuk (1968) and others have contributed to our understanding of the order of observance of distinctive features.

Prather et al. (1975) have extended our knowledge about phoneme acquisition. They studied younger children and compared their results to Sander's (1972) reinterpretation of the classical studies as well as the results of Menyuk's (1968) analysis of distinctive feature development. From their study it appears that children may be acquiring significant aspects of the phonologic system at earlier ages than once thought. Fig. 6-3 is their comparative chart.

There are vital methodologic differences between the Prather et al. (1975) study and the classical studies as reviewed by Sander (1972). How might these differences account for the variability in age of sound acquisition presented on the chart (Fig. 6-3)?

Syntactic level

A description of the syntactic level usually includes two major aspects: *word order* and *morphology*. Word order incorporates the development and use of phrase structure rules and transformations. Phrase structure rules pertain to the expansion and description of noun phrases and verb phrases, while transformations change the phrase structures to produce the surface form of the sentence. Formally, transformations are rules that add, delete, substitute, or reorder constituents in a sentence. Morphology is primarily concerned with markers indicating, for example, plurality and possession for nouns, comparison for adjectives and adverbs, tense for verbs, and derivations for words. Some writers also include the development of some free morphemes such as the copula and the auxiliary.

A number of linguists have presented descriptions of the mature, idealized syntactic system, although Chomsky (1957, 1965) has undoubtedly had the greatest impact on our view of syntax in recent years. During the past 20 years, psycholinguists also have been relating formal linguistic theory to both adults' and children's actual use of syntax. Notable among those who have addressed syntax as used by adults are Bever (1968), Fodor and Garrett (1967, 1968), Miller (1962), Miller and McKean (1964), and Slobin (1966).

By 4 or 5 years of age a language learner has acquired most of the syntactic forms commonly used, although some syntactic learning has been shown to continue until as late as 10 years of age or older (Chomsky, 1969). In general, children seem to pass through several stages of syntactic growth: the holophrastic, two-word utterances, development of phrase structure rules, modulation of basic sentences, and transformational development. Most writers are reluctant to attach ages to these stages, noting the variability in acquisition and stressing the importance of sequential stages rather than age expectations.

Table 5 presents a gross summary of the ages and stages of syntactic development, although it must be kept in mind that such a summary is of only very limited usefulness. Rather, the diagnostician needs to draw from his broader fund of knowledge concerning syntactic development.

The *holophrastic*, one-word utterance, is generally regarded as a period in which the child uses a single word to denote an entire thought. Some authors (McNeill, 1970) report that most one-word utterances are noun forms, while others (Menyuk,

1971) maintain that children use a variety of parts of speech, including nouns, verbs, adjectives, and adverbs.

Two-word utterances have been analyzed into the syntactic relations they represent. McNeill (1966) maintains that two-word utterances of English-speaking children provide evidence for basic universal grammatical relations, the most common being V + N (main verb + object), then N + N (modifier + head noun or subject + predicate), followed by N + V (subject + predicate) and finally P + N (modifier + head noun). Other writers (Bloom, 1970; Brown, 1973a), however, question McNeill's (1966) contention that all two-word utterances express these basic grammatical relations. Brown (1973a) has presented a detailed discussion of this period of early language acquisition.

The use of early complete sentences requires *development of phrase structure rules* and *morphologic modulations of the basic sentences*. Phrase structure development centers on expansion and differentiation of the noun and verb phrases. Noun phrase expansion allows for sequential ordering of adjective and noun modifiers. For example, where at the two-word stage a child might produce "white cat" and "big cat," further expansion of the noun phrase permits utterances such as "big white cat."

Verb phrase expansion is primarily concerned with development of the auxiliary (be, have, etc.) and modal verbs (can, will, must, etc.) as well as development of morphologic markers for tense (want*s*, want*ed*) and number (he want*s*, they want). The development of these auxiliary and modal verbs is very basic to later transformational development.

Concomitant with development of phrase structure rules is the development of morphologic inflections. In addition to development of inflectional markers for verbs, as noted previously, children also learn inflectional noun markers (book*s*, Mary*'s*) and grammatical morphemes such as articles (a, an, the). Brown (1973a) ranked

Table 5. Basic ages and stages of syntactic development

Age	Stage of development
12 mo	Holophrastic stage; begins single-word utterances
18-24 mo	Two-word utterances; begins joining two words together
2-3/3½ yr	Development of phrase structure rules; modulation of basic sentences; early transformational development
5 yr	Acquires most sentence structures used in adult speech
5-10+ yr	Perfects refined aspects of grammar

the order of acquisition of 14 morphemes in three children, obtaining an order that was generally compatible with other studies of morphologic development.

Later syntactic development is primarily distinguished by the *learning of transformational rules* and *selectional restrictions;* however, there is no single ordering of later transformational development. The general order of transformational emergence depends on several considerations. First, the easy transformations—additions, substitutions, and deletions occur before the hard types—embedding and permutations (Menyuk, 1969). Second, the fewer the number of transformations required, the earlier the sentence form appears. Third, the specific transformational rule influences the stage of appearance. Fourth, the greater the number and the more refined the selectional restrictions on use are, the later the correct observance of all the selectional restrictions inherent within the transformation. Finally, the more useful a transformation in terms of communicative function, the earlier it will appear. Brown and Hanlon (1970), Chomsky (1969), and Menyuk (1969) have all studied the emergence of these late-appearing transformations.

Lee (1974) and Miner (1969) have developed procedures for viewing syntactic development at various ages. Lee's work (Lee, 1966, 1974; Lee and Canter, 1971; Koeningsknecht and Lee, 1971) is a comprehensive presentation for analyzing the developmental aspects of syntax. Lee (1974) first presents a compact discussion of grammatical structure with references to early development. She then presents a classification of developmental sentence types (DST), procedures for collecting spontaneous language, and elaborate procedures for scoring and analysis. The developmental sentence scoring (DSS) analysis gives the diagnostician information as to the developmental order of pronouns, verbs, negatives, conjunctions, yes/no questions, and "wh" questions.

Prior to the development of procedures such as Lee's that have a basis in psycholinguistic theory, developmental language measures were more concerned with counting the types of responses made, for example, the number of one-word responses. Johnson et al. (1963) present a series of such measures that have been used to analyze the language utterances of children.

In evaluating the syntactic performance of clients the diagnostician will also want to consider if the presented syntactic pattern is delayed, deviant, or represents a quantitative difference in terms of the frequency with which various structures are used. Leonard (1972), Menyuk (1964), and Morehead and Ingram (1973) have all addressed these issues. Lee's (1974) and Miner's (1969) procedures are also important for this task.

Semantic level

The semantic level of language is concerned with meaning, with the use of agreed on symbols of a given language that represent things, concepts, attributes, actions, feelings, etc. The study of semantics usually includes the *lexicon* (vocabulary), *semantic features,* and *semantic relations*. While vocabulary growth is well documented, study of the development of semantic features and semantic relations is still in its infancy.

The primary focus on semantics, particularly at a concrete level, has been the lexicon, the relationship between words and their external representation (Fig. 6-4). Numerous studies, normative data, and tests have been published that aim to describe and measure vocabulary growth and breadth. Probably the most reported data regarding vocabulary growth in children are given by Smith (1926). An adaptation of that data can be found in Dale (1972).

Investigators are now attempting to describe semantic features. Just as phonemes are seen to be bundles of distinctive features, so also are lexical items seen to be

FUNKY WINKERBEAN　　　　　　　　　　　　　　　　**By Tom Batiuk**

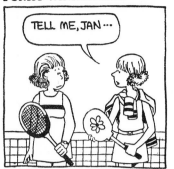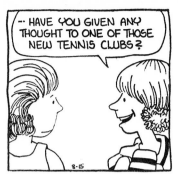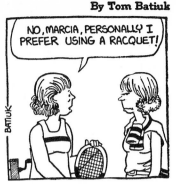

Fig. 6-4. Semantics in need of a referent? (FUNKY WINKERBEAN by Tom Batiuk; courtesy Field Newspaper Syndicate.)

bundles of semantic features. Attempts are being made to identify a comprehensive inventory of these semantic features, although to date, no one system of features has been widely adopted or gained wide clinical application.

When a child first begins to use words, he most likely does not know their full adult meaning. Rather, semantic development is a process of adding more and more semantic features until the child's meaning matches that of the adult. Clark's semantic feature hypothesis (1973) holds that children's first words are overextended categories based on perceptual experience of characteristics such as shape, size, sound, and texture. The child then forms more restricted word categories through a narrowing down process in which he observes and adds additional features to the words he uses. Clark (1973) also notes that children differentiate various areas of experience or "semantic domains" by learning the most superordinate general features before the more restricted and specific features.

Corlew (1971) has studied word variables related to naming performance in the aphasic client. Does her information about the relationship of the variables to naming performance by aphasics provide us with any information about semantic features?

The semantic roles or semantic relations between words in sentences have also been the subject of considerable theorizing. Bloom (1970), Bowerman (1973), Brown (1973a, b), Schlesinger (1971), and others have presented schemata for viewing the semantic relations expressed in sentences. Drawing from a number of sources, Miller and Yoder (1974) have presented a table that outlines these early semantic relations and shows their developmental progression.

Even though theoretical frameworks are still under development, the diagnostician should not be content to collect only vocabulary information, but he should try to describe the semantic features observed in lexical items and the semantic relations expressed in utterances.

Pragmatic level

Pragmatics concerns the speaker's functional use of language; that is, how and why does the speaker use language; what are his purposes; and what does he accomplish through different utterances? For example, a reticent adult may simply reply to questions, rarely initiating communication, while an aggressive communicator may issue forth many commands. Or perhaps young children may use language for self-stimulation or to direct their motor behavior.

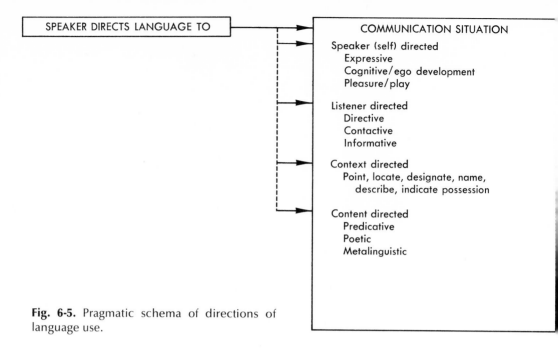

| SPEAKER DIRECTS LANGUAGE TO | COMMUNICATION SITUATION |

COMMUNICATION SITUATION

Speaker (self) directed
    Expressive
    Cognitive/ego development
    Pleasure/play

Listener directed
    Directive
    Contactive
    Informative

Context directed
    Point, locate, designate, name,
        describe, indicate possession

Content directed
    Predicative
    Poetic
    Metalinguistic

Fig. 6-5. Pragmatic schema of directions of language use.

At present there exists no unified framework that has gained general acceptance for viewing the various pragmatic uses of language. Fig. 6-5 presents a schema we have developed and find useful for representing a speaker's many uses of language. Following Hymes (1967) and Williams and Naremore (1969), we see language as being directed to some aspect of the communication situation: speaker directed, listener directed, content directed, or context directed. By directed we mean the focus, aim, or intent of the particular utterance. It is suggested that the reader also review the material presented regarding human communication and communicative interaction in Chapter 2. There may be only a fine line of difference, if any, between what are considered the roles and purposes of human communication and the pragmatic level of language. Therefore we would suggest as further reading the material presented by Mortensen (1972).

Speaker-directed language includes that language used by the speaker for his own cognitive or ego development, for pleasure and self-stimulation as in babbling or ego-

centric monologue, or as a "reflexive" expression of emotion such as "ow."

Listener-directed language may be directive, that is, commands aimed at producing a response in the listener ("Close the door."); contactive, the purpose of which is to establish a relationship between the speaker and listener ("Hello, how are you?"); or informative, aiming to provide the listener with information ("The paper you asked me about is in the office.").

Typically, *context-directed* language concerns some object or person present in the communication situation and is used to point out, locate, designate, name, describe, and indicate possession. Context-oriented comments tend to be concrete and to deal with the here and now.

Content-directed language is more abstract and removed from the here and now context. It has as its subject some idea or message that is expanded on. Predicative comments, where some subject is elaborated on, fall within this use of language. For example, "Amy is the tallest girl in the third-grade class." Poetic and metalinguistic utterances are also considered content oriented here, where the content is the message or language itself.

Besides language being directed toward these four aspects of the communication situation, the mode or manner in which language may be selected for any one direction may be either *formal* or *informal*. For example, one might direct an utterance in a formal mode ("Would you please be a little quieter?") or in an informal mode ("Shut up!"). Thus in addition to aiming language toward a specific focus of the communication situation, the speaker also selects whether or not to present the message in a formal or informal mode.

In Chapter 2 we presented a model by Schein (1969) (Fig. 2-5) as an example of an interpersonal model of speech and language. How would you fit our schema for the pragmatic level of language into this interpersonal model?

By about 1 year of age children have been reported to use their language in the following manner: pointing and naming, requesting, predicating, playing with speech, and influencing the social reactions of others (Ervin-Tripp, 1971). Other writers refer to the referential, expressive, and conative role of language at the one-word utterance stage (McNeill, 1970). Slobin (1970) presents the following functions of two-word sentences used cross-culturally by children: to locate and name, demand and desire, negate, describe, indicate possession, modify and qualify, and question. Bloom (1970) notes that children's early two- and three-word utterances function as comments, reports, directions, questions, and as having paralinguistic purposes.

Piaget (1955) has studied the development of children's use of language from an egocentric orientation to a more predominantly socialized form achieved around 7 years of age. Hymes (1962) and Williams and Naremore (1969) have presented systems for categorizing the dominant functional uses of language for the mature language user. Hymes (1962) lists the expressive, directive, poetic, contactive, metalinguistic, referential, and contextual roles of language. Williams and Naremore (1969) include the impulsive, contactive, conversative, descriptive/directive, and elaborative functions in their schema.

Relating these disparate studies to the framework for pragmatic usage of language presented in Fig. 6-5, we may make several observations regarding the development of the pragmatic uses of language. Initially in prelinguistic utterances the infant's first uses of "language" are for his own purposes, as in expressive cries and calls and in pleasurable production of oral movements and sound. During this early prelinguistic period, children also presumably use nonmeaningful utterances to attract the attention of the listener and direct others to attend to his needs. Therefore prelinguistic utterances serve at least the functions of self-gratification, directiveness, and control toward a listener.

With the onset of meaningful speech from the one-word stage on, language begins to refer to the context of the speaker. For example, at this stage children begin to name, point out, describe, and indicate possession of objects and qualities in their environment. Expanded also is a child's continued use of his language to direct his own activities and to support his cognitive development as well as increase control in using language directed toward listeners such as in commanding and questioning another.

Although all of these primary directed uses of language continue in sophistication through development, probably the latest appearing pragmatic function of language is directed toward amplification of the message content. While elaboration on a subject (predication) presumably develops quite early, certainly functions such as the poetic and metalinguistic uses of language, which focus on the message itself rather than on external reference, are later achievements in the use of language.

The following sources among others have provided us with a basis for organizing the pragmatic level of the language product. Would you organize this level in the same way or would these sources lead you to another organization? See Luria, 1961; Piaget, 1955; Skinner, 1957; Slobin, 1970; and Williams and Naremore, 1969. Rees (1973) discusses the relevance of what she calls "noncommunicative functions of language" as sources of the child's motivation for learning language. She considers the concept-formation function, the directive function, the magic function, and the establishment of self-image function. How do Rees' noncommunicative functions of language correspond to our discussion of the pragmatic level of language?

SUMMARY

A framework has been presented for organizing the verbal output of a speaker. Our framework presents two major divisions: the speech product and the language product. The speech product includes *vocal tone, resonance, voice, phonetic structure,* and *prosody*. These parameters of the speech product have been related to the physical processes in the speech production segment from which they arise. The language product has been broken down into the *phonologic, syntactic, semantic,* and *pragmatic* parameters that are created by the physical processing that occurs in the central language segment. We have suggested that a framework such as the one presented here, aids the diagnostician in conducting comprehensive observations of the speech and language product and in relating what he observes to behavioral correlates and physical processes.

REFERENCES

Berry, M., *Language Disorders of Children: The Bases and Diagnoses*. New York: Appleton-Century-Crofts (1969).

Bever, T. G., Specification and utilization of a transformation grammar. Final Report, Contract No. AF 19 (628)-5127 Awarded to Warren J. Plath, International Business Machines Corporation (1968).

Bloom, L., *Language Development: Form and Function in Emerging Grammars*. Cambridge, Mass.: The M.I.T. Press (1970).

Boone, D. R., *The Voice and Voice Therapy*. Englewood Cliffs, N.J.: Prentice-Hall, Inc. (1971).

Bowerman, M., *Early Syntactic Development: A Cross-Linguistic Study with Special Reference to Finnish*. Cambridge, England: Cambridge University Press (1973).

Bronstein, A., and Jacoby, B., *Your Speech and Voice*. New York: Random House, Inc. (1967).

Brown, R., *A First Language: The Early Stages*. Cambridge, Mass.: Harvard University Press (1973a).

Brown, R., Development of the first language in the human species. *Am. Psychol.*, **28**, 9-106 (1973b).

Brown, R., and Hanlon, C., Derivational complexity and order of acquisition in child speech. In J. R. Hayes (Ed.), *Cognition and the Development of Language*. New York: John Wiley & Sons, Inc. (1970).

Chomsky, C. S., *The Acquisition of Syntax in Children from Five to Ten*. Cambridge, Mass.: The M.I.T. Press (1969).

Chomsky, N., *Syntactic Structures*. The Hague: Mouton Publishers (1957).

Chomsky, N., *Aspects of the Theory of Syntax*. Cambridge, Mass.: The M.I.T. Press (1965).

Chomsky, N., and Halle, M., *The Sound Patterns of English*. New York: Harper & Row, Publishers (1968).

Clark, E., What's in a word? On the child's acquisition of semantics in his first language. In T. E. Moore (Ed.), *Cognitive Development and the Acquisition of Language*. New York: Academic Press, Inc. (1973).

Compton, A., Generative studies of children's phonological disorders. *J. Speech Hearing Dis.*, **35**, 315-339 (1970).

Compton, A. J., Generative studies of children's phonological disorders: A strategy of therapy. In S. Singh (Ed.), *Measurement Procedures in Speech, Hearing, and Language*. Baltimore: University Park Press (1975).

Corlew, M. M., Word variables and confrontation naming in aphasic patients. Doctoral dissertation, Case Western Reserve University (1971).

Counihan, D. T., Oral and nasal airflow and air pressure measures. In W. C. Grabb, S. W. Rosenstein, and D. R. Bzoch (Eds.), *Cleft Lip and Palate: Surgical, Dental, and Speech Aspects*. Boston: Little, Brown & Co. (1971a).

Counihan, D. T., Oral and nasal airflow and sound pressure measures. In W. C. Grabb, S. W. Rosenstein, and D. R. Bzoch (Eds.), *Cleft Lip and Palate: Surgical, Dental, and Speech Aspects*. Boston: Little, Brown & Co. (1971b).

Dale, P. S., *Language Development: Structure and Function*. Hinsdale, Ill.: The Dryden Press (1972).

Daniloff, R. G., Normal articulation processes. In F. D. Minifie, T. J. Hixon, and F. Williams (Eds.), *Normal Aspects of Speech, Hearing, and Language*. Englewood Cliffs, N.J.: Prentice-Hall, Inc. (1973).

Daniloff, R. G., and Moll, K., Coarticulation of lip

rounding. *J. Speech Hearing Res.*, **11**, 707-721 (1968).

Darley, F. L., *Diagnosis and Appraisal of Communication Disorders*. Englewood Cliffs, N.J.: Prentice-Hall, Inc. (1964).

Darley, F. L., Aronson, A. E., and Brown, J. R., Differential diagnosis patterns of dysarthria. *J. Speech Hearing Res.*, **12**, 246-269 (1969).

Darley, F. L., Aronson, A. E., and Brown, J. R., Clusters of deviant speech dimensions in the dysarthrias. *J. Speech Hearing Res.*, **12**, 462-496 (1969).

Darley, F. L., Aronson, A. E., and Brown, J. R., *Motor Speech Disorders*. Philadelphia: W. B. Saunders Co. (1975).

Emerick, L. L., and Hatten, J. T., *Diagnosis and Evaluation in Speech Pathology*. Englewood Cliffs, N.J.: Prentice-Hall, Inc. (1974).

Ervin-Tripp, S., Language development. In L. W. Hoffman and M. L. Hoffman (Eds.), *Review of Child Development Research*. (Vol. 2) New York: Russell Sage Foundation (1966).

Ervin-Tripp, S., Social backgrounds and verbal skills. In R. Huxley and E. Ingram (Eds.), *Language Acquisition: Models and Methods*. New York: Academic Press, Inc. (1971).

Fant, G., *Acoustic Theory of Speech Production*. The Hague: Mouton Publishers (1960).

Fisher, H. B., *Improving Voice and Articulation*. Boston: Houghton Mifflin Co. (1966).

Fodor, J. A., and Garrett, M., Some syntactic determinants of sentential complexity. *Percept. Psychophys.*, **2**, 289-296 (1967).

Fodor, J. A., and Garrett, M., Some syntactic determinants of sentential complexity. *Percept. Psychophys.*, **4**, 304-306 (1968).

Francis, Q. N., *The Structure of American English*. New York: The Ronald Press Co. (1958).

Heinz, J. M., and Stevens, K. N., On the properties of voiceless fricative consonants. *J. acoust. Soc. Am.*, **33**, 589-596 (1961).

Hymes, D., The ethnography of speaking. In T. Gladwin and W. C. Sturtevant (Eds.), *Anthropology and Human Behavior*. Washington, D.C.: Anthropological Society of Washington (1962).

Hymes, D., The functions of speech. In J. D. De Cecco (Ed.), *The Psychology of Language, Thought and Instruction*. New York: Holt, Rinehart & Winston, Inc. (1967).

Ingram, D., Phonological rules in young children. *J. Child Lang.*, **1**, 49-64 (1974).

Jakobson, R., Concluding statement: Linguistics and poetics. In T. A. Sebeok (Ed.), *Style in Language*. Cambridge, Mass: The M.I.T. Press (1960).

Jakobson, R., and Halle, M., *Fundamentals of Language*. The Hague: Mouton Publishers (1956).

Jakobson, R., Fant, C. G. M., and Halle, M., *Preliminaries to Speech Analysis*. Cambridge, Mass: The M.I.T. Press (1963).

Johnson, W., Darley, F. L., and Spriestersbach, D. C., *Diagnostic Methods in Speech Pathology*. New York: Harper & Row, Publishers (1963).

Klatt, D., The duration of /s/ in English words. *J. Speech Hearing Res.*, **17**, 51-63 (1974).

Koeningsknecht, R. A., and Lee, L. L., Validity and reliability of developmental sentence scoring: A method for measuring syntactic development in children's spontaneous speech. Paper presented at the Annual Convention of the American Speech and Hearing Association, Chicago (1971).

Lee, L. L., Developmental sentence types: A method for comparing normal and deviant syntactic development. *J. Speech Hearing Dis.*, **31**, 311-330 (1966).

Lee, L. L., *Developmental Sentence Analysis*, Evanston, Ill.: Northwestern University Press (1974).

Lee, L. L., and Canter, S. M., Developmental sentence scoring: A clinical procedure for estimating syntactic development in children's spontaneous speech. *J. Speech Hearing Dis.*, **36**, 315-340 (1971).

Leonard, L. B., What is deviant language? *J. Speech Hearing Dis.*, **37**, 427-446 (1972).

Luchsinger, R., and Arnold, G. E., *Voice-Speech-Language: Clinical Communicology: Its Physiology and Pathology*. Belmont, Calif: Wadsworth Publishing Co., Inc. (1965).

Luria, A. R., *The Role of Speech in the Regulation of Normal and Abnormal Behavior*. New York: Liveright (1961).

McNeill, D., Developmental psycholinguistics. In F. Smith and G. A. Miller (Eds.), *The Genesis of Language: A Psycholinguistic Approach*. Cambridge, Mass.: The M.I.T. Press (1966).

McNeill, D., *The Acquisition of Language: The Study of Developmental Psycholinguistics*. New York: Harper & Row, Publishers (1970).

McReynolds, L. V., and Huston, D., A distinctive feature analysis of children's misarticulations. *J. Speech Hearing Dis.*, **36**, 155-166 (1971).

McReynolds, L. V., and Engmann, D. L., *Distinctive Feature Analysis of Misarticulations*. Baltimore: University Park Press (1975).

Menyuk, P., Comparison of grammar of children with functionally deviant and normal speech. *J. Speech Hearing Res.*, **7**, 109-121 (1964).

Menyuk, P., The role of distinctive features in children's acquisition of phonology. *J. Speech Hearing Res.*, **11**, 138-146 (1968).

Menyuk, P., *Sentences Children Use*. Cambridge, Mass.: The M.I.T. Press (1969).

Menyuk, P., *The Acquisition and Development of Language*. Englewood Cliffs, N.J.: Prentice-Hall, Inc. (1971).

Miller, G. A., Some psychological studies of grammar. *Am. Psychol.*, **17**, 748-762 (1962).

Miller, G. A., and McKean, K., A chronometric study of some relations between sentences. *Quart. J. exp. Psychol.*, **16**, 297-308 (1964).

Miller, G. A., and Nicely, P. E., An analysis of perceptual confusions among some English consonants, *J. acoust. Soc. Am.*, **27**, 338-352 (1955).

Miller, J. F., and Yoder, D. E., An ontogenetic language teaching strategy for retarded children. In R. L. Schiefelbusch and L. L. Lloyd (Eds.), *Language Perspectives—Acquisition, Retardation, and Intervention.* Baltimore: University Park Press (1974).

Miner, L. E., Scoring procedures for the length-complexity index: A preliminary report. *J. Commun. Dis.,* **2,** 224-240 (1969).

Minifie, F. D., Speech acoustics. In F. D. Minifie, T. J. Hixon, and F. Williams (Eds.), *Normal Aspects of Speech, Hearing, and Language.* Englewood Cliffs, N.J.: Prentice-Hall, Inc. (1973).

Moncur, J. P., and Brackett, I. P., *Modifying Vocal Behavior.* New York: Harper & Row, Publishers (1974).

Morehead, D. M., and Ingram, D., The development of base syntax in normal and linguistically deviant children. *J. Speech Hearing Res.,* **16,** 330-352 (1973).

Mortensen, C. D., *Communication: The Study of Human Interaction.* New York: McGraw-Hill Book Co. (1972).

Netsell, R., Speech physiology. In F. D. Minifie, T. J. Hixon, and F. Williams (Eds.), *Normal Aspects of Speech, Hearing, and Language.* Englewood Cliffs, N.J.: Prentice-Hall, Inc. (1973).

Perkins, W. H., *Speech Pathology: An Applied Behavioral Science.* (2nd ed.) St. Louis: The C. V. Mosby Co. (1977).

Peterson, G. E., and Shoup, J. E., A physiological theory of phonetics. *J. Speech Hearing Res.,* **9,** 5-67 (1966a).

Peterson, G. E., and Shoup, J. E., The elements of an acoustic phonetic theory. *J. Speech Hearing Res.,* **9,** 68-99 (1966b).

Peterson, G. E., and Shoup, J. E., Glossary of terms from the physiological and acoustic phonetic theories. *J. Speech Hearing Res.,* **9,** 100-120 (1966c).

Piaget, J., *The Language and Thought of the Child.* Cleveland: Meridian Books (1955).

Pollack, E., and Rees, N. S., Disorders of articulation: Some clinical applications of distinctive feature theory. *J. Speech Hearing Dis.,* **37,** 451-461 (1972).

Poole, I., Genetic development of articulation of sounds in speech. *Elemen. Eng. Rev.,* **2,** 159-161 (1934).

Prather, E. M., Hedrick, D. L., and Kern, C. A., Articulation development in children aged two to four years. *J. Speech Hearing Dis.,* **40,** 179-191 (1975).

Rees, N. S., Noncommunicative functions of language in children. *J. Speech Hearing Dis.,* **38,** 98-110 (1973).

Sander, E. K., When are speech sounds learned? *J. Speech Hearing Dis.,* **37,** 55-63 (1972).

Schane, S. A., *Generative Phonology.* Englewood Cliffs, N.J.: Prentice-Hall, Inc. (1973).

Schein, E. H., *Process Consultation: Its Role in Organization Development.* Reading, Mass.: Addison-Wesley Publishing Co., Inc. (1969).

Schlesinger, I. M., Production of utterances and language acquisition. In D. I. Slobin (Ed.), *The Ontogenesis of Grammar.* New York: Academic Press, Inc. (1971).

Schwartz, M. F., Acoustic measures of nasalization and nasality. In W. C. Grabb, S. W. Rosenstein, and K. R. Bzoch (Eds.), *Cleft Lip and Palate: Surgical, Dental, and Speech Aspects.* Boston: Little, Brown & Co. (1971).

Skinner, B. F., *Verbal Behavior.* New York: Appleton-Century-Crofts (1957).

Slobin, D. I., Grammatical transformations in childhood and adulthood. *J. verb. Learning verb. Behav.,* **5,** 219-227 (1966).

Slobin, D. I., Universals of grammatical development in children. In G. B. Flores D'Arcais, and W. J. M. Levelt (Eds.), *Advances in Psycholinguistics.* Amsterdam: North Holland Publishing Co. (1970).

Smith, M. E., An investigation of the development of the sentence and the extent of vocabulary in young children. *University of Iowa Studies in Child Welfare.* No. 3 Iowa City: University of Iowa (1926).

Strevens, P., Spectra of fricative noise in human speech. *Language and Speech,* **3,** 32-49 (1960).

Templin, M. C., *Certain Language Skills in Children, Their Development and Interrelationships,* Institute of Child Welfare, Monograph Series 26, Minneapolis: University of Minnesota Press (1957).

Van Riper, C., and Irwin, J. V., *Voice and Articulation.* Englewood Cliffs, N.J.: Prentice-Hall, Inc. (1958).

Walsh, H., On certain practical inadequacies of distinctive feature systems. *J. Speech Hearing Dis.,* **39,** 32-43 (1974).

Wellman, B. L., Case, I. M., Mengert, I. G., and Bradbury, D. E., Speech sounds of young children. *University of Iowa Studies in Child Welfare.* No. 5 Iowa City: University of Iowa (1931).

Williams, F., and Naremore, R. C., On the functional analysis of social class differences in modes of speech. *Speech Monogr.,* **36,** 77-102 (1969).

Winitz, H., *Articulatory Acquisition and Behavior.* New York: Appleton-Century-Crofts (1969).

Speech and language disorders: historical heritage

The study of speech and language disorders stems from a long historical heritage. *Speech Pathology* (Rieber and Brubaker, 1966) includes two interesting historical review chapters based on European and American literature.

Since classification of speech and language disorders is basic to delimiting information for purposes of professional communication, the diagnostician must come to grips with the diverse nomenclature, classification systems, and causes that have been proposed for speech and language disorders. It is essential that the diagnostician understand how and why classification systems developed, what their points of comparison and contrast are, and how they can be used if he is to understand the speech and language disorders he must describe and interpret.

Thus Chapters 7 and 8 will focus on classifications of speech and language disorders and their causes. Chapter 7 concentrates on current practices in speech pathology—the state of the art concerning classification, nomenclature, and causal factors. Chapter 8 focuses on the development of a detailed cause-effect classification schema based on the SLPM.

CLASSIFICATION AND NOMENCLATURE: STATE OF THE ART

A practical approach to the organization of a classification system for use by the diagnostician would seem to be a search and analysis of systems used in the last quarter century. However, it becomes readily apparent that there has been a proliferation of nomenclature and classification systems derived from many professional viewpoints.

As we look at the various books and articles written in our profession, we can see the effects that different professional views had on current classification systems. Many of these systems were erected on foundations where speech and language were not the primary concern. Because of this, classification systems employ nomenclature that often is not of maximal utility for the diagnostician. In addition, these systems are often not internally consistent; one disorder might be termed from an etiologic point of view, whereas another disorder in the same classification system might carry a behavioral label.

In our review of classification systems and nomenclature, we have cast the information into the following classification systems: etiologic classifications, behavioral description classifications, processing classifications, and clinical problem–type classifications.

Etiologic classification systems

Because of our medical heritage, etiologic considerations have formed the basis for a preponderance of the classification systems developed in speech pathology.

The following causal factors are usually represented in etiologic classification systems: cleft lip and palate, cerebral palsy, mental retardation, brain injury, emotional disturbance, deafness, and hearing loss. This set of circumscribed etiologic factors is repeatedly presented, and we hear speech and language disorders discussed as "cerebral palsied speech," "cleft palate speech," "deaf speech," etc.

Do each of the preceding etiologic categories signal to you a specific set of speech and language characteristics (behaviors)? Write a brief summary statement of the speech and language behaviors you would expect in each of the categories.

The study of developmental language disorders provides an example of the development and use of an etiologic classification system. Early workers in the field of developmental language disorders established their classification system based on the supposed etiology of the child's more general problem, of which disordered language was but one facet. The focus of attention became fixed on general patterns of behavior and away from specific descriptions of language behavior. Thus the curious practice arose of classifying types of language disorders with little reference to the language behavior itself.

Myklebust, in his classic work *Auditory Disorders in Children* (1954), proposed that children with language disorders be "differentially diagnosed" into four syndromic etiologic categories: (1) mental retardation, (2) peripheral deafness, (3) psychic deafness, and (4) aphasia. He proposed that such a differentiation be achieved largely by a comparison of non-linguistic characteristics rather than the child's actual language performance. For example, among other factors, he suggested that a child's use of gestures, laughing, smiling, and crying, sensitivity to movement and other visual stimuli, attention to facial clues, motor behavior, social perception, etc. serve as criteria for deter-

mining into which of his four etiologic categories a child's behavior falls.

These four etiologic categories have been maintained. Adler (1964), McGrady (1968), Morley (1967), and Wood (1964) all continued the practice of classification by etiology, although variations in terminology are employed. A fifth etiologic category, the culturally disadvantaged, has been added by others (McGrady, 1968; Raph, 1967; Wood, 1964).

Even though this development of etiologic classification systems has been helpful in understanding the causal basis for speech and language disorders, there have been several unfortunate outcomes resulting from an etiologic emphasis.

First, emphasis on etiology has resulted in inappropriate management issues. Issues such as who should see which children became prevalent. For example, if a child is mentally retarded, does he become the sole province of the educator/psychologist; if emotionally disturbed, the psychologist; if deaf or hard-of-hearing, the deaf educator; etc.? Fortunately, these practices are breaking down, and more true interdisciplinary management programs are being put into effect.

Second, emphasis on etiology has impeded the development of classification systems based on careful analysis of speech and language behavior. When the cause is considered as the disorder rather than speech and language, it leads to such diagnostic statements as "Arik is autistic," "Roberta is retarded," and "Trisha is emotionally disturbed" rather than "Byron's language disorder is related to his mental retardation."

Marge (1972) strongly opposes this common practice of classifying by etiology. He believes that etiologic classification systems have not helped to describe the speech and language behaviors that make up the disorder and thus do not assist greatly in management considerations. We (Aram, 1972; Aram and Nation, 1975) have presented similar objections to etiologic classification systems. Our evidence strongly suggests that similar patterns of disordered language behavior may occur in children with varying etiologic histories.

Therefore, even if at times we see characteristic patterns of speech and language behaviors related to certain etiologies, the emphasis on classification should still be on disordered speech and language. Etiologic considerations are best kept in causal relationship to descriptions of disordered speech and language behavior—the first concern of the diagnostician.

Third, emphasis on etiologic classification has resulted in a simplified view of cause-effect relationships. We feel that emphasis on etiologic categories makes diagnosticians assume that single causes may explain speech and language disorders. A classification system based on a specified set of etiologic categories "sets us up" to believe that a speech and language disorder that has been seen resulted from one of the specified categories.

Even though we believe that definitive cause-effect relationships exist, an etiologic approach to classification of speech and language disorders restricts rather than broadens the cause-effect perspective needed by the diagnostician. When we carefully examine the causal basis for speech and language disorders, we see many factors coming into play, either singly or in multiple interactions. For example, consider the etiologic basis for the voice disorder that exists because of the presence of contact ulcers, which developed because of vocal abuse, which occurred because the basketball coach wanted to project a more masculine image to the boys on his team. If diagnosticians are constrained by classification systems, then their ability to formulate diagnostic hypotheses will also be constrained.

Since classification of speech and language disorders based on etiology has been so strongly entrenched in speech pathology, particularly for the purposes of "differential diagnosis," there must be some clinical usefulness to this system. We too see etiology as an important fund of knowledge for the diagnostician; he must understand the wide range of causal factors responsible for speech and language disorders. However, again we want to emphasize that causal factors should be viewed in relationship to speech and language disorders and not as classification systems for the disorders.

Behavioral description classification systems

As a reaction to the use of etiology for classifying speech and language disorders, a movement toward descriptive classification occurred. In such systems a phrase or paragraph described a client's speech and language strengths and limitations.

Milisen's early classification (1957) was instrumental in shifting the speech pathologist's attention to description. His system of classification was based on behavioral observations of comprehension and expression and included four categories: (1) communication that involves no comprehension of, or expression through, oral language; (2) communication that involves comprehension of, but little or no expression through, oral language; (3) communication that involves deteriorated comprehension and/or expression through oral language; and (4) communication that involves comprehension of, and expression through, oral language with the pattern of expression being unacceptable to the listener and/or the speaker.

Descriptive classification systems were intended to reduce examiner bias; that is, they alerted the diagnostician not to expect a certain behavior because of a certain etiologic factor. These systems were also designed to discourgage personification on the basis of a disorder; that is, the practice of labeling a person a "stutterer" was supplanted with descriptions of his speech behavior, recognizing that the stuttering behavior was but one part of the total person.

Descriptive classification systems such as Milisen's have not found wide adoption in speech pathology even by Milisen in his later writing (1971). Probably their major importance was in moving our field away from etiologic classification systems into behavioral and processing systems.

Processing classification systems

Most processing classification systems developed as extensions of behavioral systems. The intent of processing classification systems was to relate speech and language behavior to basic "communication" processes (Darley, 1964). Some variation exists among the processes specified in the classification systems but many include phonation, resonation, articulation, prosody, and symbolization. There appears to be a division implicit in this classification system; symbolization is used to consider language disorders, and the remaining processes are concerned with the production of speech.

The developers of these classification systems suggest that the diagnostician can examine each of the processes to discover the basis of the speech and language disorder. A number of subcategories of disorders were developed for each process. For example, disordered phonation would lead to the general behavioral classification of voice disorders that could then be divided into a number of subcategories such as pitch, quality, and loudness disorders or into problem types such as falsetto, diplophonia, ventricular phonation, etc.

The development of processing classification systems for speech and language disorders assisted the diagnostician in drawing better relationships between the behavioral disorders observed and disrupted speech and language processes. These systems went beyond describing the characteristics of the disorder; they provided insight into the basis of the behavioral disorder. Thus processing classification systems were a significant step forward in the speech pathologist's view of speech and language disorders.

Clinical problem–type classification systems

One of the most common approaches to classification is that which attempts to specify problem types encountered in speech pathology. What usually results in these problem-type classifications is a mixture of etiologic, behavioral, and processing terms. Little internal consistency of classification is seen. For example, Erikson and Van Riper (1967) use the term "clinical type" and include within this classification the following disorders: stuttering, misarticulation, dysphonia, cerebral palsy, aphasia, postlaryngectomee, delayed language, and hearing loss. While some of these terms may have clinical usefulness and there may be some truth to their being "clinical types," this system does not present us with a consistent basis for classification. It is a "mixed-up" system, employing medical, etiologic, processing, and behavioral nomenclature. In addition to lacking internal consistency, these clinical problem–type classifications often assumed a common understanding of such disorders as cerebral palsy, and that given such a condition, a particular speech and language disorder would be observed. These are both questionable assumptions.

Commonality of classification

None of the systems discussed are consistent classification systems based entirely on etiology, description, or processing. Each system included aspects of the others, although some were more consistent than others. From all these various attempts to classify speech and language disorders there is still little commonality in classification systems used in our current literature. For example, Emerick and Hatten (1974) follow *primarily* a clinical problem–type system and discuss diagnosis of language disorders, articulation disorders, stuttering, aphasia in adults, and voice disorders. Perkins (1977), on the other hand, follows *primarily* a processing system and discusses disorders of language, disorders of articulation-resonance, disorders of phonation, and disorders of speech flow.

Table 6. Classification and nomenclature in speech and language disorders

Reference	Author's primary system[*]	Terminology	Classification of nomenclature			
			Etiologic	Behavioral description	Processing	Clinical problem type
Emerick and Hatten (1974)	Clinical type	Aphasia Voice Stuttering Language Articulation	Aphasia	Aphasia Voice Language	Articulation	Aphasia Voice Stuttering Language Articulation
Perkins (1977)	Processing	Language Articulation-resonance Phonation Speech flow		Language Speech flow (?)	Articulation-resonance Phonation Speech flow	Language
Dickson (1974)						

[*] Either from the author's statement or from your interpretation of the basis of his classification system.

Variable and inconsistent classification systems do not provide the diagnostician or the student in training with a logical system for classifying speech and language disorders. A meaningful way for the student to explore the commonalities among the various classification systems would be to develop a comprehensive classification table from various literature resources. Table 6 provides headings for the four major classification systems we have discussed. As examples, we have plotted the basic nomenclature of Emerick and Hatten (1974) and Perkins (1977). The student should explore many writings about nomenclature and classification and plot them on the table. For example, Dickson (1974) represents another current resource. How are "communication disorders" classified in this book?

You will also see that some of the terminology is not mutually exclusive, but fits into several systems. For example, inherent in the term "aphasia" is both an etiology (brain dysfunction) and a behavior (language disorder). Thus you will have to discover the meaning of the author's nomenclature, since terminology in our profession has been quite "mixed up."

Along with this project we are incorporating an extensive list of terms used to talk about speech and language disorders. What do these terms mean and where would you plot them on the table?

Adenoidal speech
Agnosia
Anomia
Apraxia
Cerebral palsy speech
Cleft palate speech
Cluttering
Comprehension disorder
Delayed articulation
Delayed language
Denasality
Dysarthria
Echolalic
Esophageal speech
Expressive language
Falsetto
Fluency
Guttural speech
Harshness
Hypoprosody
Infantile perseveration
Interdental lisp
Internalized stuttering
Lalling
Lambdacism
Lisping
Misarticulation
Monopitch
Muffled voice
Nasality
Nasal twang
Phonetic disorder
Phonologic disorder
Pitch breaks
Rate
Receptive aphasia
Rhinolalia clausa
Rhotacism
Semantic disorder
Sensory aphasia
Slow speech
Stereotyped inflections
Stuttering
Substitution
Ventricular phonation
Vocabulary disorder

Your development of the nomenclature and classification table should help you discover the bases for much of the terminology as well as its commonality. Having completed such a project should leave you with an awareness that we need a consistent classification system that allows for quick and easy reference by the diagnostician as well as for purposes of professional communication.

CAUSAL FACTORS: STATE OF THE ART

Speech and language disorders result from many disrupting factors and conditions occurring at different times throughout life. Because so many factors can be disruptive, the understanding of causal factors for speech and language disorders has taken on a complexity sometimes beyond the diagnostician's comprehension. Although the focus has been on our medical heritage, causal factors have been presented from variable viewpoints, resulting in a literature that is difficult to assimilate and organize.

In addition, settings in which speech pathologists train or work promote different approaches and biases to the study of causal factors. Different positions are taken about the need to understand the causes of speech and language disorders. Probably the least emphasis is given to causation by those who profess to be interested in behavioral symptoms only, as in behavior modification. At the other end of the continuum are those whose orientation justifies working only with the "underlying" or "overriding" cause for the disordered behavior. Thus the causal emphasis for almost any speech and language disorder can vary significantly from one professional to another.

These diverse orientations to causation have resulted in inconsistent and often confusing approaches to causal factors for speech and language disorders. In our state-of-the-art review we identify three persistent and, to us, dead-end practices that have evolved: cataloging of etiologies, development of etiologic classification systems, and dichotomizing functional-organic etiologies.

Myklebust (1954) discusses three reasons for interest in etiology. How does he view etiologic concerns in relationship to prevention, remediation, and differential diagnosis?

Cataloging of etiologies

Authors in speech pathology and audiology have produced numerous catalogs of potential etiologies. For example, *Human Communication and Its Disorders: An Overview* (1969) provides a series of etiologic factors related to cochlear pathology, resulting in hearing disorders. Such factors as prenatal disorders and neonatal disorders (time of onset factors) are listed along with such factors as infectious diseases and ototoxic disorders. The difficulty with such catalogs is their lack of a consistent basis from which to explore etiologic factors. Frequently, no superordinate organization is evidenced. Are such catalogs derived from considerations of time of onset, disease, trauma, or what? Such lists prevent convenient use by the diagnostician.

Listing and cataloging of etiologic factors is not always without some organization. "Organic" etiologies are often structured from a medical focus. Catalogs of organic factors incorporate headings such as diseases, trauma, cerebrovascular accidents, structural defects, tumors, genetic factors, and chemical-metabolic factors. Sometimes within these headings we also see a time of occurrence breakdown, looking at the etiologic category from a prenatal, natal, and postnatal time of occurrence. Medical texts, such as that by Chusid (1970), have provided the background for catalogs such as these in speech pathology.

Listing and cataloging etiologic factors is not in and of itself an inappropriate approach to causal factors for speech and language disorders. Instead, it is the diagnostician's use of the list, leading to a search for *the* cause of *the* disorder. The emphasis has been on each potential etiologic factor rather than on learning logical cause-effect relationships. Instead of learning lists of etiologic factors, the diagnostician should be concerned with how, when, and why etiologic factors have the potential for causing speech and language disorders.

Review a number of books with the intent of developing a comprehensive list of potential etiologic factors for speech and language disorders. On what basis can you organize (catalog) these lists?

Etiologic classification systems

In speech pathology any number of etiologic classification systems have been developed, as was discussed earlier in this chapter. These etiologic classification systems are basically extensions of etiologic cataloging. Their intent is to provide a set of etiologies that potentially encompass and explain all speech and language disorders. For example, Perkins (1977) develops a series of chapters termed the "disabilities of speech": disabilities that have disruptive effects on speech and language. They are neurologic disabilities, peripheral sensory disabilities, laryngeal and lower respiratory disabilities, orofacial and upper respiratory disabilities, learning and intellectual disabilities, and personality and emotional disturbances.

Dichotomizing functional-organic etiologies

A major practice evidenced for some time in speech pathology has been the development of the functional-organic dichotomy for organizing etiologic factors. This dichotomous view of etiology carries the implication that all causes of speech and language disorders can be classified as either functional or organic. This practice tended to separate the human organism from his environment, and thus, at times, the dichotomy is expressed as organic versus environmental causes. Most traditionally used etiologic schemata reflect this functional-organic dichotomy (Berry and Eisenson, 1956; Van Riper, 1972; West and Ansberry, 1968; Wood, 1964).

Exactly how has the dichotomy of functional-organic etiologies been used in the speech pathology literature? What are the different ways the term "functional" has been defined? What has added to the confusion surrounding this dichotomy? How did this dichotomy grow out of the use of these terms in medicine? As a start, use any good medical dictionary as a source.

The use of the functional-organic dichotomy seems, in many ways, to have had a retarding rather than a facilitating effect

on understanding causal factors. First, dichotomizing etiologic factors did not increase our ability to communicate with one another about causes of speech and language disorders. The use of a dichotomous system is only helpful if each person using the classification system fully understands its intent. Often this is not the case.

Second, the functional-organic dichotomy did not concern itself greatly with the relationship between the etiology and its effect on the speech and language process. It seemed enough to say that the functional or organic etiologic factor existed and that its existence served in some self-explanatory way. Little search was given into the mechanics by which a given etiologic factor resulted in the specific speech and language disorder under consideration. The dichotomy basically served as an impetus to "hunt for" some historical factor "lurking in the background" of the client that could be considered as the etiology, and then the speech and language disorder could be categorized as functional or organic.

Third, this etiologic dichotomy tended to emphasize discovery of an organic etiologic basis. If an organic factor could not be found, the speech and language disorder would be automatically diagnosed as having a functional basis. Several writers (Perkins and Curlee, 1969; Powers, 1957; Sommers and Kane, 1974) have pointed out how the term "functional disorder" became a catchall, a wastebasket term for speech and language disorders that could not be explained on an organic basis. We feel that Bzoch (1971), for example, perpetuates the dichotomy as well as the wastebasket use of functional when he classifies the causes of "communication disorders" in persons with cleft palate into (1) an organic category, that is "diagnosable structural abnormalities which when changed by physical management result in a direct measurable improvement in speech behavior . . ." and (2) a functional category, that is "all other presumed causes which are not directly treatable by physical management. . . ."

Meyers (1965-1966) in a critical article discussing the functional-organic dichotomy in medicine argues that this dichotomy is "neither a 'fact' nor a 'self-evident truth,' but a high-order, uncritically-arrived-at, deeply internalized, linguistic-cultural habit." In his criticism of the use of the term "functional" he proposes that the causal dichotomy may result more from our methods of discovery than from reality, a point also made by McDonald (1964). In many instances the measuring instruments used may not be sensitive enough to detect organic factors; thus historically, a disorder might be classified as functional; whereas later, with changes in measuring sensitivity, the organic basis may be discovered.

Diagnosticians need to recognize that the functional-organic dichotomy may more accurately represent two sides of the same coin. Perkins and Curlee (1969) and Kessler (1971) remind us that for something to function it must exist as an organic structure, and that in the final analysis all behavior is organically based. For example, knowing that certain types of environmental deprivation can have effects on central nervous system functioning similar to the effects of certain organic factors, the dichotomy between functional and organic breaks down. It makes us aware that there may be no simple dichotomous explanation of either organic or functional etiologic factors but rather interactions of the organism with his environment in the presence of the etiologic factor. The diagnostician must account for these interactions when he views the disordered behavior that the client presents to him.

Using the previous catalog of etiologic factors you developed, organize them into a functional-organic dichotomy. What difficulties arise when you do this?

Limited understanding of etiology

These three persistent practices that have evolved around causation have re-sulted in a limited understanding of causal factors for speech and language disorders. They often lead the diagnostician toward a simplistic view of causation rather than a dynamic interactive view. Emphasis was placed on finding a cause rather than discovering a cause-effect relationship. Diagnosticians searched the client's history to see if it revealed a causal factor that is on the etiology "list." These diagnostic practices seem to arise because the diagnostician somehow feels obligated to tie a cause to a disorder or to label the disorder as functional or organic, but he does not feel the obligation to discover how and if the causal factor is important to management decisions that need to be made.

Lists and catalogs of etiologic factors have little explanatory power; they do not automatically reveal the interactions that existed between the causal factors and the speech and language disorder. Thus it is of limited value in diagnosis to gather historical data of etiologic significance without considering how the causal factors interacted with speech and language processing to result in the disordered speech and language behavior. Multiple causation, chains of cause-effect relationships, time of occurrence, severity, and the direct-indirect nature of causation must be evaluated.

Fortunately, more professionals are rethinking causation in relationship to diagnosis and treatment of speech and language disorders. They are recognizing the presence of multiple causation and different levels of causal description (Perkins and Curlee, 1969). From this, new schemata are being developed out of the old. Better insights into the complexities of causation for speech and language disorders are being sought.

How useful has our professional literature been in developing consistent, useful classification systems? How many articles can you find that devote themselves to this topic? As a beginning, see Laguaite et al. (1965).

SUMMARY

Chapter 7 has presented the "state of the art" in speech pathology regarding classification and nomenclature applied to speech and language disorders and practices employed for viewing causal factors for speech and language disorders.

We have pointed out that classification systems have been developed from varying points of view, have not been internally consistent, and have tended to emphasize etiologic classification. Thus there is little commonality among the classification systems in current use.

We have reviewed the major approaches to causation. These approaches have led to a limited understanding of cause-effect relationships seen in speech and language disorders. The emphasis seems to be on searching for a cause rather than understanding the dynamic interactions that exist between causal factors and the processes responsible for speech and language disorders.

Therefore our historical heritage has not always resulted in a consistent viewpoint of classification and causation helpful to the diagnostician. In the next chapter we will develop a schema for classifying speech and language disorders as well as a schema for exploring cause-effect relationships that we believe will assist the diagnostician in developing a more consistent viewpoint.

REFERENCES

Adler, S., *The Non-verbal Child.* Springfield, Ill.: Charles C Thomas, Publisher (1964).

Aram, D. M., Developmental language disorders: Patterns of language behavior. Doctoral dissertation, Case Western Reserve University (1972).

Aram, D. M., and Nation, J. E., Patterns of language behavior in children with developmental language disorders. *J. Speech Hearing Res.*, **18**, 229-241 (1975).

Bangs, T. E., *Language and Learning Disorders of the Pre-Academic Child.* New York: Appleton-Century-Crofts (1968).

Berry, M. F., *Language Disorders of Children: The Bases and Diagnosis.* New York: Appleton-Century-Crofts (1969).

Berry, M. F., and Eisenson, J., *Speech Disorders: Principles and Practices of Therapy.* New York: Appleton-Century-Crofts (1956).

Bzoch, E., Etiological factors related to cleft palate speech. In W. C. Grabb, S. W. Rosenstein, and K. R. Bzoch (Eds.), *Cleft Lip and Palate: Surgical, Dental, and Speech Aspects.* Boston: Little, Brown & Co. (1971).

Chusid, J., *Correlative Neuroanatomy and Functional Neurology.* (14th ed.) Los Altos, Calif.: Lange Medical Publications (1970).

Darley, F. L., *Diagnosis and Appraisal of Communication Disorders.* Englewood Cliffs, N.J.: Prentice-Hall, Inc. (1964).

Dickson, S. (Ed.), *Communication Disorders: Remedial Principles and Practices.* Glenview, Ill.: Scott, Foresman & Co. (1974).

Eisenson, J., *Aphasia in Children.* New York: Harper & Row, Publishers (1972).

Emerick, L. L., and Hatten, J. H., *Diagnosis and Evaluation in Speech Pathology.* Englewood Cliffs, N.J.: Prentice-Hall, Inc. (1974).

Erikson, R., and Van Riper, C., Demonstration therapy in a university training center. *Asha*, **9**, 33-35 (1967).

Human Communication and Its Disorders: An Overview. Bethesda, Md.: National Institute of Neurological Disease and Stroke, U.S. Department of Health, Education and Welfare (1969).

Kessler, J. W., Nosology in child psychopathology. In H. E. Rie (Ed.), *Perspectives in Child Psychopathology.* Chicago: Aldine Publishing Co. (1971).

Laguaite, J. K., Riviere, M., and Fuller, C. W., Problems in terminology. *Asha*, **7**, 152-155 (1965).

Marge, M., The general problem of language disabilities in children. In J. V. Irwin and M. Marge (Eds.), *Principles of Childhood Language Disabilities.* New York: Meredith Corp. (1972).

McDonald, E., *Articulation Testing and Treatment: A Sensory-Motor Approach.* Pittsburgh: Stanwix House, Inc. (1964).

McGrady, H., Language pathology and learning disabilities. In H. Myklebust (Ed.), *Progress in Learning Disabilities.* (Vol. 1) New York: Grune & Stratton, Inc. (1968).

Meyers, R., On the dichotomy of organic and "functional" diseases. *Gen. Seman. Bull.*, Nos. 32 and 33, 21-37 (1965-1966).

Milisen, R., Methods of evaluation and diagnosis of speech disorders. In L. E. Travis (Ed.), *Handbook of Speech Pathology.* New York: Appleton-Century-Crofts (1957).

Milisen, R., Methods of evaluation and diagnosis of speech disorders. In L. E. Travis (Ed.), *Handbook of Speech Pathology and Audiology.* New York: Appleton-Century-Crofts (1971).

Morley, M., *The Development and Disorders of Speech in Childhood.* (2nd ed.) Baltimore: The Williams & Wilkins Co. (1967).

Myklebust, H., *Auditory Disorders in Children.* New York: Grune & Stratton, Inc. (1954).

Northern, J. L., and Downs, M. P., *Hearing in Chil-*

dren. Baltimore: The Williams & Wilkins Co. (1974).

Perkins, W. H., *Speech Pathology: An Applied Behavioral Science*. (2nd ed.) St. Louis: The C. V. Mosby Co. (1977).

Perkins, W. H., and Curlee, R. F., Causality in speech pathology. *J. Speech Hearing Dis., 34,* 231-238 (1969).

Powers, M. H., Functional disorders of articulation—Symptomatology and etiology. In L. E. Travis (Ed.), *Handbook of Speech Pathology*. New York: Appleton-Century-Crofts (1957).

Raph, J. B., Language and speech deficits in culturally disadvantaged children: Implications for the speech clinician. *J. Speech Hearing Dis., 32,* 203-214 (1967).

Reiber, R. W., and Brubaker, R. S., *Speech Pathology*. Philadelphia: J. B. Lippincott Co. (1966).

Sommers, R. K., and Kane, A. R., Nature and remediation of functional articulation disorders. In S. Dickson (Ed.), *Communication Disorders: Remedial Principles and Practices*. Glenview, Ill.: Scott, Foresman & Co. (1974).

Van Riper, C., *Speech Correction: Principles and Methods*. (5th ed.) Englewood Cliffs, N.J.: Prentice-Hall, Inc. (1972).

West, R. W., and Ansberry, M., *The Rehabilitation of Speech*. (4th ed.) New York: Harper & Row, Publishers (1968).

Winitz, H., *Articulatory Acquisition and Behavior*. New York: Appleton-Century-Crofts (1969).

Wood, N., *Delayed Speech and Language Development*. Englewood Cliffs, N.J.: Prentice-Hall, Inc. (1964).

Speech and language disorders: speech and language processing model schema

Our historical heritage leaves the diagnostician with a fragmented view of speech and language disorders and their causes; a view that emphasizes labeling a disorder and classifying it into some etiologic category.

We do know that many causal factors both within and outside the individual can affect his ability to learn and use speech and language appropriately. The diagnostician must have a schema by which he can explore these dynamic relationships and go on to develop consistent, useful nomenclature and classification systems.

This chapter develops and expands the use of the SLPM as a consistent organizing schema for naming and classifying speech and language disorders, searching out and classifying causal factors, and interpreting cause-effect relationships. We consider the information presented in this chapter to be of major importance to the diagnostician for developing an understanding of the complex cause-effect relationships that exist—information that is vital to both diagnosis and remediation of speech and language disorders.

SLPM SCHEMA FOR CLASSIFYING SPEECH AND LANGUAGE DISORDERS

Nomenclature and classification systems should expedite and facilitate professional communication. One diagnostician should know what another means when he receives a report that says, "Carl has an articulation disorder." Used appropriately, a classification system can help the diagnostician delineate the essential disorder, discover cause-effect relationships, suggest a course of remediation, and even suggest the eventual outcome, all in keeping with the overall purposes of diagnosis.

Basis of classification

Classification of speech and language disorders should have its primary basis in observation and measurement of behaviors presented by the client. This essential point forces diagnosticians to develop systematic methods for describing and classifying behavior that achieve a high level of agreement among diagnosticians. Operational definitions of the behaviors observed can provide a framework to ensure that the classification terms used have been explicitly defined. We must use terms appropriate to our profession; medical, psychiatric, psychological, and other terms may be valid in some instances but should only be used in their appropriate place and time.

The following, among others, have devised behavioral systems for analysis and treatment of speech and language disorders: Brutten and Shoemaker (1967), Darley et al. (1969a, b, 1975), Miller and Yoder (1972), and Sarno et al. (1970). Are their terms internally consistent, and are they consistent with the SLPM view of classification to be discussed?

We offer the following list of principles as a basis for diagnostic classification systems.

1. For a classification system to be useful it must be agreed on by the individuals who may use it.
2. Classification systems are abstractions that are meaningful to the observer.
3. The terminology used in classification systems must be operationally and precisely defined.
4. Classification systems for speech and language disorders must grow out of knowledge about the normal speech and language process.
5. The primary speech and language information available for classification is the speaker's verbal output.

These five principles for developing a classification system could be further refined. What other considerations do you feel are important for the development of classification systems in speech and language disorders? What important points about classification would you draw from the general semanticist's tenets (Korzybski, 1948)?

Levels of classification

From the SLPM, internally consistent classification systems can be developed. The model provides for three levels of classification and specifies measurement considerations for each level. They are the product level disorders, the behavioral correlate level disorders, and the internal physical processing level disorders.

All that was discussed in Chapters 3 through 6 regarding the construction of the SLPM is applicable to this current discussion of classification and nomenclature. Therefore a protracted discussion of classification levels based on the SLPM is not needed here. Instead, we will briefly develop the use of each level of classification and refer the reader back to previous chapters for needed details.

Product level disorders

In a behavioral science the first and foremost basis for a classification system should stem from the most observable set of behaviors. Since speech and language behavior is the diagnostician's major interest, the product level of classification reflects this primacy. The product level of classification specifies the observable parameters of disordered speech and language that are heard when a client speaks. As described in Chapters 3 and 6, the product level has two divisions: the speech product and the language product. Within each of these divisions a set of observable parameters is specified to which the diagnostician directs his measurement strategies.

■ Classify the following client's behavior on the product classification level. When Mrs. Weiss was asked to define words, she defined *have* as "to have and to hold." When asked to try again she said, "What all of us have we should appreciate [long pause] the best." For the word *bridge* she responded, "Access over the river —little more than access because you [not completed]." When asked to describe a picture of a boy flying a kite she said, "He's holding the— that's attached to the flying object—the kite; yes, he's holding the ribbon."

Behavioral correlate level disorders

The SLPM provides a second level, the behavioral correlate level, for classifying speech and language disorders. Based on sets of observable behavior that are operationally defined by tasks, this level tells the diagnostician about a client's auditory reception, central language, and speech production abilities. Chapters 3 and 5 provide a detailed discussion of behavioral correlates as externalized behaviors, hypothesized as reflective of internal physical processes.

With the addition of the behavioral correlate classification level, greater insights can be gained into speech and language disorders. For example, through the behavioral correlate level the diagnostician can specify if the language disorder is one of comprehension or formulation. Or he can specify the speech disorder as primarily one of sequencing or motor control. As well, through task specification he could determine if the comprehension disorder was related primarily to the pragmatic, semantic, syntactic, or phonologic aspects of message comprehension. Many such insights are gained through task specification and classification on the behavioral correlate level.

As has been stated, the behavioral correlates are hypothesized as externalized behaviors to physical processes. This gives the diagnostician another dimension of classification of behavior. The disruptions of the behavioral correlates provide him with information about potentially disrupted physical processes as a basis for the disorders he observes. Thus the diagnostician could cite behavioral correlates as contemporary causal factors for the speech and language disorder. For example, the diagnostician could cite disruptions of sensation or perception as the basis for the current comprehension disorder.

Therefore having the behavioral correlate classification level along with the product classification level gives diagnosticians a better grasp of cause-effect relationships. In essence, the behavioral correlate level of classification can help diagnosticians explain the products they observe or it can help them infer disrupted physical processes.

■ Classify the following client's performance on the behavioral correlate level of classification. Chapters 3 and 5 will be essential in doing this. When asked to point to pictures of a dog, a cat, and a chair, 7-year-old Janet pointed incorrectly to all of them. When asked her name, she responded, "No—no." When asked if she wanted a cookie, she shook her head in a positive manner but did not reach out for the cookie held before her. When the examiner was behind her and called out her name in a whisper, she turned to face the examiner. Two bells were placed before her of the same size. One bell rang; the second did not. The examiner "rang" the two bells and replaced them before Janet. She responded by picking up the bell that rang, holding it to her ear, and shaking it.

Physical processing level disorders

In addition to the speech and language product and the behavioral correlates, a classification system based on internal physical processing can be devised. When using this system, we must keep in mind its highly theoretical, inferential, basically nonobservable basis as discussed in Chapters 3 and 5.

This classification level does not tell diagnosticians what the disordered speech and language behavior is. It does not describe speech and language disorders. Rather, its primary usefulness resides in ordering underlying disrupted processes and therefore contributing to discovering cause-effect relationships.

If the diagnostician can infer disrupted processes from the disordered product, or if he can predict disordered products from knowledge about disrupted processes, he can develop more sophisticated hypotheses about cause-effect relationships. It is the diagnostician's knowledge of the relationships among the physical processes, the behavioral correlates, and the speech and language products that allows for this sophistication.

■ Classify the following client on the physical processing classification level. You will need to consider carefully the measurement considerations discussed earlier, particularly the use of the inferential strategy. Four-year-old Paxton was seen by the diagnostician to determine why he was using only one-word responses. At 4 months of age he sustained a severe blow to the left side of the head resulting in a skull fracture; he was hospitalized for 1 month under careful observation following procedures for removal of a hematoma that had spread over a large portion of the temporal lobe. His subsequent physical development was almost within normal limits; however, speech and language were as stated: when he responded, it was with single words, not always intelligible. He did not always follow directions appropriately, but he did point to some pictures that were named at the 3-year level.

These three classification levels have distinct advantages for the diagnostician.

First, because levels of classification stem directly from the SLPM, they have a built-in consistency that is logical, understandable, and practical to the the diagnostician. Each of the levels are internally consistent; the terminology at each level was specified and defined in the construction of the SLPM and, as well, was derived from measurement considerations. Thus the use of this nomenclature and these classification systems reveals how the diagnostician arrives at the diagnostic labels he uses. Also, the levels of classification allow the diagnostician to represent the difference between what was observed and what was inferred.

Second, the diagnostician does not need a special set of nomenclature to specify the disorders he encounters. The SLPM nomenclature can be used simply by applying the noun "disorder" or the adjective "disordered." For example, the product, voice, can be discussed as a voice disorder or disordered voice; the behavioral correlate, formulation, can be discussed as a formulation disorder or disordered formulation; and the physical process, speech programming, can be discussed as a speech pro-

gramming disorder or disordered speech programming.

Third, these classification systems allow diagnosticians to incorporate other nomenclature without undue difficulty. It requires knowing how a specific term used to specify a disorder came about, but in most instances its relationship to the SLPM classification system is apparent. True, certain labels for disorders will probably remain for many years to come; for example, stuttering has a strong historical reference and implies to many people a specific type of speech behavior. This term can retain its clinical usefulness, but at the same time it can be incorporated into the SLPM as a disorder of prosody. It may be doubtful whether the term "prosody" will ever be favored over the tradition-bound term "stuttering"; but we also must remember that in the past stuttering was once called "psellismus" (Rieber and Brubaker, 1966).

Fourth, each of these levels provides the

Table 7. SLPM as a basis for classification and nomenclature in speech and language disorders

Terminology	Level of classification		
	Product level	**Behavioral correlate level**	**Internal processing level**

Classification of nomenclature is dependent on how each term has been defined and used in the literature; in the two examples below can you justify our classification?	Speech product
	  Vocal tone
	  Resonance
	  Voice
	  Prosody
	  Phonetic structure
	Language product
	  Phonologic
	  Syntactic
	  Semantic
	  Pragmatic
		Sensation
		Perception
		Comprehension
		Formulation
		Repetition
		Sequencing
		Motor control
			Auditory acceptance-transduction
			Auditory analysis-transmission
			Auditory reception-analysis
			Auditory programming
			Language representation
			Auditory programming
			Speech programming
			Speech initiation
			Speech coordination-transmission
			Speech production
			  Breathing for speech
			  Phonation
			  Resonation
			  Articulation
			  Prosodation

EXAMPLES Apraxia	Phonologic	Formulation/sequencing (?)	Speech programming (?)

Articulation	1. Phonologic
	
	2. Phonetic structure
		1. Formulation/sequencing
		
		2. Sequencing/motor control
			1. Language representation
			    Auditory programming
			    Speech programming
			2. Speech initiation/speech coordination-transmission/speech production (articulation)

diagnostician with different information about the speech and language disorder he is investigating. How he uses each level of classification depends on his diagnostic emphasis and the data made available to him. Thus these levels help the diagnostician to determine the relationships among behaviors, processes, and causal factors.

At this time the student would benefit from practice with the levels of classification derived from the SLPM. Classify the various terms from your earlier nomenclature and classification table (Table 6) into the SLPM classification schema. Table 7 plots the basic terminology from the SLPM and demonstrates several examples.

SLPM SCHEMA FOR CLASSIFYING CAUSAL FACTORS

As discussed in Chapter 7, our historical heritage has left the diagnostician with a limited view of causation, focusing on sets of causal factors rather than providing a dynamic view of complex cause-effect interactions. A consistent schema must be developed for diagnostic use, emphasizing the diagnostician's search for and interpretation of cause-effect relationships, not a search for a causal factor in and of itself.

Basis for classification

It becomes quickly obvious that the number of interacting factors that could affect speech and language learning and usage is innumerable. In fact, it may not be inaccurate to say that any identifiable factor, extrinsic or intrinsic to the human, has the potential of becoming causally related to the speech and language disorder. As well, a factor that may be causally related to a disorder in one individual may have no relationship to a similar disorder seen in another client. Many clients are seen with "a causal factor" in their history, but that factor has no bearing on their speech and language disorder. So no assumptions can be made that a given set of causal factors can account for or encompass the range of speech and language disorders seen. It is likely that the study of causal factors may defy any single organizational attempt at cataloging, nor will any organizational attempt satisfy all segments of the profession.

However, some guidelines for organizing a schema for causal factors are essential. The schema should:

1. Stress discovering cause-effect relationships, not just causal factors
2. Delimit the number of causal categories needed for a causal search mechanism
3. Demonstrate how a specific causal factor exerts its primary effect
4. Facilitate the diagnostician's purposes
5. Accommodate the current and future literature about causal factors
6. Be open-ended to allow for development of future perspectives regarding causation

Essentially, then, diagnosticians need a means of reviewing the vast range of potential causal factors and demonstrating how any specific factor exerts its influence on speech and language. The emphasis must be on a consistent schema that facilitates the diagnostician's search for causation, allowing for appropriate interpretation of cause-effect relationships. The diagnostician needs to know how the causal factors have interacted with the human being and/or his environment to create the behavioral disorder seen. The diagnostician must stress the effect of the causal factor, not the causal factor in and of itself.

To this end, we will first present a *scanning mechanism* based on the SLPM for searching out and classifying causal factors. Once this has been developed, we will then present the SLPM schema for interpreting cause-effect relationships, including perspectives on causation and the impact causal factors have on speech and language development and usage.

Scanning mechanism for causal factors

The scanning mechanism emphasizes causal factors that primarily affect the speech and language environment component and causal factors that primarily affect the internal speech and language processing component. The following outline presents the scanning categories developed within each of these components; it is a mechanism for classifying and searching out causal factors for speech and language disorders.

I. Factors primarily affecting the speech and language environment component
   A. Interpersonal factors
      1. Parents and parenting
      2. Sibling relations
      3. Other significant relationships
   B. Sociocultural factors
      1. Income, economic status
      2. Education-occupation of parents and client
      3. Racial, ethnic practices
   C. Physical-technologic factors
      1. Physical environment
      2. Technologic possessions and use
   D. Experiential factors
      1. Significant abrupt changes
      2. Sensorimotor stimulation and exploration
II. Factors primarily affecting the internal speech and language processing component
   A. Given biological makeup
   B. Structural defects and growths
   C. Nutrition
   D. Diseases, infections, and allergies
   E. Physical traumas and accidents
   F. Drugs and irradiation
   G. Psychological-emotional mechanisms

Within each component we attempted to "factor analyze" causal factors cited in the literature, looking for the commonalities among factors that could be grouped and meaningfully related to the speech and language environment and internal processing. From this "factor analysis" we developed major scanning categories for causal factors; although not mutually exclusive, redundancy among the categories was kept to a minimum. These are superordinate categories that can be subdivided into increasingly more specific factors. Using this scanning mechanism the diagnostician can search for factors known and unknown that have adversely affected his client's speech and language environment, internal physical processing system, and the interactions among the factors and components needed to explain the speech and language disorder.

The following discussion is designed to demonstrate the use of the scanning mechanism by the diagnostician, not as an exhaustive discussion of causal factors. Our intent is to provide an organizational schema for later use in analysis and interpretation of cause-effect relationships.

Factors primarily affecting the speech and language environment

To begin this discussion a word of caution is important. Little is known about how speech and language environment factors act as "causes" of speech and language disorders. What is known comes mostly from analyses of environmental variables that have been correlated with the speech and language product of children at various ages and stages of development. Therefore we suggest when the diagnostician considers causal factors primarily affecting the speech and language environment component that he study these factors emphasizing their correlational aspect rather than their causal aspect.

Speech and language environment factors are considered as extrinsic to the individual and are viewed in the SLPM primarily in terms of their effect on the quality and quantity of speech and language input (Fig. 4-1). To some degree an individual may create part of his own speech and language input through external feedback, for example, when an infant's babbling acts as a stimulus to continued babbling or when a child engages in a dialogue with himself, being both listener and speaker. For the most part, however, the speech and language environment is largely established by others, imposed on an individual by someone or something in his environment.

The preceding outline presents the major categories in the scanning mechanism for environmental causal factors. These categories are necessarily interdependent; for example, sociocultural influences are primarily executed through interpersonal relationships. Similarly, experiential factors are largely provided by the interpersonal and physical-technologic influences. As well, physical-technologic factors are often concomitants of sociocultural factors. The reader should review the material presented in Chapters 3 and 4 that discussed the speech and language environment component of the SLPM.

Interpersonal factors. Interpersonal factors are probably the most important influences on speech and language input. Here the concern is directed toward the *parents and parenting*—their psychological and physical characteristics, attitudes, behaviors, and child-rearing practices. Consideration of *sibling relations* is also included in interpersonal factors, including such influences as numerical birth order, multiple births, and sex of siblings. Finally, the diagnostician will want to consider *other significant interpersonal relationships* that the individual has such as with a spouse, a caretaker other than the parent, teachers, and extended family members.

In 1956 Beasley hypothesized certain relationships between parental attitudes and the development of speech disorders. At that time little experimental evidence was available to support many of her contentions. Is there any evidence now that gives credence to her hypotheses? (See Ling and Ling, 1974; Marge, 1965; Rebelsky and Hanks, 1971; Yarrow et al., 1973.)

Sociocultural factors. The sociocultural factors may function through individual interpersonal relationships, notably the family, or as the result of more general ethnic and cultural influences. Such immediate factors as the *income* and *economic status* and the *educational-occupational status* of an individual and his family may contribute to the amount and kind of speech and language used in the environment. Similarly, *racial and ethnic practices* in terms of verbal behavior and value attached to speech and language differ.

Socioeconomic status has frequently been implicated as a causal factor for speech and language disorders. It seems that this term is being supplanted by terms such as cultural disadvantage, economic disadvantage, and social-racial class differences. How have the following sources treated this causal factor? (See Gerber and Hertel, 1969; Raph, 1967; Shriner and Miner, 1968; Zigler et al., 1973.)

Physical-technologic factors. Probably the most "concrete" set of factors affecting the multisensory context of the speech and language environment are those relating to the physical-technologic environment. How an individual is influenced by the *physical environment* may aid or abet appropriate speech and language development. The physical characteristics of the immediate environment may include such factors as available space, cleanliness, and diversity. *Technologic possessions* and *use* relate to industrial and mechanical means of expanding and altering the immediate environment such as televisions, radios, and cars. While these technologic possessions may change the immediate environment, the changes are not necessarily in the direction of providing appropriate speech and language experiences.

What information can you discover that relates the effect of heavy television viewing on a child's speech and language development? Consider both the child and his parents as heavy viewers, that is, 5 to 7 hours a day.

Experiential factors. The final category, experiential factors, may have an effect on speech and language input and/or internal processing because of their effect on the multisensory environmental context. Included within the experiential factors are *significant abrupt changes* (hospitalization, deaths, divorces, etc.) and *sensorimotor stimulation* and *exploration*. While these experiences occur as well within the interpersonal context, the importance of these experiences for speech and language development and use is highlighted in our scanning mechanism by considering them independently. These factors affect the individual's interpersonal and multisensory environmental contexts, thereby influencing speech and language input and experiences.

Recall that we suggested that environmental factors be analyzed in terms of their effects on the parameters of speech and language input. After the diagnostician has identified any potential causal factors, he must explain how the factor exerted its influence on the quantity and quality of the input, which parameters have been affected, and how this might account for the observed speech and language disorder.

For example, twinning may present a situation where the primary companionship is each other. Each child's predominant phonologic and syntactic input may come from one another rather than from more mature older siblings or parents. However, these twins may be given adequate opportunity for sensorimotor stimulation and exploration that contributes to their semantic development. Thus twinning as a "causal factor" may differentially affect the speech and language input parameters, not necessarily reducing input "across the board." In another example set of twins there may be other siblings or playmates close to their age, providing them with normal speech and language input on all levels. Therefore a particular factor identified (in this example, twinning) does not have an automatic influence on the speech and language input. Instead, the influence depends on the particular multidimensional enviornmental context created.

The following is only a partial list from many "environmental" factors that have been cited as having an influence on speech and language development and use. Place these factors into our scanning mechanism for factors primarily affecting the speech and language environment component. Search the literature for support and details on these factors. What others might you add? Literature from child

growth and development is particularly helpful here.

Absence of father	Number of siblings
Amount of social contact	Overprotection
Bilingualism	Parental age
Birth order	Parental aspirations
Child-rearing practices	Parental attitudes
Divorce	Parental rejection
Economic deprivation	Parental standards
Educational background	Peer influence
Emotional deprivation	Personality disorders
Ethnic background	Poor family constellation
Hospitalization	Poor speech models
Improper teaching methods	Racial group
	Religious conflict
Institutionalization	Sensory deprivation
Lack of reinforcement	Severe discipline
Lack of stimulation	Sibling conflict
Mixed cultural expectations	Siblings talk for child
	"Silent" environment
Multiple births	Social class
New birth in family	Socioeconomic status

Factors primarily affecting internal speech and language processing

Many causal factors can disrupt the biological basis for language. These factors, directly or indirectly, affect the internal physical processing system for language. For example, direct damage to the left cerebral cortex can have a direct effect on the client's ability to comprehend and formulate language. However, a disease such as diabetes may be more indirect. The illness may be so physiologically debilitating that many biological systems of the body are affected, including the speech and language processing system.

When the diagnostician analyzes and interprets causal factors affecting physical processing, he will have to know if and how the factor affected one or more of the three segments of the internal processing component. Was it a direct effect, or did the causal factor affect another bodily system, which then exerted an affect on speech and language processing? Therefore the diagnostician must have specific knowledge about the physical basis for speech and language as well as more general knowledge about human biological systems. The reader should review Chapters

3 and 5, which discuss the internal speech and language processing component of the SLPM.

The outline on p. 124 presents the scanning mechanism for classifying the major categories of causal factors affecting the physical basis for speech and language. Again, as with environmental factors, the categories are interdependent. For example, a child born with a cleft lip and palate has a structural defect as a part of his given biological makeup. Although a specific causal factor may be placed into more than one category in the scanning mechanism, we believe that by the use of these categories the diagnostician will not overlook significant causal factors affecting internal processing.

Given biological makeup. An individual is born with, and continues to have, a basic biological makeup. This biological makeup consists of a number of bodily systems that constitute the individual's anatomy and physiology. There are many ways these bodily systems can be organized; for example, they can be divided into motor systems, skeletal systems, neurologic systems, vascular systems, etc., depending on the professional specialty viewing the individual. The internal speech and language processing component of the SLPM is our organizational view of the bodily system of most importance to the diagnostician of speech and language disorders. Of course, this system incorporates many of the same structures that make up other bodily systems, for example, the neurologic system. Therefore, when viewing given biological makeup as a potential causal factor for speech and language disorders, the diagnostician may have to consider the effects of disruptions in any bodily system on the internal speech and language processing system.

The causal factor, given biological makeup, is viewed as that anatomy and physiology present at the time of birth. The basis of this category is the belief that all individuals have an inherited (innate) set of anatomic and physiologic characteristics—some good, some unfortunate—that are his given biological makeup. As well, this category includes those conditions that occurred during gestation and conditions that occurred because of the birth process. Thus this category has potential overlap with all other categories of our scanning mechanism, particularly the factors of structural defects and growths and physical traumas and accidents. This overlap of categories, for example, categorizing cleft lip and palate as both a given biological makeup factor and as a structural defect factor, maintains focus both on the condition and the time of occurrence.

Within this category the diagnostician would be concerned with all the normal and abnormal structural and functional (physiologic) conditions of the client that may affect the client's ability to develop and use speech and language. The given biological makeup factor helps the diagnostician maintain an important perspective on biological conditions he sees; a perspective that says all these conditions are not necessarily "abnormal." For example, mental retardation is generally interpreted as "abnormal." Remember, however, that mental retardation is a definition based primarily on an IQ score. Given that mental abilities are presumably variations from a mean and range of mental abilities, we should expect in our general population a certain number of individuals who biologically fall below the range of the defined "normal IQ." These individuals then would have a given biological makeup that becomes defined as mental retardation—usually for educational purposes because these children cannot respond to the same methods of teaching as "normal" or "bright" children. However, are they "abnormal?" It may be more appropriate to consider them as having the potential to learn within their given biological makeup. If they are acquiring speech and language within their ability levels, then children defined as mentally retarded do not constitute children with speech and language disorders; mental retardation in these instances would not be an abnormal biological causal factor.

There are other instances where variations in structure and function are viewed in the same way, for example, dental variations, physical development, tongue size and shape, palatal dimensions, and diadochokinesis of the oral structures; all of these and many others can be examined in light of the causal factor, given biological makeup. This view helps diagnosticians determine if the condition has a relationship to the speech and language disorder, if the client has compensated or can compensate for the variation, or whether other types of management may be required.

Structural defects and growths. The individual may incur a structural defect or growth. He may be born with a congenital malformation such as a cleft palate or congenital atresia or he may acquire structural alterations later in life, as occurs with a laryngectomy, vocal nodules, or removal of brain tissue. Depending on which segment of the internal processing system is affected, the diagnostician will expect different processing disruptions with resultant disorders of the behavioral correlates and the speech and language products.

Nutrition. During the course of development the biological individual will be influenced by the quantity and quality of the food intake both pre- and postnatally.

Diseases, infections, and allergies. The biological individual may be invaded by virus, bacteria, and allergies that interfere with development and ongoing functioning. These diseases could be contracted via the mother during pregnancy or during the course of the individual's life.

Physical traumas and accidents. The individual may experience physical traumas or accidents that disrupt functioning. These traumas or accidents may be created by external agents as in birth injuries and skull fractures or occur as abrupt internal disruptions as in a cerebrovascular accident.

Drugs and irradiation. The individual may ingest drugs or be exposed to excessive radiation, which may have an adverse effect on biological structure and functioning.

Psychological-emotional mechanisms. Finally, the individual's intrinsic psychological and emotional mechanisms also influence his internal processing of speech and language. Included within the psychological-emotional mechanism category of causal factors are intrinsic processes that are often thought of as more behavioral than biological. Psychological mechanisms such as attention, motivation, and memory affect the individual's ability to process speech and language. Similarly, emotional factors such as emotional lability and self-concept influence how an individual will receive and create language. We are placing psychological-emotional mechanisms into factors primarily affecting internal processing since we view these mechanisms as a part of the individual's makeup, even though these mechanisms may be disrupted by factors extrinsic to him, that is, environmental causal factors.

Again, we present another partial list of many factors that have been cited as having an influence on speech and language development and usage. Place these factors into our scanning mechanism for factors primarily affecting the internal speech and language processing component of the SLPM. Search the literature for support and details on these factors. What others might you add?

Agenesis of brain structures	Circulatory disease
Alcoholism	Cleft lip and palate
Aneurysms	Contact ulcers
Athetosis	Diseases
Atresia of ear	Drugs
Autism	Encephalitis
Blood clots	Endocrine disorder
Brain injury	Forceps delivery
Breech birth	High arched palate
Cancer of larynx	Huntington's chorea
Car accidents	Hyperactivity
Carbon monoxide poisoning	Intracranial hemorrhage
Cerebral palsy	Malocclusion
Cerebral thrombosis	Maternal anoxia
Cerebrovascular accident	Maternal rubella
	Meningitis
	Mental retardation
	Metabolic disorder

Minimal brain damage	Sensorineural hearing
Multiple sclerosis	loss
Neoplasms	Short lingual frenum
Otitis media	Skull fracture
Parkinson's disease	Syphilis
Paralysis	Thyroid deficiency
Placenta previa	Tongue thrust
Precipitous birth	Treacher-Collins
Prenatal injury	syndrome
Radiation	Tumors
Reverse breathing	Uterine trauma
Rh incompatibility	Vitamin deficiency
Schizophrenia	

Conclusions

Diagnosticians must have knowledge of the potential causes of speech and language disorders as a first step in discovering and interpreting cause-effect relationships. The viewpoint they develop should emphasize how the factor was responsible for the speech and language disorder rather than on the causal factor (etiology) in and of itself. In this view the diagnostician searches his client's history for factors that may have influenced the learning and use of speech and language rather than searching the history for an etiology. When he is trying to answer cause-effect questions, the diagnostician can use the SLPM scanning mechanism for causal factors to determine how the factors uncovered may have primarily affected the speech and language environment and/or primarily affected the internal speech and language processing system.

The use of this SLPM-based scanning mechanism for causal factors has several distinct advantages.

1. The causal factors are not considered as specific etiologic categories. They are superordinate categories and serve as a search mechanism for any number of specific causal factors that could affect the speech and language environment and/or the internal speech and language processing system. Therefore the categories are flexible and open-ended.
2. The emphasis of the scanning mechanism is on what is affected rather

than on the causal factor. Therefore the diagnostician is not impelled to learn long lists of etiologic factors. Instead, he searches for any factors or determinants that may help explain the speech and language disorder. The focus is on the interaction of causal factors with the components of the SLPM.

3. The traditional functional-organic dichotomy is de-emphasized. Even though the scanning mechanism is built around environmental and internal processing factors, the intent is to discover the interactions of causal factors. Our subsequent discussion will point out how factors that primarily affect speech and language input may in turn affect the internal processing system and vice versa.
4. The scanning mechanism provides a useful and flexible aid for the diagnostician for hypothesizing, analyzing, and interpreting dynamic cause-effect relationships rather than proposing static etiologies for speech and language disorders. It should force the diagnostician to consider a wide range of potential causal factors, thus reducing the myopia of each diagnostician's causal biases.

How do Perkins' (1977) chapters on disabilities of speech relate to our scanning mechanism for classifying causal factors?

SLPM SCHEMA FOR INTERPRETING CAUSE-EFFECT RELATIONSHIPS

As a first step in interpreting cause-effect relationships we have developed a consistent schema based on the SLPM that allows the diagnostician:

1. To classify speech and language disorders on three levels
2. To scan the range of potential causal factors that may affect the client's speech and language environment and/or his internal processing system

In this section we will develop the SLPM schema for assisting the diagnostician in his interpretation of these complex cause-effect relationships.

Basis of cause-effect schema: complex, dynamic interactions

It is vital to client management that the diagnostician appreciate and understand the range and complexity of cause-effect interactions. Rather than search for a cause of each specific disorder he sees, the diagnostician must shift his concern to the interaction of causal factors with the speech and language learner and user. He needs to explain how the causal factors and determinants interacted to produce the disorder that he is currently seeing. Most speech and language disorders are not direct cause-effect relationships; by the time the diagnostician sees the client, multiple factors must be accounted for. The diagnostician needs a perspective that addresses questions such as, How did this disorder come to be? What went wrong? When did it happen? How long did it last? How severe was it? Was anything done about it? What's going on now?

One of the major stumbling blocks to developing mutual professional understanding of cause-effect relationships is the diverse levels of abstraction used to predict and explain causality. For example, different diagnosticians all noting Trisha's inability to produce speech sounds requiring the use of the tongue might ascribe the following causes: she cannot move her tongue; her tongue muscles are not functioning properly; her genioglossus and styloglossus muscles are impaired in their functioning; she has paralysis of tongue musculature. All of these causal explanations refer to the same behavior, Trisha's lack of tongue movements to produce sounds. What may be noted here is that the observer's level of information and point of view can influence the way in which he abstracts.

Perkins and Curlee (1969) have discussed levels of abstraction. They note that no one level of abstraction is necessarily any more "correct" than another; the preference for a level of abstraction should be determined by its relevance to the stated questions. They suggest that for speech pathology the behavioral level may be most appropriate since the questions asked in diagnosis of speech and language disorders are too complex to be answered at any other level of abstraction. We would agree with Perkins and Curlee (1969) that the behavioral level may be very appropriate in many instances; however, it is not the only level that will explain satisfactorily all the complex cause-effect relationships seen in speech and language disorders. More complex views of cause-effect relationships that go beyond the behavioral level of abstraction are needed by the diagnostician. What is important is that the diagnostician be able to explain the cause-effect relationships he develops, including the level of abstraction he chose for explaining causality.

Cause-effect relationships: SLPM perspectives

The diagnostician must develop perspectives that allow him to interpret the complexities of the cause-effect interactions—perspectives emphasizing that:

1. Cause-effect relationships are multidimensional, complex, and dynamic, not static and unidimensional
2. Contemporary disorders seen are a reflection of all that has come before

To do this the SLPM schema for interpreting cause-effect relationships develops three major perspectives, as represented in Fig. 8-1. They are the causal factor perspective, directness perspective, and timing perspective. Using this diagram the diagnostician can maintain a focus on the multidimensional interactions that occur over time.

Causal factor perspective

Earlier in our discussion of causal factors we developed a scanning mechanism that classified causal factors as (1) primarily affecting the speech and language environ-

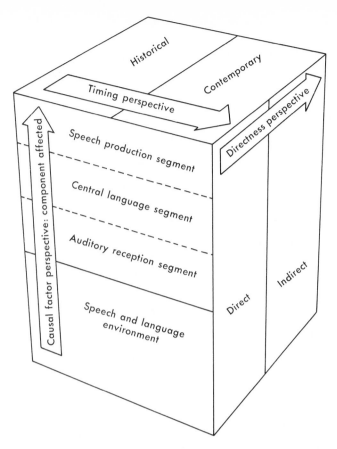

Fig. 8-1. Three-dimensional schema for causal factors of speech and language disorders. Causal factors are plotted according to time, directness, and component affected by causal factor.

ment and (2) primarily affecting the internal speech and language processing system. This scanning mechanism is the first dimension of our causal factor perspective. Now we will expand our perspective to consider two other important dimensions, the multiple nature of causation and the chains of cause-effect interactions.

Multiple nature of causation. We in the speech and language disorder field have a problem common to other behavioral sciences, that of attempting to explain complex behavior with simple answers. What frequently results is a search for the cause of a speech and language disorder rather than undertaking the more complex task of recognizing multiple causation and interactions. Much of the thrust behind "dif-

ferential diagnosis," as so often used in speech pathology, emanated from or resulted in this search for *the* cause (Adler, 1964; Myklebust, 1954).

While multiple causation is discussed frequently, it seems to be given little more than lip service. After accepting the idea of the complexity of causation in speech and language disorders on an idealized level, the diagnostician then proceeds to look for *the* cause. Like the blind men describing the elephant, he reports his partial experience as if it is the total picture (Kessler, 1971).

Perhaps it has been easier to look for a specific cause of a speech and language disorder than it has been to look for the multiplicity of factors that may account for the sequelae of behavior that truly confront us. For example, knowing that Jack was born with a cleft palate may be directly relatable to his resonance and phonetic structure disorder; but does it account for all of his speech and language abilities? There may be other factors in Jack's history that have to be considered in a multiple causation hypothesis. In children born with cleft palates the literature cites other factors as potentially causal, some of which have more clinical and research support than others. In Jack's case we would want to consider hearing loss (Hayes, 1965), dental and occlusal deviations (Starr, 1971), hospitalization (Nation, 1970), and other psychosocial factors (Goodstein, 1968). Besides these primary causal considerations, the diagnostician would also consider other experiences Jack has encountered, many which may have nothing to do with the fact that he was born with a cleft palate. For instance, Jack resides within a certain family constellation and a certain sociocultural setting, all of which contribute to the speech and language input he receives. These multiple causal factors and their interactions account for the differences diagnosticians see among clients defined as the same "problem type," in this example, cleft palate.

It is only from attempting to identify the multiple-sided nature of causation that diagnosticians can obtain fuller understanding of the presented disorder, leading to more effective remedial plans. Thus in his consideration of cause-effect relationships the diagnostician should be searching for causes, not *the* cause. As Kessler (1966) has stated:

> . . . all behavior, whether normal or abnormal is overdetermined; no single act can be explained in terms of one determinant or one variable. . . . Diagnostic formulations are likely to be in paragraph form, rather than in single terms, describing both the strengths and the problems of the child and postulating the major contributing factors, usually several in number.[*]

---

[*]From Kessler, J. W., *Psychopathology of Childhood.* Englewood Cliffs, N.J.: Prentice-Hall, Inc., 87 (1966).

■ Analyze this client from a multiple causation view. Fred was born after a prolonged labor; he weighed 8 pounds and 14 ounces. Bruises were apparent on his head, and he was slow to begin breathing. At 6 months of age a medical diagnosis of cerebral palsy was made. Now, at 6 years of age, he speaks in unintelligible "one-word" responses and seems to comprehend little of what is said to him. His hearing has been tested; he responded at 500, 1,000, and 2,000 Hz at 50 dB HL. His IQ score obtained from the Cattell (1969) was 50.

Chains of cause-effect interactions. Probably a dimension most apparent within the complexity of causation is that one cause causes a second cause, which causes yet another cause, etc. Causal factors are frequently seen as a part of a chain, or series, of cause-effect relationships.

We often see confusion in placing a causal factor within its relative position in a series of cause-effect relationships. As Kessler (1971) has pointed out, the behavioral outcome does not always reveal which cause came first. Diagnosticians sometimes find themselves tracking down a chain of original causation. For example, the cause for Philip's inability to elevate his tongue may be muscular paralysis; the cause for the paralysis may have been fetal anoxia; the cause of fetal anoxia may have been maternal toxemia; the cause of maternal toxemia may have been poor nutritional health of the mother; the mother's poor nutritional health may have been caused by an inadequate income; etc.

In such a chain of cause-effect relationships it may not be possible, practical, or useful to arrive at the ultimate causation. The diagnostician's concern is in recognizing the relationships among all these causes, some currently operating and some of only historical significance. Which causes, in such a series of cause-effect relationships, are of importance to the diagnostician? Can we ever truly arrive at the ultimate causation, and even if we do, what difference does it make? These are issues that the diagnostician must face in searching out the complexities of chains of cause-effect interactions.

■ What might the series, or chain, of cause-effect interactions be in the following client? Darrell, 3 years of age, has virtually no comprehension or formulation of language. His only output is an occasional use of jargon sound sequences seldom used in a communication situation. His history reveals an alcoholic, syphilitic mother (both conditions present during her pregnancy with Darrell). When he was born, Darrell was jaundiced and required an immediate blood transfusion. He remained hospitalized for over 2 months; on several occasions he almost died. He was removed from his home at 1 year of age because of parental neglect. At that time he weighed only 16 pounds. He is now in a state institution for the retarded. When he was admitted, the diagnosis was profound mental retardation.

Directness perspective

Any given causal factor may have both *direct* and *indirect* effects on speech and language learning and use. Consider, for example, the causal factor of Down's syndrome or other genetic factors known to cause significant mental retardation. While the mental retardation accompanying Down's syndrome may be seen to be directly responsible for much of the language delay presented, this same causal factor, Down's syndrome, may also account for other less direct influences on a child's language. For example, a parent's inability to accept such a child may result in limited verbal interaction between the parent and child. The child may be provided with little opportunity for sensorimotor exploration and learning in his environment. Thus the causal factor of Down's syndrome may both directly contribute to reduced language learning and also indirectly influence the amount of speech and language input provided.

In another example the causal factor of chronic otitis media would directly affect the auditory reception segment of the internal speech and language processing component, affecting the physical process of auditory acceptance-transduction and the behavioral correlate of sensation. This direct disruption, if severe enough, could also result in significant perception, com-prehension, and formulation difficulties by limiting the auditory information needed by other physical processes. Thus otitis media as a disease has a direct, primary effect in the reception segment as well as indirectly affecting other segments of the processing system. Still another indirect effect of the disease could be on the speech and language input provided by the mother. If the child is not responsive to auditory stimulation, the mother might unconsciously reduce the amount of talking she does to the child, completely unaware that she has done so.

Similarly, causal factors more directly affecting the amount and type of speech and language input may have an indirect effect on the internal processing system. An extreme example is seen in the reported cases of the so-called feral children (Lenneberg, 1967) who, after several years of living with wolves and presumably being exposed to no speech and language stimulation, were unable to learn to talk beyond a very basic level. Here the absence of speech and language input apparently led to an inability to process speech and language at a later age. A less extreme example of a similar effect is the reported results on speech and language development of children living in institutions (Brodbeck and Irwin, 1946; Goldfarb, 1945-1946; Mussen et al., 1969).

Thus mere specification of a causal factor does not ensure the directness or potency of its effect on the individual. The point here is that a particular causal factor does not always have a known, invariant effect on an individual. Rather, in one instance a factor may be direct *or* indirect in its effect, while in another instance it may be *both* direct and indirect.

■ Consider this client from a direct-indirect causal view. Robert, 5 years old, has a significant phonologic disorder. He primarily uses vowel sounds, although the phonemes /p, b, t, and d/ are heard with some frequency. His history reveals mildly slow physical development, visual acuity that borders on legal blindness that was not discovered until he was 2 years of age, and a bilingual background—his parents speak English, but his grandparents who live with the family generally speak German. After his visual problem was discovered, his mother seldom left him alone; she became quite anxious and fearful of what might happen to him.

Timing perspective

The variable effect of time is a major perspective through which causal factors must be interpreted. It is one thing to propose a direct cause-effect relationship that specifies what causal factor might have resulted in the onset of a speech and language disorder. A question of greater priority is how the disorder developed. A speech and language disorder does not come into existence and develop in a unidimensional manner. From the time of onset to the time of diagnosis, many influences have come to bear on the client's speech and language behavior.

Diagnosticians need to view causal factors in terms of when they happened, how severe they were, how long they persisted, and what has been done about them. Timing considerations are our way of maintaining a "developmental viewpoint" about speech and language disorders. What is seen when a client appears is a result of interactions over time. Some of these interactions have been positive, for example, the mother who might increase her verbal stimulation to a child who is retarded. Others are negative influences, for example, the mother who rejects her child who has a cleft lip and palate, thus spending little time with him.

Some exceptions to this point could be raised. Certain disorders seem more direct and unidimensional, for example, the adult who sustains brain injury resulting in a language disorder (aphasia). This language disorder is a direct concomitant of a causal factor—brain damage. However, by the time the diagnostician sees this client for diagnosis and therapy he is no longer seeing a direct effect. True, the basic language disorder is because of the brain damage, but by now there will be other dimensions to consider regarding the aphasic's language usage. The spouse may reject the aphasic and not provide speech and language interaction. The client may be so depressed that he withdraws and refuses to communicate. These are some of the potential concomitants that may be seen; again, they make the diagnostician's causal interpretation of the client's disorder multidimensional rather than unidimensional. Thus, even when the cause-effect relationship seems direct, the diagnostician must always remember that timing considerations can affect the speech and language disorder he eventually sees.

Basic to our timing perspective is a time continuum, ranging from the distant past to contemporary events, a concept presented in Chapter 1 and expanded in Chapter 4. From this time continuum we discuss causal factors as historical causation and contemporary causation. Viewing causation as historical or contemporary allows us to interpret causation in two important senses: causation as historical events that have affected speech and language and causation as seen in current input and processing deviations.

Historical causation. Historical causation refers to any past events that have affected either the speech and language environment component or the internal speech and language processing component, and it essentially demonstrates the interactions between causal factors and the components of the SLPM over time.

Plotting causal factors from a timing perspective forces the diagnostician to consider the *time of occurrence* of any causal factor. For example, maternal rubella in the first trimester produces a more generalized and devastating effect on the central nervous system of the embryo than in later pregnancy. A moderate sensorineural hearing loss acquired at 8 years of age will not have the same effect on speech and language that it would if acquired at 11 months of age. Similarly, the addition of a new sibling may characteristically create feelings for a 2 year old that are not experienced by an 8 year old.

Plotting historical causal factors from a

timing perspective also allows the diagnostician to examine causal interactions over time, highlighting multiple causation, chains of cause-effect interactions, and direct-indirect effects of causal factors.

For example, while a child may have been born with a cleft lip and palate, his structural and psychological condition at 5 years of age is quite different. At birth the child may have a cleft palate (biological makeup–structural defect) that "causes" repeated middle ear infections (diseases) as well as repeated hospitalizations (experiential restrictions) during the early language-learning years. Not only has he probably had numerous surgical and therapeutic procedures but also time to develop an attitude about himself and his condition (psychological-emotional mechanisms). Therefore in considering causal variables diagnosticians are concerned not

only with occurrences that clearly are past history such as pre-, para-, and postnatal factors but also occurrences that, while part of the client's history, may continue. For example, chronic medical conditions, emotional instability, and many other dimensions of the client's life-style may be ongoing influences.

To visually represent these historical interactions we suggest that the student plot scattergrams of causal factors as shown on Fig. 8-2. The causal factor, the SLPM component, and time should be represented. From this the details of the interactions can be interpreted.

Contemporary causation. Contemporary causation in our timing perspective is concerned with the client in the here and now. As well as knowing and understanding historical causation we also want a clear

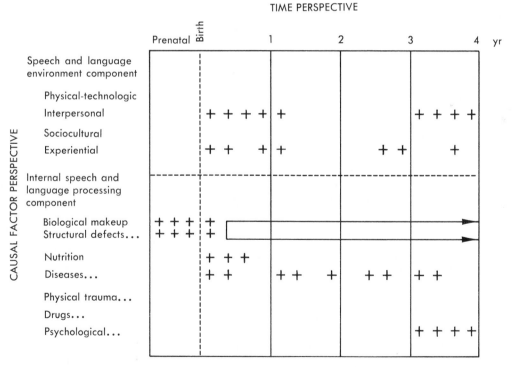

Fig. 8-2. Plotting causal factors of hypothetical client. Client: Celeste, 4 years of age, was born with bilateral cleft of primary and secondary palates. A study of speech and language disorders of children with cleft lip and palate will assist you in interpreting this figure. + = An adverse condition suggested as being present within a 3-month time period.

understanding of the client's current status. In addressing contemporary causation the diagnostician searches for the presently existing input and processing deviations that may account for the observed speech and language disorder. The presumption, of course, is that contemporary causation may have its basis in historical causation. For example, a client's current hearing loss, disrupting physical processing, may well have been present for some time.

Contemporary causation emphasizes disrupted physical processes and behavioral correlates as causal factors, which may explain the disordered product. For example, a disruption in speech programming (physical process) or sequencing (behavioral correlate) could be cited as the contemporary causation for a child's phonologic disorder. Or paralysis of the tongue (historical and contemporary cause) prevents the articulation process (physical process as a contemporary cause) from taking place and is observed in poor motor control (behavioral correlate as a contemporary cause). This poor motor control results in many phonetic structure errors (speech product disorder). Thus poor motor control, a behavioral correlate, can be cited as the contemporary cause of the phonetic structure disorder.

We could even go so far as to say that a child's comprehension and formulation problems (behavioral correlates) are the contemporary causes for his language product disorder. In some ways this is a departure from frequent diagnostic practice. Sensation, perception, sequencing, and motor control (behavioral correlates on the SLPM) are cited often as causes for speech and language disorders; however, seldom would comprehension or formulation be considered as causes, contemporary or otherwise. We do not really advocate the use of comprehension as a cause but do want to make the point that current processing deficits measured as behavioral correlates can be profitably considered as contemporary causation.

Distinguishing contemporary causation in our timing perspective is vital to the diagnostician for the following reasons.

1. It more closely ties what is going on currently with the speech and language disorder.
2. The speech and language disorder cannot be accounted for just on the basis of historical causation.
3. At times, even though historical causation has been relevant for understanding the speech and language disorder, it is no longer particularly relevant for management.
4. Contemporary causation may be available for change, whereas historical causation may not.

■ Bertheva, 5 years of age, has a moderate sensorineural hearing loss present since she was 3 years of age. Develop a summary cause-effect statement from our historical-contemporary time perspective.

Viewing causation for speech and language disorders from the causal factor, directness, and timing perspectives gives diagnosticians a more complete picture of the complex, dynamic basis for cause-effect relationships. The diagnostician will arrive at much better solutions to his diagnostic problems by taking this complex route through causation than by using lists of causal factors or etiologic classification systems as his means of explaining how a speech and language disorder came to be. In something as complex as speech and language behavior diagnosticians cannot expect to arrive at a static, stable picture of causation. Instead, they must appreciate the complexities of interactions that take place over time.

How do Johnson et al. (1963) consider history data of causal significance? Do they offer ways of interpretation for speech and language disorders?

Impact of causal factors on speech and language behavior

Now that we have presented the various perspectives of our causal schema for speech and language disorders we want to demonstrate generally the impact that causal factors can have on speech and language processing and behavior. Through our examples we intend to illustrate the complex, dynamic interactions that go on to create a speech and language disorder. Our purpose is to provide a means for analysis and interpretation of the cause-effect relationships of importance to the diagnostician, not to discuss specific causal factors that have been cited as causes of speech and language disorders.

Fig. 8-3 represents a set of basic interactions that can exist between causal factors and components of the SLPM. From this figure the diagnostician can draw any number of example cause-effect relationships. The timing perspective in Fig. 8-3 is represented simply by a two-directional

arrow; its purpose is to focus the diagnostician's attention on the fact that these multidimensional causal interactions are always occurring over time.

Interaction number 1 states that there is an adverse causal factor affecting the speech and language environment component that can result in a speech and language disorder. For example, a child exposed for the major portion of his time to parents who are deaf (interpersonal factor) may receive little oral language input stimulation. The child's speech and language product will most likely be reduced, dependent on how much stimulation he has received from other significant relationships in his speech and language environment (interpersonal factor). Thus in this interaction the characteristics of the speech and language product reflect the

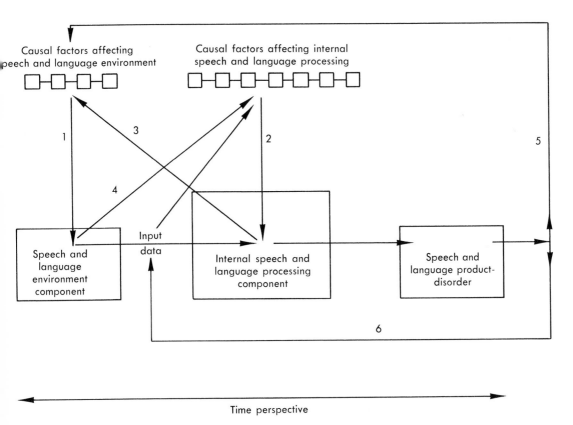

Fig. 8-3. Schematic of basic causal interactions.

quantity and quality of the speech and language input stimulation.

How would you interpret black dialect as an example of interaction number 1? First, you would have to take a position on dialectal divergence from a sociocultural interpretation. (See Baratz, 1969; Fasold and Wolfram, 1970; Houston, 1970; Shuy, 1972.)

Interaction number 2 states that there is an adverse causal factor affecting internal processing that can result in a speech and language disorder. For example, an adult who sustains brain injury (physical trauma and accident factor) to the central language segment may present a language disorder termed aphasia. The specific characteristics of his language disorder will be related to the location and severity of the brain injury. Thus in interaction number 2 the speech and language disorder is reflective of the disrupted physical processes and behavioral correlates within the segments of the internal processing component of the SLPM. A second example could be of a child born with damage to the cerebellum (given biological makeup and structural defect factors). In a direct relationship, speech characteristics reflective of disruptions in the speech production segment might be seen—disruptions of the physical process of speech coordination-transmission and the behavioral correlates of sequencing and motor control. (Of course in children born with such conditions entire chains of cause-effect interactions are likely to be seen.)

Whenever causal factors that affect the internal processing component are considered by the diagnostician, he is concerned with the effects the disrupted system has on the client's ability to derive information from input stimulation and his ability to formulate and produce messages. In management considerations the diagnostician will want to know if he can alter the way in which the client processes the speech and language data to effect better speech and language behavior (contemporary causation viewpoint).

Which of the segments of the internal speech and language processing component do you think each of the following specific causal factors may affect most directly? What physical processes and behavioral correlates would be affected?

Bell's palsy	Hypertrophied adenoids
Cerebral arteriosclerosis	Myasthenia gravis
Cerebral hemorrhage	Occlusion of middle
Cholesteatoma	cerebral artery
Conductive hearing loss	Sensorineural hearing
Contact ulcers	loss
Deviated nasal septum	Submucous cleft palate

Would you interpret these causal factors as a direct cause of a specific speech and language disorder?

Interaction number 3 states that there is an adverse causal factor affecting the internal processing component that in turn creates an adverse factor affecting the speech and language environment component, resulting in a speech and language disorder. For example, a child may be born with significant mental retardation (given biological makeup factor). The mother is unable to accept the retardation (interpersonal factor) and provides the child with little speech and language stimulation (interpersonal factor) and little opportunity to explore and learn from his environment (experiential factor). As a result, his speech and language behavior is disordered, that is, not commensurate with his mental abilities. This example also provides an illustration of multiple causation and chains of cause-effect relationships over time.

Interaction number 4 states that there is an adverse causal factor affecting the speech and language environment component that in turn creates an adverse factor affecting the internal processing component, resulting in a speech and language disorder. For example, a mother who is mentally retarded (interpersonal factor) may not know how to care for her child. As a result, in his early life he is not fed properly (nutrition factor), which affects his ability to process speech and language information, resulting in a speech and language disorder. Another example that may not fit some people's interpretation as an adverse environmental causal factor could be the instance of the abusive parent (interpersonal factor) who beats her child and causes brain injury (physical trauma factor). This brain injury results in internal processing deficits that are seen as a speech and language disorder.

What does Birch (1971) say can result from inadequate nutrition? How strong of a case does Lewin (1975) make for malnutrition as a potential cause for speech and language disorders?

Interaction number 5 states that the speech and language output product (whether normal or disordered) creates an adverse factor affecting the speech and language environment component, resulting in a speech and language disorder. For example, a child may be mentally retarded and yet developing speech and language within his abilities (normal speech and language product), but his parents cannot accept the level of development (interpersonal factor) and begin to put excessive demands (interpersonal factor) on the child for "better" speech and language. As a result, the child withdraws (psychological-emotional mechanism factor) from interpersonal communication, using less speech and language than before. In this example we reintroduced interaction number 4 to complete the series of cause-effect relationships.

Interaction number 6 states that the speech and language output product (whether normal or disordered) serves as input data to the speaker creating an adverse factor affecting the internal processing component, resulting in a speech and language disorder. For example, an adult male coach has a normally high pitch (normal speech output product) but does not like the way it sounds; it does not fit his self-image (psychological-emotional mechanism factor). In order to project a "masculine image" he lowers his pitch (disordered speech product), which results

in contact ulcers on the vocal folds (physical trauma factor), resulting in a more pervasive voice disorder.

These are the six basic interactions demonstrated in Fig. 8-3. Any number of other interactions can be illustrated by following the arrows in the directions indicated as many times as needed to explain the multiple, serial, direct-indirect interactions that may have occurred in the development of the speech and language disorder. All six of the basic interactions or any combination of the six over time could apply to a client being seen for diagnosis. For example, a child born with a cleft lip and palate (given biological makeup and structural defect factors) will encounter other causal factors as a result of this condition and its treatment. During his early life he may have had difficulty feeding (nutrition factor). He will certainly undergo surgery (experiential and physical trauma factors), perhaps require orthodontia (physical trauma factor), may have a number of x-ray studies done (irradiation factor), undoubtedly sustain middle ear infections (disease factor), and be treated for them (physical trauma and drugs factor). Later in life he may be seen for speech and language diagnosis and treatment (interpersonal factors). All these factors in interaction would seem to be enough to result in a speech and language disorder even though many of them are rehabilitation procedures utilized to prevent such a disorder. However, with this child the diagnostician may also see a mother who is rejecting, guilty, and overprotective (interpersonal factor), who does not stimulate the child verbally (interpersonal factor), who will not let him out of her sight (experiential factor), and who does not have the income to care for the child properly (sociocultural and physical-technologic factors). At the same time the father blames the mother for the birth of this child (interpersonal factor), begins to drink excessively (interpersonal factor), abuses both the mother and child (interpersonal and psychological-emotional mechanism factors), and finally leaves the home for parts unknown (interpersonal

Table 8. Cause-effect relationships as viewed from the SLPM

Causal factor	Component part affected (can be considered from all aspects)	Normal functions	Resulting disruptions		
			Processes		Products
			Physical	Behavioral correlates	
Cerebrovascular accident	Central language segment	Processes speech and language data for comprehension and formulation; turns auditory data into symbolic, representational form; turns representational data into speech data; overall process of language representation	May affect auditory programming, language representation, and speech programming	Could affect perception, comprehension, formulation, repetition, and sequencing	Could affect language product on all linguistic levels; could be no language behavior, or what occurs could be use of stereotyped sounds, words, and phrases; what would be observed depends on site and extent of damage to central language segment
Institutionalization in a nonstimulating environment	Speech and language stimulation	Provides child with input data on all linguistic levels from which he derives language code of his language community	May not affect physical processes and behavioral correlates directly but will not have information to process; processes ultimately affected if deprivation prolonged over critical periods of time during learning of speech and language		Reduced amount of language output; probable that speech product not too involved; that is, phonetic structure, voice, and prosody might be appropriate; language on all linguistic levels affected in terms of quantity and sophistication for age of child; again, depends on degree of deprivation
Cerebrovascular accident: occlusion of prerolandic branch of middle cerebral artery	Central language segment: Broca's area	Involved in behavioral correlate of formulation; turns auditory pattern of language received into motor pattern of language by physical process of speech programming; programs series of muscular activities needed in carrying out speech production	Speech programming affected	Formulation and sequencing	Spontaneous speech nonfluent and lacking some syntax, many phonologic errors; difficulty in transition from one sound to another; in severe form not able to initiate speech
Damage to recurrent laryngeal nerve during thyroidectomy resulting in unilateral recurrent nerve paralysis; adductors and abductors both affected	Speech production segment: vocal folds	Vocal folds vibrate to produce vocal tone	Speech production: phonation	Motor control	Voice hoarse and breathy; may begin to sound better over time (depending on compensation by unaffected vocal fold)

and experiential factors). The child may have a severe reaction to his own disordered speech (disordered speech product) and develop feelings of insecurity, anxiety, and worthlessness (psychological-emotional mechanisms) and then give up trying to make his speech sound any better. This example would seem to take into account all the basic causal interactions and then some.

It is now suggested that the student work with and develop Table 8 to gain still greater insight into specific causal factors that can disrupt components of the SLPM, resulting in speech and language disorders. On the table we have provided several minimal, nondetailed examples to demonstrate the use of the table as a way of abstracting essential information about cause-effect relationships. The student should develop the table as a continuing project, adding, deleting, and reinterpreting as he gains more and more sophistication about cause-effect relationships in speech and language disorders. The student should consider all the material and pursue the references presented thus far in this book as a beginning source of pertinent material available in our literature. The table then can serve as a ready reference for reviewing potential cause-effect relationships the diagnostician may see.

SUMMARY

Chapter 8 has focused on developing consistent schemata based on the SLPM for the diagnostician's use in classifying, discovering, and interpreting cause-effect relationships. The three schemata developed were as follows:

1. *Schema for classifying speech and language disorders at three levels*
   a. Speech and language product disorders
   b. Behavioral correlate disorders
   c. Physical processing disorders

   These three levels of classification work together and are particularly useful for specifying contemporary cause-effect relationships.

2. *Schema for classifying causal factors emphasizing a scanning mechanism for isolating causal factors*
   a. Causal factors primarily affecting the speech and language environment component

b. Causal factors primarily affecting the internal speech and language processing component

   Again, this classification schema assists the diagnostician in discovering and interpreting cause-effect relationships, being particularly useful for viewing historical causation.

3. *Schema for interpreting dynamic, complex, multidimensional cause-effect relationships, emphasizing three perspectives*
   a. Causal factor perspective considering the preceding scanning mechanism, multiple nature of causation, and chains of cause-effect interactions
   b. Directness perspective considering the many direct and indirect effects of causal factors
   c. Timing perspective emphasizing the historical and contemporary nature of causation, incorporating the other two perspectives

Thus Chapter 8 focuses on an integrative view of cause-effect relationships as essential study for the diagnostician rather than a static unidimensional study of speech and language disorders and their causes.

REFERENCES

Adler, S., *The Non-verbal Child.* Springfield, Ill.: Charles C Thomas, Publisher (1964).

Baratz, J. C., Language in the economically disadvantaged child: A perspective. *Asha,* **11,** 143-145 (1969).

Beasley, J., Relationship of parental attitudes to development of speech problems. *J. Speech Hearing Dis.,* **21,** 317-321 (1956).

Birch, H. G., Functional effects of fetal malnutrition. *Hosp. Prac.,* **6,** 134-148 (1971).

Brodbeck, A. J., and Irwin, O. C., The speech behavior of infants without families. *Child Develpm.,* **17,** 145-156 (1946).

Brutten, G. J., and Shoemaker, D. J., *The Modification of Stuttering.* Englewood Cliffs, N.J.: Prentice-Hall, Inc. (1967).

Cattell, P., *Cattell Infant Intelligence Scale.* New York: The Psychological Corporation (1969).

Darley, F. L., Aronson, A. E., and Brown, J. R., Differential diagnostic patterns of dysarthria. *J. Speech Hearing Res.,* **12,** 246-269 (1969a).

Darley, F. L., Aronson, A. E., and Brown, J. R., Clusters of deviant speech dimensions in the dysarthrias. *J. Speech Hearing Res.,* **12,** 462-496 (1969b).

Darley, F. L., Aronson, A. E., Brown, J. R., *Motor Speech Disorders.* Philadelphia: W. B. Saunders Co. (1975).

Fasold, R. W., and Wolfram, W., Some linguistic features of Negro dialect. In R. W. Fasold and R. W. Shuy (Eds.), *Teaching Standard English in the Inner City.* Washington, D.C.: Center for Applied Linguistics (1970).

Gerber, S. E., and Hertel, C. G., Language deficiency of disadvantaged children. *J. Speech Hearing Res.,* **12,** 270-280 (1969).

Goldfarb, W., Effects of psychological deprivation in infancy and subsequent stimulation. *Am. J. Psychiat.,* **102,** 18-33 (1945-1946).

Goodstein, L. D., Psychosocial aspects of cleft palate. In D. C. Spriestersbach and D. Sherman (Eds.), *Cleft Palate and Communication.* New York: Academic Press, Inc. (1968).

Hayes, C. S., Audiological problems associated with cleft palate. *Asha Monogr.,* **1,** 83-90 (1965).

Houston, S. H., A re-examination of some assumptions about the language of the disadvantaged child. *Child Develpm.,* **41,** 947-963 (1970).

Johnson, W., Darley, F. L., and Spriestersbach, D. C., *Diagnostic Methods in Speech Pathology.* New York: Harper & Row, Publishers (1963).

Kessler, J. W., *Psychopathology of Childhood.* Englewood Cliffs, N.J.: Prentice-Hall, Inc. (1966).

Kessler, J. W., Nosology in child psychopathology. In H. E. Rie (Ed.), *Perspectives in Child Psychopathology.* Chicago: Aldine Publishing Co. (1971).

Korzybski, A., *Selections from Science and Sanity.* Lakeville, Conn.: Institute of General Semantics (1948).

Lenneberg, E. H., *Biological Foundations of Language.* New York: John Wiley & Sons, Inc. (1967).

Leonard, L. B., What is deviant language? *J. Speech Hearing Dis.,* **37,** 427-446 (1972).

Lewin, R., Starved brains. *Psychology Today,* **9,** No. 4, 29-33 (1975).

Ling, D., and Ling, A. H., Communication development in the first three years of life. *J. Speech Hearing Res.,* **17,** 146-159 (1974).

Marge, M., The influence of selected home background variables on the development of oral communication skill in children. *J. Speech Hearing Res.,* **8,** 291-312 (1965).

Miller, J. F., and Yoder, D. E., A syntax teaching program. In J. E. McLean, D. E. Yoder, and R. L. Schiefelbusch (Eds.), *Language Intervention with the Retarded: Developing Strategies.* Baltimore: University Park Press (1972).

Mussen, P. H., Conger, J. J., and Kagan, J., *Child Development and Personality.* (3rd ed.) New York: Harper & Row, Publishers (1969).

Mykelbust, H., *Auditory Disorders in Children.* New York: Grune & Stratton, Inc. (1954).

Nation, J. E., Determinants of vocabulary development of preschool cleft palate children. *Cleft Palate J.,* **7,** 645-651 (1970).

Perkins, W. H., *Speech Pathology: An Applied Behavioral Science.* (2nd ed.) St. Louis: The C. V. Mosby Co. (1977).

Perkins, W. H., and Curlee, R. F., Causality in speech pathology. *J. Speech Hearing Dis.,* **34,** 231-238 (1969).

Raph, J. B., Language and speech deficits in culturally disadvantaged children: Implications for the speech clinician. *J. Speech Hearing Dis.,* **32,** 203-214 (1967).

Rebelsky, F., and Hanks, C., Fathers' verbal interaction with infants in the first three months of life. *Child Develpm.,* **42,** 63-68 (1971).

Reiber, R. W., and Brubaker, R. S., *Speech Pathology.* Philadelphia: J. B. Lippincott Co. (1966).

Sarno, M. T., Silverman, M. G., and Sands, E. S., Speech therapy and language recovery in severe aphasia. *J. Speech Hearing Res.,* **13,** 607-623 (1970).

Shriner, T. H., and Miner, L., Morphological structures in the language of disadvantaged and advantaged children. *J. Speech Hearing Res.,* **11,** 605-610 (1968).

Shuy, R. W., Language problems of disadvantaged children. In J. V. Irwin and M. Marge (Eds.), *Principles of Childhood Language Disabilities.* Englewood Cliffs, N.J.: Prentice-Hall, Inc. (1972).

Starr, D. C., Dental and occlusal hazards to normal speech production. In W. C. Grabb, S. W. Rosenstein, and K. R. Bzoch (Eds.), *Cleft Lip and Palate: Surgical, Dental, and Speech Aspects.* Boston: Little, Brown & Co. (1971).

Yarrow, L. J., Rubenstein, J. L., Pedersen, F. A., and Jankowski, J. J., Dimensions of early stimulation and their differential effects on infant development. Reprinted in S. Chess and A. Thomas (Eds.), *Annual Progress in Child Psychiatry and Child Development.* New York: Brunner/Mazel, Inc. (1973).

Zigler, E., Abelson, W. D., and Seitz, V., Motivational factors in the performance of economically disadvantaged children on the Peabody Picture Vocabulary Test. *Child Develpm.,* **44,** 294-303 (1973).

B.C.   **By John Hart**

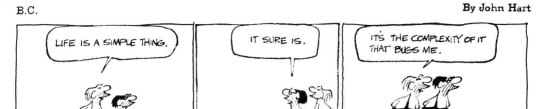

Fig. 9-2. In life, what is the canon of parsimony? (By permission of John Hart and Field Enterprises, Inc.)

The application of these steps in a rigorous fashion allows the scientist to identify, organize, control, and predict the occurrences in his field of study. The state of knowledge in any given area of study may vary; however, the method of science remains constant.

The scientist *first confronts a problem;* that is, he isolates and defines the limits of the problem. He can only confront his problems by having a firm grasp of the subject matter of his discipline—its facts and theories. It is from his fund of knowledge, interest, and curiosity about his discipline that questions arise, forming the basis of scientific intuition.

From the questions he asks about his subject matter, the scientist next *formulates hypotheses for study.* His hypotheses may be developed to verify, predict, discover, confirm, control, etc.

The scientist then *designs some type of investigation to study his hypotheses,* be it a survey, an experimental study, or a case history analysis. The intent of the scientist's design is to collect data in some systematic, objective way that will help him to determine the "truth" of his hypothesis; that is, *he collects data that are pertinent to the hypothesis* under test. To do this the scientist must have knowledge about the methodologies of importance to him, what they will and will not do and how to apply these methodologies to collect his data. While collecting his data, the scientist focuses on systematic observation.

He must know what variables exist or interact with his observations, which then affect the results obtained. He must be concerned about the accuracy, reliability, and validity of the measurements he has taken. Only by knowing what has affected his measurements will he be able to analyze and interpret his data.

The scientist goes on to *order, analyze, and interpret the data* in relationship to the hypothesis. He is interested in determining the existence, strength, and direction of the relationship he is studying. Interpretation of the information collected in relationship to the hypothesis formulated is a "tricky" part of the method of science. Here the scientist is dependent on the funds of knowledge available to him, his interpretations and understandings of that knowledge. In a sense the interpretation-generalization step of the method of science becomes one of the most subjective steps. The scientist must adhere to the facts he has obtained and still discover how these facts may be related to the body of knowledge in his discipline, a task that is never free from pitfalls and ambiguity. Given the same facts, different scientists may interpret them differently. Smith's (1970) canon of parsimony appropriately applies at this difficult step. This canon basically states that given two theories, each having equal predictive power, it is best to use the theory that makes the fewest assumptions; that is, "least is best if it does as well." However, in the behavioral sciences there is often confusion over what is simple and what is complex (Fig. 9-2).

From his analysis and interpretations the scientist finally *draws conclusions, generalizing those conclusions* to the problem area and adding, deleting, or changing the facts and theories in his field of study as warranted by the findings.

This series of steps, which define the method of science, can be applied to "thinking through" a problem in a logical way or can be applied in an experimental sense, that is, through the development of a research study. It is not a method exclusive to the researcher dealing with "hard data," rather it is a method that has as its basis the systematic, logical application of the thinking process of man.

What do human beings do in order to solve problems and make decisions? See the interesting approach to this question developed by Lindsay and Norman (1972).

APPROPRIATENESS FOR DIAGNOSIS

Diagnosis of speech and language disorders is a problem-solving skill; therefore the steps of the method of science should be appropriate to this clinical process. The diagnostician is a clinical scientist; he is attempting to predict and understand the cause-effect relationships of his client's problem in order to change the future state of the client. In our view the diagnostician of speech and language disorders does fulfill Brown and Ghiselli's (1955) concepts of a scientist.

He who rigorously applies the scientific method is a scientist. . . . The scientist acts as a probe; his task is to prod nature into displaying her workings. His search, then, must be an active one. He is not a mere passive recorder, registering successions of sensory impressions as events occur before him, but he busies himself in devising all manner of procedures, gadgets, and techniques by means of which he can push into the greater vistas that lie beyond the scope of superficial observation.[*]

---

[*]From Brown, C. W., and Ghiselli, E. E., *Scientific Method in Psychology*. New York: McGraw-Hill Book Co., 10 (1955).

Using the method of science requires the diagnostician to be rigorous in his approach to diagnosis, following a logical, orderly process of decision making. If the method of science organizes the diagnostician's thoughts and knowledge, is rigorous, systematic, and demands planning; is efficient and economical; gives control and precision; reduces error and bias; and allows for more appropriate prediction, then its appropriateness to the problem-solving skill of diagnosis becomes self-evident.

Using the method of science also has the advantage of helping the diagnostician realize what he knows and what he needs to learn. Information in our profession is continually changing and growing. Realizing that he may never know all he needs to know for the solution of his daily professional problems, the diagnostician applies his present knowledge with the intention of testing and increasing this knowledge. He engages in a continual search for information that allows him to better carry out his professional responsibilities. Thus in addition to providing a logical guide to diagnosis, using the method of science enables the diagnostician to augment his knowledge. Therefore the method of science is not just simply *appropriate for the diagnostician;* it is *highly significant* for his development as a professional problem solver.

Perkins (1977) provides a good source of information for an orientation to the scientific method as it relates to speech pathology. McDonald (1964) was among the first of speech pathologists to present the steps of the scientific method for use by the clinician.

Diagnostician-researcher: alike or different?

A tendency to dichotomize the researcher and the clinician has occurred in our profession, as if there were absolute distinguishing characteristics that separated these professionals into two distinct groups. "Hard data," quantification and science, were supposedly the researcher's way of life; whereas "soft data," subjectivity and art, were the clinician's way of life.

As pointed out by Ringel (1972), the clinician-researcher dichotomy may be quite artificial. In his article, along with editorial comments by Shriberg and Prather (Ringel, 1972), important parallels were drawn between the clinician and the researcher. A crucial point, of course, is that nothing precludes one from being the other. There are many examples of people in our profession who are successful at both research and clinical work. Once we view the researcher and the clinician as behavioral scientists, the dichotomy may disintegrate. Both, in fact, may be scientists and artists.

Palmer (1970) has developed the method of science as an approach to the psychological assessment of children. See his discussion of the scientist-clinician.

General characteristics

A professional in the field of speech pathology, whether a researcher or a diagnostician, must bring to his field of study a genuine interest and motivation to understand the subject matter and its conceptual context. In order to understand the field of study, both must be broadly trained in human behavior with special and specific consideration for the normal human communication process and its disorders.

In the previous chapters of this book we have discussed the funds of knowledge and conceptual frameworks needed by the diagnostician; we feel that the researcher in speech pathology needs similar background and training. There are bound to be variances in the emphasis and extent of training, depending on interests and work speciality; however, the broad-based knowledge of the communication sciences and speech and language disorders is needed by both. Each, through his experiences in conjunction with his reasoning abilities, develops sophistication in his special approach to the study of speech and language disorders.

Again, Schultz's (1972) work regarding the clinician as an "information processor–decision maker" is relevant.

The diagnostician and the researcher must have intellectual flexibility, the ability to use inductive and deductive reasoning in a logical way. They must be motivated to solve problems, to have the desire and curiosity to want to know, and to expand their areas of expertise. Both must develop what might be called *scientific intuition,* that is, the ability to relate information and experiences in a meaningful way. This all comes about from the training they receive both in the academic world and in the world of practice.

A common purpose

The common purpose that is shared between researchers and diagnosticians in the field of speech and language disorders should ultimately be the same: *to provide solutions for the speech and language disorders that confront human beings.*

The diagnostician is specifically interested in each client's disorder: its symptoms, causes, and management. The diagnostician hopes to use the information he obtains on a single client to generalize to other clients with similar problems. Each client tells the diagnostician more about the nature of disorders, what they are, how they are caused, and how they affect the human being who has them. These data then add to his skill and effectiveness as a diagnostician.

The researcher's interest lies more with the state of knowledge in his field: what the facts, hypotheses, and theories are that form the basis of his profession. He conducts research studies on "subjects" (representative samples); his focus is more on the knowledge gained than on the subject. By studying the effects of several treatment approaches on a representative group of subjects, he is able to generalize his data to a larger population. Each study contributes to the overall theories that help to form the information base in speech and language disorders. At one level the researcher may be trying to identify the characteristic behavior presented by individuals with language disorders, a cataloging study; at another level he may be trying to discover the causes of the language disorders, cataloging and establishing relationships; at still another level he may develop a predictive study, given cause A he would expect language behavior A to be present.

Read Moll's (1975) presidential address to the American Speech and Hearing Association. Do you agree or disagree with the common goal he sets forth for the professions of speech pathology and audiology?

In experimental research there has been much emphasis on the size of the number (N) needed in a sample to allow for appropriate generalizations. However, there is a movement in the medical and behavioral sciences toward accepting as experimental research the in-depth study of an individual or a few individuals. In many instances the in-depth study of several individuals, in the long run, may teach us more about speech and language disorders than a superficial study of large, controlled samples of subjects. Sometimes in large studies the attempt to control so many of the human variables may, in fact, obscure the results that could be of most importance.

The diagnostician studies an individual; however, that does not mean he does not generalize and apply the knowledge he has gained from past clients who were similar to the client he is currently seeing nor to clients he will see. The diagnostician is involved in "research" with an N of 1, the single individual with all his variability from other individuals. Thus the diagnostician can study his clients in great depth. In this way he can contribute to the researcher by feeding him information about the variables of importance in speech and language disorders. The diagnostician is

dealing with human beings with all their foibles rather than with a set of characteristics that must be controlled.

The skills of both the researcher and the diagnostician are embedded in the application of the method of science. Using these skills to provide solutions to speech and language disorders is the essential parallel between the researcher and the diagnostician.

As professionals, each has much to share and much to say to the other; the day-to-day observations and problems of the diagnostician become the day-to-day problems of the researcher. The findings of the researcher in turn become applications by the diagnostician. For example, a diagnostician may be confronted by a client with hypernasality with no readily apparent cause. However, the facial configuration of the client leads the diagnostician to hypothesize deviant nasal-oral cavities. He can provide the researcher with his observations and questions. The researcher can then consider a series of investigations regarding the relationship between nasal-oral cavities and hypernasality. The researcher may first conduct a normative anatomic study; second, he may conduct a study of individuals with known abnormalities of the oral-nasal passageways; then, he may devise analogue studies varying the components of the analogue to determine what degree of change would lead to hypernasality. This accumulation of data by the researcher, which stem from a clinical problem, then serves the common purpose of both the researcher and the clinician: to solve the speech and language problems presented by specific clients.

See Sidman (1960) for more advanced reading about methodologic problems in scientific research. He presents many concepts that are appropriate to diagnosticians who are interested in controlling the situations under which they work.

While we have tried to develop the viewpoint that diagnosticians and researchers have many commonalities, particularly their overall purpose in studying speech and language disorders, we do not intend to overemphasize or insist that the two professionals are entirely alike. We, like Schultz (1972), feel there are essential differences in their orientation, this orientation being reflected in the professional tasks they undertake. The diagnostician solves the individual's problem; the researcher gathers data from larger groups of people from which he makes generalizations regarding the larger population of speech and language disorders.

Unfortunately, we are frequently at different points in the continuum of concern. The diagnostician must do something about a problem that may not have been sufficiently explored by experimentation, so he works "in the dark." At the same time the researcher, who may have little involvement or interaction with clinical workers, may not be aware of important clinical questions and thereby may not be doing research of most significance to the clinician. This is not by way of saying that a researcher must always care about the immediate concerns of the diagnostician. There is a need for basic scientific information about speech and language disorders, information that may at one point seem to have no relevance to clinical work. However, there are interactions that should exist between the researcher and the diagnostician engaged in solving the problems of the person with a speech and language disorder.

The reader who is interested in pursuing some of the arguments and positions regarding the researcher and the clinician can consider the following from journals of the American Speech and Hearing Association: Hambre (1972), Ringel (1972), Schultz et al. (1972), "Viewpoint" (1963), and "Viewpoint" (1964).

Diagnostician-researcher: steps of the scientific method

We have discussed our view that the researcher and diagnostician have many commonalities. Our conclusion is that the diagnostician should be considered a clinical scientist—no contradiction in terms. The researcher and diagnostician of speech and language disorders have a common purpose: to understand, solve, and prevent the occurrence of speech and language disorders. They each go about their jobs using the method of science.

We would like to further the comparison-contrast by presenting in chart form the roles played by the diagnostician and the researcher at each step of the scientific process.

The *seven steps of the scientific method* presented in the chart on p. 150 are a distillation from a number of ways they have been expressed. The exact number of steps of the process varies in the texts and articles discussing the scientific method, but the order and intent of the steps remain similar and delineate the constancy of the method. The seven steps are as follows:

1. Definition and delimitation of the problem area: understanding the subject matter
2. Development of hypotheses to be tested
3. Development of procedures for testing the hypotheses: research design
4. Collection of the data
5. Analysis of the data
6. Interpretation of the data: support or reject the hypotheses
7. Generalizing from the data: conclusions

Compare the steps of the method as presented by Brown and Ghiselli (1955), Smith (1970), and Williams (1968).

The comparison-contrast chart provided will only summarize in outline form the essential considerations of the researcher's role at each of the steps. Notations, primarily in question form, will be presented in the columns for the diagnostician. Our intent here is to have the student think through and reflect on the purposes of diagnosis and the role the diagnostician

Text continued on p. 154.

Researcher	Diagnostician

Step I: Definition and delimitation of the problem area: understanding the subject matter

Fund of knowledge
    Broad general background in field of study
    Comprehensive and integrated knowledge of the facts and theories in his area of expertise: conceptual frameworks
        Identification
        Organization
        Classification
        Principles
        Generalizations

Diagnostician column:
What is our problem?
What are we diagnosing?
What fund of knowledge do we need as diagnosticians?
How do we acquire the knowledge we need to do diagnoses?
How may this knowledge be organized by the diagnostician?
How much does theory rule our jobs as diagnosticians?
Since the diagnostician is confronted with so many different speech and language disorders, do you think he needs a broader base of knowledge than the researcher?

Command of information
    Specific knowledge in the problem area
    Ability to selectively recall relevant information
    Reasoning abilities
        Relationship among events
        Scientific intuition and inquiry
        Develops questions about his problem area
    Ability to use language to convey information

Diagnostician column:
How does the diagnostician use his general fund of knowledge for the purpose of diagnosing an individual client?

- The theories from which the researcher operates must have predictive power. The researcher who is developing hypotheses from theoretical constructs is concerned about how well the theory will predict the behaviors he may be studying. Faulty theory leads to faulty hypotheses, which lead to faulty experimentation; the results obtained may have no value.

References: Brown and Ghiselli (1955), Chapter 7; Smith (1970), Chapters 2 to 6.

References: Previous chapters in this book; Perkins (1977), Chapters 3 to 14.

Step II: Development of hypotheses to be tested

- From his definition and delimitation of the problem areas the researcher formalizes his problem by stating it as a hypothesis.

Analysis of available information
    Facts
    Theories

Diagnostician column:
What are the purposes of diagnosis?

Conceptualizes relationships into a hypothesis
    Constituent analysis
    Strength of the relationships

Diagnostician column:
How can hypotheses be formulated by the diagnostician that fit the concept of the use of the hypothesis in research or in the use of the method of science?

States the hypothesis
    Often stated in null form—there is no relationship
    Stated to explain, predict, and control

Diagnostician column:
Are statements of hypotheses appropriate for studying the individual?
How do we state a clinical hypothesis?

Researcher	Diagnostician

Step II: Development of hypotheses to be tested—cont'd

States the hypothesis—cont'd

Stated to determine variables to be studied
Stated in terms of alternate hypotheses
Stated to keep experiment free of bias

How do our hypotheses relate to the problem presented by the client, by the referral source?
What relationships should be expressed in a clinical hypothesis?
Can clinical hypotheses be unbiased?
A researcher is generally free to study hypotheses of specific interest to him; hypotheses that are as narrowly defined as he feels warranted for predicting events in his field of knowledge. Does the diagnostician have this freedom?

References: Brown and Ghiselli (1955), Chapter 8; Smith (1970), Chapter 8.

References: Previous chapters in this book; Perkins (1977), Chapter 2.

Step III: Development of procedures for testing the hypotheses: research design

• The researcher designs and controls an empirical testing situation to estimate the degree and the reliability of the relationship expressed in the hypothesis. Research design becomes, as Perkins (1977) says, the "blueprint" of the study to be carried out. The research is only as good as the design. The design must fit the hypothesis that has been developed; the hypothesis frequently determines the methods that will be developed. The procedures must fit the problem.

Subjects
  Sampling
Methods
  Selection of testing procedures to test the hypothesis
    Criteria for selection
    Strengths and weaknesses
  Measuring instruments
    Precision
    Reliability
    Validity

What are the clinical tools needed by the diagnostician?
How are the tools of diagnosis selected for the purposes of diagnosis for the individual client?
How does the diagnostician evaluate the appropriateness of his tools?

Can the diagnostician exert control in his testing sessions by selection of his tools?
Do we have tools for diagnosis that meet the requirements for measuring instruments that are so important for research? Do we have to be concerned about precision, reliability, and validity?

Control
  Experimental and statistical design
    A researcher conducting an experimental study would be concerned about objectivity. If another person were to conduct the same experiment, his results, the data, should be the same. Objectivity allows for replication of the data.

Since the diagnostician does not know his client personally before the time of the diagnosis, how can he consider control over the variables that may be present?
How much time should be allotted for testing procedures?
Is there an order for presenting testing procedures in diagnosis? Are we concerned about the effect one procedure may have on another?

Continued.

Researcher	Diagnostician

Step III: Development of procedures for testing the hypotheses: research design—cont'd

Control—cont'd
  Variables
    Stimulus variables   Independent variables
    Response variables   Dependent variables
  Bias
    Something in the experiment that tends to give a consistently wrong result; often cannot eliminate, but must keep it as small as possible.
  Practical considerations

Reference: Brown and Ghiselli (1955), Chapter 9.	References: Previous chapters in this book; Perkins (1977), Chapter 2; Emerick and Hatten (1974), Chapter 3; Darley (1964), Chapters 2 to 6; Sanders (1972).

Step IV: Collection of the data

• The design of the research dictates the basis on which the data is collected. The subjects, methods, and control over the variables all enter into the actual collection of the data.

What are the clinical procedures of diagnosis?

Systematic observation
  Objective of research
    The objective of research, as recognized by all sciences, is to use observation as a basis for answering questions of interest.
  Formulation of questions
    One or more questions are formulated; systematic observation is then made of things believed to be relevant to the questions; whether the observations to be made in a given research problem are relevant to the questions they are supposed to answer must always be given serious consideration in the planning of the research. Do not haphazardly make observations of any and all kinds; attention is directed to those observations that answer the questions that have been formulated.
  Controlled presentation
    Controlled presentation of the measurement procedures selected.

Can the diagnostician control all the variables during the testing session? How does he account for variables that he cannot control?

What happens if the diagnostician is not able to use the procedures he initially selected? Does this invalidate the diagnosis?

Young children present significant testing problems? What can a diagnostician do during the testing session to assure that the data that is obtained is accurately recorded?

Can the diagnostician be as systematic in collecting the data needed for diagnosis as the researcher who has control over his experiment? Can the word systematic be interpreted in such a way as to apply to the diagnostic process?

Recording the observations
  Comprehensive and accurate recordings of the data are needed. Any biasing effects or researcher observational limitations are important to note.

How can the diagnostician observe and record verbal information objectively?

Reference: Brown and Ghiselli (1955), Chapter 9.	References: Emerick and Hatten (1974), Chapter 3; Sanders (1972); Palmer (1970), Chapters 10 and 11.

Researcher	Diagnostician

Step V: Analysis of the data

• The researcher organizes and analyzes his results in a way that allows him to interpret the results meaningfully. He organizes his results in relation to the hypothesis that is being studied.

Results

Descriptive statistics (e.g., means, standard deviations)

Having made a systematic series of observations, the observer then reduces these to a limited number of statistical measures that provide a summary description of the complete set.

Statistically significant

By means of further operations on the descriptive measures, the evaluation of the data is placed on an objective basis.

Predictive statistics

Predict what would be true of an entire group on the basis of your sample; make inference about people you have not studied. To use predictive statistics sample must be representative.

How is the information obtained ordered for analysis?

How does the diagnostician score the information?

How do we analyze the information obtained in the diagnostic process?

Do we have measures that are descriptive and predictive?

Can the results obtained in diagnosis be quantified?

Reference: Brown and Ghiselli (1955), Chapter 10.

Reference: Perkins (1977), Chapter 2.

Step VI: Interpretation of the data: support or reject the hypothesis

• The researcher orders his results in relationship to the hypothesis he is studying. He views them to see if his hypothesis is confirmed or denied. In doing this he must review all the results, those that are positively related to his hypothesis as well as those that may be negative to his study.

How does the diagnostician interpret the results obtained in the diagnosis?

Indicate nature and amount of relationship

Evaluate strength of agreement between results and original hypothesis

Results must be interpreted in terms of the effect that was measured; results must be looked on as an estimate, not the same as the true effect; it is an estimate of the true effect; estimates, then, have an element of error.

How can we know if our results are close to the true behaviors we set out to study?

When interpreting the findings of the diagnosis, do we rely only on the specific test findings?

How is the information organized in relationship to the hypothesis?

How is the information synthesized and summarized?

Reference: Brown and Ghiselli (1955), Chapter 10.

References: Previous chapters in this book; Perkins (1977), Chapters 11 to 14.

Continued.

Researcher	Diagnostician
Step VII: Generalizing from the data: conclusions	
The decision process 　Considers value of results 　Considers how results indicate solutions to the 　　problem 　　List of actions—applications 　　List of outcomes of actions *Considers how results relate to other unsolved problems* 　Implications for further research 　Modification of theories *Communication* 　Communicate information regarding findings 　Communicate implications of findings and 　　potential applications	How does the diagnostician interpret and com- municate the findings of the diagnosis? What applications to other clients can be made from the interpretations made on the client seen? Can this or should this be done? In what forms is the information from the diag- nosis communicated? Does diagnosis stop at this point? How does the diagnostician determine appro- priate management plans?
Reference: Brown and Ghiselli (1955), Chapter 11.	References: Previous chapters in this book; Emerick and Hatten (1974), Chapter 9; Johnson et al. (1963), Chapters 10 and 11; Palmer (1970), Chapter 17.

might perform at each of the steps in the method. We want the student to develop a scientific orientation to the clinical process by comparing diagnostic tasks to those of the researcher. The student can ask more clinical questions, adding comparative, contrastive information at each of the steps. By filling in the role of the diagnostician and the researcher at each of the steps, the student will be able to see how a diagnostician approaches clinical problems in a scientific manner.

Now that you have studied the relationships between the researcher and the diagnostician as reflected in the steps of the scientific method, write a short summary paper on your conclusions about the relationship. Have you found any exceptions, activities performed by the diagnostician that do not fit within the steps of the scientific method?

Application to diagnosis

In our view the method of science can be applied to the case of the individual client who presents a speech and language dis-order. Our client can be studied as if he constituted a "mini research project." Our study of the diagnostician's purposes and functions revealed that using the method of science adds certain advantages to his professional skills. The method forces diagnosticians to be rigorous, systematic, and organized. It helps to plan diagnoses more efficiently and economically, essential ingredients in the diagnostic process. Diagnosticians seldom have the luxury of doing diagnoses leisurely over long periods of time.

Through the appropriate application of the method of science, diagnosis should be more precise and more controlled, evidencing less bias and error, thereby allowing for more appropriate interpretations and predictions of behavior. The diagnostician can learn to sharpen his skills of observation and reasoning abilities by applying the scientific method. Greater sophistication and confidence should come as the method is applied, although at first, deliberate thought is needed until the method becomes the diagnostician's habitual way of thinking through the diagnostic problems he sees. From using the method he will be able to develop greater insights into the accuracy of his decisions. The more questions he asks about the conclusions he makes, the greater will his powers of observation become. His failures should be less frequent, since the method allows for correction of error. Hopefully, the constant use of the method of science in his diagnostic practice will prevent him from having unwarranted biases; therefore inappropriate recommendations for treatment and referral will be prevented.

The adaptation and application of the method of science should provide the diagnostician with an approach useful for all diagnostic problems he confronts. Rather than diagnostic procedures for voice problems, articulation problems, etc., he has an approach that is applicable to all disorders. The method of science should prevent the reliance on the "problem-type" diagnosis, which amounts to little more than a testing approach for a disorder rather than a diagnosis. As Darley (1964) states:

The clinician devoted to the methodology of science will come at each new patient afresh, bringing his most lively curiosity and careful critical analysis to bear upon the problem. He will not shackle himself to a previously developed conviction of what he will find nor be overly influenced by the connotations of whatever labels come already affixed.[*]

CONCLUSIONS

This chapter has developed our view that the method of science can be applied rather directly to the diagnostic process. The researcher and the diagnostician have many commonalities in purpose and approach to their jobs. We have drawn comparisons between the researcher and the diagnostician with the intent of demonstrating how the diagnostician can apply the method of science to the specific instance of the individual client; the client becomes his N of 1. The method of science gives the diagnos-

tician a systematic, orderly approach to diagnosis. His problem-solving and decision-making abilities are enhanced.

Besides serving as a guide for diagnosis of speech and language disorders, the method of science provides an approach for teaching and learning the diagnostic process. Part II of this book aims to teach the diagnostic process through an adaptation of the scientific method. Throughout the remainder of this book, we will use a case-method approach to demonstrate the diagnostic adaptation and application of the scientific method. Through this varied case approach, we hope to capitalize on the individual essence of diagnosis, while continuing to retain the overriding constancy and direction of the method of science.

REFERENCES

Brown, C. W., and Ghiselli, E. E., *Scientific Method in Psychology*. New York: McGraw-Hill Book Co. (1955).

Darley, F. L., *Diagnosis and Appraisal of Communication Disorders*. Englewood Cliffs, N.J.: Prentice-Hall, Inc. (1964).

Emerick, L. L., and Hatten, J. T. K., *Diagnosis and Evaluation in Speech Pathology*. Englewood Cliffs, N.J.: Prentice-Hall, Inc. (1974).

Hambre, C. E., Research and clinical practice: A unifying model. *Asha*, **14**, 542-545 (1972).

Johnson, W., Darley, F. L., and Spriestersbach, D. C., *Diagnostic Methods in Speech Pathology*. New York: Harper & Row, Publishers (1963).

Lindsay, P. H., and Norman, D. A., *Human Information Processing: An Introduction to Psychology*. New York: Academic Press, Inc. (1972).

McDonald, E., *Articulation Testing and Treatment: A Sensory-Motor Approach*. Pittsburgh: Stanwix House, Inc. (1964).

Moll, K. L., A focus on our common goal: Presidential address—1974 National Convention. *Asha*, **17**, 3-8 (1975).

Palmer, J. O., *The Psychological Assessment of Children*. New York: John Wiley & Sons, Inc. (1970).

Perkins, W. H., *Speech Pathology: An Applied Behavioral Science*. (2nd ed.) St. Louis: The C. V. Mosby Co. (1977).

Ringel, R. L., The clinician and the researcher: An artificial dichotomy. *Asha*, **14**, 351-353 (1972).

Sanders, L. J., *Procedure Guides for Evaluation of Speech and Language Disorders in Children*. (3rd ed.) Danville, Ill.: The Interstate Printers & Publishers, Inc. (1972).

Schultz, M. C., *An Analysis of Clinical Behavior in Speech and Hearing*. Englewood Cliffs, N.J.: Prentice-Hall, Inc. (1972).

---

[*]From Darley, F. L., *Diagnosis and Appraisal of Communication Disorders*. Englewood Cliffs, N.J.: Prentice-Hall, Inc., 10 (1964).

Schultz, M. C., Roberts, W. H., and Fairi, E., The clinician and the researcher: Comments. *Asha*, **14,** 539-541 (1972).

Sidman, M., *Tactics of Scientific Research: Evaluating Experimental Data in Psychology*. New York: Basic Books, Inc., Publishers (1960).

Smith, R. G., *Speech Communication: Theory and Models*. New York: Harper & Row, Publishers (1970).

Williams, F., *Reasoning With Statistics: Simplified Examples in Communications Research*. New York: Holt, Rinehart & Winston, Inc. (1968).

Viewpoint. *J. Speech Hearing Res.*, **6,** 109-110, 203-206, 301 (1963).

Viewpoint. *J. Speech Hearing Res.*, **7,** 3-6, 207-208 (1964).

Part II

APPLICATION OF
THE SCIENTIFIC METHOD

Chapter 10

The diagnostic process

The complete scope of the diagnostic process takes into account two major considerations. First, and of most importance, is the diagnostician's professional activity. Using his funds of knowledge, problem-solving skills, and client concern the diagnostician provides his clients with help for their specific speech and language problems. The second major consideration is the administrative support necessary for the diagnostician to efficiently and economically carry out his professional functions.

The diagnostician does not work in an administrative vacuum. Someone must attend to a range of administrative matters that ensure smooth scheduling, follow-up, and information flow into and out of the work setting. In some circumstances these administrative matters fall to the diagnostician and in some they do not. In any event, diagnosticians must know about and understand the administrative procedures of their work setting. Even when not directly responsible for administration, the diagnostician certainly influences and is influenced by the administrative personnel and practices in his job setting.

In this chapter we present an overview of this complete scope of the diagnostic process. First, we present the professional activity of the diagnostician as reflected in the steps of the method of science. Second, we present information about administration to develop an awareness and understanding of basic administrative procedures of importance to the diagnostician.

DIAGNOSIS: AN APPLICATION OF THE SCIENTIFIC METHOD

In Chapter 9 we concluded that the steps of the scientific method can be adapted and applied to each diagnosis. Following the method of science establishes a logical organization to diagnosis. At the same time it allows for flexibility in meeting the needs of any client in any setting. The scientific method can guide the diagnostic process and at the same time allow the diagnostician to exercise his individual professional decision-making abilities.

The diagnostic model

Fig. 10-1 presents our model for adapting the steps of the method of science to the diagnostic process. As in the method of science, our diagnostic model presents a series of steps that the diagnostician must systematically consider as he solves the clinical problems presented in each diagnosis. The seven steps of the diagnostic model are (1) definition and delimitation of the clinical problem: constituent analysis; (2) development of the clinical hypothesis: cause-effect relationships; (3) selection and development of the clinical tools: design of the diagnosis; (4) collection of the clinical data: systematic observations; (5) analysis of the clinical data; (6) interpretation of the clinical data: clinical evaluation; and (7) conclusions: management considerations, interpretive conference, and follow-up.

These seven steps outline and organize the primary functions the diagnostician

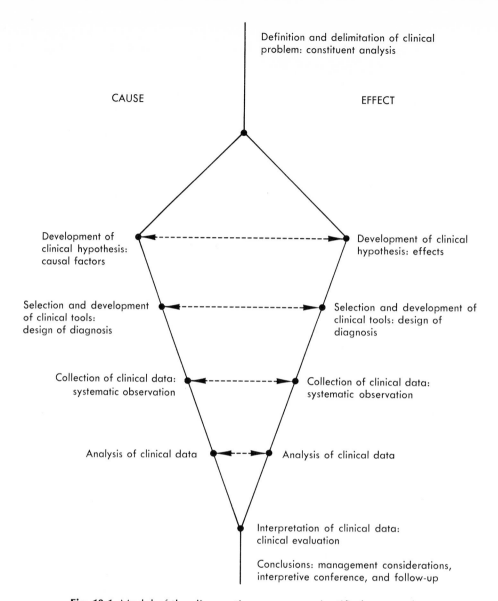

Fig. 10-1. Model of the diagnostic process: a scientific framework.

performs during a diagnosis. The steps are discrete in that at each step the diagnostician has certain specifiable tasks to perform. The steps, however, are also interactive and cyclic. What occurs at one step influences all others. This interaction is depicted in the model by a converging diamond-shaped figure, showing the cumulative convergence of all steps into conclusions, the tentative solution to the clinical problem.

In addition to outlining the major steps in diagnosis and showing their interaction, the model also illustrates that we can separate the diagnostic process into two major halves, one concerned with causal factors and the other with effects. Thus, if the diagnostician's primary concern for a certain client is about causal factors, he can proceed to follow the steps on the left-hand side under *cause,* somewhat independent of the *effects* on the right-hand side.

In other situations, for example, when the diagnostician knows the cause of the speech and language problem as in an adult with aphasia resulting from a cerebrovascular accident (CVA), he may want to concentrate his efforts on the effect steps. By allowing concentration on both cause and effect, or either one, the model shows how the diagnostic adaptation of the scientific method can be directed to the diagnostic needs of the specific client or referral request.

Definition and delimitation of the clinical problem: constituent analysis

The first step of the diagnostic process, definition and delimitation of the clinical problem, can be considered somewhat analogous to the literature review that precedes a research project. It is from studying the information available about a particular subject matter that a researcher develops questions he wishes to address. Similarly, in diagnosis it is from studying what is known about a client that the diagnostician develops his initial clinical questions.

The definition and delimitation process, the constituent analysis, is a thorough, systematic analysis of each bit of information (*constituent*) that has been made available about the client. The diagnostician's ability to perform this analysis is dependent on two primary sources of information.

1. The client information he has available to him from any source prior to actual client contact
2. His organized funds of knowledge about normal and disordered speech and language

At this first step of the diagnostic process, the diagnostician reviews the client information made available from a number of sources: the referral source, case history forms, and medical records among others.

The diagnostician then analyzes and interprets each of the constituents in light of his funds of knowledge to determine if they are relevant and important for asking appropriate clinical questions. It is on the basis of his constituent analysis that the diagnostician determines what his specific job will be with each client he sees.

The constituent analysis, then, integrates two important ingredients: what the diagnostician knows about the client and what the diagnostician knows about normal and disordered speech and language. This step readies the diagnostician for the remainder of the diagnostic process.

■ Analyze the following constituents. What are the relevant and important constituents? Robert is a 4-year-old child who was referred by his pediatrician against the wishes of his mother. She is bringing Robert only because she wants to prove the pediatrician wrong. Robert, as far as she is concerned, does not have the speech disorder the pediatrician hears. The pediatrician in his referral letter has stated, "This boy's speech is so difficult to understand that I believe something is significantly wrong with his speech development. The mother is against this referral but will follow through with the evaluation. We need to get this boy some help." What process will you go through to analyze the constituents? If you were able to obtain a history on this child prior to his appointment, what might you want to explore?

Development of the clinical hypothesis: cause-effect relationships

At the second step of the diagnostic process the diagnostician formulates a working clinical hypothesis expressing a cause-effect relationship.

Derived from the constituent analysis, the hypothesis is a statement of the *most likely* cause-effect relationships. Hypotheses can be stated with varying degrees of specificity and assurance, depending on the significance and validity of the constituents used for analysis. For example, from a neurologist's referral stating that James Burcham suffered a severe cerebrovascular accident affecting the left cerebral hemisphere, the diagnostician probably would be more assured that this causal factor contributed to the language disorder than a mother's report that "my neighbor thinks Bryon's tongue is lazy."

Although in diagnosis we are generally concerned with both causes and effects, we have noted (Fig. 10-1) that the diagnostic process can diverge into a causal (left side) or an effect (right side) emphasis. This divergence develops an important diagnostic perspective; that is, the diagnostician can pursue cause and effect either separately or simultaneously. If he wishes to view the problem in terms of the behaviors that are disordered, the model allows him to develop hypotheses regarding the behavioral (effect) disorders independent from concerns regarding causal factors. Or he may want to explore only causal factors through developing causal hypotheses.

Because of the incomplete state of knowledge regarding causal factors of speech and language disorders, diagnosticians must be cautious about making causal hypotheses. We therefore want to present the independence of cause and/or effect hypotheses while at the same time emphasizing their interdependence. The dotted lines and arrows on the model are our way of showing the interrelationships of cause and effect throughout the diagnostic process. The convergence of these two aspects throughout the remainder of the steps indicates that we are striving to bring together information about causal factors and observed speech and language disorders while at the same time continuing to demonstrate both the dependence and independence of some aspects of cause-effect relationships.

The cause-effect hypothesis, then, is the diagnostician's best statement or question about the causal factors and presented speech and language disorders of the clients he sees. While these hypotheses are initially formulated on the information available prior to client contact, they may be reformulated or revised as further information is made available throughout the complete diagnostic process. The hypothesis is the diagnostician's tentative solution to the client's problem.

■ What hypothesis would you derive for Robert? What support would you use to convince another professional that you have developed the most likely hypothesis? Does this hypothesis seem meaningful: "Robert has a severe voice disorder related to vocal abuse?" Why or why not?

Selection and development of clinical tools: design of the diagnosis

In the third step of the diagnostic process the diagnostician plans the diagnostic session in order to test his clinical hypothesis. He designs the diagnosis. He wants to gain information about the client's hypothesized speech and language disorder and its causes. The diagnostician in this phase selects and develops needed tools to fit his design, and he plans his testing strategy to optimize data collection.

In designing the diagnosis for a particular client, an overriding concern is the plan for systematically observing the client's behavior. In his planning for systematic observation, the diagnostician draws on the countless tools and procedures available. The interview is a major source of information. The diagnostician must decide what he wants to learn in the interview and how he is going to learn it. Besides the interview, the diagnostician may plan for unstructured situations in which to observe spontaneous behavior, develop his own testing protocols for eliciting desired behavior, or choose from the array of commercial or experimental tools available.

Whatever the specific tools selected, the diagnostician evaluates their usefulness to him for gathering information about the cause-effect relationships he has hypothesized. He must evaluate the importance of each tool he wants to use in relationship to all other tools and procedures considered. How important will the information gained from each tool be for understanding the clinical problem?

Also, in designing the diagnosis, the diagnostician must plan his testing strategy to optimize his data collection. For example, in the interview, how might he best frame his questions to gain the most complete and valid information? In testing, in what order will he present his procedures to best capitalize on his client's abilities and personal characteristics: which would be best to start with and end with? How does he plan to record his observations?

Just as well-executed research studies come from well-designed research plans, so also do successful diagnoses follow carefully conceived diagnostic plans.

■ With Robert what tools would you consider because he is 4 years old? Why would age be a consideration for selecting and developing clinical tools? What tools would you consider for the mother? If she is resistant to this referral, does that make a difference?

Collection of the clinical data: systematic observation

The fourth step of the diagnostic process starts the actual face-to-face contact with the client and his family. It is here that the diagnostician gains his interview information and administers the tools he has selected to test his clinical hypothesis. He collects his data by systematic observation.

A major concern in data collection is control over the stimuli, responses, and reinforcements. As well, the diagnostician is concerned with the appropriateness of the tools. Will he have to adapt the format of the tool to fit the client? Will he have to adapt the order in which he presents each of the procedures he has selected? He must also determine if all the procedures selected are needed.

The diagnostician has to understand that many adaptations of the tools and procedures will be made during the actual examination of the client. Even though he has carefully selected the procedures he wants to use and has a good understanding of the potential clinical problem, he still will have to adjust to the specific and actual behaviors of the client. No diagnostician's anticipatory design will ever come completely true. This flexibility is of major importance, especially when testing young children who do not always behave in a way that facilitates the diagnostician's testing and observations.

Besides his presentation of the tools selected, the diagnostician must be concerned with factors that are a major part of any interview and testing situation. He must be able to relate to each client, keeping in mind the various background experiences and needs that both he and his clients bring to the diagnostic situation.

The collection of clinical data step also includes recording of the data as it occurs. The diagnostician must capture the data in a form that he can analyze and reflect on at a later time. In effect, he needs some means of making permanent his evidence about his cause-effect hypothesis. Some test procedures provide scoring forms that assist in this process; others do not.

■ Let us suppose that Robert was very uncooperative. From the moment you introduced yourself to him and his mother he developed clinging behavior, seemed resistant, and would not speak; and when you attempted to take him and his mother to your testing room, he began to scream and throw himself on the floor. What does this do to your selection of clinical tools? How would you manage a situation like this? What tool would you need most at this time?

Analysis of the clinical data

In the fifth step of the diagnostic process the diagnostician analyzes the data he has collected. He does this by scoring, categorizing, and ordering all the information obtained in the interview and testing sessions in relation to the clinical hypothesis he has formulated.

Scoring of the data is done, basically, to determine how well or how poorly the client performed in reference to some standard criteria. This standard criteria may be normative data as specified by the test instrument used. Or the standard may be in terms of intragroup comparisons, that is, comparing the client being seen with other clients with similar problems. In many instances, particularly when "scoring" spontaneous behavior, the standard derives from the diagnostician's background information on normal use of speech and language and his information about the characteristic speech and language behavior in disorders that have been profiled in the literature.

After scoring and comparing the obtained data, the diagnostician then needs to order the data in relation to the cause-effect hypothesis. He must order and categorize the data that provides causal information and the data that provides information about the characteristics of the speech and language disorder. At this time the diagnostician must consider the validity, reliability, and completeness of the data obtained. This step in the diagnostic process is meant to be an objective scoring and ordering of data, not an interpretive step. It should be viewed as a prelude to the next step, interpretation of the data. Incidentally, as a discrete step in the diagnostic process, analysis of the data is one of the more arbitrary steps. The same is true in research studies. Seldom is analysis of the data truly separated from either data collection or, more important, from data interpretation. However, we feel the objectivity implied in this analysis step is important enough to make it explicitly separate, especially for the student learning the diagnostic process. We must learn to look at the results of our data collection apart from the interpretation we may then give them.

■ Information concerning Robert was collected using the screening portion of the *Templin-Darley Tests of Articulation* (Templin and Darley, 1969), the *Northwestern Syntax Screening Test* (Lee, 1969), the *Peabody Picture Vocabulary Test* (Dunn, 1965), an audiometric screening test (Northern and Downs, 1974; *Asha* Committee on Audiometric Evaluation, 1975), and the *Goldman-Fristoe-Woodcock Test of Auditory Discrimination* (Goldman et al., 1970). First, looking backward from the tools used, what would you think the clinical hypothesis for Robert might have been? Next, how would you analyze the information from these

tests? How do you go about analyzing data from tests such as these?

Interpretation of the clinical data: clinical evaluation

After he has analyzed the data, the diagnostician proceeds to an interpretation of the clinical data, the sixth step on the diagnostic model. In this step the diagnostician uses all the information now available on the client, from all sources, to determine its meaning and significance. He now wants to know if the data confirms or denies his original hypotheses or if it suggests other interpretations. If it is supported, he will have to determine what management alternatives will be needed. If it is not supported, he will need to determine whether the data suggests an alternative hypothesis that needs testing or if he already has enough data to support an alternate hypothesis, in which case he again proceeds to provide management alternatives. The interpretation of the information is of extreme importance in diagnosis: it sets the course for future management of the client.

The diagnostician undertakes at least three major tasks in the interpretation of the clinical data. He must first determine the significance of the results of the clinical analysis. Here he takes all the data available to him and determines what it means in relationship to his cause-effect hypothesis, to the general purposes of diagnosis, to the referral request, and to the statement of the problem as seen by the client.

The second major task of interpretation is to formulate and state the diagnosis. After logically interpreting his data, the diagnostician has to finally arrive at some conclusion to his thoughts, however tentative they may be. Thus he is called on to state succinctly what the disorder may be and to implicate probable causal factors.

The final task in the interpretation step is to provide the formal support to the diagnosis that has been succinctly stated, the overall clinical evaluation. This step of the diagnostic process is not merely an objective scoring or summary of the data. Rather, it is the diagnostician's creative act of putting the pieces together, an attempt to understand the whole without necessarily having all the pieces. The diagnostician must use his problem-solving abilities to present the most logical interpretation of the available data. Note that we have said the information available; however, missing information may be as important to interpretation as the information that has been obtained.

The diagnostician in the interpretation phase is exercising his highest degree of professionalism. He must be aware of all the variables that have entered into the diagnostic process for each client, keeping his interpretations within these boundaries, while at the same time using his knowledge and problem-solving skills to arrive at his best answers to the clinical problems presented.

■ In our analysis of Robert's responses to the testing tools presented in the last step, we discovered that he fell below the mean or average on all of the tests. How might you interpret the meaning of this data? Interpretations, remember, are in terms of your working hypothesis and should take into consideration cause-effect relationships.

Conclusions: management considerations, interpretive conference, and follow-up

At the seventh and final step on the diagnostic model, conclusions are drawn by the diagnostician that revolve primarily around management considerations. The diagnostician's primary tasks at this point are to formulate a management proposal, present his findings and management proposal to the client complex,* and follow up on the diagnostic decisions. He must decide what is to be done and how it is to be done.

The interpretation of the clinical data from the previous step allowed the diagnostician to identify the nature of the speech

and language disorder and its probable causal factors. Now he must decide if the disorder constitutes a problem that needs attention and, if so, what can be done about it. He must formulate a management proposal. The diagnostician must know what management alternatives are appropriate for the disorder and its contributing causal factors. He also must consider the best alternatives considering age, family concerns, other factors, and probable prognosis. He must not arrive at merely an ideal plan but must have practical knowledge of the options available to him in his community within the cost and time restrictions of the client. All phases of the diagnostic process enter into making these decisions, including how the client may be able to follow through with any management decisions made.

After arriving at a mangement proposal, the diagnostician's next task is to communicate the findings of his diagnosis and his recommended management plan to the client. The diagnostician must know how to interpret the diagnostic findings to the client complex so that they understand what has been said and what implications the findings have for them. The diagnostician must be able to engage in a two-way consideration of his recommended management proposal. He must determine if his plan is realistic and will be supported by the client complex or if alternative plans need to be implemented. At this phase the diagnostician must demonstrate competence in interpersonal communication, being able to transmit his findings and plan of action and being able to listen to the questions, concerns, and viewpoints of the client and his family. As well as communicating with the client and his family, the diagnostician must be able to communicate his findings and plans to other professionals involved with the client. This includes reporting the findings to the original referral source and making the diagnostic findings available to others concerned with the proposed management of the client.

---

*Client complex means all those persons concerned or involved with the management of the client's speech and language problem.

As the final task of the diagnostic process, the diagnostician must follow up on the diagnostic decisions that have been made. He must follow the recommendations that have been developed in the management proposal to ensure implementation. This may include referrals, scheduling for therapy, or whatever steps need to be taken.

Step seven, then, focuses on an action plan for the client. Here, at last, the diagnostic process has payoff for the client complex. They are helped in developing an understanding of the disorder and its probable causes and join with the diagnostician in determining what can be done about it.

■ From your interpretation of Robert's problem, you decide that therapeutic intervention is necessary as well as further testing by an otolaryngologist. Knowing the mother's initial resistance, how might you interpret your findings and recommendations for her, helping her gain the perspective she needs to get something done for the child? As we indicated at the beginning of this example on Robert, the mother was expecting you to prove her right and the pediatrician wrong.

These seven steps of the clinical adaptation of the method of science illustrate the functions of the diagnostician throughout the diagnostic process. All diagnoses require the use of these steps in various degrees of specificity. We have listed each step of the process as a discrete stage in diagnosis. We do this, not because this reflects how diagnoses are "really" performed, but because we feel these steps are necessary components for all diagnoses and can be isolated to some degree for teaching purposes. While the tasks embodied in the seven steps occur in all diagnoses, they may not always happen exactly as listed; steps may reoccur more than once within a single diagnosis. What is important here, however, is to show how an application of the scientific method can guide our diagnostic process as well as guide the teaching of that process.

In conclusion, by following the seven steps of the diagnostic process, the diagnostician should have a comprehensive understanding of diagnosis as it applies to the individual client, regardless of the type of speech and language disorder presented. As a clinical scientist, the diagnostician should arrive at reasonable solutions to the clinical problems and at the same time know the weaknesses inherent in each diagnosis he performs. Following this method we would expect the diagnostician to:

1. Demonstrate his reasoning abilities for deriving an appropriate clinical hypothesis.
2. Be familiar with the literature and current thinking on the clinical problem he has hypothesized.
3. Be able to present supporting evidence for the logic of his clinical hypothesis, including any contradictory evidence.
4. Give careful thought to the best way the client should be approached in terms of testing procedures.
5. Be aware of the inherent difficulties in his approach to the clinical problem and make educated and judicious decisions about his testing procedures.
6. Give thought to the potential results when he selects his tools and procedures.
7. Develop suitable methods of description and analysis.
8. Know how well the results of his approach and analyses will apply to the solution of the speech and language disorder.
9. Be able to cope with future difficulties and carry out his proposed plans in an acceptable manner.

How do the evaluation process concepts Schultz (1973) has derived from information theory parallel those we have derived from the scientific framework? Are the two compatible?

Setting and referral modifications

In Chapter 1 we discussed how the diagnostician's job functions vary depending on their work setting and the intent of the referral. These two factors frequently require the diagnostician to alter the general purposes of diagnosis to fit the special circumstances of each referral and each work setting. Regardless of the circumstances, however, the diagnostic process following from the method of science allows the diagnostician to adapt the steps of the method to the specific needs of his specific job function.

Setting modifications

Various amounts of time are allotted to the diagnostic process in different settings. Time, therefore, becomes an important practical consideration in using the steps of the method. In one setting the entire process may be restricted to an hour's duration; in others, several hours or repeated sessions may be permitted. In many school settings and some inpatient facilities, the diagnostic process may extend over many short time periods. With restricted time limits, the diagnostician may emphasize one step of the process more than another. For example he may be called on to "screen" a large preschool population. In this setting he probably would focus more on the speech and language behavior than on causal factors; his hypotheses and diagnostic design would be developed for the group served rather than individuals, and most of his allotted time with each individual would be devoted to data collection.

The type of client seen in each setting also determines how the steps are used. If, for example, the entire client population is adult aphasics, the steps would be adjusted to account for the specific needs of this population. The diagnostician would probably specify to a greater extent the speech and language testing procedures for data collection, as the cause-effect relationships would be clearer. A diagnostician in a setting where only trainable mentally retarded children are seen may again primarily be concerned with the speech and language behavior of the children rather than causation. (Of course, this depends on the security of the diagnosis of mental retardation.) His job may be to specify the amount and type of speech and language behavior the children use with the purpose of providing baselines of behavior for designing language and speech therapy. The diagnostician working in a setting with deaf and severely hard-of-hearing children may again be mostly concerned with the development of speech and language behaviors. Or his purpose in this setting may be to determine each child's ability to process auditory information with emphasis on the amount of amplification that may be needed. In settings such as these the diagnostician may be primarily involved with determining how a client may best learn speech and language rather than in establishing cause-effect relationships.

Referral modifications

In addition to the modifications dictated by the various work settings, the purpose of the referral may require the diagnostician to modify the diagnostic process. Diagnosticians are not always asked to provide an intensive cause-effect workup of an individual client. Some referrals are for the purpose of screening large groups of individuals; others may ask for a consultation regarding a likely cause for an already specified speech and language disorder; others may ask for a definitive analysis of the speech and language behavior; still others may ask for the diagnostician's expertise with a specific testing tool. These represent only some of the referral requests that require the diagnostician to modify his use of the steps of the diagnostic process.

Even in screening procedures, although often not thought of as a diagnostic function, all aspects of the model are being used. The intent of speech and language screenings is generally to discover who has a variation and who does not. During his screenings the diagnostician may employ tools for both cause and effect. A screening articulation test may provide information about both phonetic structure and speech mechanism function. A routine speech mechanism examination certainly is used to discover any causal relationship between errors in sound production and deviations of the speech-producing mechanism. The audiometric screening test functions both to detect hearing problems in and of themselves or as potential causes for any speech and language variation that may be discovered. From the information obtained during screening procedures the diagnostician may recommend a more complete diagnostic workup. At times enough information is obtained during the screening to warrant recommendations for immediate therapeutic intervention. Thus in many instances "screening" procedures encompass the entire set of steps in the diagnostic process.

If the referral source has asked for a detailed specification of the speech and language behaviors, the diagnostician may emphasize the effect side of the diagnostic model. He would select tools to give him detailed information to report back to the referral source. Or the referral source may be more interested in the information the diagnostician may be able to supply about suspected causal factors. The referral source may give detailed information about the speech and language characteristics but wants the diagnostician's opinion about the relationship these characteristics may have to various underlying causal factors. Thus the diagnostician would study the speech and language characteristics, emphasizing the causal side of the diagnostic model. His clinical question might be, "What are the potential causes for the specified set of speech and language symptoms?" Again, he would devise testing procedures to uncover the relationship between the effects and the potential causes.

Referrals such as these examples require the diagnostician at times to focus on a certain aspect of the total diagnostic process. Even though the diagnostician's job varies depending on referral requests, he still maintains a focus on all the steps of the diagnostic process. In his verification of another professional's hypothesis he looks at the data that tell him whether the initial referral statement is consistent with his own analysis of the data. If not, he can set up alternate hypotheses for testing or for suggestion to the referral source.

In Chapter 1 we discussed terminology related to diagnosis as well as "types of diagnoses." Review these concepts as they now relate to the diagnostic model presented in this chapter. The model should help to clarify the terminology often used to signal various job functions of the diagnostician.

Adaptation of diagnostic process to setting and referral requirements

Following the diagnostic model gives the diagnostician the flexibility for fulfilling all his job functions regardless of his setting and the intent of the referrals he receives. The examples on p. 169 present a series of potential job functions a diagnostician may have relative to both his work setting and the intent of the referral. The examples illustrate how the diagnostician would focus on different aspects of the diagnostic model, maintaining his overall view of the purposes of diagnosis—to offer tentative solutions to clinical problems.

These are only several among many of the referrals for diagnosis that come to the diagnostician in different work settings. The constancy of the diagnostic model as an adaptation of the scientific method assists the diagnostician in handling the variability that occurs.

Palmer (1970) discusses important information about referrals as they affect the specific purposes of psychological testing. Are his ideas compatible with those expressed here?

ADMINISTRATION AND THE DIAGNOSTICIAN

The scope of the diagnostic process goes beyond the specifics of what the professional does to prepare for and perform a diagnosis with a given client. In conjunction with the professional diagnostic ser-

"Devin has a severe articulation problem. I have not been able to determine the extent of his articulatory pattern to plan treatment."

"My son Devin has a speech problem. We want to know if it is significant."

"Devin cannot make the s, sh, ch, z, and j sounds. Should he have therapy now?"

In this referral the diagnostician would most likely initially emphasize the effect side of the diagnostic model. An effect hypothesis has been stated: "articulation problem." The diagnostician has been asked to assist in clarifying the articulatory pattern to assist in treatment. He would consider the products of phonetic structure and phonology for emphasis. However, since no causal factors are stated, the diagnostician would probably design his diagnosis within a causal framework. In a referral like this the chances that the pattern of articulation is related to something other than development are likely. Still his emphasis, as requested, will be the analysis of the articulatory pattern.

He would design his diagnosis to discover as much as possible about the characteristics of Devin's sound system. He would select tools to gain details about the sounds he can produce, which sounds are in error, how the sounds are in error, where they are in error, etc. Because of the causal aspect, he would probably do this with a careful view of Devin's speech production abilities.

He would analyze and interpret his data in terms of the referral and provide the referral source with information that might assist with treatment planning.

If he discovered other information about the child's speech and language system, he would convey this to the referral source, particularly if other important causal factors have been uncovered.

This is a wide-open referral with any number of possibilities. The diagnostician would have to consider both the cause and effect aspects of diagnosis. He would have to do a constituent analysis at the time the client came for his appointment and set up tentative hypotheses for testing.

All the steps of the diagnostic model would be used. However, the diagnostician might have to consider the use of tools that sample a wide range of behaviors since so little is known. He would surely want to obtain a good spontaneous speech sample early in the testing to see if he could isolate the basic area of variation. The mother has indicated there is a problem, but she is unsure if it is significant. Therefore the diagnostician must consider as well that the child's speech may be normal for his age.

The diagnostician would select tools and order them in such a way that each tool adds more information and allows the diagnostician to disregard certain cause-effect relationships.

Throughout, he is attempting to discover if there is a problem and what may be causally related in order to analyze and interpret this information to the mother in light of her referral question, "Is the problem significant?"

In instances like these the diagnostician may have to be quite tentative. Much information may be missing. He may have completed the diagnostic session with only a more secure hypothesis that needs further exploration.

Let's presume in this setting the therapist usually does not see kindergarten children except on special referral. His first reaction may be that the child is developing these sounds late. But teachers often know the difference; so, is something else going on? The diagnostician in this instance may want to emphasize the causal side of the diagnostic model. There may be something about the child's speech mechanism that prevents him from producing these sounds correctly.

The diagnostician may elect, first, to sit in the classroom and listen to the child to verify his sound errors. From what he hears he may go no further. He may hear a typical sound substitution pattern that he will reevaluate at the end of the school year. However, he may hear production errors that suggest a closer look. He then may have the child come to his therapy room at another session and select tools that emphasize speech production abilities. His emphasis would be on the why—why these sound errors exist.

He would select procedures that test the articulation process as used in the production of the sound classes in error—affricate and fricative production.

He may select tools to analyze tongue function and dentition. He would most likely be interested in a kinesiologic analysis, how the articulators function in production of these sounds.

From his analysis and interpretation the diagnostician should be able to answer the referral question, "Is therapy needed now?" Or he may have discovered an underlying cause that needs other types of attention.

vices offered a client comes "paperwork." Paperwork is euphemistically used to mean the administrative procedures necessary to process a client for diagnostic services. Procedures used are developed primarily as a means for the client to gain diagnostic services and as record-keeping mechanisms.

When a client or professional seeks service from an agency, his first contact is usually administrative. If the administrative face of the agency is ambiguous, cumbersome, or "sloppy," the public may develop a faulty impression of the professional activities of the agency, which will be reflected in their use of the agency. Clear, concise processing procedures focusing on the individual requesting service and not on the needs of the agency are essential. Both must be served, but the primary focus should be on the client. If the client is required to go through extensive, and to him irrelevant, procedures to obtain an appointment for a speech and language diagnosis, he may arrive on his appointment day with resentments toward the agency or may not show up at all. These situations must be circumvented. This is not to say that certain paperwork procedures cannot be instituted and used as long as the client understands how these procedures facilitate the professional services he receives. What people seeking professional services want is someone who perceives their needs and responds to them as directly as possible. Thus explanations about the required administrative procedures may be needed to alleviate much of the frustration some clients feel.

The administrative procedures designed for record keeping gather information pertaining to who the client is, where he lives, his problem, how he came to the diagnostic setting, what his current status is, whose responsibility it is for follow-up, etc. These records have numerous intra-agency purposes, designed often for statistical reasons and to "keep track" of the clients seen. Records are often necessary for use by other community and governmental agencies. Record keeping has become an absolute necessity in a setting offering diagnostic services to the public, whether in a community agency, a hospital, a school system, private practice, or elsewhere.

Weed (1970) has pointed out how careful and systematic record keeping that has its first concern in patient care is important in the medical profession. How might the procedures he has developed be adapted for speech and hearing services?

Administrative components

The three major administrative components of diagnosis include *intake procedures* (the procedures that are followed for processing information about a client prior to his appointment), the *diagnostic session* (what occurs from the time the client arrives for his appointment until the diagnostic "day" is over), and *follow-up* (involvement with the client complex following the diagnostic session).

We offer a flowchart (Fig. 10-2) that represents the service performed within each component. We will briefly discuss each of the components and then provide an outline for the reader's consideration. Our intent is to give the student an understanding of the importance of administration to the diagnostic process and the different functions he may have to perform in his work setting.

Our development of the three administrative components may fit some settings better than others. However, we feel the flowchart and outlines can be adapted to the specific needs of any work setting. We have also included in Appendix I a set of forms that can be reviewed in conjunction with the flowchart. Each form represents a different administrative function and is designed to assist the agency in carrying out these functions. The forms are not intended to be used as they are by any specific agency; rather they are representative of forms designed to facilitate client service.

From the outset it is important to keep in

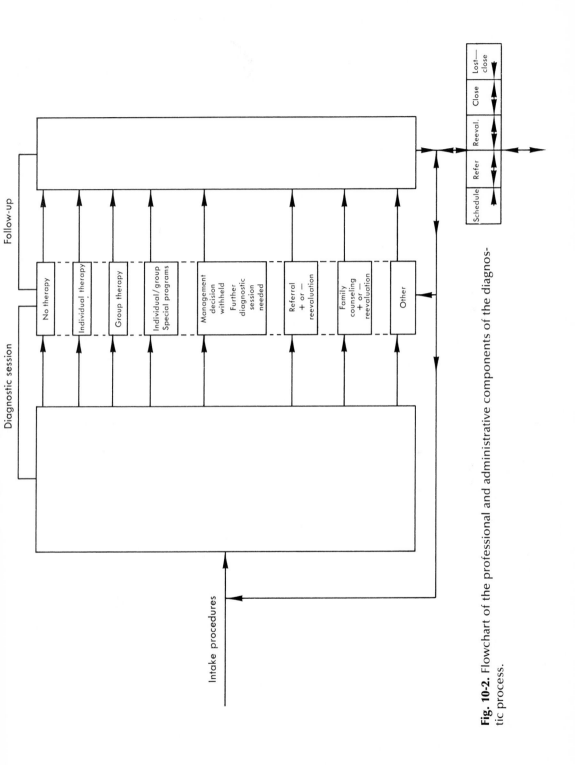

Fig. 10-2. Flowchart of the professional and administrative components of the diagnostic process.

mind that many or all of the details within each administrative component may be handled by the diagnostician rather than by supportive administrative personnel. Some settings use administrative personnel, whereas other settings, for example, private practice, require the professional staff member to handle all aspects of the processing of clients for diagnosis. Our use of the words "professional" and "administrative" in this discussion refers primarily to functions rather than people. For example, the individual who takes incoming referral calls may well be either a diagnostician or a scheduling secretary.

Intake procedures

Intake procedures and policies include the client-processing activities from the time of the initial referring contact until the time the client is scheduled for an appointment. Within this administrative component a system would be instituted for taking information about the client, the referral source, the problem, client concerns, etc.

It is of great importance that the client knows what is going to happen at this initial stage. Information that allows the client to feel secure that the agency understands his needs and will follow up as efficiently as possible should be provided. This is relatively easy if an appointment for diagnosis is given at the time of initial contact. Then the client knows when he is to come and when something will be done. However, if appointments are not given until later, the client must know when and how the appointment is to come. The use of a follow-up acknowledgment letter (Appendix I) is a useful device in providing information like this. The letter can state the conditions of the scheduling process and any other information that may be useful to the client. A brochure or letter that describes the agency, its services, and its costs also can be useful for providing a basic understanding of the services offered by the speech and hearing agency.

Another aspect of intake procedures is the intra-agency processing needed to keep track of the client until he is scheduled for his diagnostic appointment. There is usually no excuse for losing a client in the "administrative mill." If paperwork is necessary for providing services to human beings, then the process should be as efficient and economical as possible; clients should not be "mislaid" and costs should not skyrocket because of extensive administrative processes and personnel.

The information that is made available to the diagnostician prior to actual client contact is a part of intake procedures. How much client information is needed prior to client contact and what administrative procedures are established for receiving, accepting, and processing referrals vary from setting to setting and are more or less dependent on the professional philosophy of the setting. For example, the diagnostician working in a hospital setting may receive the referral (consult request) in the form of a telephone call from the duty nurse who is transmitting the physician's orders for a speech evaluation. In this instance the diagnostician has available to him the patient's medical chart. Whatever is in that chart in terms of general, developmental, and medical history as well as the patient's current medical status is data the diagnostician can use prior to contact with the patient. He will know a great deal about the patient, including whether he is healthy enough to respond to a speech and language evaluation. The diagnostician can also contact the physician for further information and discuss the patient with the nursing staff. Thus considerable information is available.

Another example is the public school setting where the diagnostician receives a referral from the classroom teacher stating that a child seems to have a speech problem that is interfering with his classroom performance. In this setting the diagnostician may have available the school records on the child, which may be extensive or minimal, depending on the philosophy of the school. At the least the child's records will usually include his academic performance, teacher reactions to him, and perhaps an academic profile, how well he does in what subjects. In some instances intelligence test results are available, some health records, and family information that may have been filed by the school nurse or psychologist. Again, the diagnostician may have a good bit of information to use unless it is the policy of the school system not to make pupil records available to the diagnostician, a practice in some systems as well as in some agencies.

A question that sometimes arises about intake procedures is with whom the client should have his first contact. Should it be a professional or can other administrative personnel function in this manner? It is of prime importance that the first person a client makes contact with is someone who demonstrates knowledge of the agency and its procedures. If the initial contact person is not a speech pathologist, he should know what questions he can answer and when the assistance of a professional is needed. This initial contact person begins the client's contract with the agency and should handle this situation sensibly and sensitively. Whoever assumes this role must project warmth, sincerity, and knowledge, especially since this first, crucial contact is usually by telephone. These administrative concerns are of particular importance in large agencies serving many individuals with speech and language problems.

Can a secretary be trained to handle the complexities of taking referral information? How much can administrative personnel other than the diagnostician say to a mother who has immediate questions about her child's problem?

The following outline presents the major considerations within the intake procedures component of the administration flowchart (Fig. 10-2).

Administrative
Staff responsibilities and roles
   Professional
   Administrative
Initial referral contact
   Procedures for processing
      Referral data forms
      Processing flow
      Follow-up
         Letters and forms
Information gathering
   Types of information
      Histories
      Other professional services performed
   Procedures for processing
      Requests for information
   Follow-up
      Forms and letters
Appointment scheduling
   Criteria for scheduling
      Client needs
      Professional staff availability
      Individual
      Teams
      Space and time allocations (see diagnostic session)
   Scheduling procedure
      Client contact
      Procedures for processing
      Forms and letters
      Follow-up
Professional
Steps 1, 2, and 3 of the diagnostic process

Diagnostic session

The second administrative component (Fig. 10-2) begins at the time the client arrives for his appointment with the diagnostician. There are both administrative and professional aspects to this component.

Someone within the diagnostic setting needs to attend to the practical details of where, when, and with what material the diagnostic sessions will be performed. In a smoothly administered setting these decisions are made well in advance of the diagnostic day so that time and space problems are circumvented and needed diagnostic materials are available. When the client arrives at the agency, it should be made clear to him where he is to go. Even if he has been given a room number when he was scheduled for his appointment, there should be clearly visible information as to the location of the diagnostic setting within the building. There should be someone to greet the client when he arrives—in large settings this may be the function of a receptionist; in other instances the professional staff member is present. Just as important as the beginning of the diagnostic session is its ending. The client may need directions for leaving the setting. In some agencies the client must go to a business office for fee arrangements, but even in a one-person private practice the client will want to know fee payment procedures. This information should be given to the client; he should not have to ask.

The primary activity of the diagnostic session is to conduct the diagnosis. These professional services are achieved through the seven steps of the diagnostic process. Therefore the professional service aspect of the diagnostic session will not be expanded on here.

The following outline presents the major aspects of the diagnostic session component of the administrative flowchart (Fig. 10-2).

Administrative
Staff responsibilities and roles
  Professional
  Administrative
Space allocation
  Room availability
  Observation facilities
  Specially equipped rooms
    Audiologic
    Videotape
    Others
  Waiting rooms
  Playrooms
Time allocation
  Unit of time for a diagnostic session
  Block or staggered scheduling
Materials and equipment
  Specially equipped rooms
  Availability of diagnostic tools
    Acquisition of needed materials
    Location of materials
    Procedures for use of materials
Initial client contact
  Waiting room location
Business procedures
  Fees
  Method of payment
Professional
Steps 4, 5, 6, and 7 of the diagnostic process; reconsideration of steps 1, 2, and 3 as needed

Follow-up

The third component of the administrative flowchart is concerned with those administrative and professional services provided for clients after they have completed the initial diagnostic session. Once the client has been diagnosed and management proposals have been offered, the primary concern of the diagnostician and the agency is the follow-up needed to see that whatever continued services the client needs are obtained. These services may include scheduling for therapy, referrals to outside agencies, parental conferences and assistance, etc. Again, we provide an outline of the major aspects of the follow-up component, and Appendix I provides some forms that are useful for these purposes.

Administrative
Staff responsibilities and roles
  Professional
  Administrative
Referral processing procedures
  Letters and forms
  Follow-up
Therapy scheduling
  Client assignment
    Needs of client—diagnosis
    Staff availability
    Space and time allocations
  Scheduling procedures
    Forms and letters—scheduling form
    Follow-up
Record keeping
  Reports
  Procedures for maintaining records
    Active
    Inactive
    Accessibility
Professional
Step 7 of the diagnostic process

Setting and administration

The specifics of intake procedures, diagnostic session, and follow-up may differ considerably in a nursing home, a public school, or a community hearing and speech agency. For example, a particular agency may have a multidisciplinary diagnostic clinic staffed by speech pathologists, audiologists, psychologists, social service workers, etc. The procedures for administration would have to reflect how all personnel interact with one another to perform all the services that might be needed. On the day of the diagnosis there would be a need to establish the leader of the diagnostic team, which might vary from client to client depending on the nature of the clinical hypothesis. Or the agency might always use several sessions for each diagnosis, particularly for children. The flowchart could reflect this two-session policy for diagnostic procedures. A second block could be added to indicate the follow-up that was to occur in the second session. This type of organization would be more reflective of a team approach or a staffing approach to the diagnosis of clients with speech and language disorders. A staffing approach to diagnosis is frequently instituted in agencies where the primary client is the young child who may be severely involved emotionally, mentally, psychologically, or physically.

The flowchart (Fig. 10-2), the outlines, and the appendix of forms (Appendix I) can be adapted for use in any diagnostic setting.

As we stated at the beginning of this administration section, clients should not be lost because of lack of concern over administrative structure. What was done at the speech and hearing clinic of the Mount Sinai Medical Center to decrease their no-show rate (Bar, 1975)?

REFERENCES

Asha Committee on Audiometric Evaluation, Guidelines for identification audiometry. *Asha,* **17,** 94-99 (1975).

Bar, A., Decreasing the no-show rate in an urban speech and hearing clinic. *Asha,* **17,** 455-456 (1975).

Dunn, L. M., *Peabody Picture Vocabulary Test: Manual.* Circle Pines, Minn.: American Guidance Service, Inc. (1965).

Goldman, R., Fristoe, M., and Woodcock, R. W., *Goldman-Fristoe-Woodcock Test of Auditory Discrimination.* Circle Pines, Minn.: American Guidance Service, Inc. (1970).

Lee, L. L., *Northwestern Syntax Screening Test.* Evanston, Ill.: Northwestern University Press (1969).

Northern, J. L., and Downs, M. P., *Hearing in Children.* Baltimore: The Williams & Wilkins Co. (1974).

Palmer, J. O., *The Psychological Assessment of Children.* New York: John Wiley & Sons, Inc. (1970).

Schultz, M. C., The bases of speech pathology and audiology: Evaluation as the resolution of uncertainty. *J. Speech Hearing Dis.,* **38,** 147-155 (1973).

Templin, M. C., and Darley, F. L., *The Templin-Darley Tests of Articulation: Manual.* Iowa City: University of Iowa Press (1969).

Weed, L. L., *Medical Records, Medical Education, and Patient Care.* Cleveland: The Press of Case Western Reserve University (1970).

Chapter 11

Definition and delimitation of the clinical problem: constituent analysis

Clients request services to obtain help. They present problematic situations, and the diagnostician must provide solutions to their problems. The constituent analysis is the diagnostician's first step in his quest for a solution; that is, he must define and delimit the clinical problem brought to him. His goal is to differentiate each client's specific speech and language concerns from all others. From his constituent analysis the diagnostician then establishes his overall diagnostic approach to the client's stated problem.

As diagnosticians, we start defining and delimiting our client's problem from the variable amount of information obtained prior to the client's appointment. What usually is available, at the very least, is a referral statement. At other times extensive information is available, including history forms filled out by the client or his family and other medical, psychological, and educational information.

Whatever the amount of information, the diagnostician analyzes and interprets the constituents in reference to his funds of knowledge about normal and disordered speech and language. For example, if Mrs. Braverman requests a speech and language diagnosis for her 3-year-old daughter Julie who "does not talk yet," the diagnostician interprets this statement in reference to normal language acquisition: what language patterns do most 3-year-old children have? Thus at the heart of the constituent analysis is the juxtaposition of specific client information against the diagnostician's fund of knowledge about speech and language. Through this systematic analysis, the specific cause-effect constituents gain relevance.

The constituent analysis becomes the blueprint for planning the remainder of the diagnostic process. From it, all the other steps emanate: the clinical hypothesis, the selection of tools and procedures, the collection of data, the analysis of data, the interpretation of the data, and the conclusions. Inquiry starts with the definition and delimitation of a problem, not a method for solving a problem. As Brown and Ghiselli (1955) put it, "So much is known about methodology that the solution of many new problems seldom demands a radical change in method. Even research findings of 'world shaking' proportions have arisen from only slight alterations in already well-established and familiar methods."

Thus the diagnosis that is performed will end up being only as good as the constituent analysis. If the diagnostician makes errors in his analysis, he will likely make errors in the remaining steps of diagnosis, unless he can apply corrective procedures during the ongoing diagnostic process. The constituent analysis is as objective and systematic as possible, thereby minimizing diagnostician error.

THE CONSTITUENT ANALYSIS: HOW IT IS DONE

In reality a constituent analysis is continuously performed throughout the diagnostic process, culminating in a final interpretation at step 6, interpretation of the clinical data. For teaching purposes, however, we will use the term "constituent analysis" to refer to those tasks the diagnostician performs before the client's appointment. This section now aims to teach this first step of the diagnostic process—how to do a constituent analysis. We will first discuss the information base needed, followed by the tasks that the diagnostician must perform with that information.

Information bases

To do his constituent analysis the diagnostician uses information from two sources: his professional funds of knowledge and the information gathered about the client.

Funds of knowledge: the foremost base

The diagnostician comes to the diagnostic process with his professional area of expertise, his knowledge about normal and disordered speech and language. The only way the diagnostician can adequately define and delimit potential clinical problems is by filtering client information through his constantly growing and changing fund of knowledge. This knowledge, as detailed in Part I, is what allows him to understand and analyze the history and current status of the client he will be seeing.

Client information base: nature and sources

Besides his fund of knowledge, the diagnostician starts the diagnostic process by having to deal with new information, the specific constituents about a client whose speech and language disorder he is to diagnose. Generally, information becomes available to the diagnostician from one or more of the following sources: (1) a referral either received verbally or in writing, (2) a history questionnaire sent out to the client or parents by the agency and returned prior to the diagnosis, and (3) letters and reports from other professionals and agencies.

The information the diagnostician gathers about his client from these sources provides the case history background on the client, the basis for what some writers call the *case study* (Dickson and Jann, 1974). This client history information is used by the diagnostician to discover past and present events, facts, attitudes, situations, and conditions that relate to the speech and language disorder. The information is used to determine the way other people or the client himself views the problem.

The type of information that the diagnostician receives reflects the professional concerns of the people from whom it is obtained. For instance, physicians generally provide medical history; teachers provide educational information; and psychologists provide behavioral, emotional, and intellectual information. Of course, any referral source might provide the diagnostician with much broader information. The physician might also include his findings about speech and language development. The psychologist might provide information about the medical history of the client. The teacher most probably will give a good bit of information about general behavior. All professionals acquire information beyond their specific professional bounds; but, to some extent, the source from which information is obtained specifies the type of information obtained. Thus no single source usually provides the diagnostician with all the types of information he may want for fully understanding the client's need for a speech and language diagnosis. So the information gathered from the different sources must be collated; each bit of information must be analyzed against all other bits of information. Gaining information from multiple sources increases the reliability and validity of the information made available prior to contact with the client.

As part of the typical case study approach, the information obtained by the diagnostician can be categorized by subject matter over time. The medical history, social history, family history, speech and language history, emotional history, developmental history, educational history, etc. are examples of subject matter categories. These and other potential categories are obviously not mutually exclusive. The information within each subject category can also be viewed chronologically. A typical example would be information that expresses the physical development of a child, the so-called motor milestones—when did he hold his head erect, when did he roll over, when did he sit unsupported, when did he crawl, when did he take his first steps, when did he hop, skip, and jump, etc.? From information of a developmental nature, the diagnostician can make comparisons between his client's development and expectations from normative data, as well as gain more insight into the interactions of various aspects of the client's history.

The types of useful information that could make up the case history of any client are different depending on the client being seen. An obvious example would be the use of birth history information. For a young child, information about his birth may be instrumental in determining a cause-effect relationship. However, for a 53-year-old man who became aphasic after a cerebrovascular accident or a normal 17-year-old boy who sustained brain injury in an auto accident with subsequent dysarthria, the need for birth history information most likely would not be useful. The diagnostician is interested in gathering data of relevance to the diagnosis of his client, not simply an accumulation of data.

In order to capitalize on potential sources of information, the diagnostician will want to be familiar with the various sources and types of information he may be able to acquire prior to the scheduled appointment with the client. At this time we will present a discussion of the types of information that might be obtained from the three primary sources of information: the referral, the history questionnaire, and letters and reports from other professionals and agencies who have been involved with the client.

Referrals. Referrals come in many forms. In some settings a person may simply call and request an appointment for a diagnosis and may be asked to give little information other than the prospective client's name, age, address, and telephone number. Other settings may require that the referral for services come only from a physician or other recognized professional. Such "official" referrals range from a brief note on a prescription pad, "I recommend evaluation of Janet for a speech problem," to detailed descriptions of the presenting problem. In some settings the referral may be quite informal, as when the classroom teacher stops the speech pathologist in the hall and asks him to "look at Philip; his voice has been hoarse for a month." Other settings may require elaborate intake procedures before services can be obtained (see discussion of intake procedures Chapter 10).

Whatever the policy for receiving referrals, there is certain basic information the diagnostician should have. He should know how the referral came to him, what is wanted by the referral source, and, of course, basic identifying information about the client and his suspected problem.

The diagnostician must have a clear understanding of the origin of the referral; it is important to know how a client comes for service in order to provide appropriate follow-up. The diagnostician must verify whether he is receiving a direct or an indirect referral. Who does the client feel was the primary referral? There is a difference between asking for diagnostic services at someone's suggestion versus being referred directly for diagnostic services. For example, a mother who calls for diagnostic services on the suggestion of the pediatrician may herself be the direct referral source. The pediatrician's suggestion to the mother may only have been to alleviate her undue concern about the child although he felt all along that nothing was wrong. If, however, the diagnostician receives a letter, report, or call from the pediatrician concerning services for the child, the pediatrician becomes the direct referral source and most probably will become directly involved with the overall management of the child. How the referrals come requires the diagnostician to follow up in different ways.

The referral source should provide at the minimum his intention for making the referral. Sometimes the referral source will provide detailed causal information and minimal descriptions of the speech and language behavior. For example, a physician referring a child with a medical diagnosis of cerebral palsy may give detailed information about physical growth and development, the type of cerebral palsy, the etiology of the condition, and then say only that the child does not talk. From this the diagnostician may not know the specific intent of the physician's referral. Yet the physician may be interested specifically in the capabilities of the child to develop speech or if muscle function is sufficient to produce speech. Not knowing the physician's specific intent, the diagnostician, in turn, may not provide the physician with the information he wanted.

■ How would you proceed on the basis of the following two different referrals? Is it clear what the referral source is asking for in each case?

1. Dr. David Link referred Mr. Howard Hardee, a 58-year-old white male, who has been diagnosed as having multiple sclerosis. Dr. Link has asked if Mr. Hardee can be taught to compensate for his deteriorating speech-producing abilities.
2. Dr. Joe Deli referred Mrs. Ann Rome, a 32-year-old white female, for a voice evaluation. In his letter of referral Dr. Deli stated that Mrs. Rome has been hoarse for about 2 months.

At times the referral source does not have a specific intent for his referral but, instead, is asking for a diagnosis and recommendations at the discretion of the speech and language diagnostician. Implicit in such a referral is the referral source's interest in knowing if a problem exists and what to do about it. In these instances the diagnostician proceeds to provide services in line with the overall purposes of diagnosis.

The diagnostician must also be aware that at times referrals will come that are not entirely appropriate. He then must decide how to handle the referral. Sometimes the inappropriate referral is not discovered until the case history questionnaire is returned by the family; at other times it is recognized when the referral letter arrives. For example, in speech and language settings it is not uncommon to receive a referral to help someone with their public speaking skills. At other times the referral may be from someone who thinks the speech pathologist can diagnose mental retardation or emotional disturbance. When it is discovered that the primary problem is not a speech and language disorder but an educational, emotional, psychological, medical, or other problem, the diagnostician must know what to do with these referrals. Often there is a speech and language disorder associated with the individual's more pervasive problem that has led to referral to the speech pathologist. In some of these instances the diagnostician may follow through with the diagnostic process in order to effect a more appropriate referral, to assist the client in obtaining more appropriate services. At other times he will have to discuss his concerns with the referral source and assist in redirecting the referral.

Along with his intent, the referral source should provide basic information about the client. Identification data is crucial. Without the name, age, address, telephone number, etc. a referral is difficult to follow up. It is amazing how many referrals do come without this basic identifying information. The referral source should, if possible, provide his impressions of the client's speech and language disorder and causal factors related to it as well as any other information about factors that, to him, are important to the client's problem.

■ Consider this referral from a physician: Maurice Redlands has had a speech disturbance since birth. He has had no serious disease in the past. He does have congenital esotropia and secondary diplopia in the right eye. What are your reactions to this referral? What do you think the significance of the information about the right eye might have? How would you interpret a speech disturbance that has been present since birth?

■ The following referral was received from a clinical psychologist. Analyze it in terms of the type of information provided. How are subject matter and time presented? What would you do from this point? What is not included in the referral letter that you might like to know before proceeding?

On February 19, 1975, Lee Newton was seen at the psychological clinic in regard to his slow development. Lee obtained an intelligence score of 67 and a mental age of 3 years, 3 months on the *Stanford-Binet Intelligence Scale.* Lee has a vocabulary age of approximately 2½ years. His best subtests were memory (for hidden objects) and identification of objects. No other tests were passed at the 4-year level.

On March 19, 1975, Dr. Anthony administered an EEG to Lee who was 4 years, 10 months of age. I have seen the record, and it shows a low degree of abnormality with irregular diffuse delta activity. Another EEG has been administered recently, but I have not yet seen the results.

I would appreciate a report of your evaluation of Lee. If I can be of further help to you, please do not hesitate to contact me.

History questionnaire. A history questionnaire in this context refers to a questionnaire completed by the client, his family, or agency personnel prior to the client's initial meeting with the diagnostician. The use of case history forms is particularly common in settings that do not have immediate access to client information. Thus we find history questionnaires particularly common in university speech and hearing centers, community agencies, and private practice. Hospitals, other inpatient settings, and multidisciplinary agencies often make less use of questionnaires in advance, as much of the requested information becomes available in the medical or intra-agency records.

The use of questionnaires to gather historical information for case studies has been standard practice in our profession (Johnson et al., 1963; Milisen, 1971), although professionals may differ in the value they place on such tools. Some prefer to gain historical information only in a face-to-face interaction with the client, feeling that they can then better judge the importance and accuracy of the information they obtain. Other limitations have been pointed out in gaining information via questionnaires: not allowing the client to state what may be most important to him, wording questions in such a way that the informant does not understand nor know how to respond, and the difficulty of adapting a form suitable to clients of all ages with varying problems. A further problem with the history questionnaire is the client's lack of understanding of why certain information is requested. Often a parent has no idea why a form asks for birth information and may simply choose not to answer such questions. Finally, one of the chief criticisms of questionnaires is the questionable accuracy of the information obtained.

Our view about the use of questionnaires is that they provide a primary source for gaining vital information prior to client contact. In addition, we do not suggest that questionnaires be used in place of client or parental interviews or as a form to be followed and filled in during an interview. Rather, questionnaires provide preinformation for the purpose of planning the diagnostic session.

In the context of the total diagnostic process, questionnaires have several distinct advantages. In general, they increase the overall efficiency of diagnosis. They provide routine facts that can be recorded in advance. They allow the diagnostician to identify areas of missing information and particular problem areas around which he can focus his constituent analysis and subsequent interview. The questionnaire serves as a springboard for the interview, helping to establish rapport since the client feels the diagnostician already knows something about the problem. We also find that completing a questionnaire at home often gives the parent time to think about the questions asked and allows him to consult sources such as the baby book or pediatrician's record for specific information.

We like to view questionnaires as a primary source of information for the constituent analysis. However, we must accept that some of the information may be inaccurate. If approached from this critical viewpoint, it should help the diagnostician be more cautious regarding the use of the information obtained. All in all, we maintain that the advantages of questionnaires outweigh the disadvantages. If it is used in interaction with the interview, the reliability and validity of the information can be cross-checked. The client can then expand on and qualify the information he has provided.

Many of the criticisms can be overcome by carefully designed questionnaires. Questions can be framed and vocabulary selected in a straightforward manner that can be understood by most people without offending their sense of privacy. To circumvent the need for lengthy responses and to increase the reliability of responses, questions can be framed that require checking an appropriate blank, yes or no responses, or minimal written responses. Leaving space at the end of the questionnaire for open-ended responding allows the respondents to discuss any aspects of their problem not covered by the questionnaire. Cover letters can also accompany the questionnaire to explain its purposes and to alleviate a client's concern about not understanding all aspects of the questionnaire. If the questionnaire is presented as being helpful to the diagnostician in doing a more thorough job, it will be acceptable to most people asked to respond.

A difficulty encountered in questionnaire construction is in making them appropriate for the many different clients serviced by the speech and hearing setting. In an agency serving large numbers of clients, of all ages and with all types of speech and language disorders, it would be quite impossible to develop anything suitable for all the clients except the most general of questionnaires. For example, how could a form be constructed that would be appropriate for a 3-year-old child with a suspected language disorder and a 23-year-old person suspected of a prosody disorder? Thus in some settings more than one case history form must be constructed to use with the different clients to be seen.

In each instance, however, the guideline for construction should be that the questionnaire serves the greatest number of clients. Therefore the development of a children's case history questionnaire should be able to provide the essence of the information needed, regardless of whether the disorder is phonetic structure, prosody, language, or voice and regardless of the potential causes of the disorder. An "all-purpose" questionnaire finds the greatest applicability.

Since a case history questionnaire is a collection of data usually by unsupervised written response, it should be designed not only to motivate the informant or to gain specific subject matter but also to assist in the steps of the diagnostic process, particularly the constituent analysis. Does the history questionnaire give sufficient information as to the client's identity: Who he is and where he fits in the world? What is his world like? What has he got going for him? Against him? What has already been determined about the problem and its causes? What has the family been told? How do they and others perceive the problem? What importance do they give it? What do they want from the diagnostician?

Some settings choose to send out questionnaires that have been devised for specific "problem types." For example, if it is known that the child referred has a repaired cleft palate, a history form designed for that potential causal factor may be used rather than a general history form. There are instances where this could be appropriate, but it requires immediate verification of the special "problem type" before the questionnaire can be sent. Johnson et al. (1963) suggest supplementary case history information for a number of problem types including cerebral palsy, cleft palate, dysphasia, and postlaryngectomy. Notice how these supplementary histories tend to be organized around etiologic factors (see the discussion in Chapter 7). If such etiologic information is known at the time of referral and is considered valid and reliable, there may be justification for sending specific history questionnaires related to these causal factors. In most instances, however, a general history form, perhaps one constructed for children and one for adults, would serve the setting most efficiently. Even this division may cause some difficulty; most children's case history forms do not seem appropriate for the adolescent, nor does the adolescent fit into many of the adult histories. The adolescent and the geriatric client are often "in limbo" when it comes to the construction of case history questionnaires.

If it is kept in mind that the case history questionnaire is used in conjunction with an interview, the general information can be supplemented when the diagnostician has the opportunity to interview the client complex. The detailed information about specific causal factors can be added to the general information obtained just as we add more information about the speech and language disorder in the interview.

We will now discuss in some detail an example children's case history questionnaire to demonstrate how and what information can be obtained from this source. The case history form is a general questionnaire useful through the early teenage years, but perhaps most useful for preschool children and children up to 10 years of age. This case history form has been developed over a number of years. It has met with both success and failure, revisions being made over time to combat the failures. Its construction allows for gathering in some detail information about the many types of children's speech and language disorders stemming from many different causal factors. Each item on the form has been found useful for doing the constituent analysis.

The children's case history form asks for several major categories of information and, where possible, develops questions

---

FORM 1

Identification section of the children's speech, language, and hearing history

Date _____

Person completing this form _____ Relationship to child _____

I. IDENTIFICATION

Name _____ Birth date _____ Sex ____ Age ____

Address _____ Phone_____

Mother's name _____ Address _____ Age ____

Father's name _____ Address _____ Age ____

Referred by _____ Address _____

Family doctor _____ Address _____

Child's pediatrician _____ Address _____

chronologically. The categories of information are identification, statement of the problem, speech, language, and hearing history, general development, medical history, behavior, educational history, and home and family information. For each category we will discuss the subject matter and its ordering, suggesting ways it might be useful to the diagnostician for doing his constituent analysis. For the reader's convenience we will reproduce each of the sections of the case history form as it is being discussed. For a completed history form see Appendix II.

Identification information (Form 1), including the referral source, is presented first on the children's case history. It gives the diagnostician immediate information about the informant, the child, his parents, and medical supervision. He will know if the informant is the mother, father, another family member, or perhaps the physician, social worker, or other agency personnel.

From these items the diagnostician can begin to analyze the environmental background of the child. This section, used in conjunction with the home and family section of the history, provides insight into causal factors that may have affected or be affecting the speech and language environment component (see Figs. 4-1, 8-3, and the outline on p. 124). Such information as parental addresses and ages tells us about the family structure: is the family unit intact; are both parents living together; is there a wide age discrepancy between the parents; are these young or old parents? If the person completing the form is the father rather than the mother, is this important? Perhaps it is a social worker or a physician. What do these constituents tell the diagnostician about the family? The address begins to provide information helpful for socioeconomic considerations. Of course, the diagnostician will have to know his own community before an address registers any information about style of living for the family. As depicted in Fig. 4-1, we are trying to assess the sociocultural con-

text, the multisensory context, and the interpersonal context that make up the speech and language environment of the child being seen—what effects causal factors (see outline on p. 124) have on the past and contemporary speech and language input received by the child.

The identification section does not give direct information about speech and language products. However, if the child is a 4-year-old girl, the diagnostician would immediately have an expectation reference point. He knows what speech and language normal 4-year-old children should have acquired. So knowing only the age and sex of the child being referred, the diagnostician could infer about expected speech and language products.

If there is both a pediatrician and a family doctor, or neither, it gives data about the general health care provided for the child. The information about the referral source, as seen by the informant, gives the diagnostician information for doing a reliability check on the source of referral.

In the statement of the problem section (Form 2) the family, early in the history form, is asked to present their perceptions of the speech and language problem and its causes. Presenting this section early on the history form allows the family to present their basic concerns about the child prior to having to respond to questions that may not seem as relevant, for example, birth history.

The informant is asked to describe the problem somewhat chronologically—at the present time, when first noticed, how it has changed, and what caused it. This time dimension, which creates some redundancy, may help to validate the perceptions of the family. The items in this section would provide what could be considered as the most general of general case history questionnaires. These items could serve all populations of speech and hearing disorders.

If this section is filled out completely by the informant and if the diagnostician considers it as reliable and valid, he begins to obtain a good representation of possible

---

FORM 2

**Statement of the problem section of the children's speech,
language, and hearing history**

II. STATEMENT OF THE PROBLEM

Describe as completely as possible the speech, language, and hearing problem. _____

_____

_____

_____

When was the problem first noticed? _____

How has the problem changed since you first noticed it? _____

What has been done about it? Has this helped? _____

What do you think caused the problem? _____

Are there any family members or relatives who have or had speech, language, or hearing
problems? _____

---

cause-effect relationships. Depending on the responses made to these open-ended questions, the diagnostician should also gain significant insight into the informant's ability to describe the child's speech and language disorder. Any type of problem stemming from any type of cause may be presented here. The diagnostician may also discover that the informant is only presenting another's impressions of the child's problem; quite often a parent will report information gained from the child's pediatrician or his teacher. Thus the diagnostician may obtain information here about the speech and language product, the speech and language environment, and the internal speech and language processes as well as causal factors that affect the various components of speech and language processing (Chapters 3 through 8).

If the parent reported, "My son cannot be understood when he talks," the diagnostician would suspect something different than if the parent reported, "My son doesn't understand what is said to him." If the informant has indicated the child does not comprehend what is said to him and also states that it is because of a hearing loss, the diagnostician can begin to establish certain potential cause-effect relationships. He might, in this instance, implicate the behavioral correlate of comprehension, inferring that the physical process of language representation is affected due to an auditory processing deficit. Likewise, he might also begin to infer speech and language products affected, knowing from his fund of knowledge what effects hearing loss has on speech and language development and usage.

The speech, language, and hearing history (Form 3) follows immediately after the statement of the problem section. This section allows the informants to continue providing information that they can easily see is directly relevant to the problem with which they are concerned. This section then continues to build motivation for completing the remainder of the history form. The speech, language, and hearing history section is developed with a time dimension in mind—from past development to current

FORM 3

Speech, language, and hearing section of the children's speech, language, and hearing history

III. SPEECH, LANGUAGE, AND HEARING HISTORY

How much did your child babble and coo during the first 6 months? _____

When did he speak his first words? _____ What were the child's first few words? ____
_____

How many words did the child have at 1½ years? _____ When did he begin to use two-word sentences? _____

Does he use speech? Frequently _____ Occasionally _____ Never _____

Does he use many gestures? (Give examples if possible.) _____
_____

Which does the child prefer to use? Complete sentences _____ Phrases _____

One or two words _____ Sounds _____ Gestures _____

Does he make sounds incorrectly? ____ If so, which ones? _____
_____

Does he hesitate, "get stuck," repeat, or stutter on sounds or words? _____

If so, describe. _____

How does his voice sound? Normal ____ Too high ____ Too low ____ Hoarse ____ Nasal ____

How well can he be understood? By his parents _____ By his brothers and sisters

and playmates _____ By relatives and strangers _____

Did your child ever acquire speech and then slow down or stop talking? _____
_____

Does he imitate speech but not use it? _____

How well does he understand what is said to him? _____
_____

Does your child hear adequately? _____ Does his hearing appear to be constant or does

it vary? _____ Is his hearing poorer when he has a cold? _____

Has your child ever worn a hearing aid? _____ Which ear? _____ How long? _____

Hours per day? _____ Does it seem to help him? _____

NOTE: If the child has a hearing aid, please bring it and the earmold along with you when you come in for your appointment.

use of speech and language. Adding this section to the statement of the problem, the diagnostician begins to get more details about the specific speech and language disorder and when it occurred. As well, he develops more insight and confidence into possible cause-effect relationships.

From the additional information provided in this section the diagnostician can better specify the product that may be dis-ordered. There are specific items about voice, prosody, phonetic structure, and all the parameters of language. Knowing the history of speech and language development not only gives information about the characteristics of the speech and language product, but, depending on the analysis of the information provided, it can give clues as to possible causal factors and underlying speech and language processes. If, for example, speech and language development is significantly delayed, a question that would arise for the diagnostician is the possibility of slow mental development. The information about hearing provides essential data both about hearing loss as a problem and as a probable cause of a speech and language disorder. The diagnostician also might infer about the speech and language environment from such items as, "How well can he be understood by his parents, by his brothers and sisters, by his playmates, and by relatives and strangers?" If the child cannot be understood by those around him, it may tell us something about his overall communicative interaction with people in his environ-

---

FORM 4

General development section of the children's speech, language, and hearing history

IV. GENERAL DEVELOPMENT
A. Pregnancy and birth history

Total number of pregnancies _____ How many miscarriages, stillbirths? _____
Explain. _____
Which pregnancy was this child? ____ Length of pregnancy? ____ Was it difficult? ____
What illnesses, diseases, and accidents occurred during pregnancy? _____
Was there a blood incompatibility between the mother and father? _____
Age of mother at child's birth _____ Age of father at child's birth _____
What was the length of labor? _____ Were there any unusual problems at birth (breech birth, caesarean birth, others)? If so, describe. _____
_____

What drugs were used? _____ High or low forceps? _____ Weight of child at birth _____
Were there any bruises, scars, or abnormalities of the child's head? _____
Any other abnormalities? _____
_____

Did infant require oxygen? _____ Was child "blue" or jaundiced at birth? _____
Was a blood transfusion required at birth? _____
Were there any problems immediately following birth or during the first 2 weeks of the infant's life (health, swallowing, sucking, feeding, sleeping, others)? If so, describe.
_____
_____

At what age did infant regain birth weight? _____

B. Developmental

At what age did the following occur? Held head erect while lying on stomach _____
Rolled over alone _____ Sat alone unsupported _____ Crawled _____ Stood alone _____
Walked unaided ____ Fed self with spoon ____ Had first tooth ____ Bladder trained ____
Bowel trained ____ Completely toilet trained: Waking ____ Sleeping ____ Dressed and undressed himself ____ What hand does he prefer? ____ Has handedness ever been changed?
_____ If so, at what age? _____ How would you describe your child's current physical development? _____

ment. The question "Does he imitate speech but not use it?" is intended to help discover if a child may be repeating but not comprehending or formulating speech and language. Other questions are also designed to provide information about speech and language processes. Again, Chapters 3 through 8 are important for analyzing the information provided in this section.

A two-part section on general development (Form 4) follows the speech, language, and hearing history. The first part is

---

FORM 4—cont'd

Check these as they apply to your child.

	Yes	No	*Explain: give ages if possible.*
Cried less than normal amount			
Laughed less than normal amount			
Yelled and screeched to attract attention or express annoyance			
Head banging and foot stamping			
Extremely sensitive to vibration			
Very alert to gesture, facial expression, or movement			
Shuffled feet while walking			
Generally indifferent to sound			
Did not respond when spoken to			
Responded to noises (car horns, telephones) but not to speech			
Difficulty using tongue			
Difficulty swallowing			
Talked through nose			
Mouth breather			
Tongue-tied			
Difficulty chewing			
Drooled a lot			
Food came out nose			
Constant throat clearing			
Difficulty breathing			
Large tongue			
Difficulty moving mouth			

concerned with the pregnancy, birth, and first few weeks of life of the child—the prenatal, perinatal, and immediate postnatal history. The second part continues the general physical development of the child, including more specific information relevant to the auditory reception and speech production aspects of speech and language. Again, this information is ordered or asked for within a time-dimension framework. For the informants it is still apparent that these items are relevant to their primary concern, their child's speech and language problem.

The general development section is primarily causally oriented. These items assist the diagnostician in determining if there are any causal factors that may have primarily affected the internal speech and language processing component (Fig. 8-3 and the outline on p. 124). From his funds of knowledge the diagnostician knows that a child who had a difficult birth or is having physical development problems also may have associated speech and language disorders. Therefore these items can particularly assist in uncovering potential structural and neurologic deficits that may be causally related to the speech and language disorders. From this section the diagnostician should discover such potential factors as the presence of a cleft lip and palate, cerebral palsy, other neurologic problems, and mental retardation.

The chart presented in this section is more specific to the auditory reception segment and the speech production segment of the internal speech and language processing component of the SLPM. Items here are designed to "look at" certain behaviors that often reflect underlying hearing and speech mechanism disruptions. For example, the items "Talked through nose" and "Food came out nose" obviously relate in some way to palatal function; whereas the items "Difficulty using tongue" and "Difficulty moving mouth" relate to lip, jaw, and tongue activity. From certain constituents provided in this section, the diagnostician again will be able to infer certain disordered speech and language products. An obvious example would be if the informant checked that the child "talked through nose," the diagnostician should immediately suspect that the resonance product may be disordered.

Tying all this information together assists the diagnostician significantly in hypothesizing causal factors for speech and language disorders.

The next category of information presented on the case history form is medical history (Form 5). The concern of this section is additional specific data on the health status of the child, including information about the general medical care the child received in the past and currently. The items are asked in a way that the informant supplies the time dimension. They give information about the ages, times, and severity when certain medical events took place in the child's life.

The medical history section continues to add more information concerning possible causal factors for the speech and language disorder. The list of diseases and illnesses incorporates those that may be directly or indirectly related to speech and language disorders. A series of, or even single, illnesses, diseases, operations, and hospitalizations can account for certain speech and language disorders. As discussed in Chapter 8, speech and language disorders result from the interactions of multiple potential causal factors over time (Figs. 8-2 and 8-3). Knowing when these events occurred and for how long gives the diagnostician a time perspective on interacting situations in the life of the child that may be causally related to the speech and language disorder.

This section, again, assists in determining the validity and reliability of other data previously presented. If, for example, the child had tonsillitis, a tonsillectomy, and ear infections in the medical history, we could then refer back to the general development section to see if he may have been a mouth breather or if he may have been indifferent to sound for a period of time. Thus certain aspects of the data reported can be verified and cross-checked.

The behavior section of the case history

FORM 5

Medical history section of the children's speech, language, and hearing history

V. MEDICAL HISTORY

Is your child now under the care of a doctor? _____ Why? _____

Is he taking medication? _____ Type? _____ Why? _____

At what ages did any of the following illnesses, problems, or operations occur? Please indicate how serious they were.

	Age	Mild	Mod.	Severe		Age	Mild	Mod.	Severe
Adenoidectomy					Heart problems				
Allergies					High fevers				
Asthma					Influenza				
Blood disease					Mastoidectomy				
Cataracts					Measles				
Chickenpox					Meningitis				
Chronic colds					Mumps				
Convulsions					Muscle disorder				
Cross-eyed					Nerve disorder				
Croup					Orthodontia				
Dental problems					Pneumonia				
Diphtheria					Polio				
Earaches					Rheumatic fever				
Ear infections					Scarlet fever				
Encephalitis					Tonsillectomy				
Headaches					Tonsillitis				
Head injuries					Whooping cough				

Has the child ever fallen or had a severe blow to the head? _____ If so, did he lose consciousness? _____ Did it cause a concussion? _____ Did it cause: Nausea _____ Vomiting _____ Drowsiness _____ Describe any other serious illnesses, injuries, operations, or physical problems not mentioned above. _____

_____

What illnesses have been accompanied by an extremely long, high fever? _____

Temperature _____ How long did the fever last? _____

Which of the above required hospitalization? _____

Where was the child hospitalized? _____ For how long? _____

Who was the attending physician? _____

FORM 6

Behavior section of the children's speech, language, and hearing history

VI. BEHAVIOR

Check these as they apply to your child.

	Yes	*No*	*Explain: give ages if possible.*
Eating problems			
Sleeping problems			
Toilet training problems			
Difficulty concentrating			
Needed a lot of discipline			
Underactive			
Excitable			
Laughs easily			
Cried a lot			
Difficult to manage			
Overactive			
Sensitive			
Personality problem			
Gets along with children			
Gets along with adults			
Emotional			
Stays with an activity			
Makes friends easily			
Happy			
Irritable			
Prefers to play alone			

How do you discipline your child? _____

_____

What are the child's favorite play activities? _____

_____

form (Form 6) is a chart asking the informant to respond to a series of items that can describe the essential aspects of the child's behavior, both from an intrapersonal and an interpersonal viewpoint. The time-dimension framework is built in by asking the informant to specify the ages at which any of the items (behavioral signs) may have been significant.

From the responses to these items the diagnostician gets information about the social, emotional, psychological, and behavioral aspects of the child's life. These behaviors may signal an associated problem often seen in children with speech and language disorders. Sometimes these problems are causally related to the speech and language disorder; at other times they are only coincidental with the speech and language disorder, both existing side by side. Still at other times both the behavioral disorder and the speech and language disorder stem from the same underlying causal factor. At any rate, by the time the diagnostician sees the child the two are interacting in the total intra- and interpersonal life of the child.

Associated behaviors, as well, give indications of various underlying causal factors for speech and language disorders. They may provide a direct link to psychological-emotional mechanisms as well as to certain mental and neurologic conditions. For example, mental retardation and brain injury tend to produce certain types of behavioral responses as do hearing loss and deafness. Or the behavioral information provides added ingredients for the diagnostician's interpretation of the child's speech and language environment. For example, if he discovers that the child is happy, laughs easily, gets along with other children and

---

FORM 7

Educational history section of the children's speech, language, and hearing history

VII. EDUCATIONAL HISTORY

Did child attend day care or nursery school? _____ Where? _____ Ages _____

Kindergarten? _____ Where? _____ Ages _____

School now attending _____ Address _____

Grade he is now in _____ Grades skipped _____ Grades failed _____

What are his average grades? _____ Best subjects _____ Poorest _____

Is the child frequently absent from school? _____ If so, why? _____

How does child feel about school and about his teacher? _____

_____

What is your impression of your child's learning abilities? _____

_____

_____

Has anyone ever thought he was a slow child? _____

_____

Describe any speech, language, hearing, psychological, and special education services that have been performed including where this was done. How often was your child seen in this service? _____

_____

_____

adults, and makes friends easily in spite of a reported severe speech and language disorder, it tells the diagnostician something about the child's overall communicative interaction, his overall intra- and interpersonal relationships. Again, Fig. 8-3, which depicts the interactions of multiple causal factors, can assist the diagnostician in interpreting the significance of the information provided in the behavior section of the children's case history form.

The educational history (Form 7) provides information about educational experiences that add to the child's environmental background. Knowing if he is in school, how he is doing, and how he feels about school tells us more about him as an individual within an environmental context. As in all the sections, these items give information to the diagnostician about cause-effect relationships as well as potential management concerns.

Of significance from this section is information obtained about mental abilities, learning abilities, and overall intellectual abilities of the child that may have a bearing on the speech and language disorder. For example, knowing that a child is in a special class for the retarded, the diagnostician would develop expectations about the speech and language products that may be disordered. His funds of knowledge about mental retardation as a causal factor for speech and language disorders allow him to infer potential problems he may encounter. Tying the information obtained in this section with previous sections, the diagnostician might also learn the basis for the child's mental retardation; for example, it may have resulted from brain injury sustained at birth or in utero rather than being familial.

Again, certain items can be used for a reliability-validity check. For example, the information provided about adjustment to school can be related to previous information about the behavior of the child. This section, like others, also provides the diagnostician with sources from which to obtain further information.

The home and family section (Form 8)

adds to the information provided in the identification section, giving more insight into the family life-style. This section continues to provide information about cause-effect relationships. The emphasis here is on environmental factors that, in some way, may have affected the child's learning of speech and language—causal factors that affect the input stimulation received by the child. The occupation of the parents, the home and neighborhood, levels of education, source of income, and the address of the family can provide the basis for estimating socioeconomic status using the Warner et al. (1960) scale (see Johnson et al., 1963). Knowing the number, ages, and health status of the siblings and other members of the home as well as other languages spoken adds information about family living conditions. Interpersonal interactions and sociocultural information can be interpreted from these items. If there are other normal siblings, the parent's statement of the problem gains validity since they do have points of comparison, that is, the other children who have developed normal speech and language. Knowing as much as possible about the life-style of the family assists in planning the interpersonal approach to the diagnosis; diagnosticians must adapt their personal approaches, depending on the background of the families that seek their services. If financial considerations are important, the information provided in this section can be useful for determining the family's ability to pay for the services requested.

The student should now review several case history questionnaires using a similar type of analysis. He should determine how the history form has been constructed and what it offers for use in the constituent analysis. Barsch (1968) presents much useful information that assists the diagnostician in case history analysis and interpretation. Since a children's history form was discussed here as an example, we would suggest the student start with an adult case history form for comparative purposes.

FORM 8

**Home and family section of the children's speech,
language, and hearing history**

VIII. HOME AND FAMILY INFORMATION

Father's occupation _____ Last grade completed in school _____

Mother's occupation _____ Last grade completed in school _____

Brothers and sisters:

Name	Age	Sex	Grade in school	Speech, hearing, or medical problem
1.				
2.				
3.				
4.				
5.				
6.				
7.				
8.				

Are there any other languages spoken in the home? _____ If so, by whom and how often?

_____

Home and neighborhood (check all that apply): Residential _____ Business area _____
House ___ Rural ___ Above average ___ Housing development ___ Excellent condition ___
Apartment area ____ Average ____ Crowded ____ Suburban ____ Number of rooms? ____
Members of household other than family? _____
Primary source of income (check the appropriate blanks): Salary ___ Hourly wages ____
Commission _____ Welfare _____ Profits and fees _____ Savings and investments _____
Other _____
Please add any additional information you feel will help us in understanding your child
and his problem: _____

_____

_____

_____

_____

Letters and reports from other professionals. A final major source of information for the diagnostician is from other professionals who have had contact with the client. This source of information is usually the primary one in inpatient settings and other multidiscipline agencies. Often these reports are maintained in an intra-agency file, for example, a medical chart accessible to any professional in that setting. At other times letters or written reports are sent directly to the diagnostician. This information may accompany the professional referral as requested by the client, or the request for such information is initiated by the diagnostician, usually requiring client permission.

The responses the diagnostician receives from his requests understandably reflect the specialty of the professional or agency contacted. For example, if information is requested from a neurologist, he will most likely provide data about the medical status of the patient, emphasizing the neurologic disease or condition. He may also present some information about the speech behavior and, perhaps, indications of management and prognosis. Or if information is requested from hospital records, a duplicate copy of the medical charts of the patient during his hospitalization may be received, sometimes including the day-to-day nursing chart.

Since the diagnostician is requesting information from other involved professional sources, he can specify, to some extent, the information that he feels has a specific bearing on the client's speech and language disorder. A form letter can be constructed to serve this purpose; however, at times a personalized letter of request will be needed. This procedure varies with the diagnostician and the work setting (see request for information form in Appendix I).

Verbal reports and consults may also be obtained. Often when the diagnostician has an ongoing relationship with another professional who has seen the client, information is exchanged over the telephone. These phone contacts are initiated by either professional. In multidiscipline settings information is often transmitted verbally. For example, the diagnostician in a school setting may informally talk with the classroom teacher about the problems of a particular child.

Reliability and validity of the information base

Since the information used in the constituent analysis comes from these various sources, diagnosticians must consider how reliable and valid the information may be. The diagnostician must take into account the biases of the reporter, the memory of the reporter, the accuracy of the reporter, etc. All the information available must be viewed as just what it is—the perceptions of one or more people about another person, the client, reported to a third person, the diagnostician. This information contains all the flaws that exist in human perception—biases, inaccuracies, loss of details, judgments, overextensions, etc. Since the diagnostician only has some of the information important for diagnosing the client's speech and language disorder, he must evaluate it carefully. He knows that the data is second hand, filtered through other people, parents and professionals.

Information reported by parents may be about events that occurred some years before. The diagnostician can presume that the parents made the observations at the time they occurred, but how well can they recall the events that took place? At times this depends on the significance of the event in the parents' and client's life. For example, parents usually remember fairly accurately when their child took his first steps, an event that is awaited by parents. But all developmental events are not reported with such accuracy. Do the parents recall when the child said his first word, spoke in two-word sentences, and other details of their child's growth and development? Parents may also present certain biases when they report information about their child. Do they want us to believe that the child is more able than he is and, in some instances, less able than he is?

As well, professionals from whom information is obtained are not immune to perceptual inaccuracies. They too make errors in observing, measuring, and reporting information about their clients. The reports that are written are sometimes a recollection from sketchy notes of a visit that took place some time before. As much as we would like to, we do not always write reports immediately following contact with the client. Professionals, too, have biases and make errors of judgment. For example, a physician may have a bias for viewing all language-delayed children as aphasic.

If the diagnostician is to develop an accurate interpretation of the information available, he must recognize all these possible sources of distortion. The sources of error must be checked out by the diagnostician when doing his constituent analysis, since the constituent analysis and resulting hypotheses can only be as sound as the data from which they arise.

Varying amounts of information

The amount of data the diagnostician gathers about his prospective client can vary greatly. The variations generally reflect the needs the diagnostician has for the information and the policy established by the setting in which the diagnostician works. We have also encountered diagnosticians who do not want any previous information because "it can be biasing!"

Given sufficient time there is no limit to the amount of information the diagnostician can acquire prior to the diagnosis. He can gather information from the referral source, send out a case history questionnaire to be returned, ask for letters of information from sources that have been in contact with the client, and telephone and discuss the client with other professionals; he could also call the client or his family to gain more information regarding the problem and their intents and purposes for being seen. Of course, this must all be done judiciously, considered in terms of time, usefulness, and professional relationships.

In many settings the information commonly available consists of a referral and a case history form filled out by the client. However, there are many settings in which the information may be only in the form of a referral, often by telephone. This makes it important for the person who takes referral information to have a set of questions of primary significance to be asked. Ideally, he should obtain identifying information, the referral source, and ask the following basic questions: What is the problem? What do you think caused it? What has been done about it?

The diagnostician's tasks

In teaching the diagnostic process we will proceed throughout this book from the position that the diagnostician has several sources of information available to him, usually a referral statement, a completed case history questionnaire, and at times letters and reports from other concerned professionals. We feel that a student who masters the diagnostic process in this comprehensive manner will be far better prepared to perform diagnoses in settings where only minimal information is obtained.

From the client information base that he has gathered the diagnostician performs the two tasks specified in the constituent analysis. First, he lists and categorizes the available constituents and, second, he determines the significance of the constituents. It should be made clear that these two tasks are not distinct, separable entities but, more realistically, occur simultaneously. However, to facilitate learning to do the analysis and demonstrate its relevance to the overall planning of the diagnosis, we are treating these tasks as if they were distinct.

Lists and categorizes available constituents

The client information base provides the diagnostician with many constituents. A constituent is any piece or pieces of information or any relationship drawn by the diagnostician among the pieces of information. There is no single way to view constituents. The constituents come in many forms: reliable, personal, theoretical, situational, inferential, factual, abstract, meaningful, nonmeaningful, explanatory, valid, unreliable, etc.

The diagnostician must ascertain what each constituent reveals to him and how valid and reliable it is. For example, a constituent may be factual and reliable (Pamela is 3 years old), theoretical and explanatory (Fred does not talk because

FORM 9

Constituent analysis form

	SLPM: Cause-effect categorization			
	Speech and language environment component—causal factors affecting	*Internal processing component—causal factors affecting*	*Speech and language product component—variations/disorders*	
Client identification				*Management consideration*
Purpose of diagnosis	(Consider speech and language input, total environmental context, and causal factors)	(Consider anatomy, physical processes, behavioral correlates, and causal factors for all segments)	(Consider levels and characteristics of speech and language products affected)	(Consider information that leads you to think about possible management needs)
General (Diagnostician's job)				
Referral (Consider purposes asked by referral source)				*Behavioral consideration*
Statement of problem				(Consider information that may help you manage the client's behavior during the diagnostic session)
(Consider how the problem has been stated by different people concerned with the client)				
Further information needed				*Incidental information*
Interview (Consider questions you may want to ask to gather more information)				(Information that may be useful but is not categorized elsewhere)

To use this form for doing his constituent analysis, the diagnostician should be completely familiar with the material presented in Part I of this book.

he doesn't want to), abstract (Judy has a speech disorder), personal and situational (Todd talks like his father), and non-meaningful and unreliable (Aiko's speech problem started at birth). Of course, no constituent is only in one form; the same constituent could be abstract, reliable, personal, and situational. All constituents require examination and validation; the diagnostician must sort out all the constituents that come to him in their many forms.

The diagnostician's first task in the constituent analysis, listing and categorizing the constituents, can be thought of as taking an inventory of the available information. As in all inventories, the diagnostician must develop a format for taking his inventory. His inventory should reflect the purposes of his job—to define and delimit the client's clinical problem from all other speech and language disorders. Therefore his inventory should be listed within categories relevant to this job.

To facilitate listing and categorizing constituents we have devised a format represented in Form 9, a constituent analysis form. The form is designed to integrate

Table 9. Categorization of selected constituents from the information available about Katherine Compardo*

Constituent	Categorization
Four older siblings with no speech, hearing, or medical problems	Speech and language input
Gets along with other children and adults	Speech and language input Behavioral considerations Speech and language product (?)—what role does her speech and language play in getting along with others?
Family lives in a residential, average, suburban neighborhood in a six-room house	Speech and language input—environment
Pediatrician listed as the referral source	Further information needed Cause-effect—if pediatrician referred, there is reinforcement for the presence of some type of speech and language disorder
Understands everything she is told	Internal processing—comprehension and language representation Further information—interview Behavioral considerations
Only speaks a few words	Speech and language product—language product Cause-effect Internal processing—formulation and speech production segment; language representation and speech programming
Makes most sounds incorrectly	Speech and language product—phonetic structure and phonology Internal processing—speech programming and remainder of speech production segment; behavioral correlates and physical processes
When baby was infant, I questioned her hearing because she was so quiet; now I am sure she can hear; I have just convinced myself there was nothing wrong; now I have to start thinking otherwise	Internal processing—auditory reception segment Further information—interview Purpose of diagnosis Statement of problem

*The student should complete this categorization of Katherine Compardo's constituents.

client constituents into the framework developed in this book, emphasizing the SLPM and cause-effect relationships. The student must continuously refer back to Chapters 3 through 8 and the figures and tables provided in those chapters to fully utilize the approach presented here. Form 9 assists the diagnostician in keeping in mind a number of important considerations for defining and delimiting his client's clinical problem.

1. Identification data
2. General purposes of diagnosis
3. Specific purpose of each diagnosis
4. Characteristics of the speech and language disorder
5. Causal factors to be considered
6. Management considerations
7. Sources and types of further information that may be needed
8. Information that may assist in controlling behavioral problems that might occur during the diagnostic session
9. Incidental information that might prove relevant but cannot be categorized elsewhere on the form.

The diagnostician should remember that any single constituent might be categorized in more than one place; a causal constituent can also be used as an effect constituent. For example, a 4 year-old child who is only speaking in one-word sentences is obviously having trouble with language (an effect constituent). This extremely slow language development might also be signaling a causal constituent— mental retardation, hearing loss, etc.

■ At this point we will introduce our demonstration client, *Katherine Compardo*. Katherine will be used throughout the remainder of the book as our primary example for illustrating the diagnostician's tasks at each of the steps of the diagnostic process.

Katherine Compardo was referred to a community speech and hearing agency by her mother at the suggestion of Katherine's pediatrician. The information obtained was the telephone data on the request for service form and a children's case history questionnaire that was sent out, completed by the mother, and returned to the agency. No further information was received or requested prior to the diagnosis. This client information is reproduced in Appendix II.

From this information certain constituents have been selected to demonstrate the diagnostician's task of categorization. Following the recommendations on Form 9, the constituent analysis form, Table 9 presents the selected constituents and their categorization.

Determines significance of the constituents

Once the diagnostician has listed and categorized the constituents according to the format provided, he is ready for the second task, determining the significance of the available constituents. The diagnostician wants to find out if he has relevant and secure constituents (theoretically and factually) for defining and delimiting his clinical problem. He does this by examining the constituents in relationship to his professional funds of knowledge and experience.

■ $Constituent_1$ "Bruce's father died when he was 3 months old and that is why he doesn't talk."

That Bruce's father died is factual; however, as a cause for Bruce's not talking, it is not theoretically secure. We would be hard pressed to discover either from our clinical experience or from the literature such a direct cause-effect relationship. We would have to approach this constituent from a more indirect route; for example, did the death of the father create other problems, which in turn more directly affected Bruce's speech and language development?

The diagnostician must develop the relations that exist among the constituents. This lets him see how the parts relate to the whole. He must develop a unitary picture of the constituents that encompasses all the relationships among the pieces of information. He must extract as much meaning as possible from each bit of information relative to every other bit of information if he is to gain a clear perspective of his clients' clinical problem.

■ $Constituent_2$ "Gretchen did not walk until she was 20 months old."
  $Constituent_3$ "Gretchen did not say her first word until she was 24 months old."

$Constituent_4$ "Gretchen is now 6 years old."

$Constituent_5$ "Gretchen only has 50 words that we understand."

These constituents could be analyzed as a group. Each offers important information, but as parts of a whole, the diagnostician can draw a better analysis of their significance. A child who does not walk until this age is quite late in motor development. What are the potential reasons for such late development? How can this information be related to the data about speech and language development that were also quite late (the normal age of the first word is more like 10 to 12 months, and at 6 years of age normal children have a relatively complete, sophisticated use of language)? Since these constituents are factual and some describe the speech and language characteristics, how can they be used by the diagnostician to infer certain causal factors? What literature might he want to explore to secure his inferences?

When determining the significance and relevance of the constituents, the diagnostician proceeds to designate the strength each constituent has for explaining the clinical problem. Within a given category he may "rule in" and "rule out" certain constituents. Those constituents that appear to bear no explanatory relationship to the problem are disregarded (ruled out), while those that appear to demonstrate a relationship are retained (ruled in) for further investigation. The constituents retained are those that offer a more secure explanation of the speech and language disorder.

■ $Constituent_6$ Mother: "Dorothy isn't talking well because her two older sisters talk for her."

$Constituent_7$ Teacher: "Dorothy doesn't talk much because she is shy and doesn't want to talk."

$Constituent_8$ School psychologist: "Dorothy's speech is difficult to understand because she talks softly."

$Constituent_9$ Dorothy: "I don't talk much because I'm afraid I will stutter."

How many of these statements of the problem constituents are factual and theoretically secure? Each source of information provides different reasons for what they all agree on—something seems to be wrong with Dorothy's speech. How would the diagnostician go about ruling in and out these various constituents? Can any literature support be found for the causal factors stated in these constituents? For example, what role do older siblings play in the development and use of speech by a younger sibling? Would a series of interacting factors rather than a direct cause-effect relationship be more likely?

The diagnostician must constantly return to the professional literature if he is to keep abreast of information that helps explain the significance of the constituents he is examining. It is in this task, the determining of significance of the constituents, that the diagnostician continues to expand his professional knowledge and, in turn, his expertise as a diagnostician. This constant expansion of clinical expertise keeps the diagnostic error rate down; it helps prevent misdiagnoses from occurring, jumping to unwarranted conclusions about cause-effect relationships.

■ $Constituent_{10}$ "My boy Maury stutters because his father does."

This is an inferential constituent, an explanation provided presumably by the mother. This constituent also has potential factual data; that is, "my boy stutters." This could be an accurate behavioral observation based on the mother's ability to observe and know what stuttering is in children. To give significance to this constituent, the diagnostician could explore his professional literature to answer such questions as What is stuttering in children? How is it misperceived by parents? What is the occurrence of stuttering in children? At what age is it seen? Also of importance is the direct cause-effect relationship stated by the mother. Is it probable that a child learns to stutter because his father does? How would Maury's stuttering behavior be similar to, or different from, his father's? Can stuttering be learned? Or is something else learned; that is, does the child learn from his father that speech is difficult? What do the theories say about stuttering as a learned behavior? All of this information must be considered regarding this constituent to determine how secure it may be for clinical purposes.

Errors in diagnosis can occur. The only way to circumvent these errors and potential misdiagnosis is to develop our funds of knowledge to the greatest extent possible, knowing what we know and what we don't know, making it our professional responsibility to learn what we need to know. For example, if a diagnostician is confronted with a child who, unknown to him, is mentally retarded, and the diagnostician has little information about the relationship between mental retardation and speech and language, he may miss mental retardation as a causal factor. But he may go on and make a diagnosis since that is his job. Thus he may come up with a misdiagnosis. For him, the child might be deaf, emotionally disturbed, or brain injured—whatever seems to best tie the client's behavior to the diagnostician's fund of knowledge.

The constituent analysis step of the diagnostic process helps circumvent these diagnostic errors. This step requires the diagnostician to constantly review the constituents presented about his client and to seek out information from the literature that helps him determine the significance of the constituents. The exacting use of this step should prevent the occurrence of too many misdiagnoses.

■ *Constituent*₁₁ "Mrs. Metz has aphasia." This constituent would most likely come from a physician who has made a medical diagnosis of aphasia. It is a constituent that is both factual and inferential but highly theoretically secure. A cause-effect relationship is stated in the constituent. Aphasia is a language disorder due to brain injury. But the diagnostician should not be completely secure. In our experience we have received referrals like this only to discover that the client was not aphasic but rather dysarthric. There are many considerations that go into an analysis of this constituent. What is aphasia? What causes the aphasia? For this client, we would want to consider how the aphasia is manifested; does it need to be differentiated from other speech and language disorders resulting from neurologic damage? Undue assumptions about a referral constituent can lead to misdiagnosis.

If the diagnostician has categorized all the constituents according to the format presented (Form 9), it becomes most efficient for him to determine their significance and examine their relevancy according to the categories on the constituent analysis form. He can choose to examine the significance of individual constituents within a category, look at groups of constituents within a category, or examine the entire category simultaneously.

■ Turning to our example client, Katherine Compardo, we again present a selection of constituents accompanied by a discussion of their significance (Table 10). We present them in different ways to demonstrate this task. Some will be individual constituents and others constituents grouped within categories. The way we have chosen to group certain constituents within categories is in no way meant to be standard practice. Constituents can be grouped in any number of ways, using the SLPM for grouping and determining the significance of the constituents. Grouping can be based on single behavioral correlates, a series of physical processes, combinations of physical processes and behavioral correlates, specific causal factors affecting one of the components of the SLPM, etc. The diagnostician is assisted in his delimitation of the clinical problem by viewing the constituents within a variety of categories; however, no categorization will answer all the clinical questions.

Because the constituent analysis as a part of the scientific framework must be adaptable to varying amounts of information, we also want to briefly discuss how the diagnostician might proceed to think through a constituent analysis with only a referral statement as his source of information. In instances where little information is available on which to do a constituent analysis, the diagnostician must rely completely on his funds of knowledge and clinical experience.

For example, consider the following referral statement from a mother about her 4-year-old boy, "Devin has a speech problem." Depending on how this referral is viewed, there is either a single constituent (Devin has a speech problem) or five constituents (name, age, sex, speech problem, and referral from the mother). How can this be analyzed? The referral statement

Table 10. Determination of significance of selected constituents from client information available about Katherine Compardo[*]

Constituents	Significance
Only speaks a few words	Katherine is now 27 months of age. The following sources indicate that a child this age should have a vocabulary of 300 to 400 words and be speaking in two- or three-word phrases, using nouns, prepositions, verbs, adjectives, and pronouns (Anderson et al., 1963; Dale, 1972; Hopper and Naremore, 1973; Lee, 1966; Lenneberg, 1967).
	With this constituent we can at least say that Katherine is far behind the normal in use of words. There is much more that could be discussed regarding the significance and relevance of this single constituent as it relates to the SLPM. Of relevance is what the constituent says about Katherine's language formulation and, by inference, the physical process of language representation.
	Berry (1969), Eisenson (1972), Irwin and Marge (1972), and Morley (1972) consider that such a delay may signal the disorder labeled childhood aphasia.
Makes most of her sounds incorrectly	Children Katherine's age usually have a fairly well-developed repertoire of speech sound usage (Menyuk, 1971; Sander, 1972; Templin, 1957; Winitz, 1969).
	This constituent also adds to our information about late acquisition of the speech and language system. Again, Katherine appears to be far behind what would be expected. This constituent should be considered for its relevance to the speech production segment of the SLPM, beginning with the physical process of speech programming as well as to the speech and language product component. Eisenson (1972), McCarthy and McCarthy (1973), Morley (1972), Perkins (1971), and Yoss and Darley (1974) discuss late acquisition and difficulty with speech sounds as a characteristic of the disorder labeled apraxia of speech in children.
Sensation, perception, comprehension	
Some of the constituents that help determine if Katherine hears and comprehends speech and language using behavioral correlates as a basis for grouping	From these constituents we can determine some things about Katherine's ability to hear, perceive, and comprehend. A variable history is presented, the mother at one time seeing signs that made her believe Katherine was not hearing as an infant. However, the constituents indicate that she hears appropriately at this time. (See constituents about her responses to sound and ability to comprehend.) We might be able to conclude from this that Katherine's hearing mechanism is intact—the physical processes of auditory acceptance-transduction, auditory analysis-transmission, and perhaps auditory reception-analysis. Thus the behavioral correlates of sensation and certain aspects of perception may be relatively intact. There may be a question about the behavioral correlate of perception as it relates to the physical process of auditory programming. Katherine's difficulties with developing language and producing speech sounds may signal problems in auditory processing. The literature on the relationship of speech and language acquisition to auditory perception is equivocal, depending on the studies read (Rees, 1973). What do our constituents offer us in regard to auditory perception?
Hears adequately now but mother concerned about hearing as an infant; quiet as an infant	
No lack of response when spoken to; responds to noises and voice	
Responds to telephone and car horn	
Not indifferent to sound	
Yelled and screamed to attract attention	
Alert to gesture, facial expression, movement	
Did not babble and coo much during the first 6 months	
Did not imitate sounds during the first and second years	
Had no words at 1½ years of age	

[*] These examples in no way reflect all the constituents available on Katherine Compardo nor their examination for significance and relevance. Many more clinical questions need to be asked. The student should continue the examination of the constituents available until they feel they are ready to derive and support a clinical hypothesis.

Continued.

Table 10. Determination of significance of selected constituents from client information available about Katherine Compardo—cont'd

Constituents	Significance
Sensation, perception, comprehension— cont'd	
Spoke her first word at 2 years of age Understands everything she is told Currently prefers to use one or two words Makes most of her sounds incorrectly Uses speech occasionally; prefers to use gestures	The report that Katherine, although responsive to sound, did not babble and coo, was a quiet infant, did not imitate sounds, was late in language acquisition, and makes many sounds incorrectly, indicates that the behavioral correlates of perception of the language stimulus may be a problem. Lack of speech and language development may occur because of auditory processing deficits even when there is no hearing loss. Eisenson (1972), McReynolds (1966), Morley (1972), Myklebust (1954), and Yoss and Darley (1974) all point to auditory processing problems in children labeled as aphasic children who have a significant delay in speech and language acquisition. However, the constituent that Katherine understands everything she is told looms in front of us. Does she really comprehend everything? What is she asked to comprehend? So the question regarding auditory processing, the relationship between the behavioral correlates of perception and comprehension, should remain open.
Language representation—speech programming	
Constituents that help us determine if Katherine can formulate and sequence speech and language using physical processes as a basis for grouping	Many of the constituents listed within this category are the same as used for demonstration in the previous category. How might these constituents be used to examine the relevancy and significance for language formulation and sequencing?
Quiet as an infant Did not babble and coo much during the first 6 months Did not imitate sounds during the first and second years Had no words at 1½ years of age Spoke her first word at 2 years of age; first words were "here," "daddy," and "hi" Currently prefers to use one or two words—only speaks a few words Uses speech occasionally; prefers to use gestures Just isn't talking Makes most of her sounds incorrectly Difficulty using her tongue and moving her mouth when she talks	
Mother reports Katherine understood by parents etc., response is "everything" to all the items	We would question the validity of this response by the mother. It seems as if she interpreted the question to mean How well does Katherine understand these people? See mother's responses elsewhere that Katherine "understands everything."
Causal factors affecting internal processing system	
See outline on p. 124 for the rationale for grouping the constituents under this category; for this grouping we will not include any constituents about the speech and language product, physical processes, behavioral correlates, or speech and language	First, as mentioned, there are many other constituents that may tell as much if not more about disruptions of the internal processing system than those categorized here. We are simply providing another example of how constituents can be examined for relevancy to a client. Each client requires different forms of categorization for delimitation.

Table 10. Determination of significance of selected constituents from client information available about Katherine Compardo—cont'd

Constituents	Significance
Causal factors affecting internal processing system—cont'd	
environment that might be relevant to causal factors for Katherine's speech and language disorder; our interest in this categorization is the relationship between certain causal factors and bodily systems that can have an effect on the internal speech and language processing system	
Length of pregnancy, 9 months	Each of the constituents listed here can be fitted into the categories given in the outline on p. 124, factors primarily affecting the internal speech and language processing system. Each of them can be reviewed in relationship to the professional literature. For example, Katherine did not walk until she was 15 months of age. From Church and Stone (1973), Frankenburg and Dodds (1967), and Mussen et al. (1969), we get a range for onset of walking from 12 to 18 months. Therefore walking as an isolated constituent may give little information and must be examined in relationship to other physical development. What do these same sources give as an age for crawling?
No accidents or illnesses during pregnancy	
No blood incompatibility	
Five pregnancies; no history of miscarriages or stillbirths	
No problems with delivery; no drugs or instruments used	
Mother 36 years of age at time of birth	
Length of labor, 5 hours	
No unusual problems at birth	
No oxygen required for infant	
No immediate postnatal problems	
Held head erect (2 to 3 weeks); sat alone (3 months); crawled (10 months); walked unaided (15 months); fed self with a spoon (1½ years)	Review the constituents presented here in light of the information about physical development, birth history, and general behavior of children classified as aphasic and apraxic. (See Chase, 1972; Eisenson, 1972; Johnson and Myklebust, 1967; McCarthy and McCarthy, 1973; Morley, 1972; Yoss and Darley, 1974.) What would these constituents offer regarding mental retardation? (See Lillywhite and Bradley, 1969.)
Seems much slower (physically) than my other children	
Prefers both hands	
Difficulty using her tongue and mouth when she talks	
Mild case of chickenpox	
No serious medical history	
No severe blows to the head	
Quiet as an infant	
No eating, sleeping, toilet training problems	
Not difficult to manage	
Yelled and screeched to attract attention (all along)	
Alert to gesture, facial expression, and movement since she was a baby	
Difficulty concentrating—runs around a lot	
Overactive—runs around a lot	
Makes friends easily; plays both alone and with other children; gets along with other children and adults	
Mother's nephew did not start talking until he was 29 months old	

says speech rather than language. But do referral sources make a differentiation between these two as the professional diagnostician might do? How do parents make referral statements?

In our experience, parents, using their own terminology, often do state different problems in different ways. For example, in terms of speech versus language problems we have received statements that do lead in one direction or another such as: "He doesn't understand what I say to him." "He doesn't talk good." "He doesn't make his sounds right." "I can't understand him when he talks." "He can't say anything like he should." "He doesn't move his tongue when he talks." An interesting statement of the problem was presented by one mother about her daughter. She stated, "Sandy uses nasal sounds and puts an *e* on the ends of words." Puts an *e* on the ends of words did not mean much for the constituent analysis at the time. However, after the diagnosis the accuracy of the mother's description was noted. The child was extremely unintelligible, producing strings of vowel sounds with glottal stops to signal syllabic production. Many of the vowels were produced nasally, increased in duration, and the final vowel of the string was a prolonged /i/. A transcription of several words would look something like this: /æ:ʔĩ:/ for rabbit and /ũ:ʔĩ:/ for music.

Devin's referral constituent requires the diagnostician to review the types of speech and language disorders that occur in children and how often they occur. From this he could list in order the most probable areas of disorder. The incidence data available might lead him to first expect a disorder in phonology, in our framework a language disorder on the phonologic level, and in more general terminology an articulation disorder. However, since so little is known, alternative potentials must be developed. Devin might have a language disorder on more than the phonologic level. From incidence data the diagnostician might expect a language disorder at the next highest level of incidence. Thus from his funds of

knowledge the diagnostician can determine the significance of this referral constituent and develop from it a series of hypotheses from most to least likely. How likely would it be that Devin stutters or has a voice disorder? In our experience it would not be too likely, since parents tune into stuttering and voice, and seldom express it simply as a speech problem; rather they come right to the point of their concern, "Devin stutters."

So even if limited information is available prior to diagnosis, the diagnostician can develop an approach to the constituent analysis that would be more efficient than if he just waited until the person came. Another way of viewing the constituent analysis when no other information comes would be to order the analysis to tap all the probabilities that may exist. From knowledge about speech and language as reflected in the SLPM a constituent analysis could be set up that leads to a global hypothesis: all behaviors and processes may be affected, which would require systematic sampling of the various speech and language behaviors and processes.

■ What might you consider the general problem to be in the following referrals? What are the constituents? (1) From the second-grade teacher, "Sue isn't doing well in my class because of her speech problem. Will you see her for me?" (2) From the pediatrician, "Mrs. Starr will be calling you about her daughter Brenda who isn't talking. Please see her as soon as you can." (3) From the neurologist, "Mr. McGee has a strange speech pattern, but we haven't found any neurologic basis for it. Does he need speech therapy?"

In these referrals a number of clinical questions can be developed and examined for relevancy. For example, from Mr. McGee's referral we can assume that we are going to be seeing an adult (why?) who for some reason went to a neurologist. The speech pattern has been described as strange. Does this mean the neurologist has never heard speech like this? Surely if Mr. McGee was stuttering, the neurologist would have recognized that pattern of speech behavior, but perhaps not; it may be a very atypical pattern of nonfluency. If the speech pattern were neurologically based, would the neurologist not have recognized it? Not necessarily, since speech sometimes deteriorates in neurologic disease before the disease can be diagnosed by neurologic testing. Could Mr. McGee have sustained a minor cerebrovascular accident that went undetected except for this speech pattern, which the neurologist did not recognize as related to a possible cerebrovascular accident? These are only some of the constituents that can arise from the diagnostician's fund of knowledge about this specific referral. What are others you may want to examine in this referral as well as in the other examples?

SUMMARY

The constituent analysis, the first step of the diagnostic process, consists of two major tasks performed by the diagnostician.

1. He lists and categorizes the bits of information he obtains about his client.
2. He determines the significance of these constituents for defining and delimiting his clinical problem.

The diagnostician's overall goal in this step is to develop a baseline of relevant information about the client he is to see. To do this he uses two primary sources of information—his professional knowledge and the specific client information he has gathered. Available to him for gathering information are referral sources, case history questionnaires, and letters and reports from other professionals.

When he has completed the constituent analysis, the diagnostician knows what relevant information he has available about his client's speech and language disorder—its characteristics and its potential causes. From this he is now ready to derive his clinical hypothesis, his clinical perspective on the most likely cause-effect relationship. He has begun to meet the goals of diagnosis—to determine the nature of the speech and language disorder, to understand its causes, and to propose appropriate client management.

A CLIENT PROJECT
William Gafford

The student should now do a detailed constituent analysis on a client following the guidelines and procedures set forth in this chapter. The client for this project is 46-year-old Reverend William Gafford. Reverend Gafford called the clinic on October 17, 1975, immediately following his ear, nose, and throat examination. Information was obtained from Reverend Gafford and recorded on the request for service form. His physicians, Drs. Gershon and Lefkoff, made the recommendation. Because of his chief complaint of hoarseness that was affecting his occupation as a pastor, he was given an immediate appointment 2 days later. A call was placed to Drs. Gershon and Lefkoff who provided verbal information that was then included in a referral letter that arrived on the day of the diagnosis. No history questionnaire was sent out. The information available on Reverend Gafford can be found in Appendix II.

Because of the limited amount of information available on Reverend Gafford, the student will have to explore the literature carefully and develop many of his own constituents for exploring potential cause-effect relationships. The following could serve as primary resources (Boone, 1971; Brodnitz, 1961; Cooper, 1973; Greene, 1964; Moore, 1971; Van Riper and Irwin, 1958).

REFERENCES

Anderson, R. M., Miles, M., and Matheny, P. A., *Communicative Evaluation Chart from Infancy to Five Years.* Cambridge, Mass.: Educators Publishing Service, Inc. (1963).

Barsch, R. H., *The Parent of the Handicapped Child.* Springfield, Ill.: Charles C Thomas, Publisher (1968).

Berry, M. F., *Language Disorders of Children: The Bases and Diagnosis.* New York: Appleton-Century-Crofts (1969).

Boone, D. B., *The Voice and Voice Therapy,* Englewood Cliffs, N.J.: Prentice-Hall, Inc. (1971).

Brodnitz, F. S., Contact ulcer of the larynx. *Arch. Otolaryng.,* **74,** 70-80 (1961).

Brown, C. W., and Ghiselli, E. E., *Scientific Method in Psychology.* New York: McGraw-Hill Book Co. (1955).

Chase, R. A., Neurological aspects of language disorders in children. In J. V. Irwin and M. Marge (Eds.), *Principles of Childhood Language Disabilities.* New York: Appleton-Century-Crofts (1972).

Church, J., and Stone, L., *Childhood and Adolescence: A Psychology of the Growing Person.* New York: Random House, Inc. (1973).

Cooper, M., *Modern Techniques of Vocal Rehabilitation.* Springfield, Ill.: Charles C Thomas, Publisher (1973).

Dale, P., *Language Development Structure and Function.* Hinsdale, Ill.: Dryden Press (1972).

Dickson, S., and Jann, G. R., Diagnostic principles and procedures. In S. Dickson (Ed.), *Communication Disorders: Remedial Principles and Practices.* Glenview, Ill.: Scott, Foresman & Co. (1974).

Eisenson, J., *Aphasia in Children.* New York: Harper & Row, Publishers, (1972).

Frankenburg, W. K., and Dodds, J. B., *Denver Developmental Screening Test.* Denver: University of Colorado Medical Center (1967).

Greene, M. C. L., *The Voice and Its Disorders.* (2nd ed.) Philadelphia: J. B. Lippincott Co. (1964).

Hopper, R., and Naremore, R., *Children's Speech: A Practical Introduction to Communication Development.* New York: Harper & Row, Publishers (1973).

Irwin J., and Marge, M. (Eds.), *Principles of Childhood Language Disabilities.* Englewood Cliffs, N.J.: Prentice-Hall, Inc. (1972).

Johnson, D. J., and Myklebust, H. R., *Learning Disabilities: Educational Principles and Practice.* New York: Grune & Stratton, Inc. (1967).

Johnson, W., Darley F., and Spriestersbach, D., *Diagnostic Methods in Speech Pathology.* New York: Harper & Row, Publishers (1963).

Lee, L., Developmental sentence types: A method for comparing normal and deviant syntactic development. *J. Speech Hearing Dis.,* **31,** 311-330 (1966).

Lenneberg, E., *Biological Foundations of Language.* New York: John Wiley & Sons, Inc. (1967).

Lillywhite, H. S., and Bradley, D. P., *Communication Problems in Mental Retardation: Diagnosis and Management.* New York: Harper & Row, Publishers (1969).

McCarthy, J. J., and McCarthy, J. F., *Learning Disabilities.* Boston: Allyn & Bacon, Inc. (1973).

McReynolds, L. V., Operant conditioning for investigating speech sound discrimination in aphasic children. *J. Speech Hearing Res.,* **7,** 519-528 (1966).

Menyuk, P., *The Acquisition and Development of Language.* Englewood Cliffs, N.J.: Prentice-Hall, Inc. (1971).

Milisen, R., Methods of evaluation and diagnosis of speech disorders. In L. E. Travis (Ed.), *Handbook of Speech Pathology and Audiology.* New York: Appleton-Century-Crofts (1971).

Moore, G. P., Voice disorders organically based. In L. E. Travis (Ed.), *Handbook of Speech Pathology and Audiology.* New York: Appleton-Century-Crofts (1971).

Morley, M., *The Development and Disorders of Speech in Childhood.* (3rd ed.) Baltimore: The Williams & Wilkins Co. (1972).

Mussen, P. H., Conger, J. J., and Kagan, J., *Child Development and Personality.* New York: Harper & Row, Publishers (1969).

Myklebust, H. R., *Auditory Disorders in Children: A Manual for Differential Diagnosis.* New York: Grune & Stratton, Inc. (1954).

Perkins, W. H., *Speech Pathology: An Applied Behavioral Science.* (2nd ed.) St. Louis: The C. V. Mosby Co. (1977).

Rees, N. S., Auditory processing factors in language disorders: The view from Procrustes' bed. *J. Speech Hearing Dis.,* **38,** 304-315 (1973).

Sander, E., When are speech sounds learned? *J. Speech Hearing Dis.,* **36,** 55-67 (1972).

Templin, M. C., *Certain Language Skills in Children, Their Development and Interrelationships.* Institute of Child Welfare, Monograph Series 26, Minneapolis: University of Minnesota Press (1957).

Van Riper, C., and Irwin, J. V., *Voice and Articulation.* Englewood Cliffs, N.J.: Prentice-Hall, Inc. (1958).

Warner, W. L., Meeker, M., and Eells, K., *Social Class in America.* New York: Harper & Row, Publishers (1960).

Winitz, H., *Articulatory Acquisition and Behavior.* New York: Appleton-Century-Crofts (1969).

Yoss, K. A., and Darley, F. L., Developmental apraxia of speech in children with defective articulation. *J. Speech Hearing Res.,* **17,** 399-416 (1974).

Chapter 12

Development of the clinical hypothesis: cause-effect relationships

The development of the clinical hypothesis, done prior to client contact, is the second step of the diagnostic process as outlined in Fig. 10-1. The clinical hypothesis is a formal statement by the diagnostician of the cause-effect relationship he derives from his constituent analysis. He uses his best reasoning abilities to arrive at a statement that offers a logical explanation of the clinical problem.

In the constituent analysis the diagnostician categorized and determined the significance of the constituents. To derive the clinical hypothesis, the diagnostician must now draw together causal constituents and effect constituents and integrate these constituents into cause-effect relationships. He narrows down the number of possible explanations for the clinical problem, forming priorities among the potential cause-effect relationships until he has derived his most likely explanation of the speech and language disorder and its causes.

The derivation of the clinical hypothesis serves several purposes for the diagnostician. Hypothesis statements are attempts to clarify the clinical problem by expressing potential cause-effect relationships. The hypothesis implies a level of understanding rather than a level of knowing. The hypothesis is not a statement of facts, nor is it a "dead-end" statement; it is a tentative statement of understanding.

The hypothesis also offers a tentative solution to the speech and language problem. The hypothesis is inferential and predictive; it has a forward reference in that it expresses a relationship that requires further examination. The role of hypothesis formulation is to derive a dynamic cause-effect relationship used for exploring the client's problem, remembering the complex interactions between speech and language disorders and their potential causes. In general, the clinical hypothesis provides a thrust and an organization for the completion of the diagnostic process. Therefore the hypothesis is always under scrutiny, and in the practical world of diagnosis it may change during the diagnostic process. It undergoes modification as more insight is gained into the clinical problem. Hypothesis derivation, as expressed by Schultz (1973), is a continuous recycling process as more data are gained about the client.

THE CLINICAL HYPOTHESIS: HOW IT IS DONE
Information bases: nature and sources

In order to perform the tasks for deriving the clinical hypothesis the diagnostician relies on three fundamental sources of information. First, he has the client information from his constituent analysis. Second, he returns to his funds of knowledge, particularly those that emphasize cause-effect interactions within the SLPM framework. Third, he relies on his knowledge of problem solving and his ability to reason logically. All of these information bases have previously been discussed in some detail. Here we will only make minor comments and refer the reader back to appropriate sections of this book.

The constituent analysis was discussed in Chapter 11, step 1 of the diagnostic process. In this step the diagnostician analyzed the client information. He categorized the information in reference to the SLPM and examined its significance for explaining the clinical problem. These constituent analysis data now represent the client data needed for deriving a clinical hypothesis.

In addition to the constituent analysis information the diagnostician must return to his fund of knowledge, emphasizing cause-effect interactions within the SLPM perspective. Chapters 7 and 8 in Part I detailed causal factors and their relationship to speech and language disorders. The complexity of causation seen in different levels of abstraction, multiple causation, direct-indirect effects, chains of cause-effect interactions, and variables of time and severity were stressed. The diagnostician must keep in mind that cause-effect relationships are complex interactions taking place over time. They are not static factors found in the history of clients with speech and language disorders. An extensive literature search is often necessary to discover how a suspected causal factor might be related to the speech and language disorder. In deriving his clinical hypothesis the diagnostician must apply the information and theory presented in Chapter 8. He should pay particular attention to the framework for interpreting causal factors that affect the various components of the SLPM, the SLPM now representing the client being diagnosed. Fig. 8-3, which schematizes the basic causal interactions, and the project developed in Table 8 will be instrumental in achieving sophistication in deriving clinical hypotheses.

To derive the "best" clinical hypotheses the diagnostician must be skilled in problem solving. This information was detailed in Chapter 9 and presented as the scientific method, the diagnostician's major tool. Because so little is known about cause-effect relationships for speech and language disorders, and because at times there is so little information available about clients, diagnosticians often work inferentially. The diagnostician must recognize the strengths and weaknesses of the inferences he makes, using his deductive and inductive reasoning abilities in the most logical way for deriving appropriate hypotheses for testing.

Diagnostician's tasks

Our focus in this second step of the diagnostic process—development of the clinical hypothesis—is on ordering and integrating the constituents from the first step into expressed cause-effect relationships. What causes go with what effects?

To complete step 2, three tasks are required of the diagnostician. First, he derives the clinical hypothesis by examining the various relationships that exist between causes and effects, thereby developing a hierarchy of probable cause-effect explanations. Second, he states the clinical hypothesis as a cause-effect relationship, considering the most likely hypothesis as well as alternate hypotheses. Third, he evaluates the quality of the hypothesis, formalizing this process by presenting the arguments for his position.

As pointed out in the constituent analysis, the steps of the diagnostic process must be adaptable to varying amounts of information. This is also true of developing the clinical hypothesis. We are presenting this step as taking place prior to client contact; however, during the diagnostic session new information about the client will be obtained that requires the diagnostician to constantly reevaluate his original hypothesis. Reformulations take place frequently, from minor modifications of the hypothesis to completely new derivations.

Derives the clinical hypothesis

The diagnostician derives a clinical hypothesis by examining the relationships between causes and effects that have been revealed in the constituent analysis. From his mental operations he draws together relevant cause-effect relationships, develops new relationships through his ability to infer cause from effect and effect from cause, and identifies missing pieces of information needed to verify his expressed relationships. From this derivation task the diagnostician arranges his priority of probable explanations for the speech and language disorder.

Examines the relationships among causes and effects. The diagnostician examines the inventory of constituents, looking for links between causal factors and disordered speech and language. When the diagnostician examines the relationship among his cause and effect constituents, he goes through a process of aggregation and delimitation. He "computes" the information, looking at all the constituents in all their interrelationships. He wants to identify those that have a past and a current effect on the speech and language disorder. The process of aggregation requires integrating all the constituents that in some way make up the client as a human being. The process of delimitation is like a progressive approximation toward those constituents bearing the most significance for explaining the cause-effect relationships.

For example, if a series of constituents about physical growth and development reveal that all motor milestones are within normal limits, the chances are that the diagnostician will rule out retarded physical development as a potential explanatory factor. The information has offered him no assistance in determining the nature and cause of the speech and language disorder. On the other hand, the diagnostician must ask himself if he has sufficient information about physical growth and development to rule it out as a causal factor. The information he has may be limited, may be wrong, or may be inaccurately reported.

Or suppose we have examined a set of product constituents and have tentatively concluded that Lucia has either a prosody or a severe phonologic disorder. The strength of these conclusions rests with the interpretation of the constituents as examined in relation to each other; it may not be an either/or situation. Lucia's deviant phonologic formulation may make her so unintelligible that she has developed a number of starts and stops to get her parents to understand her. Add to this her age; she is not quite 4 years old—an age when speech and language usage may not be easy for a child. Her speech is filled with whole-word and phrase repetitions. Thus what may be occurring is not a prosody disorder but normal nonfluencies exacerbated by a significant deviation in the use of the phonologic system. Her parents may be reacting more to the nonfluencies as the basis for the unintelligibility than to the sound deviations. Then, just to add to the mix, the parents were told by Lucia's pediatrician "not to worry about the way she produces speech sounds; that's normal for her age." Therefore the diagnostician's interpretation of constituents as a group changes the clinical questions he might ask about cause-effect relationships.

The diagnostician must review all the information to develop an overall perspective. Since his constituent analysis has been performed within the SLPM framework, this same framework is used to derive his clinical hypothesis. From the SLPM he examines his cause-effect relationships in terms of speech and language products affected, behavioral correlates, and physical processes disrupted. He views causal factors in terms of their affect on the speech and language environment and the internal speech and language processing system. In essence, the diagnostician places the client into the SLPM; in each diagnosis the client "becomes a *mini slpm*."

The SLPM also provides the diagnostician with his basis for drawing inferences about the constituents when supporting information is not available. From this orientation the diagnostician may infer certain causal factors for the speech and language characteristics that have been revealed, or he may infer certain speech and language product disorders from available causal information. His power of inferential reasoning, spoken of before as a measurement strategy, becomes a major tool for deriving his clinical hypothesis—sometimes the entire basis of the clinical hypothesis.

All the cause-effect relationships examined are potential explanations for the client's speech and language disorder, whether they are revealed in the constituent analysis or the diagnostician develops them from his inferential strategies. For example, he may have discovered in his analysis that Trisha, referred for a "speech disorder," had serious chronic bouts of otitis media from the age of 8 to 20 months. His analysis leads him to suspect that associated with the otitis media were significant temporary hearing losses, even though this was not reported. From his knowledge and inferential reasoning he might develop a relationship between the bouts of otitis media, the hearing losses, and a presumed phonologic variation. That is, a causal constituent has led him to a particular language product effect—an explanation he could arrive at only by using his knowledge and inferential strategy. Then, of course, in his diagnosis he would have to "fill in" this relationship if it becomes part of his clinical hypothesis. Knowing that this hypothesis was derived inferentially should keep the diagnostician cautious and conservative about the diagnosis he makes from it.

Develops a hierarchy of probable cause-effect explanations. From his integration of cause-effect relationships the diagnostician hopes to arrive at some conclusions that potentially explain the client's clinical problem. The chances are there will be more than a single relationship revealed, and the diagnostician will then develop a hierarchy, a set of priorities for explaining the client's speech and language disorder. If, for instance, the integration of the constituents indicates that Aiko has severely delayed language on all linguistic levels but no causal information has been provided, the diagnostician will have to recall and research the most likely causes for severe language delay in children and order his set of explanations accordingly. He might infer a number of causal factors: mental retardation, childhood aphasia, or deafness. From a disrupted processing viewpoint he might infer language representation or speech production. Or he might infer that Aiko just arrived from Japan and has not had enough exposure to the English language.

The diagnostician rules in and out the various interactions until he arrives at a set of relationships he feels will explain the speech and language disorder. This set is ordered in terms of the diagnostician's reasoning that one expressed relationship explains the disorder better than another. The more closely related the explanation is to the time of onset of the disorder and of expected disruptions in speech and language processing, the more likely it may be as a potential explanation (Table 8).

In developing his set of probable explanations the diagnostician may put at the top of his list a cause-effect relationship that has less information from the constituent analysis than another; however, it may be more theoretically secure because of the diagnostician's inferential strategy. His explanation for the disorder may be better, more appropriately computed, than the explanation offered by the constituents. Or the diagnostician may develop a relationship that has led him to different explanations than those provided by the referral source or the parent in the statement of the problem on the case history questionnaire. There will be many such statements of the problem offered that are not theoretically secure, particularly as they relate to causal factors, for example, when a parent states that "Chloe does not talk because she doesn't eat right." Even if he hypothesizes a different causal route, the diagnostician still has to account for these other statements and referrals in his overall planning.

So at times he will derive not only his own clinical hypothesis but also pose clinical hypotheses ordering the cause-effect relationship in the way it is viewed by the referral source or the parents.

For example, suppose that the constituent analysis has indicated that Ellen has disordered phonetic structure. When she produces the /s, z, ʃ, and dʒ/ phonemes, they are distorted by lateral emission of air. The only causal constituents that were available came from the mother's statement. Mrs. Wirley felt that Ellen's speech problem was due to her inattentiveness. "When I tried to show Ellen how to say the sounds, Ellen wouldn't pay attention and do it." Now this constituent might be important to the overall analysis of Ellen's problem; however, it is not very secure theoretically as a causal factor and could not be placed at the top of the diagnostician's list of potential explanations. Instead, his inferential strategy may lead him to consider a different set of explanations: (1) disrupted articulation process—a contemporary causal explanation; (2) maturation—Ellen is not ready to produce these sounds; (3) dental deviations—malocclusion; and (4) mislearning—she is now maintaining these sound productions through habit strength. These may be only some of the inferences the diagnostician makes for this example, which represents only one possible ordering of the explanations. How the set is ordered depends on the strength and support for each cause-effect relationship expressed, including the the one presented by Mrs. Wirley.

Any inappropriate referrals and associated problems should be revealed during this hypothesis task if not before. The diagnostician should discover them when he examines the relationships between causes and effects. Associated problems that are not causally related cannot be integrated into a cause-effect relationship. At times a client will be seen who has a significant history of emotional difficulty, but the emotional difficulties are not responsible for the speech and language disorder; nor is the speech and language disorder necessarily related to the emotional difficulty. Clients who are seen with stuttering behavior sometimes represent this complex relationship. The diagnostician will have to sort out the relationship of the stuttering behavior to the client's personality, his emotional difficulties. Each problem may need to be explored and treated but not necessarily by the speech pathologist. The diagnostician must be aware when he examines cause-effect relationships that not all the problem areas he views in a given client will have causal relationships, even though they may have an effect on the client's overall communicative interaction—his adjustment to life.

Thus throughout this first task the diagnostician is looking for the *most to the least likely potential explanations*, his own explanation perhaps being more likely than the explanations offered by others. At times the diagnostician may develop his list of priorities based on the preponderance of the information he has available, whereas at other times he must rely more heavily on his inferential strategies. Sometimes his inferences take precedence over the specific information available. In either instance he must offer his reasoning for the explanations he is offering. As a result of his ability to derive potential clinical hypotheses, the diagnostician will arrive at a set of explanations ordered in a most likely to a least likely hierarchy.

■ Again, we turn to our client example, Katherine Compardo, to demonstrate how the diagnostician derives his clinical hypothesis. At this point we will assume that the constituent analysis from the previous step has been completed and documented where necessary. Therefore we now know which categories of constituents are significant for drawing out important cause-effect relationships. In this demonstration, once again, we will not present all of the details that would go into the derivation of Katherine Compardo's clinical hypothesis. Our intent is to demonstrate how the task works; the student should explore this derivation in greater depth. First, we will present a table that explores some of the relationships revealed in the constituent

Table 11. Derivation of the clinical hypothesis—examining and integrating selected, significant constituents about Katherine Compardo

Effect significance	Causal significance
	Speech and language environment component
	The general environmental background does not offer much information that may be causal; rather, it suggests a relatively normal environment and family structure, providing adequate speech and language input stimulation.
	Internal speech and language processing component
	There is little direct information to support any causal factors affecting the internal processing component. Pregnancy and birth history and immediate postnatal period are reported as normal. Age of mother at this last birth and the three children in close succession might be relevant but highly inferential. Would Katherine's borderline, slow physical development be indicative of any causal factor? Slow mental development?
	Central language segment
Language product	→ *Formulation: language representation*
We have a good bit of information that supports a disorder of language. Katherine has been very slow in the onset and development of all aspects of the language product. Language usage is characterized by a minimal vocabulary; few two-word combinations are used, thus both syntax and semantics are delayed. She also tends to prefer gestures over the use of the speech she has. Might this be because she is unintelligible? Or do we have reason to question as well the pragmatic level of speech and language usage.	Formulation is disrupted as evidenced by the speech and language product, thus inferring that language representation is disrupted. Unless, of course, the reason for the defective product is in the speech production segment.
The constituents indicate that the phonologic level is also delayed or deviant. Katherine makes most sounds incorrectly. She should have many correct sounds by this age.	→ *Formulation: speech programming* → *Perception: auditory programming* There is some information here. Questions can be raised about auditory programming on the basis of her speech and language behavior. Perhaps her problem with speech sounds relates to problems of auditory programming—a disruption of some aspects of the behavioral correlate of perception—perhaps sequencing and discrimination of speech sounds are disrupted.

analysis, and then we will present a hierarchical ordering of these relationships, from most to least likely.

Table 11 is constructed to reveal how the cause-effect relationships were derived within the SLPM framework. The left-hand column presents conclusions that have effect significance, and the right-hand column presents conclusions that have causal significance. Through the use of arrows, where relevant, we will show the direction of inference that might occur in establishing the cause-effect relationship. The student should review Chapters 3 through 8 for assistance in interpreting our demonstration of this first task in developing the clinical hypothesis.

States the clinical hypothesis as a cause-effect relationship

Now that the cause-effect relationships have been derived, the diagnostician's second task at this step is to formally state his

Table 11. Derivation of the clinical hypothesis—examining and integrating selected, significant constituents about Katherine Compardo—cont'd

Effect significance	Causal significance
Language product	←*Comprehension: language representation*
	Comprehension is reportedly intact. May want to question this conclusion. If comprehension of language is present at age level, it would be difficult to conclude that a perceptual problem—a disrupted auditory programming process—could account for Katherine's deviant language product, unless auditory programming acts differently at the semantic and syntactic levels than at the phonologic level. She reportedly does not imitate speech, although she does understand it.
	Speech production segment
Speech product	→*All behavioral correlates and physical processes*
But are her sound errors more a speech product deviation than a phonologic deviation?	It would seem that if these processes were affected, we might have received reports of greater difficulties in the speech musculature—the behavioral correlate of motor control. We do have a few comments regarding Katherine's difficulty with the tongue and mouth when she talks. "When she talks" is a significant aspect of this constituent. If we were to see a motor control problem, it would most likely be seen at times other than when she talks.
There is no information about prosody or sound patterns. This would be helpful if we had it. The only clue is the late development of two-word combinations. Could this be evidence for difficulty putting sounds or words together?	*Auditory reception segment*
	Some confusion from the constituents, but it seems most likely that hearing is intact; the processes up to auditory programming will not provide much secure information for causal factors.

POINT: Katherine's information does not point to clearly established causal factors for the significantly delayed speech and language. The diagnostician may want to emphasize contemporary causation—behavioral correlates and physical processes—rather than infer a special causal factor when he formally states his hypothesis. We will not take this approach totally but will express a causal factor.

The hierarchy of cause-effect relationships from most to least likely for Katherine Compardo is stated quite broadly as follows:

1. Childhood aphasia—cause and effect implied
2. Childhood apraxia—cause and effect implied
3. Dysarthria—cause and effect implied
4. Language disorder related to auditory processing deficits
5. Language disorder related to mental retardation

most likely clinical hypothesis. Following the statement of the clinical hypothesis the diagnostician also proposes alternate hypotheses, explanations that were not considered as the most probable hypothesis but that could become a more likely hypothesis before the diagnostic process is completed.

Statement of the most likely clinical hypothesis. From the first task where he or-

dered the list of potential cause-effect relationships, the diagnostician selects the most likely to him and formally states this as his clinical hypothesis—stated as clearly as possible to reveal the potential solution to the clinical problem. It is important to remember that, unlike the researcher, the diagnostician is not stating a hypothesis that he wishes to prove or disprove. Instead, the clinical hypothesis is conceived of as a working hypothesis, a guide to his clinical design.

We want to make it clear to the student that this formal statement of the clinical hypothesis is the diagnostician's working hypothesis. It is not generally used in a discussion with parents or other professionals, nor does it appear in reports as "the statement of the problem." It is the diagnostician's diagnostic guide. At times, however, when he is talking to a parent he might say, "I'm thinking about approaching Denise's problem this way." Or to a professional referral source he might say, "It appears to me that Bonnie's stuttering might really be normal nonfluencies." These types of discussions are statements of the diagnostician's hypotheses to other sources, but they are qualitatively different than the formal statement and are used quite differently.

Even though it is a working hypothesis, the hypothesis is a statement of probability. In his formally stated hypothesis the diagnostician is inferring that the stated disorder is related to the stated causal factor. Thus the wording of the hypothesis is of prime importance. The statement gives direct evidence for the diagnostician's level of understanding and security about the clinical problem. The following two sample hypotheses reflect, through their wording, different levels of security between the stated disorder and its cause: (1) Herbert has a language disorder related to mental retardation that appears to be secondary to brain injury sustained at birth. (2) Herbert has a language disorder due to mental retardation that was caused by the brain injury he sustained at birth.

Furthermore, the way in which the hypothesis is worded will imply various interpretations of the stated cause-effect relationship. The hypothesis statement can be modified according to severity as denoted by "mild," "moderate," and "severe." In addition, they can be ordered chronologically according to time of onset as expressed by the terms "congenital," "acquired," "prenatal," "developmental," and "recurrent."

Even the general ordering of several causal factors embedded within the hypothesis has implications as to their "direct" or "indirect" importance as determiners of a particular speech disorder.

■ What is the difference in the causal emphasis placed on these two hypotheses? (1) Anthony has a voice disorder resulting from vocal abuse that caused contact ulcers. (2) Anthony has a voice disorder related to the presence of contact ulcers that stemmed from constant vocal abuse. Will these two hypotheses signal any differences in your approach to the diagnosis or to your possible management of the problem?

Of special importance to the diagnostician is the level of abstraction at which he states his hypothesis. If a hypothesis is too abstract, it becomes open-ended; everything is possible: "Pequetti has a speech disorder due to many causes." If it is too specific, it becomes subject to greater error; too little is possible: "John produces the /m, n, and ŋ/ phonemes without appropriate nasal resonance due to hypertrophied adenoids that are blocking the nasopharynx." All clinical hypotheses cannot be expressed as specific, concrete causes and effects. The diagnostician seldom has enough prior information to allow for such specificity, although he tends to know more about specific effects (behaviors) than causes. More often the hypothesis is stated abstractly, expressing a general relationship among the cause-effect factors under consideration. Further empirical testing is usually required before the hypothesis can be stated in specific terms.

Regardless of the level of abstraction, however, the diagnostician's statement of his clinical hypothesis should express a relationship that assists him in designing the diagnostic session. The broader, more abstract the hypothesis, the more open-ended the design; the narrower, less abstract the hypothesis, the more specific the design. For example, if a hypothesis were stated as: "Linda cannot say her /l, r, t, d, and n/ sounds because she can't elevate her tongue due to an extremely short lingual frenum," and this was a true hypothesis, the remainder of the diagnostic process would seem rather clearly specified.

For every client to be seen a hypothesis can be stated—even if at a high level of abstraction. The diagnostician must learn how to state his hypothesis at the most useful level of abstraction warranted by the information and still offering a potential solution to the clinical problem. He can build security into his clinical hypothesis by stating it at various levels of abstraction; that is, he can create a series of hypotheses around the same cause-effect relationship. Within this series of hypotheses he hopes to find the true hypothesis. For example, from the same information about a client the following series of clinical hypotheses might be derived—stated from the least to the most specific.

1. Rufus has a language disorder related to a hearing loss.
2. Rufus has a language disorder related to an auditory processing deficit caused by a sensorineural hearing loss.
3. Rufus has a language disorder characterized by both comprehension and formulation disruptions related to an auditory perceptual problem that is secondary to an auditory processing deficit, due to a sensorineural hearing loss resulting from eighth nerve damage.
4. Rufus has a language comprehension and formulation disorder primarily on the phonologic level related to his inability to process (discriminate) the phonemes of his language. This processing deficit is related to his sensorineural hearing loss that was caused by eighth nerve damage, etc.

This series of hypothesis statements reflects several levels of understanding the diagnostician has about the information available to him. The first hypothesis might be chosen because it is more open-ended; the diagnostician would design a more comprehensive diagnosis. However, he may feel secure with his derivation and go for the fourth hypothesis, thereby designing a more specific diagnosis. Part of this task—stating the hypothesis—is related to the diagnostician's comfort level. That is, how comfortable is the diagnostician with his understanding of the information, with his ability to use his professional knowledge at the risky inferential level?

Proposes alternate hypotheses. If there are indications from his derivation task of more than one potential cause-effect relationship, the diagnostician must now propose his alternate hypotheses. There will be as many alternate hypotheses as warranted by the cause-effect relationships revealed during the constituent analysis and the hypothesis derivation tasks. One source of a potential alternate hypothesis arises when the diagnostician's derivation does not match the statement of the problem presented by others. Earlier we presented an example client, Ellen, whose mother felt she had sound errors because of inattentiveness. On the other hand, the diagnostician may have derived a clinical hypothesis that pointed strongly to a malocclusion as responsible for the sound distortions, and he stated this formally as his clinical hypothesis. Now he can state an alternate hypothesis more in line with the mother's concern; even if he believes this not to be at all likely, he is stating it to fulfill certain purposes of diagnosis. Thus he may state an alternate hypothesis as: "Ellen has sound distortions because she is inattentive to methods of teaching her how to produce them." In his design he would then determine if Ellen could be attentive and learn the production of these phonemes. He would then be able to discuss this consideration with the mother during the interpretive conference.

Alternate hypotheses express different cause-effect relationships and purposes than stated in the first hypothesis, the original clinical hypothesis. The following examples illustrate this.

1. Alterations of the causal factor
   a. Albert has a language disorder related to mental retardation.

b. Albert has a language disorder related to brain injury.
2. Alterations of the speech and language disorder
   a. Bertha has a language disorder related to cerebral palsy.
   b. Bertha has an articulation disorder related to cerebral palsy.
   c. Bertha has a prosody disorder related to cerebral palsy.
3. Alterations of both the causal factor and the speech and language disorder
   a. Bart has a language disorder (aphasia) due to a cerebrovascular accident.
   b. Bart has a phonetic structure disorder related to an unspecified neurologic disease.
   c. Bart has a voice disorder related to Huntington's chorea.

These alternate hypotheses are ordered by the diagnostician, following the original hypothesis, in terms of probability of correctness from most to least likely. This ordering provides him with his probability estimate. His original hypothesis is his best, followed in decreasing order of probability by each of the alternate hypotheses ordered from 1 to x number of alternates. Of course, the diagnostician anticipates his original hypothesis to be the "true" hypothesis, but if not, his hope is that the "true" hypothesis is embedded within his alternates. As he proceeds with his diagnosis, his order of probability may change, his third alternate becoming the most likely, and his original hypothesis becoming his least likely. Alternate hypotheses must be incorporated into the design of the diagnosis along with the original hypothesis. Therefore they, too, must be stated with clarity, express a potential solution to the clinical problem, and be worded at an appropriate level of abstraction.

A final alternate hypothesis must be proposed by the diagnostician. He always proposes that the client may have no speech and language problem and states the alternate, the "null" clinical hypothesis: "Andrea has no speech and language disorder." Whenever the diagnostician states a possible clinical hypothesis: "Missy has a speech and language disorder related to . . . ," he automatically states the alternate: "Missy has no speech and language disor-

der." This alternate is particularly important since all speech and language disorders are comparative—compared to normal speech and language development and usage. This alternate hypothesis helps keep the diagnostician on track, that is, to focus on the distinctions between speech and language variations versus disorders. It also assists in viewing certain causal factors, and one that comes immediately to mind is mental retardation. The diagnostician must know that mental retardation can slow down a child's use of speech and language, but this slowdown may well be normal within the degree of mental retardation. So the alternate hypothesis of no speech and language disorder applies. A strange way of putting this is: "There may be a cause—but no effect."

Evaluates the quality of the hypothesis

The diagnostician's third task in developing the clinical hypothesis is to make an evaluation of the quality of the hypothesis he has stated. This task formally explicates why and how the particular hypothesis is offered and examines the strength of the hypothesis. The diagnostician must account for why he has derived one hypothesis rather than another. Even though we are presenting this quality evaluation as the third task in developing the hypothesis, it should be apparent that this task does run throughout this second step of the diagnostic process.

When he evaluates the quality of his hypothesis, the diagnostician is concerned about both the specification of his hypothesis and the support he can offer for it, that is, the arguments he might present to defend his hypothesis. To do this he must have guidelines and criteria for evaluating the quality of his hypothesis.

In specifying his hypothesis the diagnostician strives for absolute clarity of statement. He provides an unambiguous statement that includes formal propositions and specifications for testing them. In our discussion of the previous task, points were made about clarity of terms, levels of abstraction, and ways of expressing the cause-effect relationships.

Ringel (1972) suggests that the diagnostician evaluate his clinical hypothesis in terms of the following questions: (1) Is it clearly stated and pertinent to the solution of the problem? (2) Does it reflect an adequate understanding of the problem or an objective attitude? Other questions that might be asked are (3) What is the strength of the relationship expressed in the hypothesis? (4) What are the factual versus inferential aspects of the hypothesis? (5) Are the relationships expressed in the hypothesis available for testing? (6) What are the sources of error in the hypothesis? (7) What support is available for this hypothesis versus alternate hypotheses?

The diagnostician responds to these evaluative questions by presenting his arguments both in support of and in opposition to the hypothesis he has derived. For the practicing diagnostician this might be in the form of the mental process he goes through prior to the diagnostic session. In some settings staff participation may be required with the clients to be seen. In these settings the diagnostician may have to prepare a more formalized presentation. This is likely in settings where staffings form the basis of diagnosis, and it is a practice required of students in training. When supporting his hypothesis, the diagnostician presents his documentation, his arguments; he shows the evolution of the problem from his funds of knowledge and from the literature that support it. The diagnostician's supportive arguments come from his constituent analysis and hypothesis derivation, which reflect his reasoning abilities. Any errors he has made will be reflected in the quality of the hypothesis he has derived.

In teaching this task, we require the student to develop a formal written support paper emphasizing documentation from the literature since at this stage in their career they seldom have extensive clinical experience from which to draw; their professional fund of knowledge is limited.

■ As a way of demonstrating this last task, several hypotheses are stated in this project, and comments are made regarding their quality. The student should delve into these examples further. Are our comments about quality relevant? Should we have approached them differently? Is further information needed to continue the evaluation?

1. *Odvar has a language disorder due to unknown causes.* Even though clearly stated, little specific information is provided in this hypothesis. It is highly abstract and provides little information as a potential solution to the clinical problem. Some level of the language product must be affected—pragmatic, semantic, syntactic, phonologic, or perhaps all of them. The diagnostician does not know if comprehension or formulation or both are involved. Nothing is known of causal factors. The diagnostician would have to design his diagnosis primarily from inference for this hypothesis; his inferential abilities would be the sole basis for causal factors. This hypothesis reflects that the diagnostician either had little information to go on or else did not feel secure about his interpretation of available information.

2. *Gregory has a language disorder on all linguistic levels related to an emotional disturbance.* More specificity is introduced into this hypothesis. We know that the language product is affected on all levels; however, we do not know whether comprehension or formulation is disrupted. Severity might be inferred, since all levels are affected; however, it would help to specify this. The major weakness of this hypothesis is in the statement of causation. The causal factor lacks clarity; it is highly abstract and ambiguous. What does "emotional disturbance" mean? What support can the diagnostician offer that an emotional disturbance is related to the language disorder? This hypothesis may not reflect an objective and adequate understanding of the problem. An alternative hypothesis may have been more likely. The interactions between emotional problems and language disorders are difficult, at best, to discern and secure. Which comes first? Perhaps in Gregory's case the language disorder was apparent early in development and created subsequent frustration that led to significant episodes of depression. If all levels of language are affected, the probability of resultant emotional problems is a potential. For further evaluation of this hypothesis, refer to our earlier discussions about associated problems.

3. *Nancy has a formulation disorder primarily affecting syntactic development related to her learning abilities. Nancy has been classified as an educable mentally retarded child with an IQ of 75.* This hypothesis is stated clearly and provides some rather specific information. The diagnostician has stated that the language disorder is formulation of syntax. The disorder is expressed as both a behavioral correlate and product disorder. No statement of severity is provided, which would be helpful here since the diagnostician must infer the degree to which other linguistic levels are affected. A specific relationship has been expressed that provides a potential solution to the problem. In his design the diagnostician might focus on syntax to determine what might be necessary to increase Nancy's ability to formulate better syntactic structures. The hypothesis also specifies the causal factor; presumably it means Nancy has learning problems because she is an educable retarded child with an IQ of 75. This relationship provides a source of error in this hypothesis, perhaps a lack of adequate understanding of the problem. We have to assume here that Nancy has not developed syntax because of learning problems. Is this typical of a child with an IQ of 75? Perhaps an alternate hypothesis would be better: "Nancy has syntactic development commensurate with her mental age." Or perhaps there is another causal factor interacting with her mental abilities that may be a better explanation for the language disorder. There are other aspects of this hypothesis that need clarification.

4. *Joyce has a severe language comprehension and formulation disorder on all linguistic levels due to mental retardation that is secondary to central nervous system dysfunction resulting from brain injury. Joyce sustained a severe blow to the left temporal cortex when she was 3 years old.* Evaluate the quality of this hypothesis. Consider carefully the interactions of causal factors; what is stated, what is implied, and what must be inferred.

■ Now we return to our client example, Katherine Compardo, and exemplify the last two tasks of step 2 of the diagnostic process. First, we will state the clinical hypothesis and an alternate; then we will evaluate the quality of the hypothesis and present a brief support paper.

From the list of potential cause-effect relationships the most likely relationship is stated as a formal clinical hypothesis. The first relationship expressed in Table 11 was "Childhood aphasia—cause and effect implied."

Statement of the clinical hypothesis. Katherine Compardo has congenital childhood aphasia and apraxia characterized by language formulation disruptions observed on all language product levels, thus implicating the physical processes of language representation and speech programming. The cause inferred for this disorder is implied in the terms "aphasia" and "apraxia"—central nervous system dysfunction (more specifically a disruption of certain parts of the central language segment).

Statement of an alternate hypothesis. Katherine Compardo has congenital apraxia of speech that has greatly limited her use of all levels of language. The causal relationship is implied in the term "apraxia"—disruption of the central language segment (in this hypothesis more specific to the speech programming process).

The students should now try their hand at stating their hypothesis for Katherine Compardo or stating various alternates as reflected by the cause-effect relationships established earlier. They also should evaluate the quality of the specification of the above hypotheses.

Development of a support paper. We will present only a relatively brief support paper for Katherine Compardo. The student can study this position paper and add more evaluative details. Our intent is to exemplify the task, not present it in detail. We will develop our position paper in the following way. First, we will present viewpoints on the concept of childhood aphasia and apraxia. Following this, we will demonstrate briefly how Katherine's constituent analysis supports our position stated in the hypothesis.

There is not complete agreement in the literature regarding the condition so often referred to as childhood aphasia or developmental aphasia. When early attention was brought to this condition by Myklebust (1954), the current concepts of adult aphasia were simply transferred to children. Thus "aphasic children" were either receptive, expressive, or global aphasics. Since then, more attempts were made to differentiate the language characteristics seen in this group of nonverbal children. However, there is still a primary differentiation into two essential types of childhood aphasias (Eisenson, 1972; Morley, 1967) or combinations of them. Adding to this classification difficulty, the concept of childhood apraxia was introduced into the childhood aphasia schema. Again, as in adults, questions are being asked about whether apraxia is a component of "expressive aphasia," or if it can occur in isolation.

Examining Katherine's hypothesis in light of some of this information lends support to the position that she has childhood aphasia and apraxia characterized by language formulation difficulties on all linguistic levels. Katherine is a "nonverbal" child who does not present any significant sign of mental retardation, emotional disorder, hearing loss, or physical problem. These signs are in keeping with both Eisenson's (1972) and Morley's (1967) classifications, which define aphasia in children in almost this way. The characteristics presented by Morley (1967) fit Katherine: a severe delay in the onset of speech, little or no vocal play or babbling, and one or two isolated words used during the first 2 to 3 years of life. As well, she indicates that the aphasic child would be emotionally stable and have normal hearing, intelligence, and social interests—all of which seem to be the case with Katherine.

The interpretation of Katherine's ability to comprehend language is crucial to this hypothesis. Does the literature support a diagnosis of aphasia that is characterized primarily by language formulation difficulties but leaves comprehension intact? We have already mentioned the dichotomy of types of childhood aphasia that have been proffered in the literature. Morley's description would add that if comprehension was at age level, then the developmental aphasia would be considered as predominantly expressive. Eisenson concurs that this circumstance can occur; however, he might consider this type of child, the one who comprehends but does not speak, as congenitally apraxic. He indicates that this includes only a small number of nonverbal children. We are concluding that Katherine is one of these, a child who comprehends but is basically nonverbal. Her sound development "makes most sounds incorrectly," and the reported "difficulty moving her tongue and mouth when she talks" provides added evidence for both Eisenson's and Morley's concepts of apraxia.

All in all, Katherine Compardo appears to fit Eisenson's concept of congenital oral apraxia, which is rather synonymous with Morley's developmental expressive aphasia with accompanying articulatory apraxia. Katherine understands spoken language but has failed to develop formulated language appropriate for her age. She has a significant cluster of other characteristics that support this hypothesis: she responds to sounds and noises and comprehends spoken language, even though there was little early babbling, cooing, and vocal play, and she still does not imitate speech. She uses gesture for communication, although we do not know how highly developed her gesture system is. Her speech output is quite limited; she primarily uses single-syllable words composed of front consonant plus vowel combinations.

As mentioned, this support paper is intended to be brief by way of demonstration. The student should now review the criteria discussed for evaluating the quality of a hypothesis and develop a more extensive support position for Katherine Compardo, either using the hypothesis presented here, an alternate hypothesis, or his own derived hypothesis. Keep in mind that the support position can consider many aspects of the potential problem, including how the disorder may have come about, what effects it will continue to have on the client, and what management considerations might be proposed if the hypothesis were true. The position paper is an interpretation of the hypothesis, which is, in effect, a testing out of the hypothesis to determine its clinical validity.

SUMMARY

The development of the clinical hypothesis derives from the diagnostician's examination and integration of the cause-effect relationships revealed in the constituent analysis. In stating his clinical hypothesis, the diagnostician delineates the speech and language disorder he expects to see and its probable cause. The hypothesis is a working hypothesis that expresses a potential solution to the clinical problem. Once the clinical hypothesis and any alternates are stated, they are evaluated for their clarity and relevance to the clinical problem, serving to organize and design the remainder of the diagnostic process.

In developing his clinical hypothesis, the diagnostician performs three tasks:

1. *He derives the clinical hypothesis.* He performs this by drawing relationships between causes and effects, using the perspective provided by the SLPM—his inferential strategy being crucial to this task. He presents his integration of relationships as a hierarchy of most to least likely cause-effect explanations for the clinical problem.

2. *He states the clinical hypothesis as a cause-effect relationship.* This task is the formal statement of the most probable cause-effect relationship as revealed in the preceding task. In addition, he also offers alternate hypotheses—those he considers as less likely to explain the clinical problem. He always proposes the "null" hypothesis—that no speech and language disorder exists.

3. *He evaluates the quality of the hypothesis.* Here the diagnostician presents his evaluation of the specification and support for his hypothesis. He addresses the clarity of his statement and presents his arguments in support of his hypothesis, including those factors that might weaken as well as strengthen his position.

Now that this step of the diagnostic process is completed, the diagnostician is one step closer to fulfilling the goals of diagnosis. He then turns his attention to designing the diagnosis, selecting and developing the clinical tools for testing the hypothesis.

CLIENT PROJECTS
Isadore Alexander

The student should now develop a clinical hypothesis on a client following the procedures set forth in this chapter. For this purpose another client will be introduced. The client is 68-year-old Isadore Alexander. The referral was made by Dr. Jarius Lambert, Chief of Otolaryngology, University Hospitals, to the hospital's speech pathologist. When checking Dr. Lambert's consult notes, the diagnostician discovered that Mr. Alexander had been referred to Dr. Lambert by another otolaryngologist, Dr. William Fowles. Mr. Alexander had also seen Dr. Lee Uransky, a neurologist. Before seeing Mr. Alexander, the diagnostician felt it was necessary to obtain further information from Dr. Fowles and Dr. Uransky. No history questionnaire was sent. The information available on Mr. Alexander is reproduced in Appendix II.

Before the student can develop his hypothesis for Mr. Alexander, he will have to do a constituent analysis on the available client information. Some resources the student might find useful are Aronson (1971), Aronson et al. (1964, 1966), and Darley et al. (1969a, b, 1975).

Previous client: William Gafford

The student should also develop and propose a clinical hypothesis for William Gafford from the constituent analysis done in the last chapter.

REFERENCES

Aronson, A. E., Early motor unit disease masquerading as pyschogenic breathy dysphonia: A clinical case presentation. *J. Speech Hearing Dis.*, **36**, 115-123 (1971).

Aronson, A. E., Peterson, H. W., and Litin, E. M., Voice symptomatology in functional dysphonia and aphonia. *J. Speech Hearing Dis.*, **29**, 367-380 (1964).

Aronson, A. E., Peterson, H. W., and Litin, E. M., Psychiatric symptomatology in functional dysphonia and aphonia. *J. Speech Hearing Dis.*, **31**, 115-127 (1966).

Darley, F. L., Aronson, A. E., and Brown, J. R., Differential diagnostic patterns of dysarthria. *J. Speech Hearing Res.*, **12**, 246-269 (1969a).

Darley, F. L., Aronson, A. E., and Brown, J. R., Clusters of deviant speech dimensions in the dysarthrias. *J. Speech Hearing Res.*, **12**, 462-496 (1969b).

Darley, F. L., Aronson, A. E., and Brown, J. R., *Motor Speech Disorders*. Philadelphia: W. B. Saunders Co. (1975).

Eisenson, J., *Aphasia in Children*. New York: Harper & Row, Publishers (1972).

Morley, M., *The Development and Disorders of Speech in Childhood*. (2nd ed.) Baltimore: The Williams & Wilkins Co. (1967).

Myklebust, H., *Auditory Disorders in Children*. New York: Grune & Stratton Inc. (1954).

Ringel, R. L., The clinician and the researcher: An artificial dichotomy. *Asha*, **14**, 351-353 (1972).

Schultz, M. C., The bases of speech pathology and audiology: Evaluation as the resolution of uncertainty. *J. Speech Hearing Dis.*, **38**, 147-155 (1973).

Chapter 13

Selection and development of the clinical tools: design of the diagnosis

The third step of the diagnostic process, again done prior to client contact, follows logically from the constituent analysis and the development of the clinical hypothesis. This step involves the overall planning of the diagnostic session for testing the clinical hypothesis.

To design his diagnosis the diagnostician engages in three tasks. First, he plans his diagnosis around the clinical hypothesis and the specific personal characteristics of the client. The constituent analysis gives the particulars about the client such as age, expected behavioral characteristics, and possible physical and intellectual limitations. The hypothesis leads the diagnostician to expect the presence of certain causes and effects. In this first task the diagnostician now plans what he wants to do, what he wants to measure.

Second, the diagnostician selects and critically evaluates the specific tools that fit his overall plan for gathering the data. Here the diagnostician will select from the almost infinite tools available or develop his own tools for data gathering. His expertise must include knowledge of the various sources and types of tools available. He must have available a tool-retrieval system for selecting the tools he needs to fit his plan, that is, what he is going to use for measurement.

Third, the diagnostician develops his testing strategy to carry out his plans with the tools he has selected. This strategy is mapped out in advance in hopes of optimizing data collection within the practicalities of the setting and the particular client characteristics.

The design of the diagnosis gives the diagnostician control: a plan, an order, and purposes to all aspects of the actual diagnostic session that will follow. The rigor of the diagnosis depends on the quality of this overall design. It is the diagnostician's clinical methodology designed to solve the clinical problem stated in the clinical hypothesis.

DESIGN OF THE DIAGNOSIS: HOW IT IS DONE
Information bases: nature and sources

In designing the diagnosis, the diagnostician calls on information from three major sources: (1) the previous steps in the diagnostic process, (2) his knowledge about disorders and their measurement, and (3) the clinical tools available to him.

Previous steps in the diagnostic process

The constituent analysis and the clinical hypothesis direct the diagnostician's planning of the diagnostic design. His intent is to gather data to verify his hypothesis or, as the case may be, to discover alternate cause-effect relationships. If, for example, a prosody disorder characterized by sound repetitions and prolongations is hypothesized, the diagnostician's plan will take quite a different form than if a severe language problem is hypothesized. Similarly, if the hypothesis points to motor control problems as probable causal factors, he will plan his diagnostic time differently than if sensation problems are hypothesized.

The diagnostician designs the session so that he gets the data he needs for his original hypothesis as well as for any alternate hypotheses. Hypotheses based on a high degree of inference require extreme care in planning. These hypotheses have far more missing information than hypotheses derived from specific, clear information. An inferential hypothesis is more subject to error than one based on more factual data. This is more often the case in designing for causal considerations than for the speech and language characteristics. But in some instances it may be otherwise. For example, we referred in the last chapter to a child, Trisha, referred with a history of repeated otitis media. No information was available other than "speech disorder" for developing an effect hypothesis. The diagnostician inferred a phonologic variation, a product inference based on a potential cause. Without any factual support for this effect aspect of the hypothesis, the diagnostician must carefully design his approach for testing and verifying this highly inferential cause-effect relationship.

When conducting the previous two steps, the diagnostician often finds the information available incomplete and unclear, which raises many questions needing follow-up. The diagnostician carefully selects his tools to learn more about these questionable areas. For example, a physician may have reported that "Rachael was the product of a difficult labor." The diagnostician may question what "difficult" means and the effect of that labor on Rachael, exploring this information in the interview with the parent. Or a parent may have reported that "Patty is hard to manage." The diagnostician may both want to question the parents further about this problem and to observe Patty's manageability for himself. In short, all that is known about the client, the information received and the diagnostician's study of that information in the first two steps, is used in helping him formulate his diagnostic design.

Funds of knowledge

In order to design the diagnosis, the diagnostician needs to know *what he wants to measure* and *how he is going to measure it* before he selects his measurement tools. The client information has pointed the direction in which to look; now the diagnostician's knowledge as a measurement expert tells him how to study the suspected disorder—how to devise the methods he needs.

For example, having hypothesized a vocal tone disorder related to vocal nodules, the diagnostician draws from his knowledge about voice problems and vocal nodules to suggest the overall methods he may use to measure this specific cause-effect relationship. For instance, he may plan to obtain a series of measures describing pitch, such as habitual pitch and pitch range. He may also judge quality and loudness attributes. These measures would derive from what the diagnostician knows about voice problems, not from a prescription of "here is what you do for any and every voice problem." Vocal nodules as the hypothesized causal factor require the diagnostician to determine a method for verification; perhaps he already knows from his referral; perhaps he will have to find out by referral. The diagnostician's fund of knowledge tells him what behaviors are appropriate to measure and what causal factors may be expected.

In addition to amplification of what it is that he will measure in his diagnosis, the diagnostician also must know how to systematically measure whatever levels of detail he has specified—again, a quality of the diagnostician as a measurement expert. He must have facility with all aspects of measurement needed for gaining information about the components of the SLPM (Chapters 3 through 6).

In diagnosis of speech and language disorders, no matter how many techniques are developed for specifying observations, the diagnostician is still bound to his perceptual measurement abilities. It is a primary skill the diagnostician must master. We use ourselves, our *critical listening skills*, to determine if a voice is hoarse, if an /s/ sound is in error, or if there is a moment of prolongation. Techniques only help us to "organize ourselves," our systematic observations as the primary measurement tool in diagnosis. Even when the diagnostician can use certain physical measurements, he still must make a judgment about the quality of the response. Instrumentation may give information about the spectral characteristics of an /s/ sound, about a voice, or about a prolongation; however, only the diagnostician can determine if it is disordered. He makes the comparative judgment from a standard to be able to state that the /s/ is distorted, the voice is hoarse, or the prolongation is excessive.

Infinite tools

A major information base needed for completing this third step of the diagnostic process is knowledge about the tools and tests available for designing the diagnosis. The number of techniques (tools) available to the diagnostician to assist him in systematic measurement is, perhaps, infinite —what has been and what will be. All of these tools, no matter how developed, were and are intended to provide information about some aspect of speech and language disorders and their causes. Some of the tools were developed from very practical bases, others from highly theoretical bases. They have come from many sources: schools, clinics, researchers, teachers, and commercial publishers to name a few. They come in many forms: some highly structured, others very unstructured, some highly objective, and others very subjective. Many are also specified by type: lan-

guage, articulation, speech mechanism, screening, hearing, interview, and perceptual-motor. They also are scored and interpreted in a variety of ways.

From all this the diagnostician must be able to select the tools needed to fulfill his measurement design. He must be familiar with a wide range of tools and know how to use them, that is, what they will and will not do for him. He must know what the tools are designed to do and evaluate their usefulness in gaining the information he wants. Since new testing tools are being made available with great frequency, the diagnostician must also be able to evaluate and incorporate these into his diagnostic practice.

To be able to utilize all these tool resources, the diagnostician needs an orientation for learning about and selecting from the vast possibilities available. Our intent here is to point up some categories of tools, to suggest criteria for evaluating the adequacy of tools, and then to present a "tool-retrieval system" for use in selection.

Categories of tools. There have been various attempts to classify diagnostic tools into dichotomous classes such as subjective-objective, formal-informal, and structured-unstructured. These classifications have seldom been satisfactory and at times have promoted false reliance on tools described as structured and objective. At this time we will not attempt to present an encompassing classification of the tools and techniques potentially useful to the diagnostician. Instead, we will first present some rather arbitrary categories of sources, forms, and types of tools. Later, we will discuss a more systematic means of organizing tools.

Diagnostic tools may be organized into five categories; however, any specific tool might be found in any number of the categories. The five categories discussed are the interview, commercial tools, experimental tools, setting protocols, and guided observation. We consider it important to alert the student to these categorizations, as each offers useful information for selecting diagnostic tools.

THE INTERVIEW. The interview, unlike many other techniques, does not have a circumscribed use in the diagnostic process. There is no single approach to interviewing; rather, there are many approaches depending on the interviewer's purposes (Bingham and Moore, 1941; Fenlason, 1952; Garrett, 1972; Stevenson, 1971; Sullivan, 1954).

Often in the diagnosis of speech and language disorders the concept of the interview is approached from a narrow perspective, that is, a verbal exchange between a parent and a diagnostician for gaining the parent's impressions of their child's speech and language disorder. However, the interview in its more general sense is a tool that can be used with any person who can provide information about the client's speech and language disorder, including the clients themselves. Even paper and pencil tasks can be viewed as forms of interviews. For example, when the parent fills out a case history questionnaire prior to the diagnostic session, information is being exchanged between the source (the parent) and the diagnostician.

For the purposes of this book, we want to confine our view of the interview to the information exchange that takes place during the diagnostic session with any member of the client complex. The interview is used to gain information and insights about the client from whomever is interviewed—the parents, spouse, social worker, the client himself, or any other interested person. The use of pencil and paper tasks might be incorporated into the interview techniques, but it is seen primarily as a verbal exchange of information. We will introduce our basic concepts about the interview at this step of the diagnostic process; however, because we formally view the interview as data collection, the next step of the diagnostic process, we will augment interview information there.

The information obtained from an interview depends on the intents and purposes of the interview. If much client information was available prior to the diagnostic session, the diagnostician might hold "an attitude about" the problem interview designed around management concerns. If little information was available, the interview might become the primary source of data about the specifics of the disorder and thus have a constituent analysis intent. Or still again, the interview may be primarily designed to discover causal factors that were unclear, thus having primarily a hypothesis development intent. Each interview, therefore, is designed for specific purposes, assisting the diagnostician in completing any of the diagnostic tasks at any of the steps and at any time during the diagnostic process.

The interview can be used to gain both verbally reported and extraverbally observed data. Verbally reported data is that information given us in words by the informant. In gaining such information, however, we need to keep in mind the possible discrepancy between the information that the diagnostician wants to learn, the information that the informant wants to tell, and the information of real importance to understanding the true nature of the speech and language problem.

Three interrelated processes may be seen to be operant in gaining verbally reported data: *amplification, clarification,* and *verification*. If the information offered is insufficient or irrelevant, there is a need to amplify. Hopefully, an increase in quantity of data will help increase the validity and reliability of the information. Many of the diagnostician's questions will be of an amplification type. There is a need to clarify if the information offered is vague, ambiguous, or inconsistent. Ideally, a question should be worded in a way that limits the degree of ambiguity of any possible response. By doing so, there is a subsequent increase in specificity—the diagnostician gets at the details he seeks. There is a need to verify if the information offered seems unreliable. The diagnostician should be aware of inconsistencies in behaviors or verbal responses that suggest unreliability. If he suspects that the informant is offering inaccurate information, he must try to determine if these are conscious or unconscious distortions. This will help assess the informant's awareness and understanding of the problem.

All three intents—amplification, clarification, and verification—can be embedded in a single question. A question might be asked primarily to expand (amplify) information from the client history form. If the response is not clear or accurate, a question or statement to clarify or verify the response is provided, for example, "What do you mean by . . .?" or "Then, what you are saying is. . . ."

In addition to the verbal data obtained in the interview the diagnostician also gains information from extraverbal observations. He may assess the gestalt of the interview, considering what is said as well as what is not said. For example, why is there no mention of the child's relationship with the father? The diagnostician will want to note gaps in information as well as recurrent references or themes that emerge. He may be particularly alert to inconsistencies between what the informant says and how he appears to feel about what he says. For example, if the informant's words indicate concern but his voice and manner indicate indifference, the diagnostician might question the reliability of the information that is being offered. Is the informant consciously or unconsciously distorting the information? If a parent, is he trying to defend his ability to raise children or mask his fear that the child may have a serious problem?

The diagnostician may wonder what he may do with such subjective, nonexplicit observations. Such information may be particularly useful in learning the informant's real concerns and feelings about the information he is giving. Such observations also may cue topics where discussion may be very fruitful. Finally, observing the informant's extralinguistic behavior may provide a foundation for understanding that person, which would be particularly helpful when interpreting the results of the diagnosis and planning client management.

Together, verbally reported data and extraverbal observations may serve to fill in missing constituents, to support or reject the clinical hypothesis, and to assess the informant's understanding, insight, and concern relating to the client's problem.

COMMERCIAL TOOLS. At first glance this may seem an illogical category, and it is. However, we want to draw the student's attention to the wide range of tools available through the commercial publishing houses. Commercial sources of tools are more prevalent today than in the past. Perhaps it is a sign of sophistication in our profession that we now have tools available for purchase and no longer need to rely on developing our own for each client we see. There is a great surge in commercially published tools. Monthly, new tools are marketed, each vying for a place in the diagnostician's testing repertoire. Many of these tools are outgrowths of techniques first used experimentally or clinically.

Tools are commercial only in the sense that they are available for a price. Beyond that, this category of tools has little in common. Some tools are highly original; others are thinly disguised adaptations of information readily available. Some give impressive normative data; others give none. Some obtain credible validity and reliability, while others do not address these concerns. Some tools require elaborate or official training procedures before their use is authorized; others can be used by anyone who can read and follow instructions.

Many of the available tools have been designed to measure some aspect of a specific "problem type" (tests of articulation, aphasia, language) or to measure some rather specified level of speech and language behavior (morphology, speech sounds, syntax, nonfluencies); still others have been designed to measure certain defined "processes" (comprehension, sensation, perception, diadochokinesis, phonation). Other tools are available that are more appropriate to causal testing, some of which are the primary province of other professionals, some the province of the speech pathologist, for example, auditory tests, perceptual-motor tests, intelligence tests, personality tests, and projective tests. Psychology, psychiatry, neurology, medicine, education, and other professions have all contributed commercial tools useful in the diagnosis of speech and language disorders.

The student can begin to explore commercially available tools by reviewing the following books that discuss tests for diagnosis: Emerick and Hatten, 1974; Irwin and Marge, 1972; Johnson et al., 1963; Sanders, 1972.

EXPERIMENTAL TOOLS. The research literature offers another source of useful tools and procedures that can be adapted by the diagnostician for use. These tools come in all types and forms and measure many different aspects of speech and language disorders and their causes. The experimenter has developed his tool to systematically measure some aspect of his hypothesis, a situation not unlike the diagnostician confronted with a range of clinical hypotheses; therefore these tools and procedures are usually relatively objective. However, at times they may not be as reliable nor as valid as the experimenter had hoped. Many of the tools now commercially available for diagnosis were originally developed out of research projects (Carrow, 1968; Lee, 1970; MacDonald and Blott, 1974). If not commercially available, some of the tools have been presented in the literature with suggestions for their diagnostic use (Nation, 1972).

With so many potential tools available from the experimental literature, it would be helpful to have a "central" listing of applicable tools. For example, Johnson and Bommarito (1971) have developed a collection of tests and measurements in child development that appeared in the experimental literature. The

student could begin a project similar to this for his personal use in designing diagnoses. As a start, the student could review the following experimental reports to determine what tools were used that might be applicable to the diagnosis of the individual client? For what type of client might the tools be useful? (See Aten and Davis, 1968; Berry and Erickson, 1973; Deal and Darley, 1972; Labelle, 1973; Lahey, 1974; Monnin and Huntington, 1974; Schwartz and Goldman, 1974; Yoss and Darley, 1974.)

SETTING PROTOCOLS. There are any number of tools of all types and forms that have been constructed by personnel working within specific work settings. Settings may develop their own "private label" test for aphasia, articulation, stuttering, etc. For example, in most settings a format can be found directing the speech mechanism examination, a format for observing and analyzing stuttering behaviors, and a format for observing parameters of voice. Many tools such as these do not strictly fall into a test format and seldom achieve commercial publishing status; they are setting protocols.

Other setting protocol tools are highly structured; they are first developed for clinical use to fit a specific need of the diagnostician, then they may be used in experimentation, and ultimately, may end up as commercial tools. The *Minnesota Test for Differential Diagnosis of Aphasia* by Schuell (1965) basically took this route. Tests like this were originally devised to fill diagnostic and research needs in certain work settings when no tools were available.

From work settings, then, come a primary source of tools for diagnosis. Tools derived from this source often are our most practical, applicable tools even when the standardization data may be limited. There is much to be said for tools that have a professional's clinical experience guiding their construction. These tools have been worked out and "tailor-made" for disordered populations. They often may be more applicable than tools worked out on normal populations. Some of these tools gain wide distribution through the clinical literature —articles that discuss certain types of disorders and how to test for and treat them.

Besides some of the references previously mentioned, the following present tools useful for diagnostic design: Bangs, 1961; Fluharty, 1974; and Spradlin, 1963. The student should continuously seek out tools that stem from setting protocols.

GUIDED OBSERVATIONS. We have specified a final tool category for diagnostic design. For want of a better term we have called this category guided observations. This category encompasses all the observations the diagnostician wants to make that do not fall under the rubric of a test or a specific observational form. These are the tasks frequently referred to as unstructured, general, or informal observations. We prefer to think that all our observations are guided—that structure is present in the observations made of the activities and behaviors of the client. The client's behaviors may not be structured, but the diagnostician's observations should be. Observations are planned and thus constitute a tool of diagnosis. As has previously been stated, the skill of systematic observation is the primary method of diagnosis. All tools are primarily techniques for structuring and guiding our systematic observations. Thus every activity that occurs in the diagnosis serves as a source of data to be observed; no source of information should go unobserved or be wasted.

At times the stimuli presented are rigorously controlled; at other times, they are controlled only in a very general sense. For example, when a client is asked to sit down, stand up, or hop, skip, and jump, the diagnostician has controlled his stimuli to specify a response. He may want to observe the client's motor abilities and/or his ability to follow directions. Or if the plan is to obtain as much spontaneous speech as naturalistically as possible, the diagnostician's stimulus specification may be more general; that is, the diagnostician

bases his conversational stimuli on the client's spontaneous conversation. But the diagnostician's observations of this conversation may be highly planned and structured to obtain specific speech and language data. This use of planned communicative interaction between client and diagnostician in many instances becomes his only tool, developed from and based on guided observations. Even when considerable data from more specific tests are available, the diagnostician will use guided observations of these spontaneous situations to gain additional data about the client's abilities. Diagnostic design is often a balance between responses to structured tools and responses obtained in a more naturalistic activity.

Some diagnosticians develop observation forms to guide them during the diagnosis, structuring the observation form differently depending on the hypothesis and the personal characteristics of the client. These observational protocols are useful for designing the diagnostic session; they guide the diagnostician in recalling all the things he may want to note during the time he is with the client.

The five categories of tools discussed provide the diagnostician with an infinite variety of tools to use, from stringing beads to a highly formalized tool such as the *Illinois Test of Psycholinguistic Abilities* (Kirk et al., 1968). Many tools are designed to elicit only a specified set of behaviors. For example, most articulation (phonetic structure) tools sample the client's sound production within a specific context, usually at the beginning, middle, and end of a word. Rating scales for judging voice and stuttering behaviors provide the diagnostician with a systematic method for observing and recording when and how much a certain behavioral characteristic may be present. Other tools sample more than a single level of behavior. For example, some tests of language measure many language products and processes such as the *Language Modalities Test of Aphasia* (Wepman and Jones, 1961) and the *Michi-*

gan Picture Language Inventory (Wolski, 1962). Some tools have complex instructions and criteria for administration and others have simple instructions.

Compare the mechanics, the operations, for administering the following two tests of vocabulary: the *Peabody Picture Vocabulary Test* (Dunn, 1965) and the *Full-Range Picture Vocabulary Test* (Ammons and Ammons, 1948).

Adequacy of tools. As well as knowing what tools are available for use, the diagnostician must be able to evaluate their measurement adequacy. He must determine how well each tool selected assists him in his skill of systematic observation, that is, how much precision he gains from its use.

More and more reliance is being placed on the so-called objective, standardized test. Scores are often being used in place of the diagnostician's descriptive data and clinical judgments. This movement toward the use of objective tools is seen in the increased number of commercial tests that have become available. The *Porch Index of Communicative Abilities* (Porch, 1967) is an example of this movement.

Objectivity in testing and interpretation is playing a greater role in diagnostic design. While objectivity is essential in evaluating the adequacy of a diagnostic tool, determining adequacy still rests with the diagnostician: did the tool do the job for him? For example, if the diagnostician used a well-standardized test for measuring a child's phonologic errors but the items on the test did not sample this specific child's primary errors, it was not adequate for the child. As a tool, no matter how extensive its standardization, it has failed. The diagnostician must remember it is not the tool that is ultimately important; it is his use of the technique to obtain appropriate information. Even though tools are essential to the diagnostician, an accurate diagnosis of speech and language problems is the diagnostician's success, not the success of a tool, a test, or any set of tools.

We discussed in Chapter 9 that a part of the researcher's concern is the precision with which he measures the responses he wants. The same is true of the diagnostician. He must know when his tools provide him with adequate, accurate, reliable, and valid information. If the diagnostician is to design and control his diagnoses to reduce error and bias and to gain precision of measurement, he must develop an appropriate awareness and respect for measurement criteria—for objectivity.

It is not our intent to provide a detailed discussion of measurement theory, although we do believe, as pointed out in Chapter 9, that it is an essential component of a diagnostician's knowledge. Instead, we will briefly discuss certain concepts that might be considered by the diagnostician in his design of the diagnosis. Our intent is to develop an awareness and a motivation for evaluating the tools selected.

The diagnostician must have criteria for evaluating the adequacy of the tools he considers for diagnostic design. The criteria discussed are validity, reliability, and standardization. These criteria arise from measurement theory, criteria often applied to something called a "test," but it can be applied to any tool. Even when a tool does not have data reported on these criteria, it is not necessarily eliminated from diagnostic usefulness. Questions arising from these criteria can be applied: Does the tool do the job intended by the diagnostician? Is the tool consistent? If repeated, will similar results occur? Does the tool provide comparative data, intra- and intergroup comparisons?

VALIDITY. Validity is of primary concern in tool construction, but it is often one of the most overlooked criteria in terms of supporting research. In its basic form, validity states that the tool is designed to measure or sample what is intended—the behavior of interest. The diagnostician would not first choose a test of phonetic structure if he hypothesized a prosody disorder. Often, validity is assumed; a statement is made that the tool has face validity, another way of saying that it is supposed to be obvious that the tool measures what was intended. For example, if we were interested in measuring syntax, we might develop a tool that asks a client to produce verb forms, thus concluding that the tool has face validity; it generates a response about one level of syntax. Using such a tool, the diagnostician is asked to accept the rationale, the face validity, on which the tool was based. Validity in this broad sense only serves the diagnostician's general purposes for measuring dimensions of the cause-effect relationship. That is, he selects tools that appear valid for his use. He asks, Does the tool measure a specific disordered behavior? Does the tool measure some aspect of the causal factor?

However, even if a tool does have face validity, it cannot be assumed that it will differentiate among various populations. The *Northwestern Syntax Screening Test* (Lee, 1969, 1970) is an example of such a tool. In a study of its internal consistency, Ratusnik and Koeningsknecht (1975) revealed that although the test gave consistent results, it failed to differentiate among the clinical groups studied as well as among the clinical and normal groups. There were variable findings regarding the receptive and expressive portions of the test. Therefore the diagnostician could not use this tool and assume that it provides him with complete information about his client's language disorder.

Validity criteria, however, are more complex. Tools can be evaluated in terms of various types of validity: concurrent, predictive, content, and construct validity. Each of these types of validity tells the diagnostician something different about the tools he may be using, although all are bound tightly together.

When the diagnostician is choosing between two tools that were designed to measure the same thing, he is concerned with *concurrent validity*. Are the tools equivalent to one another, and will they provide him with equally adequate information? Any number of tools may be available to measure a selected aspect of speech and language performance in a client. A question that must be asked is, "How equivalent are the tools for measuring that performance?" Is test *A* for syntactic formulation equal to test *B*? Do they tell us the same thing? The evidence seems fairly clear that we would not always obtain the same information with different tools. Little has been done experimentally to determine test equivalency. Nation and Corlew (1974) pointed out that naming items in aphasia tests are not equivalent, and an article by Needham and Swisher (1972) shows that measures of auditory comprehension in aphasic clients measure that behavioral correlate differently. Thus when selecting tools, diagnosticians must always maintain an awareness that the tools used are only estimates of the client's performance and may vary depending on the tool used.

When the diagnostician chooses a specific tool in hopes that he can generalize about other aspects of the client's behavior, he is concerned with *predictive validity*. Can he estimate how intelligible a child might be on the basis of a tool that measures single-sound production in words? Will this tool be predictive of what errors the child might make in spontaneous speech production? The diagnostician is interested in predicting more general behavior from the data obtained in a specific circumstance.

Prutting et al. (1975) compared the expressive portion of the *Northwestern Syntax Screening Test* (Lee, 1969, 1970) with a spontaneous language sample. In this study it was found that the spontaneous language sample obtained by the speech pathologist gave the best information about the children's language abilities. Would findings such as these make the *Northwestern Syntax Screening Test* an inappropriate tool to use in diagnosis?

When the diagnostician is choosing a tool to provide a representative sample of a specific behavior, he is concerned with *content validity*. Are the items used and the behavioral response required representative of that class of behaviors? Should he use an articulation test that samples individual phonemes in the context of words, or should he use a test that samples syllables as the basic unit of speech? Beyond this the diagnostician should ask if the items selected provide a range of responses from easy to hard, from early to late, from concrete to abstract, etc.?

McDonald's *Deep Test of Articulation* (McDonald, 1964) tests for phonemes within syllabic contexts, whereas the *Templin-Darley Tests of Articulation* (Templin and Darley, 1969) tests phonemes within word contexts. How would you determine which test has the better content validity? If you were to use the *Templin-Darley Screening Test of Articulation* (1969) with a 3-year-old child with a severe disorder of phonetic structure, would you obtain a valid sample?

When the diagnostician is choosing between tools designed to obtain information about the same disorder, he is concerned with *construct validity* (see also concurrent validity). If his interest is in the rationale, the theory on which the tool was based, his concern is construct validity. Should he choose the *Minnesota Test for Differential Diagnosis of Aphasia* (Schuell, 1965) or the *Porch Index of Communicative Ability* (Porch, 1967)? Choices like these are especially difficult to make, since many similar tools developed from different theories have experimental literature that support them as appropriately designed tools; that is, each has construct validity. Construct validity takes into account the theory by which a test was constructed. If the theory is strong, experimentally supported, the test may be strong. But if the test is constructed on incomplete or inadequate theory, the test will be weak.

Do any tests of speech and language have a high degree of construct validity? Some of the most interesting tools to examine for construct validity are the tests designed to measure the speech and language behavior of aphasic clients. To do this requires knowledge of each test maker's approach to aphasia: what options they have taken for understanding this complex disorder. As a start, examine the following three tests for aphasia, each purported by the authors to diagnose, classify, and in some instances prognosticate recovery from aphasia: The *Minnesota Test for Differential Diagnosis of Aphasia* by Schuell (1965), the *Boston Diagnostic Aphasia Examination* by Goodglass and Kaplan (1972), and the *Porch Index of Communicative Ability* by Porch (1967). Are these tools comparable, and would you find out the same type of information on an aphasic client with each of them?

RELIABILITY. Once responses have been obtained, the diagnostician wants to know if they can be relied on. Are they reflective of true responses? Or has the diagnostician obtained spurious results? Tools that are objective, provide standard instructions for stimulation, and provide standard procedures for scoring responses have a good chance of being reliable as long as the client is responding in a typical way. Reliability, therefore, focuses on two primary concerns. First, the diagnostician needs to be concerned with the consistency of the responses offered by the client. Would the client perform the same if given the test a second time—*test-retest reliability?* Second, the diagnostician needs to be concerned with scoring consistency. Scoring reliability is frequently evaluated by *interjudge* and *intrajudge* reliability. Two diagnosticians following the same scoring protocols must achieve similar results before interjudge reliability of a tool can be established. Intrajudge reliability is established when the same diagnostician scores the tool the same at different times. Diagnosticians should occasionally check themselves for scoring consistency to prevent scoring biases from creeping into their analyses.

Reliability often is difficult to establish with tools that rely on the diagnostician's perceptual measurement abilities. For example, how could tools be developed for differentiating reliably among voice disorders? How have Wilson (1972) and his colleagues gone about this?

STANDARDIZATION. The number of tools for diagnosis of speech and language disorders that have achieved standardization status is very small. Although more objective tools with reported reliability and validity estimates are available, there are few with normative data based on large representative samples. According to Weiner and Hoock (1973), there are probably no tools exempt from serious criticism. Thus even though the diagnostician has more objective tools to select from with some "normative" data, he cannot use the normative data uncritically. To do so may result in inappropriate analysis and interpretation.

Weiner and Hoock (1973) have written a timely article about standardization of tools used in diagnosis. They present a series of criteria and criticisms that can be used by the diagnostician to evaluate the adequacy of standardization in the tools he selects. By way of example they critique the standardization of the *Peabody Picture Vocabulary Test* (Dunn, 1965), the *Illinois Test of Psycholinguistic Abilities* (Paraskevopoulos and Kirk, 1969), and the *Goldman-Fristoe-Woodcock Test of Auditory Discrimination* (Goldman et al., 1970). The student, following their example, may try the same analysis with the following tools frequently used in diagnosis: the *Auditory Discrimination Test* (Wepman, 1958), the *Fisher-Logemann Test of Articulation Competence* (Fisher and Logemann, 1971), and the *Assessment of Children's Language Comprehension* (Foster et al., 1972).

Another aspect of standardization of importance is the construction of stimulus items. For any tool to be useful the diagnostician must know if the items are appropriate to the client (see discussion of content validity). The items in a standardized tool should obtain a range of responses. Age is an important consideration. Standardized tools that measure developmental data must present items applicable to various ages. At the early years, for some language measures, this may mean items selected at 3- to 6-month intervals. As well, pass-fail criteria for each item, or groups of items, by the standardization population should be available. Diagnosticians will need this information to make comparisons with their client.

Most tools that are standardized have been developed using what is termed a "normal" population. This practice can, in a sense, reduce the usability of a tool with a disordered population, at least until "normative" data is available on the disordered population. Knowing that a client has a disorder of speech and language requires the diagnostician to view performance in light of the abnormality rather than simply normative comparisons. A standardized tool appropriate for a normal 4-year-old child may be highly inappropriate for a 4-year-old child with a severe reduction of language abilities related to central language processing disruptions. What are needed, as well, are standardized objective tools that allow the client to perform in the presence of his special disability. For example, most language comprehension tools present both an auditory stimulus, "point to transportation," and the visual representation of the auditory stimulus. If the client has a visual or auditory impairment, standard presentation of this tool could become inappropriate. The diagnostician would have to find alternate ways of providing the stimulation. Thus alterations in instructions are sometimes necessary when using objective standardized tools. Of course, any alterations must be accounted for in the analysis and interpretation of the results.

CLINICAL ADEQUACY. There are few, if any, tools that do meet all the measurement criteria discussed. These adequacy criteria are difficult, if not impossible, to meet. If, for no other reason, the time and expense involved in standardization on large representative populations are frequently prohibitive. These adequacy criteria should be regarded as guides to the development of tools for diagnosis, and test makers should work toward achieving these goals and clearly report in their test manuals which goals are not yet achieved. Until adequacy information is completely supplied for each tool, the diagnostician will have to carefully evaluate the tools he selects when designing his diagnosis. He can develop a level of confidence in their use based on his analysis of the objectivity and construct validity of the tools. As well, he can rely on his professional experience to determine if a selected tool helps him interpret the speech and language problem, that is, to determine if the tool is *clinically adequate*.

The diagnostician must be a careful reader of the literature, sharpening his knowledge about tool construction. He can study the rationale, the theoretical constructs by which the tool was designed. He can ask himself if the tool seems reasonable in light of what he knows about the behaviors being tested. He can look carefully at the operations of the technique—how it samples behavior. Is it sampled in a systematic, standard manner, or does it seem loosely constructed or haphazard?

Thus the diagnostician selecting tools for designing his diagnosis should evaluate all tools critically. This does not mean that he will only select tools that have been standardized or that are always absolutely objective; it only means that he will judiciously select tools for the individual diagnosis, knowing what each tool is capable of providing for him.

Often diagnosticians consider instrumentation as belonging in the speech scientist's laboratory. How many of the instruments discussed by Hanley and Peters (1971) could be used by the diagnostician to gain important information about their clients? As a project, we feel the student diagnostician would benefit from developing a chart that indicates the type of instrumentation that measures the physical characteristics of the speech and language product.

A tool-retrieval system: the SLPM

Darley (1964) states that the diagnostician has only two basic tools at his disposal, the test and the history. He goes on to specify a test as stimuli presented to clients to elicit some form of response—a sample of behavior. In line with this perspective we maintain that the diagnostician has only a single measurement method available to him—systematic observation. All tools, regardless of how structured, of what type, or in what form, are techniques designed to elicit responses that are to be systematically observed.

However, before he can select tools for systematic observation, the diagnostician needs a way to organize and retrieve the many available tools—a tool-retrieval system. The earlier categories of tools we presented are not a particularly helpful method of organization for the diagnostician to use for selecting measurement tools. As an alternative, the diagnostician might choose to organize his tools according to the traditional problem-type classification system, that is, tools for articulation disorders, voice disorders, etc. Although the problem-type classification has served professionally over the years, as discussed in Chapter 7 it has serious drawbacks that we feel would delimit its use for organizing and retrieving tools.

A more logical retrieval system would be one tied closely to the purposes of diagnosis and the SLPM framework presented in Chapters 3 through 8. Just as the diagnostician can view and classify speech and language disorders and their causes from the SLPM perspective, so also can he view and classify the tools needed to diagnose these disorders and their causes. A tool-retrieval system based on the SLPM focuses more on what a tool does than on what a tool is called. Using the SLPM, the diagnostician is free to study tools in relationship to his clinical hypothesis rather than simply relying on the stated purpose or theoretical orientation of a given tool.

Components. Tools can be organized around the three components of the model.

There are many tools available that directly measure some detail of the speech and language product component. These tools are designed to provide detailed information about the characteristics of the speech and language variation to determine if, in fact, it is disordered. Any tool that allows the diagnostician to systematically observe some detail of the speech and language product could be an appropriate tool to include in the diagnostician's design, dependent on the effect to be measured. Some tools are better than others for the type and amount of information offered; some provide more detailed data than others.

■ The following three tests for phonetic structure give varying amounts and quality of information: the *Developmental Articulation Test* (Hejna, 1959), the *Deep Test of Articulation* (McDonald, 1964), and the *Arizona Articulatory Proficiency Scale* (Fudala, 1972). Which might you use with 8-year-old Hildegarde who has /r, ɝ, l, and l̩/ errors?

The internal speech and language processing component is far more difficult to measure. As previously discussed, it is measured primarily through speech and language products and behavioral correlates. The diagnostician obtains a measure of some behavior that he understands to be correlated with internal processes. Thus this component is measured primarily through inference. The tools used to measure the speech and language product are often the same as those used to draw inferences about internal processes. At other times behavioral correlates are measured, for example, gestures that tell the diagnostician about certain internal processes. The inference is made that if the behavior is intact, so is the underlying process. Designing tools for this component requires careful consideration of the inferential measurement strategy discussed earlier in this book. Almost any tool provides some degree of information about internal processing.

■ What internal processes might you be "testing" if you used the following tools in your

diagnosis of 35-year-old Mrs. McWilliams: the "Rainbow Passage" (Fairbanks, 1960) and production of /a/ at three different pitch levels?

Tools to tap the speech and language environment component are used primarily to discover causal factors. Most of these tools are retrospective, trying to discover past occurrences that may be causally related to the current speech and language disorder. Case history questionnaires and direct interviews are the tools most commonly used. Of course, the diagnostician can look at the current environment of the client by "visiting" him in his various environmental circumstances: at home, on the job, at school, etc.

■ What series of questions might you devise to discover if 3-year-old Claude had and is receiving enough speech and language stimulation to compensate for his mild bilateral hearing loss, which is suspected as being responsible for his delay in language development.

Appendix III presents an alphabetical listing of many tools available for use by the diagnostician for designing his diagnosis within the SLPM framework. Instructions for use of the appendix are provided there. It is suggested to the diagnostician that this appendix be expanded on, that is, developed according to his specific needs in his work setting.

Causal factors. We have made a major point in this book that causal factors can be studied within the SLPM framework. Detailed information has been presented about causal factors, cause-effect interactions, and deriving cause-effect hypotheses to be tested. We now want to add some information vital to the diagnostician when designing his diagnosis for causal factors, for selecting tools to measure the causal aspect of his hypothesis.

When he designs his diagnosis to gain support for his causal hypothesis, the diagnostician must recognize his causal testing limitations. There are some causal factors the diagnostician can design and test for, for example, if hearing loss has been hypothesized as the basis for the speech and language disorder (auditory testing), if a short lingual frenum has been hypothesized (speech mechanism testing), or if a lack of speech and language stimulation has been hypothesized (interview testing). There are other causal factors the diagnostician can only partially design and test for, for example, if mental retardation has been hypothesized, if inadequate velopharyngeal closure has been hypothesized, or if brain dysfunction has been hypothesized. In many such instances the ultimate design and testing for causal factors must be left up to other specialists. For example, if brain damage has been hypothesized, it will be the neurologist who will make the final causal diagnosis; if it is mental retardation, it will likely be the psychologist or the educator; or if emotional disturbance is hypothesized, it will be the psychologist or psychiatrist.

Because of the nature and complexities of causal factors, the diagnostician has few tools that he can use to directly test the causal factor. Generally, the tools the diagnostician uses in his design measure certain behaviors that provide support for potential causes but do not provide direct, demonstrable proof. A major tool available to the diagnostician is the constituent analysis step from which he derived his original cause-effect hypothesis. Adding the interview to this information may give the diagnostician further insights into the validity of the causal relationship expressed. Beyond the case history analysis and the interview, the diagnostician can select and use certain tools that provide information about visual abilities, hearing status, motor performance, social development, psychological status, emotional status, and mental abilities. These tools, along with guided observations that focus on extraverbal behaviors accompanying interpersonal communication, provide information about the client's overall areas of functioning that could be causally or coincidentally related to the speech and language disorder.

Guided observation may provide one of the few avenues the speech pathologist has for gaining data pertinent to causal factors. Observations of a child's play behavior may provide much information about the child's level of intellectual and cognitive ability. The diagnostician may present a child with a certain selection of things to do such as doll furniture, dolls, and doll clothing (stimulus control) and observe how the child explores, plays with, and develops relationships among the sets of materials he has been given. Observing the child who demonstrates excessive motor activity, is unable to attend, is in leg braces, drools constantly, is highly emotional, or seems frightened or the adult who appears with a right hemiplegia, is depressed, and walks into things is one of the many observations that may lend evidence supporting certain causal factors that have been hypothesized.

There are questions that sometimes arise about the professional qualifications necessary for using certain tools, particularly if the tools are "borrowed" from another professional discipline. The use of some tools by the speech pathologist as "causal tests" raises few questions, for example, the *Oseretsky Tests of Motor Proficiency* (Doll, 1946), whereas others may raise considerable questions, the *Bender-Gestalt Test for Young Children* (Koppitz, 1964). Still others are generally considered out of bounds, for example, the *Arthur Adaptation of the Leiter International Performance Scale* (Arthur, 1952).

However, in this age of interdisciplinary training and work settings, lines of demarcation for test use are sometimes fuzzy. There are tools that are used across various professional groups, depending on the level of training and how the information from the tool is to be used and interpreted. The most frequently cited examples are intelligence and personality tests, generally considered as part of the psychologist's armamentarium. Can the speech pathologist justifiably select and use some of these tools to gain information about causal factors? Many of these tools are used in our experimental literature. As we grow and develop as professionals with greater interdisciplinary interests, there may be less concern over who uses what test and more concern over why the test is being used by the professional.

The student in training should explore the experimental literature for uses of tests that may assist him in gaining information about causal factors. How did Prins (1972) use the *California Test of Personality* (Thorpe et al., 1953), and what information does his article provide about personality as a causal factor for stuttering?

From the tools he uses the diagnostician may have arrived at strong inferences about causal factors and then must rely on other professionals to verify his causal hypothesis. When these causal circumstances exist, referrals to other specialists are needed to complete the design and testing for the causal aspect of the hypothesis. As we pointed out earlier in the constituent analysis, the diagnostician is always on the alert for a need to make referrals. So referral becomes another tool for diagnostic design. But the diagnostician has to know what other specialists do if he is to make informed referrals. The diagnostician must know what he wants, how to get it, what it means when he gets it, and what it does for him in client management. The ability to state, "I need a neurologic examination" is not enough to obtain needed answers to diagnostic questions. The diagnostician must understand the nature and intent of a neurologic examination—what information it will and will not provide that is pertinent to the client being diagnosed. So diagnosticians have an obligation to understand some of the basic tools used by other specialists. For example, the diagnostician who refers for medical information should know the essentials of what may be done by the physician. His first consideration should be referral to a physician who understands speech and language disorders. However, depending on the causal

factors of concern, different specialists will be called on. In voice disorders the otolaryngologist will be important; for children with language disorders the pediatrician or pediatric neurologist may be called on; for dysarthria due to any number of causes the neurologist or physical medicine and rehabilitation specialists will be important. Each of these specialists generally approaches the client in a similar fashion. A general examination will be done, followed by special tests for isolating causal factors for the speech and language disorder, or from their point of view, the medical or physical problems the patient may have.

Richardson (1972) presents her basis for medical diagnosis of children with language disorders. How much of what she suggests as the essentials of a medical evaluation can be understood or even performed by the diagnostician of speech and language disorders? How does knowing this information assist with making referrals?

As well as providing information about causal factors, certain tools used primarily by other professions also can provide significant data about speech and language. This is very evident in intelligence tests that require verbal performance. We (Aram and Nation, 1971) did an analysis of speech and language items on a number of frequently used intelligence tests using an earlier version of the SLPM as a framework for the analysis. It became quite clear from the analysis that a child with a significant deficit in speech and language would be greatly penalized by many of these tools because of their heavy verbal loadings. Having information like this assists the diagnostician in both making referrals and interpreting data he receives. Thus knowing tools that other specialists use is one way of making intelligent referrals, of using referrals as tools of diagnosis.

Again, in Appendix III, a number of tools that are considered primarily causal tools or tools for associated behaviors are listed. Some of these are used by diagnosticians of speech and language disorders; others are not.

• • •

In summary, knowing the conceptual orientation to the SLPM gives the diagnostician the knowledge needed to develop a tool-retrieval system for diagnostic design, regardless of the type of client, the type of speech and language disorder seen, its specific characteristics, and the many causal factors that may have been or are interacting with the speech and language disorder. The SLPM not only gives the diagnostician a frame of reference for selecting the tools appropriate to his hypothesis, but it also allows him to "plug in" new tools as they are developed. Relating tools to the conceptual framework of the SLPM forces him to question what a tool does for him. With this approach to design and selection of tools, the diagnostician can expose himself to a wide range of tests and procedures, develop his skill in using the tool when needed for a given diagnosis, and evaluate the effectiveness of the tool, thereby having available an inventory of tools for future reference.

Diagnostician's tasks

By the time he reaches the third step of the diagnostic process, the diagnostician has a firm grip on the potential clinical problem he will see. Now he must focus on methodology; he must design his diagnostic session. To complete this third step we have specified three tasks. First, he must plan for systematic observation of the clinical hypothesis. Second, he selects the specific tools he wants to use to fit his measurement plan. Third, he develops an overall testing strategy for efficiently carrying out his plan while optimizing data collection.

Plans for systematic observation

Perhaps the first question the diagnostician might ask in order to complete this design task would be, "How do I plan to accomplish what I want to do in this diagnosis, and what contingencies may occur to prevent it?" To answer this question he begins by laying his hypothesis and client knowledge "out on the table"; then he asks what he wants and needs to know and what others may want and need to know. He knows his measurement plan must be developed to determine if his clinical hypothesis is correct or if another solution (alternate hypothesis) is correct. He also knows that the specification of his plan will vary depending on how the purpose of referral lines up with his own hypothesis (see earlier discussions of referral purposes). And he also knows that he may not accomplish all he wants because of certain personal characteristics of his clients or, at times, the setting in which he works.

Cause-effect relationship expressed in the hypothesis. In his diagnostic plan the diagnostician must first determine if his hypothesis is testable. Can he measure the relationships expressed in the hypothesis? If not, he must go back to the drawing board and derive a more testable hypothesis for the client. He must determine what information may be easily obtained and what may be more difficult to measure. In general, the easiest to measure are the characteristics of the disorder, the variations in the speech and language product presented by the client. Planning for the causal factors generally presents more difficulties than does planning for the speech and language behavior; that is, language products are easier to measure than is brain injury.

As part of his planning the diagnostician considers his various alternate hypotheses, including the null hypothesis of no problem. These alternate hypotheses reflect cause-effect uncertainties on the part of the diagnostician; he must design his diagnosis to reduce these uncertainties, to determine which hypothesis may be the "best fit." One way he can facilitate the reduction of uncertainties is by planning systematic measurements that rule in and out several probabilities simultaneously. For example, he may be working from a hypothesis that states that Annie Mae has a language disorder only on the phonologic level and an alternate hypothesis that states the semantic level is disordered as well. He could plan measures that let him observe Annie Mae's use of phonology through a naming task, a task that would also estimate her vocabulary usage. If she was able to name the items but with many phonologic errors, the diagnostician gains strength for a phonologic disorder as well as strength for ruling out the hypothesized semantic disorder. When the diagnostician finishes, he wants to be able to state how strong his conclusions are; he hopes to have reached the most likely probability. Thus the diagnosis should be designed to systematically and simultaneously observe as many aspects of the alternate hypotheses as possible.

Task specification. A major part of the planning done at this stage is task specification. Let us say that the diagnostician has hypothesized a semantic disorder for Sandy May. He may specify tasks to measure the extent of her vocabulary, her use of nouns having varying degrees of abstraction, or tasks to evaluate the semantic relations signaled by her utterances. Or if he has hypothesized an auditory processing deficit as responsible for Nathan's comprehension disorder, he may specify various types of auditory measurements from audiometric tests to tests of auditory comprehension.

As well, depending on his hypothesis, the diagnostician may specify processing tasks more than product tasks. If he hypothesized a disruption of the articulation process as responsible for the phonetic errors, he may devise many tasks for measuring the functions of the articulators. Or if he were more interested in the phonetic product, he may devise many tasks measuring phonetic structure in as many contexts as possible and spend less time with the articulation process. The diagnostician has many degrees of freedom available to him for task specification as long as his tasks solve the problem and

allow him to propose appropriate management plans.

■ What would be the level of task specification for the product in this "hypothesis"? "Mr. Theisen cannot talk because his larynx was recently removed." How much detail would you want or expect to obtain about the speech product? What would be the purpose of task specification for this diagnosis?

As a part of task specification, the diagnostician is concerned about measures that give estimates of the severity of the problem and estimates of prognosis. Tools that have built-in severity and prognostic guides would be useful. Both of these aspects of diagnosis are difficult to plan since so few measurements are available to provide reliable estimates. More often the diagnostician's clinical experience guides his judgments about the severity of the disorder and prognosis for change.

Client characteristics. Sometimes it must seem that our interest is a cause-effect relationship instead of a specific client. Hopefully, in making our points about the purpose and process of diagnosis, we have not forsaken client concern; it is the client with all his personal characteristics in whom we are interested. It is the client who has the problem perceived as a cause-effect relationship. When we plan our diagnosis, we ultimately must design it around the specific needs and abilities of the client. An aphasic who is extremely depressed will not respond adequately to the measures we plan unless we first work through the depression. A child who is running around the room will not "point to the shoe" until we get him controlled. A child who will not talk cannot be expected to name the items on our language test until we are able to establish much better rapport. The examples of particular client needs, abilities, and behaviors that must be met are endless.

In his planning the diagnostician must consider what type, level, and range of tasks the client will respond to; what stimuli will motivate the client enough to elicit observable responses. The diagnostician must control all the variables that enter into the diagnostic session; he must plan for them.

The diagnostician must consider many client complex characteristics when he is developing his overall plan for systematic observation: age, sex, type of disorder, cause of the problem, personality, emotionality, physical disabilities, affect, need to communicate, parental attitudes, motivation, interests, cultural background, ability to attend, and level of concern—a few, among many. His plans for systematic observation must be considered within the abilities of the client complex to be tested. Any or all of these contingencies can arise to spoil the best laid plans.

■ The following are summary statements derived from several informant's remarks about their child's "personality adjustment." How might you use this information to plan your systematic observation? A hypothesis is provided for each child.

1. *Carl Wolpaw, aged 6 years, 3 months, stutters because of an emotionally unstable family background.*

Summary statement. Carl was described by Mr. Wolpaw as an active, healthy boy who eats and sleeps well. He plays mainly with his brothers and sisters and "gets along as well as kids ever get along." He is shy with adults and somewhat reluctant to talk to them. Mr. Wolpaw considers Carl "as easy to discipline even though he requires a lot of it." He tries to be too much like his older brother, who is a real problem.

2. *Jacqueline Smith, aged 5 years, 5 months, has a severe language disorder related to slow mental development.*

Summary statement. As reported by Mrs. Dana Faith, Jacqueline's foster mother, Jacqueline is a happy child who gets along well with both children and adults. At times Mrs. Faith has found it difficult to discipline Jacqueline, while at other times she responds immediately. Mrs. Faith noted that Jacqueline "seems inconsistent in behaving and seems to act on impulse." She seems to have difficulty concentrating, especially on directed work such as learning the alphabet, although at times "she seems to think deeply and remembers well."

3. *Tog Richards, aged 4 years, 9 months, has a severe articulation-resonation problem related to his cleft palate condition.*

Summary statement. As reported by his mother, Mrs. Leslie Richards, Tog usually plays with other children his age and gets along with both children and adults. He does not have difficulty concentrating and enjoys having books read to him. He is an active boy who likes being outdoors and doing things with his father. However, he is cooperative with other adults only when "properly motivated" and not when "pushed." Tog's schoolmates are teasing him about his speech. He reacts by ignoring them and leaving their presence, but Mrs. Richards feels Tog is hurt by the teasing.

Selects tools for measurement

The diagnostician now asks himself, "Now that I have an overall plan, what tools (techniques) will allow me to take my measurements?" The selection of tools to fit the plan is a critical task for designing the diagnosis. We have all had diagnostic failures because of poor selection of tools. Did failure occur because the tool was inappropriate for the client—the child was too young? Did failure occur because the tool was inappropriate for the hypothesis—an articulation test was chosen for a language disorder? Did failure occur because the tool was too complicated—too many behaviors were sampled? Did failure occur because the administration procedures were unfamiliar—too little practice with the tool? Careful selection of tools based on the clinical hypothesis, the characteristics of the client, and the diagnostician's skill level will reduce the number of diagnostic failures. In this task the diagnostician retrieves tools for the specific client; that is, he tailor-makes his diagnostic design.

Retrieves tools. Once the diagnostician has worked out his plan for systematic observation, he must select the specific tools by which he will carry out that plan. We have discussed the infinite number of tools available to the diagnostician, developed a tool-retrieval system through a SLPM organization, presented a selected list of available tools in Appendix III, suggested a series of criteria by which tools can be evaluated, and have indicated that the personal characteristics of the client and the work setting must be considered.

Several other considerations should be mentioned at this time. First, the diagnostician is working under time constraints; therefore the tools he selects should be accomplishable within his time limitations. Therefore he also may select a single tool to measure several things simultaneously. Second, the diagnostician should understand his own limitations—is he familiar with all aspects of the tools he has selected? Third, the diagnostician must consider some rather practical aspects of the tools. Of most importance are their portability. Carrying around suitcases of props or heavy equipment simply is not feasible in many work settings. Thus tools must be physically manageable.

Given this entire set of considerations for retrieving the specific tools needed for testing the cause-effect hypothesis, we will proceed to a set of diagnostic situations exemplifying these considerations. These situations are only schematic. They are representative of certain circumstances the diagnostician may confront in his various work settings. The student should develop the overall planning that would go into each of these situations that leads to tool selection. All the tools presented in the examples can be found in Appendix III.

■ Harriet Nordell, 4 years, 6 months, was referred to a community speech and hearing agency. Hypothesis: "Severe language problem on all linguistic levels. . . ."

The diagnostician, Ms. Seligman, has available to her a full range of tools. To observe the language product she first selects a *spontaneous speech and language sample* and the *Vocabulary Usage Test* (Nation, 1972). Diagnosticians often rely on a spontaneous speech sample to measure language performance (for example, Lee, 1974). All language products can be observed if the client offers any language output. Since Harriet has a severe language problem, Ms. Seligman may have difficulty obtaining enough of a sample for analysis or she may obtain all that the child is capable of, from unintelligible vocalizations to one- or two-word

responses. The stimuli provided by Ms. Seligman will be crucial to obtaining this sample. Ms. Seligman chose this tool because she has a firm comparative foundation—knowledge about the normal language behavior of children this age. What information, other than the language product, might you obtain with a spontaneous speech sample?

The *Vocabulary Usage Test* (VUT) was selected because it provides information about a specific language product, the semantic level. This tool was chosen based on the stages of language acquisition; semantic items (vocabulary) are seen first in a child's development. Since Harriet has a deficit on all linguistic levels, her best output performance may well be in vocabulary usage. The tool is developmental and objective although not highly standardized. Ms. Seligman also feels she will obtain some other information from this tool that allows her to distinguish between possible comprehension and formulation deficits. The *Vocabulary Usage Test* requires the child to respond to pictured items from an auditorally presented stimulus.

Ms. Seligman also selected the following tools for Harriet: the *Houston Test for Language Development* (Crabtree, 1963) and the *Verbal Language Development Scale* (Mecham, 1958). What information do you think she was trying to obtain from these tools?

The spontaneous speech and language sample ranks high among the various techniques selected to observe language products. The diagnostician is likely to obtain more typical responses with this measure than with some of the structured stimulus-response tools that may be available. From his sample the diagnostician performs various analyses on the data for comparison to normal language development. However, analysis of the data from this procedure is not easy. It is easier to record a response to a structured stimulus; for example, right or wrong, and from the derived score determine if the client's performance is above, at, or below the norms than it is to take a spontaneous language sample that, in all likelihood, will have to be tape-recorded, listened to over and over, and then apply analysis procedures to arrive at a description of the client's language behavior. However, the end result of this latter procedure may result in better management planning.

The diagnostician must remember that when a child produces language, he also reveals information about his underlying language processes. For example, if the diagnostician presents a stimulus, "Tell me what's happening in this picture," and the child responds, "Boy throw ball," the diagnostician can easily measure the semantic and syntactic levels of the language product. As well, if the response is on target, he knows something about comprehension and formulation. He can interpret aspects of the child's language rule system for formulation; in this example the child is demonstrating a relationship of agent + action + object.

MacDonald and Nichols (1974) have presented a strategy for diagnosis and treatment of children with severely delayed language called the *Environmental Language Inventory*. Its use is for children using language at the one- or two-word stage. How could you adapt this technique for children who may be using more language but are still considered to have a language disorder?

■ Ms. Marge Celeste, the kindergarten teacher, asked the speech pathologist, Mr. Jim Thorington, to see Paul Cronise who just entered her kindergarten class. Ms. Celeste thinks Paul may be retarded. Hypothesis: "Severe language comprehension disruptions. . . ."

Mr. Thorington selects the *Peabody Picture Vocabulary Test* (Dunn, 1965) and the *Assessment of Children's Language Comprehension* (Foster et al., 1972). Both of these tools are objective and in the case of the *Peabody Picture Vocabulary Test* quite well standardized, although not without criticisms of the standardization (Weiner and Hoock, 1973). Mr. Thorington selects these tools because he wants an objective baseline of Paul's ability to comprehend at the semantic and syntactic levels. Comprehension, a behavioral correlate, has always been difficult to measure. It cannot be observed directly but must be measured by observing certain responses from which the diagnostician infers comprehension abilities. Thus objective measures as selected by Mr. Thorington are ex-

tremely important to use since it is difficult to know from general conversation at what level Paul may be comprehending. For example, how would we know which of the following two stimuli would be appropriate for Paul: "Would you like to color in the coloring book?" and "Did you walk to school today?"

Typical tools of comprehension, such as those selected by Mr. Thorington, ask a client to point to a choice of pictures that correspond to the auditory stimulus presented. Stimuli may be words, phrases, sentences, and paragraphs. Foil pictures are often used to check for accuracy of response or closeness of response. Tools for comprehension of syntax have been questioned by Waryas and Ruder (1974). They have pointed out that in some of the comprehension tools used the client may not have to process all the elements of the auditory stimulus to arrive at a correct response. In order to circumvent some of these problems they have developed a technique called the grammatical preference procedure. In this procedure the client is asked to indicate which of the stimulus sentences presented is the best, thus a preference for grammaticality is measured.

•   •   •

How easy or difficult might it be to adapt the procedures suggested by Waryas and Ruder (1974) to the practicalities of the diagnostic session? Could Paul have a severe comprehension disorder as hypothesized and still perform such a task?

•   •   •

Since Ms. Celeste is concerned about mental retardation, Mr. Thorington hopes the *Peabody Picture Vocabulary Test* may provide him with useful information. But Mr. Thorington is aware of the use of verbal measures for estimating the intelligence of children with speech and language disorders, particularly in Paul's case since he has hypothesized a severe comprehension deficit. This very issue was addressed by Weiner (1971) who studied the reliability and stability of two measures of intelligence on children with language disorders—the *Peabody Picture Vocabulary Test* and the *Arthur Adaptation of the Leiter International Performance Scale* (Arthur, 1952).

•   •   •

From Weiner's information (1971), what might Mr. Thorington expect from his use of the

Peabody Picture Vocabulary Test with Paul? If he were to refer Paul for psychological testing, what justifications could he offer for the specification of an intelligence tool to be used?

• • •

Evaluate the following tools also selected by Mr. Thorington for Paul: the *Illinois Test of Psycholinguistic Abilities* (Kirk et al., 1968) and the *Flowers-Costello Test of Central Auditory Abilities* (Flowers et al., 1970).

■ Marie Shivers, aged 4 years, 9 months, has little language. She is being seen by Mr. Larry Bobkoff, speech pathologist at University Hospitals, as a part of a comprehensive inpatient work-up. Hypothesis: "Severe language comprehension and formulation disorder related to cerebral dysfunction."

Mr. Bobkoff selects guided observations of all aspects of general behavior during Marie's daily activities while in the hospital. Mr. Bobkoff has taken this approach in order to observe behaviors that may signal the presence of cerebral dysfunction as a basis for the lack of speech and language development. He is particularly interested in any direct physical signs such as gait, awkward coordination, and speech-mechanism deviations as well as behaviors that are at times predictive of cerebral dysfunction—signs such as hyperactivity, compulsivity, inability to attend, motor perseveration, emotionality, and variable, inconsistent responses to auditory and visual stimulation. His goal is to assist the team in organizing the most efficient set of tests for isolating the basis of Marie's speech and language disorder. From his findings he will provide recommendations for testing to the other team members.

Mr. Bobkoff recommended the use of the following tools: the *Arthur Adaptation of the Leiter International Performance Scale* (Arthur, 1952), *Oseretsky Tests of Motor Proficiency* (Doll, 1946), *Clinical Examinations in Neurology* (Mayo Clinic, 1971), and the *Developmental Test of Visual Perception* (Frostig, 1964). What does Mr. Bobkoff hope will be accomplished by the use of these tools? Do you see these as tools that are causally selected?

■ Dr. Maureen Whitney is seeing her first aphasic client at Springfield General Hospital. She has a range of aphasia tests accessible to her and appropriate training in their use. The hospital staff, however, has always used the *Minnesota Test for Differential Diagnosis of Aphasia* (Schuell, 1965) because of its prognostic ability. While Dr. Whitney understands the prognostic implications for using this test, her theoretical orientation to aphasia leads her to other choices of tools. She has been asked to justify her selection of the *Boston Diagnostic Aphasia Examination* (Goodglass and Kaplan, 1972) for initial diagnostic purposes followed by the *Porch Index of Communicative Ability* (Porch, 1967) for later objectification and prognostication.

Can you justify Dr. Whitney's approach to selection of tools to fulfill the purposes of diagnosis? Are these tools practical for all settings? In what type of setting might this approach be most useful? How much time would it require to administer the tools? Would Eisenson's *Examining for Aphasia* (1954) fulfill the requirements of prognostication?

Prognosis for change of disordered speech and language behavior is a major part of the diagnostician's function. Following his diagnosis, the diagnostician should be able to make tentative judgments about the client's ability to change if given the maximum therapeutic intervention needed. Aside from his clinical experience with similar clients, the diagnostician has little to guide him in making prognostic statements since only a few tools have been developed that give prognostic information. Notable among them are the *Minnesota Test for Differential Diagnosis of Aphasia* developed by Schuell (1965).

Generally, however, the diagnostician relies on *stimulability testing* to determine if a client can learn, can change his pattern of speech and language given appropriate stimulation (Milisen et al., 1954). Thus any tool or device that demonstrates that a client can learn to change his behavior has potential for prognostication. Some tools are being developed to assist the diagnostician with specific types of clients. Jacobs et al. (1970) have developed a stimulability test for children whose speech characteristics are related to a cleft palate condition. The *Miami Imitative Ability Test* (MIAT) has provided information that the cleft palate child's improvement in articulation can be occasionally prognosticated on the basis of results from the *Miami Imitative Ability Test.*

It is one thing to determine if a client can change a given speech and language pattern and quite another to know if he will "recover" from his speech and language disorder. What do causal factors tell us about chances of recovery? What does severity of a disorder tell us? What is the difference between these two types of prognostication, each type represented in the two tools mentioned above?

■ Dr. Ivan Cook is seeing Ms. Leslie Golden, who was referred for stuttering therapy. There is no doubt in Dr. Cook's mind that she is a stutterer. Thus he selects tools to determine the type, extent, and severity of her prosody disorder. He wants information that will tell him when she stutters, what type of prosody variations she is exhibiting, how often these occur, how much they interfere with communication, etc. Thus this diagnosis is concerned with a contemporary view of the disorder rather than discovering a historical cause-effect relationship.

Other than presenting various types of stimuli to Ms. Golden and organizing his observations of her responses, what can Dr. Cook do to get the information he is looking for? If you were to follow Riley's procedure (1972) using his *Stuttering Severity Instrument* (SSI), would you be able to characterize the disorder as well as determine its severity? What information would the *Southern Illinois University Speech Situations Check List* and the *Southern Illinois University Behavior Check List*, both by Brutten and Shoemaker (1974a, b), provide for systematically obtaining the information that Dr. Cook wants?

In summary, the diagnostician selects tools to assist him in observing relevant information about the cause-effect hypothesis he has formulated. The client is his ultimate concern; therefore all tools selected must be usable with each individual client. Although standardization and objectivity are important tool criteria, the diagnostician must have flexibility in his testing. He must use all manner and means of tools to get at the client's disorder. All tools have relevance as long as the diagnostician

knows what they do for him. In diagnosis he is not trying to standardize the client; he is trying to discover the nature and significance of the speech and language disorder to make decisions for management. Client concern is his primary motivation.

Interview questions. If the interview has been selected as a tool to be used in the diagnosis, the diagnostician must plan the format of that interview. While much of what happens in the interview will be dependent on interpersonal factors (Chapter 14), the diagnostician should be prepared to enter the interview situation. We suggest, therefore, that the diagnostician consider two fundamental questions in planning the interview: (1) What information does he want? (2) How does he plan to get it?

As with any tool that has been selected for the diagnosis, the interview aims at gaining data to shed more understanding about the clinical hypothesis that was formulated through the constituent analysis. The diagnostician will need to fill in missing data, and, in addition, he will need to amplify, clarify, and verify information made available to him. Some of the information he has is insufficient. For example, on the children's speech and language history questionnaire, in response to, "When did he speak his first word," a parent may have written *late*. Here the diagnostician would want to get a more refined idea of what late means. He may be able to pin down a more specific time or gain a better estimate of the time in relation to other events such as birthdays, visits to grandmothers, etc.

Often the diagnostician will want the informant to amplify on information provided prior to the interview. For example, if reference was made to the fact that a child was in "therapy," the diagnostician would want to delineate more clearly the details of that therapy. Was it speech therapy, psychotherapy, or physiotherapy? What are the goals of therapy? What was its duration and frequency?

At other times the diagnostician will

need to clarify information that is ambiguous or inconsistent. For example, a teacher may report that "Larry has trouble keeping still in class." The diagnostician will need to determine if "still" refers to Larry's verbal or activity level and what circumstances surround his difficulty "keeping still." At times information from different sources (or even from the same source) is inconsistent and contradictory. A pediatrician may report that Ruth had difficulty being toilet trained, while a parent reports no such problems; or one source may report two siblings and a second source reports three. A mother may report hemorrhaging during pregnancy, while the pediatrician's report states an uneventful pregnancy. In all such situations, further information is needed to reconcile the contradictory information.

Finally, a diagnostician may need to verify information if he questions its reliability or validity. For example, a referring social worker may suggest that family stresses, including a working mother and alcoholic father, are the basis for Victor's speech and language problems. During the interview, the diagnostician will want to explore the nature of these family stresses more thoroughly to determine if in fact the home situation does adversely affect the speech and language environment of the child.

■ In the following examples determine what missing data needs to be gained and where amplification, clarification, and verification of constituent analysis information are indicated.

1. A physician, Dr. Draeger, reports that 6-year-old Alexander has had a history of chronic otitis media.
2. The only information regarding motor milestones for 10-year-old Sarah is walking at 15 months. She has been described as clumsy by her gym teacher and is doing poorly in reading and spelling in school.
3. An adult client, Mrs. Rockman, describes her speech and language problem as "difficulty making myself understood."
4. The referring psychologist reported that 4-year-old Tommy's parents are divorced.

Tommy lives with his mother and maternal grandmother and 6-year-old sister. The father has visitation rights and spends every other Sunday with Tommy and his daughter.
5. On the children's speech and language history form, Mrs. Rupert checks *yes* to "eating problems," "difficult to manage," and "personality problem" but did not explain or give ages.

■ Turning again to Katherine Compardo, we can refer back to the children's speech, language, and hearing history questionnaire that was available prior to the diagnostic session to determine what additional data we want to get in the interview. Table 12 lists examples of the constituents available in Katherine's history and points to areas in which further information is needed. It is suggested that the student continue to evaluate the remainder of Katherine's history questionnaire information in this manner.

Having decided what information he wants, the diagnostician next needs to think through how he plans to get that information. Here he is concerned with framing his questions. Styles of eliciting information differ markedly from a nondirect approach, where the information evolves from considerable dialogue and reflection on the informant's comments—"I see that you are concerned." "You feel uncertain about Jerome's abilities." "Renee's stuttering worries you."—to a direct question-answer exchange characteristic of much political poll taking or consumer interviewing: "Do you have a dog?" "What brands of dog food have you used in the past month?" "Have you ever tried Grow-pup Super Meat?" "Is your income bracket below $10,000, between $10,000 and $15,000, or above $15,000?"

We can view most forms of interview probe questions as falling on an open-closed continuum determined by the degree of structure allowed in the informant's response. Closed questions elicit specific, relatively predictable information; the number of alternative answers or choices in answering is limited. Questions such as "How old is Lee?" "When did Jonathan

Table 12. Determination of information needed in interview

Constituent as reported by mother	Further information needed
I. Identification Address: One St. Mary's Street	Where is St. Mary's Street? What does this address tell us about the family's life-style?
II. Statement of the problem Nothing has been done about it	What does "nothing" mean to the mother? Is "nothing" consistent with her later comments about questioning hearing, convincing herself nothing was wrong, and starting to think otherwise? Have any other family members "done anything" about Katherine's problem?
III. Speech, language, and hearing history Understands everything	What specifically does Katherine understand? How does Mrs. Compardo judge Katherine's understanding?
IV. General development No information reported about toilet training	Has toilet training been started? If so, what progress has been made? If not, is this due to the mother's approach to toilet training or an indication that Katherine is not ready?
V. Medical history No illnesses indicated except chicken-pox	Verification of this information is needed. It is unusual for a child with two elementary school-aged siblings not to have had any of the other childhood illnesses? Check colds, earaches, and ear infections.
VI. Behavior Runs around a lot	What are the circumstances surrounding her "running around"? What does "running around" entail? Is this normal activity, purposeless, unrelenting?
VII. Educational history Mother left blank: "Has anyone ever thought she was a slow child."	On the developmental section of the questionnaire, the mother reported: "She seems much slower than my other children." How do you reconcile this inconsistency in information?
VIII. Home and family information—additional information "I have just convinced myself there was nothing wrong, now I have to start thinking otherwise."	Why was the mother trying to convince herself nothing was wrong? What prompted her to feel she must start thinking otherwise?

Table 13. Closed-open question continuum

Question type		Examples
Closed end	Yes/no	Did Martin require any oxygen immediately following birth? Did your husband want to come today?
	Multiple choice	Does Emory use his left hand, right hand, or both? Does Mark primarily use speech or gestures?
	Fill in the blank	John is how old? What drugs were used during delivery? Where was your husband's surgery performed?
	Circumscribed amplification	Describe Torry's speech problem. What kinds of things does Kevin play with? How have Mr. Worzella's spirits been since his stroke?
Open end	Take off anywhere	What would you like to talk about today? Is there anything you would like to talk about that we haven't already discussed? I'd like you to try to give me a picture of Sandy as you see her at home.

first begin to walk?" "Did Carter ever have any ear infections?" are examples of relatively closed questions. Open questions, at the other end of the continuum, allow for considerable choice and flexibility in the informant's responses. Such questions gain elaborated, less predictable information and are often feeling oriented (Bernstein, 1970; Richardson et al., 1965). "How does Leigh spend her day?" "How would you describe your husband's problems in speaking?" and "How did you understand the problem as Dr. Bastob explained it to you?" are such open-ended questions. Table 13 lists a number of types of questions that are arranged in terms of their degree of openness or closedness. There are many variations and additions to these types of questions, and there is nothing sacred or special about the particular list of question types in Table 13; rather, these types of questions represent a range often used in the interview.

While some writers recommend that open questions should predominate in the interview (Garrett, 1972; Richardson et al., 1965), we maintain that a range of question types are useful and that the information needed determines the type of question asked. Yes/no, multiple choice, and fill in the blank questions are direct, efficient means of gaining specific, relatively nonequivocal factual information. For example, if the diagnostician wants to know if there are any siblings in the family, a yes/no question, "Does Ramon have any brothers or sisters?" would gain the information most directly.

In using relatively closed questions, however, the diagnostician needs to guard against presenting prepackaged alternatives and specifying dichotomies when none exist. For example, "Is Sarah toilet trained?" may elicit a simple yes/no response when a range of toilet training can exist—from no control, through degrees of control, to complete control. Asking a parent if they are "relieved or unsettled" by Max's placement in a school for the retarded may in no way match their feelings

about the situation. Not all informants are secure enough to disregard the nonapplicable alternatives presented in the interview questions. Thus, in using closed questions, the diagnostician needs to be sure he furthers data collection not cuts it off or elicits invalid information. His questions should not inhibit spontaneity on the part of the informant or allow the informant to outguess him and give the "correct" rather than the accurate answer. Too many closed questions will make the interview appear rote and prefabricated. The question may make the informant feel that the only information wanted from them is the yes/no, multiple choice, or fill in the blank variety. They may interpret this as disinterest in how they really feel about the problem at hand. The diagnostician should be sure to allow for amplification and self-expression by the informant even when using closed questions. Often, for example, a yes/no question may be followed by a question asking for more information. "Does Shorty have any brothers or sisters?" If answered affirmatively, it may be followed by further fill in the blank questions: "How old are they?" or with circumscribed amplification: "What kinds of things do Shorty and his sister do together?" or "How does his sister respond to Shorty?"

Open-ended questions allow for maximal individual expression on the part of the informant. Such questions tend to let the informant say what is important to him in the way that he wants to express it, thus restricting possible bias or shortsightedness on the part of the diagnostician. The diagnostician cannot predict all that he needs to know; thus he must allow the informant room to say what he wants to say. Open-ended questions, however, are inefficient in gaining specific, nonequivocal information. If the diagnostician wants to know if Kate has had psychological testing, he does not need to go all around the barn to get an answer. A question such as "What have you done about her problem?" may not address the information wanted.

Also, at times, some informants have difficulty responding if some structure is not provided for their response. Some may feel that "there's no place to start" in describing a pervasive problem; others "don't know what to say." Such informants may respond in one or two words to "take off anywhere" questions but provide much more information to circumscribed amplification questions. In sum, the diagnostician should have a range of question types at his disposal as different information and clients will require different question types. Framing interview questions is not an either/or proposition, rather it is a purposive selection and combination of several question types.

The following sources provide additional suggestions for developing interview questions: Garrett, 1972; Johnson et al., 1963; Richardson et al., 1965; Stevenson, 1971.

■ Referring back to Table 12 where we specified further information needed for Katherine Compardo in the interview, we can now formulate questions to gain the identified information. Below we have begun to transform this information into specific questions. The reader is encouraged to continue framing questions for the remainder of the information specified in Table 12.

Further informa-tion needed	*Question framed*
Where is St. Mary's Street?	Here the diagnostician wants to gain specific location information. He may do this most directly in one of the closed-type questions. "Where is St. Mary's Street?" "What suburb do you live in?" or "Is St. Mary's Street in South Whittier?"
What does this address tell us about the family's life-style?	The diagnostician wants descriptive information that helps him understand Katherine's speech and language environment. He can best gain this in a more open question such as circumscribed amplification. "Tell me about how Katherine functions in your neighborhood. For example, how does she spend her day, where does she play, with whom does she play, etc.?"
What specifically does Katherine understand?	The diagnostician wants examples that will give him specific information about Katherine's level of understanding. He therefore asks a circumscribed amplification question. "Can you give me some examples of situations in which Katherine understands the language used?"
How does Mrs. Compardo judge Katherine's understanding?	The diagnostician wants to verify the mother's observations of Katherine's understanding. He therefore is looking for data that will allow him to judge the validity of her observations. He does not want to offensively question her statement but wants to know how the mother arrived at her conclusions. He therefore wants descriptive data. "How does Katherine let you know she understands what is said to her?" or "Sometimes it's tricky to know if a child understands the words we say to them or gets the message through our gestures or other situational clues. Can you think of any situations in which it was clear to you that Katherine understood what was said to her rather than what she saw?"

After determining the information needed and framing questions to get that information, the diagnostician will then be ready to launch his questions in the interpersonal context of the actual interview.

Tailor-makes the design. As stated, the diagnostic design must be accountable to the hypothesis and the overall plan for systematic observation. This leads us to discuss two practices that often occur in diagnosis: first, the practice of performing "routine" diagnoses or using "routine" tools and second, the practice of performing "problem-type" diagnoses. Neither of these practices fulfills the orientation developed in this book; however, both can be viewed in relationship to this orientation.

Many speech pathologists make the mistake of considering diagnosis to consist of a series of standardized routines, for example, all children with language disorders being given the same, invariant set of tools. At times, unfortunately, this is the dictate of the specific work setting. To us, this belies the diagnostician's basic problem-solving job function. Instead, it forces the diagnostician to rely on tests rather than searching for answers to clinical questions.

An invariant battery of tools for a given disorder or a given causal factor will result in the use of some tools that are inappropriate and will overlook tools that are more appropriate. Reliance on a battery of tools can create attitudes that tools in the battery, which may not reveal much information, should be eliminated. It also creates the attitude that the "new tool" must be added to the battery. No technique should be discontinued as part of the diagnostician's catalog of tools simply because it is useful only for a selected number of clients. Tool selection is based on the diagnostician's judgment of what may be needed for each specific client.

There are instances where the concept of "routine procedures" may partially apply; for instance, when the diagnostician receives little prior information beyond knowing the age and sex of the client and that some type of speech and language disorder presumably exists. If the diagnostician is confronted with many of these referrals in his work setting, he may establish what could be called a basic testing plan for beginning his diagnosis. This basic plan would be designed to measure quickly many speech and language behaviors and processes. From this, the diagnostician can isolate the problem area and establish "on-the-spot" hypotheses and then select tools for detailed analysis.

This basic plan can be considered a "screening device." Dependent on the work setting, the diagnostician may devise several of these for different populations of clients. Of course, the most basic procedure would be to engage the client in conversational speech and carefully observe the speech and language product as well as the way the client responds to the various stimuli provided. If this can be done, the diagnostician is on his way to deriving a clinical hypothesis.

How can we adapt screening tools such as that developed by Fluharty (1974) to the diagnosis of individual clients? What do Johnson et al. (1963) suggest as a "general speech behavior evaluation"?

Routine testing, the invariant selection of a tool for all diagnoses, stems from the concept of routine diagnoses. For example, all children are given a *Peabody Picture Vocabulary Test* (Dunn, 1965) whether they need it or not. A more common example is the routine use of the speech mechanism examination. The assumption apparently underlying this practice is that since we "talk with our mouths," the mouth must be examined. Similarly, we find routine use of audiometric procedures. The same type of assumption is present; since we "hear with our ears," they must be examined. Another practice that occurs is based on the dictates of a work setting or a diagnostician. Frequently we hear, "the *Illinois Test of Psycholinguistic Abilities* (Kirk et al., 1968) is given to all children with language disorders." There is no way from our orientation that we can rationalize an underlying assumption for this practice. It tends to occur most often when a new tool appears that is promoted as a well-standardized tool. An adverse result of this practice is "throwing the baby out with the bathwater." Other tools, previously used, that have been useful are discarded in favor of the new tool. The fad of "the new test" strikes us much the same as the "wayward child."

Again, the use of routine tools may have a place in diagnosis, but they should be selected and used on the basis of the diagnostician's concern about certain dimensions of his hypothesis. Routine tools are helpful in reducing uncertainties the diagnostician may have as expressed in alternate hypotheses, including the null hypothesis. For example, routine speech mechanism examinations and audiometric

Table 14. Measurement plans and tools selected for Katherine Compardo

Diagnostician's tasks	Planning

Plans for systematic observation

Cause-effect relationships

Well specified in the clinical hypothesis	Will need real skill at behavioral observations and presenting stimuli to elicit responses for support of the causal hypothesis. Must be careful not to set off unwanted or uncontrollable behaviors.
Based heavily on inference from the constituent analysis	
Expressed in problem-type, product, and processing terms	Must fully understand how childhood aphasia and apraxia manifests itself as speech and language behavior.
Causal factor not directly observable	Hypothesis is derived for formulation; but the problem type would warrant a check of comprehension (see constituent analysis). A lot of inference must go into the plans.
	What is the difference in behavioral manifestations between children with aphasia and children defined as minimally brain damaged?
	If causal factor appears to be supported, must immediately consider referral as a tool. Best source would be a pediatric neurologist who has experience with this type of child.

Task specification

Constituent analysis indicates she is not talking	What will Katherine be able to do in the way of specific speech and language tools?
All language product levels affected	Perhaps best approach would be a sequence of stimulus-response items geared to measure several things simultaneously. Perhaps consider a comprehension-imitation-formulation paradigm.
	Believe effect is most important to verify first. If the hypothesis is on target, the effects should give us support for the causal factor—at least enough to make an informed referral.
	Also, will want to look at any speech and language behaviors that isolate the difference between speech production processes and language formulation processes, particularly speech programming. Behavioral correlates of sequencing and motor control will be important.

Client characteristics

Not much to go on here that would make the situation difficult	Being young is our major concern; 27-month-old children, normal or disordered, do not respond that well to directed activities.
Katherine is young	Natural spontaneity with the mother present initially should do the trick. But start out with an "at the table" activity to keep potential overactivity down. Save more active tasks until later.
She has been around adults	
Likes picture books	
Some minimal indication of overactivity	

Selects tools for measurement

	The tools are not presented in any order. The selection is mostly task oriented rather than specific, objective tools that are standardized. The student should explore any tools that may be feasible for Katherine and that can be used at this age level with this hypothesized disorder.
	1. Guided observations throughout the diagnostic session: sandbox activity; hidden objects activity—use of *Fer-Will Object Kit* (?); fine and gross motor activities; free play activities; other activities designed to observe Katherine's visual, social, emotional, physical, and communicative behaviors, for example, imitation of gestures; *Denver Developmental Screening Test* (?)

Table 14. Measurement plans and tools selected for Katherine Compardo—cont'd

Diagnostician's tasks	Planning
Selects tools for measurement—cont'd	
	2. *Peabody Picture Vocabulary Test* and the *Vocabulary Usage Test* in a combined comprehension, formulation, imitation task
	3. Naming tasks
	4. Speech mechanism observation—direct and indirect tasks —voluntary, automatic, and speech
	5. Imitation of sounds, words, and two-word phrases (make use of "here, Daddy, and hi")
	6. Direct stimulation for teaching speech responses—emphasis on sequencing
	The student should now tie these tools selected to the plans and task specifications. Consider two factors: (1) what the tool may do for you and (2) why it was selected.

procedures assist in ruling in or out disruptions in two major segments of the internal speech and language processing component—the auditory reception segment and the speech production segment. However, there is no reason to assume that in all speech and language disorders there may be either a disrupted speech mechanism or a hearing problem. These two segments make up only a small part of the disrupted processes or damaged structures accountable for speech and language disorders. The diagnostician should be able to state the importance of any routine practice in light of each specific hypothesis; it should not be an unthinking selection, nor "we were taught to always give a hearing test."

The second routine practice, the problem-type diagnosis, is not unlike the routine diagnosis. However, the problem-type diagnosis has more important implications, since it stems generally from concern over a specific causal factor and relates to our discussion of classification by problem type presented in Chapter 7. In the problem-type diagnosis the emphasis is on a set of tools selected around the special disability, for example, a diagnosis of the cleft palate child, the child with cerebral palsy, the deaf child, or the brain-injured child. If these conditions are hypothesized as the causal basis for the speech and language

disorder, then this practice becomes more appropriate. However, the diagnostician should not assume that just because a child has cerebral palsy that the speech and language disorder is related to this physical condition. The child's physical disability may have affected only his lower extremities, and the reason he has a language disorder is because of his significant hearing loss. So the diagnostician must not draw one-to-one relationships between certain disabilities and the speech and language disorder. Jumping to these unwarranted conclusions creates unwarranted hypotheses and ultimate failure in diagnosis. Instead, even in those problems where the predicted speech and language disorder may be highly probable, the diagnostician still develops his hypothesis from all the data and tailor-makes his diagnostic design. He does not want to develop a stereotyped orientation to any specific problem type.

■ This point can be exemplified in the following two referral statements on the same child: "Darwin is a cleft palate child." "Darwin, who has a cleft palate, stutters." How does this change your thinking about selecting tools to fit the hypothesis?

The point of view that we tailor-make our diagnoses is vital if the diagnostician is to continue to improve with experience. Diagnostic skill is not something that is arrived at by learning a set of required procedures in a rote fashion. It is obvious that not all techniques are used in all instances. The diagnostician must make decisions as to what tools will be most productive of his time and energy. On the one hand, he must not leave out some areas to be tested that are important, and on the other hand, he must not waste time with many unnecessary and time-consuming tools.

■ We now return to our client example, Katherine Compardo, demonstrating in Table 14 these first two tasks of designing the diagnosis—planning for systematic observation and selecting tools for measurement. The student is encouraged to develop the information on Table 14 to a greater extent.

Develops a testing strategy

This third task of diagnostic design is a step-by-step thinking through of (1) the order in which the tools selected will be presented to establish the cause-effect hypothesis and (2) the order in which the tools will be presented to elicit the best samples of behavior from the client. The diagnostician plans his testing strategy to balance the examiner-tool-client interactions in order to optimize data collection. This advance planning helps reduce the number of diagnostic failures; the diagnostician has thought through possible testing difficulties: if Judy will not talk, the diagnostician has a plan.

In general, but not invariably, the order of tool presentation in the diagnostic session is from the effect to cause, from general to specific, from easy to hard. The diagnostician knows what his tools will do, which are complex, which are simple, which give general information, and which are tasks to obtain specific detailed information. Ordering his tools, the diagnostician obtains the most important information about his clinical hypothesis first, be it cause, effect, or both. He can then order the remainder of his tools to get the necessary details for the remainder of his diagnostic specifications.

Ordering the presentation of tools facilitates data collection; the diagnostician knows how he intends to move from one tool to the next, depending on the information he obtains with each tool. Knowing what each tool provides assists the diagnostician in first establishing some baseline of behaviors, which are followed up by the next tool; or the next tool could be eliminated if it no longer seems needed. For example, if the diagnostician started out with a spontaneous conversation with Julius and quickly discovered that he understands and creates dialogue adequately, then the diagnostician could eliminate his tools for comprehension. In this way the diagnostician alternates between causal tools and effect tools as the information accrues until he has verified and specified his cause-effect relationship.

Keeping the client-tool-examiner interaction in focus facilitates obtaining adequate and representative samples of the client's behavior, obtaining as many responses as possible within the time limitations. Following the general order from easy to hard can give the client an early opportunity for successful performance. The harder tasks that he may fail can be presented later at a time when he and the diagnostician have built up a better interpersonal relationship. By then, the client may be more willing to try difficult tasks, and at the same time, the diagnostician will know more about the manner in which to present the tasks. As the diagnostician and the client move along in the session, each will gain a better understanding of the other and of the overall purposes behind the tasks. The diagnostician can build in successes to counterbalance the failures the client may be experiencing.

Most tools are designed to provide easy tasks (basals) before more difficult ones (ceilings). However, there are some tests that present what are considered the more difficult items first (Porch, 1967). Presumably, this is done to counter the usual test procedure of ending with failure on the final test items. The diagnostician must know the order of item presentation and its effect on client performance. At the same time, the diagnostician's job is to discover the extent of the disorder, and thus he must get samples of disordered behavior and failures as well as adequate performance. The outside world of the client is not ordered in terms of easy to hard.

How might Brookshire's (1972) work on task difficulty as it affects naming performance in the aphasic individual be adapted to your testing strategy?

■ The student should now return to our client example, Katherine Compardo, and consider the overall testing strategy they might use. Develop a flowchart—how you might proceed from tool to tool, at each step gaining more information about your cause-effect hypothesis. Suppose you are to start with what we have called the hidden object activity (Table 14). In this activity objects wrapped in loose tissue paper are placed in a paper bag. Katherine is instructed to close her eyes and select one. How would you introduce this activity? What objects would you put in the bag? What type of responses might you want? How would you elicit and facilitate a response that gives you information you need? How many different types of responses would you be able to elicit and observe from this task? Where would you go next?

SUMMARY

The diagnosis is designed to test the clinical hypothesis that has been formulated from the constituent analysis. To develop such a design, the diagnostician must apply what he knows about speech and language disorders in order to specify what data he wants to obtain. His expertise in measurement of speech and language disorders tells him how to get the data he wants. He uses various tools drawn from a seemingly infinite array of available choices from various sources including the interview, commercial tools, experimental tools, setting protocols, and guided observations. The SLPM framework serves as an organizing system for easy tool retrieval. In addition, the diagnostician applies several

criteria for determining the adequacy of tools for selection. These criteria are validity, reliability, standardization, and clinical adequacy.

In designing the diagnosis the diagnostician performs three tasks.

1. He *plans for systematic observation* of the cause-effect relationships expressed in the clinical hypothesis. He does this by specifying the type of tasks necessary, considering client characteristics.
2. He *selects tools for measurement* to fit the plan he has considered in the first task. He tailor-makes the measurement design, considering the criteria for adequacy of tools. He also plans the interview he will undertake.
3. He *develops a testing strategy* with the tools selected to optimize data collection. He plans the order of presentation of his tools and anticipates client variables in order to obtain the best data within the constraints of the specific diagnosis.

These tasks accomplished, the diagnostician is ready to go to the next step—collection of his clinical data. Finally, the client becomes a real person to be met.

CLIENT PROJECTS
Derek Park

Derek Park, aged 5 years, 3 months, has just been enrolled in kindergarten at Iles Elementary School. Ms. Eckelmann has asked the speech pathologist to see Derek. Mr. Posch, the speech pathologist, is at Iles twice a week only in the mornings. Because of his case load, he seldom is able to take kindergarten children except on special referrals. On his initial consult with Ms. Eckelmann, he learned that Derek was difficult to understand and that he had a repaired cleft lip and palate. He called Mrs. Park and informed her that he was to see Derek and obtained the name of his plastic surgeon. Mrs. Park also told him that Derek had been seen by the St. John's Hospital Cleft Palate Team. Before seeing Derek, Mr. Posch obtained letters of information from both these sources. This information is reproduced in Appendix II. Given these circumstances how would you proceed to do your constituent analysis, derive your hypothesis, and then develop and select your clinical tools, that is, design your diagnosis?

Previous clients: William Gafford and Isadore Alexander

The student should now design the diagnosis for the two clients previously introduced for study purposes. The settings in which these clients are seen should be kept in mind.

REFERENCES

Ammons, R. B., and Ammons, H. S., *Full-Range Picture Vocabulary Test*. Missoula, Mont.: Psychological Test Specialists (1948).

Aram, D. M., and Nation, J. E., Intelligence tests for children: A language analysis. *Ohio J. Speech Hearing*, **6**, 22-43 (1971).

Arthur, G., *Arthur Adaptation of the Leiter International Performance Scale*. Washington, D.C.: Psychological Service Center Press (1952).

Aten, J., and Davis, J., Disturbances in the perception of auditory sequence in children with minimal cerebral dysfunction. *J. Speech Hearing Res.*, **11**, 236-245 (1968).

Bangs, T. E., Evaluating children with language delay. *J. Speech Hearing Dis.*, **26**, 6-18 (1961).

Bernstein, B., A sociolinguistic approach to socialization: With some reference to educability. In F. Williams (Ed.), *Language and Poverty: Perspectives on a Theme*. Chicago: Markham Press (1970).

Berry, M. D., and Erickson, R. L., Speaking rate: Effects on children's comprehension of normal speech. *J. Speech Hearing Res.*, **16**, 367-374 (1973).

Bingham, W. V., and Moore, B. V., *How To Interview*. New York: Harper & Row, Publishers (1941).

Brookshire, R. H., Effects of task difficulty on naming performance of aphasic subjects. *J. Speech Hearing Res.*, **15**, 551-558 (1972).

Brutten, G. J., and Shoemaker, D. J., *Southern Illinois University Behavior Check List*. Carbondale, Ill.: Southern Illinois University (1974a).

Brutten, G. J., and Shoemaker, D. J., *Southern Illinois University Speech Situations Check List*. Carbondale, Ill.: Southern Illinois University (1974b).

Carrow, M. A., The development of auditory comprehension of language structure in children. *J. Speech Hearing Dis.*, **33**, 99-111 (1968).

Crabtree, M., *Houston Test for Language Development*. Houston: Houston Test Co. (1963).

Darley, F. L., *Diagnosis and Appraisal of Communi-cation Disorders*. Englewood Cliffs, N.J.: Prentice-Hall, Inc. (1964).

Deal, J. L., and Darley, F. L., The influence of linguistic and situational variables on phonemic accuracy in apraxia of speech. *J. Speech Hearing Res.*, **15**, 639-653 (1972).

Doll, E. A., *Oseretsky Tests of Motor Proficiency*. Circle Pines, Minn.: American Guidance Service, Inc. (1946).

Dunn, L. M., *Expanded Manual for the Peabody Picture Vocabulary Test*. Circle Pines, Minn.: American Guidance Service, Inc. (1965).

Eisenson, J., *Examining for Aphasia: A Manual for the Examination of Aphasia and Related Disorders*. New York: The Psychological Corporation (1954).

Emerick, L. L., and Hatten, J. T., *Diagnosis and Evaluation in Speech Pathology*. Englewood Cliffs, N.J.: Prentice-Hall, Inc. (1974).

Fairbanks, G., *Voice and Articulation Drillbook*. (2nd ed.) New York: Harper & Row, Publishers (1960).

Fenlason, A. F., *Essentials in Interviewing: For the Interviewer Offering Professional Services*. New York: Harper & Row, Publishers (1952).

Fisher, H. B., and Logemann, J. A., *Fisher-Logemann Test of Articulation Competence*. Boston: Houghton Mifflin Co. (1971).

Flowers, A., Costello, M. R., and Small, V., *Flowers-Costello Tests of Central Auditory Abilities*. Dearborn, Mich.: Perceptual Learning Systems (1970).

Fluharty, N. B., The design and standardization of a speech and language screening test for use with preschool children. *J. Speech Hearing Dis.*, **39**, 75-88 (1974).

Foster, R., Giddan, J. J., and Stark, J., *Assessment of Children's Language Comprehension*. Palo Alto, Calif.: Consulting Psychologists Press, Inc. (1972).

Frostig, M., *Developmental Test of Visual Perception*. Chicago: Follett Publishing Co. (1964).

Fudala, J. B., *Arizona Articulation Proficiency Scale*. Los Angeles: Western Psychological Services (1972).

Garrett, A., *Interviewing: Its Principles and Methods*. (2nd ed.: revised by E. P. Zaki and M. M. Mangold) New York: Family Service Association of America (1972).

Goldman, R., Fristoe, M., and Woodcock, R. W., *Goldman-Fristoe-Woodcock Test of Auditory Discrimination: Manual*. Circle Pines, Minn.: American Guidance Service, Inc. (1970).

Goodglass, J., and Kaplan, E., *The Assessment of Aphasia and Related Disorders*. Philadelphia: Lea & Febiger (1972).

Hanley, T. O., and Peters, R., The speech and hearing laboratory. In L. E. Travis (Ed.), *Handbook of Speech Pathology and Audiology*. New York: Appleton-Century-Crofts (1971).

Hejna, R. F., *Developmental Articulation Test*. Ann Arbor, Mich.: Speech Materials (1959).

Irwin, J. V., and Marge, M. (Eds.), *Principles of Child-*

hood Language Disabilities. Englewood Cliffs, N.J.: Prentice-Hall, Inc. (1972).

Jacobs, R. J., Philips, B. J., and Harrison, R. J., A stimulability test for cleft-palate children. *J. Speech Hearing Dis.,* **35,** 354-360 (1970).

Johnson, O. G., and Bommarito, J. W., *Tests and Measurements in Child Development: A Handbook.* San Francisco: Jossey-Bass, Inc., Publishers (1971).

Johnson, W., Darley, F. L., and Spriestersbach, D. C., *Diagnostic Methods in Speech Pathology.* New York: Harper & Row, Publishers (1963).

Kirk, S. A., McCarthy, J., and Kirk, W. D., *Illinois Test of Psycholinguistic Abilities.* Urbana, Ill.: University of Illinois Press (1968).

Koppitz, E. M., *Bender-Gestalt Test For Young Children.* New York: The Psychological Corporation (1964).

Labelle, J. L., Sentence comprehension in two age groups of children as related to pause position or the absence of pauses. *J. Speech Hearing Res.,* **16,** 231-237 (1973).

Lahey, M., Use of prosody and syntactic markers in children's comprehension of spoken sentences. *J. Speech Hearing Res.,* **17,** 656-668 (1974).

Lee, L. L., *Northwestern Syntax Screening Test.* Evanston, Ill.: Northwestern University Press (1969).

Lee, L. L., A screening test for syntax development. *J. Speech Hearing Dis.,* **35,** 103-112 (1970).

Lee, L. L., *Developmental Sentence Analysis.* Evanston, Ill.: Northwestern University Press (1974).

MacDonald, J. D., and Blott, J. P., Environmental language intervention: The rationale for a diagnostic and training strategy through rules, context, and generalization. *J. Speech Hearing Dis.,* **39,** 244-256 (1974).

MacDonald, J. D., and Nichols, M., *Environmental Language Inventory.* Columbus, Ohio: Nisonger Center, Ohio State University (1974).

Mayo Clinic, *Clinical Examinations in Neurology.* (3rd ed.) Philadelphia: W. B. Saunders Co. (1971).

McDonald, E. T., *A Deep Test of Articulation.* Pittsburgh: Stanwix House, Inc. (1964).

Mecham, M. J., *Verbal Language Development Scale.* Circle Pines, Minn.: American Guidance Service, Inc. (1958).

Milisen, R., et al., The disorder of articulation: A systematic clinical and experimental approach. *J. Speech Hearing Dis., Monogr. Suppl.,* **4** (1954).

Monnin, L. M., and Huntington, D. A., Relationship of articulatory defects to speech-sound identification. *J. Speech Hearing Res.,* **17,** 352-366 (1974).

Nation, J. E., A vocabulary usage test. *J. Psycholing. Res.,* **1,** 221-231 (1972).

Nation, J. E., and Corlew, M. M., Aphasia tests: Differences among naming tasks. *Arch. phys. Med. Rehab.,* **55,** 228-231 (1974).

Needham, L. S., and Swisher, L. P., A comparison of three tests of auditory comprehension for adult aphasics. *J. Speech Hearing Dis.,* **37,** 123-131 (1972).

Paraskevopoulos, J. N., and Kirk, S. A., *The Development and Psychometric Characteristics of the Revised Illinois Test of Psycholinguistic Abilities.* Urbana, Ill.: University of Illinois Press (1969).

Porch, B., *Porch Index of Communicative Ability.* Palo Alto, Calif.: Consulting Psychologists Press (1967).

Prins, D., Personality, stuttering severity, and age. *J. Speech Hearing Res.,* **15,** 148-154 (1972).

Prutting, C. A., Gallagher, T. M., and Mulac, A., The expressive portion of the NSST compared to a spontaneous speech sample. *J. Speech Hearing Dis.,* **40,** 40-48 (1975).

Ratusnik, D. L., and Koeningsknecht, R. A., Internal consistency of the Northwestern Syntax Screening Test. *J. Speech Hearing Dis.,* **40,** 59-68 (1975).

Richardson, S. O., Medical diagnosis and evaluation of language disabilities. In J. V. Irwin and M. Marge (Eds.), *Principles of Childhood Language Disabilities.* Englewood Cliffs, N.J.: Prentice-Hall, Inc. (1972).

Richardson, S., Dohrenwend, B. S., and Klein, D., *Interviewing: Its Forms and Functions.* New York: Basic Books, Inc., Publishers (1965).

Riley, G. D., A stuttering severity instrument for children and adults. *J. Speech Hearing Dis.,* **37,** 314-322 (1972).

Sanders, E. K., When are speech sounds learned? *J. Speech Hearing Dis.,* **37,** 55-63 (1972).

Schuell, H., *Minnesota Test for Differential Diagnosis of Aphasia.* Minneapolis, Minn.: University of Minnesota Press (1965).

Schwartz, A. H., and Goldman, R., Variables influencing performance on speech-sound discrimination tests. *J. Speech Hearing Res.,* **17,** 25-32 (1974).

Spradlin, J. E., Assessment of speech and language of retarded children: The Parsons language sample. *J. Speech Hearing Dis., Monogr. Suppl.,* **10,** 8-31 (1963).

Stevenson, I., *The Diagnostic Interview.* (2nd ed.) New York: Harper & Row, Publishers (1971).

Sullivan, H. S., *The Psychiatric Interview.* New York: W. W. Norton & Co., Inc. (1954).

Templin, M. C., and Darley, F. L., *Templin-Darley Tests of Articulation.* Iowa City: University of Iowa (1969).

Thorpe, L. P., Clark, W. W., and Tiegs, E. W., *California Test of Personality.* Monterey, Calif.: California Test Bureau (1953).

Waryas, C., and Ruder, K., On the limitations of language comprehension procedures and an alternative. *J. Speech Hearing Dis.,* **39,** 44-52 (1974).

Weiner, P. S., Stability and validity of two measures of intelligence used with children whose language development is delayed. *J. Speech Hearing Res.,* **14,** 254-261 (1971).

Weiner, P. S., and Hoock, W. C., The standardization of tests: Criteria and criticisms. *J. Speech Hearing Res.,* **16,** 616-626 (1973).

Wepman, J. M., *Auditory Discrimination Test*. Chicago: Language Research Associates, Inc. (1958).

Wepman, J. M., and Jones, L. V., *Language Modalities Test for Aphasia*. Chicago: Education-Industry Service (1961).

Wilson, F. B., *The Voice Disordered Child*. St. Louis: Jewish Hospital (1972).

Wolski, W., *Michigan Picture Language Inventory*. Ann Arbor, Mich.: The University of Michigan Press (1962).

Yoss, K. A., and Darley, F. L., Developmental apraxia of speech in children with defective articulation. *J. Speech Hearing Res.*, **17,** 399-416 (1974).

Chapter 14

Collection of the clinical data: systematic observation

After his considerable preparation in the previous three steps, the diagnostician now meets his client and collects data to test his clinical hypothesis. In this fourth step he will be required to actualize what he has planned and prepared. He will now implement his diagnostic design, his testing strategy. He will present his tools, elicit responses, and observe and record the responses. As well, he must demonstrate his professional skill in working with people to gain the information he needs to help them with their concerns. At this step, the clinical scientist blends into a clinical artist.

The diagnostician and client complex are not automatons, gaining and giving data in a completely preprogrammed manner; rather, both are human. Interpersonal considerations thus become a significant new dimension to data collection, a dimension that pervades the diagnostic session. Here the diagnostician needs to draw from his knowledge about people and about himself to successfully implement data collection in this interpersonal context. He particularly needs this understanding in special testing situations such as with the "difficult child" and the "overwhelmed adult."

From his diagnostic design and his knowledge about how to implement that design in an interpersonal setting, the diagnostician performs three tasks to complete clinical data collection. First, on the diagnostic day he must prepare for the diagnostic session. Before meeting the client, he must attend to the physical arrangements for the diagnosis, including such matters as setting up the diagnostic room, being sure the tools he has selected are available, and having the appropriate forms. He then prepares himself and the client for the diagnostic session when he establishes the initial personal contact with the client complex. This initial interaction allows each to get some idea of what they may expect from the other and sets the tone for what follows.

Second, after meeting the client, the diagnostician must collect the data. The diagnostician conducts the interview and engages in clinical testing. In both the interview and clinical testing he proceeds with the systematic measurements he has planned, while adapting his plan to new information and to the needs of the interpersonal context. As part of this task, he must record his observations.

Third, as the final task in this step, the diagnostician must close the diagnostic session. He must know when to wrap up his data collection and let the client know what the next step will be. In some instances the close of the diagnostic session will lead immediately into the interpretive conference, where the client complex* learns of the diagnostic findings. Plans for the client's management are developed. In other situations the diagnostic session and interpretive conference may be separated by several days or weeks.

These three tasks (preparing for the session, collecting the data, and closing the diagnostic session) form this fourth step in the diagnostic process. Afterward, the diagnostician will be ready to enter the fifth step: scoring, ordering, and analyzing the data he has collected, which will make it ready for interpretation.

COLLECTION OF THE DATA: HOW IT IS DONE

Collection of data involves systematically observing various samples of the client's behavior, using the tools and strategies planned. Through his procedures the diagnostician provides appropriate stimulation that maximizes the clients responses. The diagnostician wants to obtain a representative sample of the desired behaviors in order to determine the reality of the clinical problem. So the diagnostician must have information about interpersonal interactions and tool administration.

Information bases: nature and sources
Previous diagnostic steps

The most immediate information that the diagnostician must use as his guide to data collection is the diagnostic design that he planned in the previous step. The diagnostician uses his planned strategy for interviewing and tool administration. All that he has considered in the design of the diagnosis becomes a source of information for understanding and implementing the collection of data. These previous steps and tasks of the diagnostic process give the diagnostician the information he needs to administer his tools in a studied, system-

---

*From this point, the word client will generally be used to refer to either the client or the client complex.

atic, purposeful manner for each specific client.

Interpersonal context

Before we proceed with the information base about tool administration, which is vital to data collection, we want to develop an information base about diagnosis in an interpersonal context. We feel that the concepts about administration of tools become more meaningful when first viewed from this other important and often understated context. No data can be collected from tools if the client does not respond to the diagnostician or the tools.

Needless to say, the many variables considered by the diagnostician when selecting tools are compounded once he begins testing a person. He must manage the chair, table, child, test, parent, and venetian blind all at the same time. He can never anticipate all the potential interactions that take place. Variables will go uncontrolled, get out of hand, not be observed, etc.—all while he is trying to go about his business of gathering data.

In implementing the diagnostic design, it is crucial that the diagnostician know how to relate to and adapt his plan to the clients he sees. Many children and adults willingly enter into the diagnostic situation, cooperatively give all the information wanted, and participate enthusiastically in all the procedures planned. Others are there against their will or have fears and behavioral problems that interfere with straightforward collection of data. At times the diagnostician is fighting against attention span, disinterest, lack of motivation, or lethargy. To be effective he must know how to modify his testing strategy to reinforce the client to continue responding. With most adults this is a relatively easy matter. The diagnostician can usually explain what is wanted and why the information is needed. With children he can only explain up to a point, and encouragement only goes so far. Children may want to do what is asked, but often their good will gives way to fatigue, boredom, or distraction. How can young children be encouraged to participate? What will bring out their best responses? What can the diagnostician do in the face of a severe behavior problem? How does he handle fear and anxiety? How does he react to the emotionality presented by an aphasic or his spouse? What does he do with the anger expressed by the client's mother during an interview? Collection of data thus requires an understanding of people, their problems, their concerns, their hopes, their guilt, their anxieties—the whole of what makes them human.

Even though the diagnostician's job is to elicit and observe appropriate responses, the client does not necessarily know or care about the diagnostician's job—he acts like he is going to act. A child who is out of control does not care if the diagnostician wants him to point to the picture of a cat. During data collection the diagnostician must know how to move with his client. If the child is very active, then the diagnostician must pursue his testing actively; if the child is a plodder, then plod along. Work with the client, not against him. Backup procedures become essential; change the stimuli presented, ask for responses in a different manner, rearrange the seating arrangement, or if necessary, go for a walk with the client. Quiet conversation may have to take the place of the structured language test. The diagnostician must be able to change his design if need be. He may not be able to adhere to the tools selected. Unlike the researcher studying a representative sample, he cannot "throw out" his nonrepresentative client. He must get the best data he can, in whatever way is necessary.

While we usually think of adults as presenting fewer behavioral problems than children, diagnosticians who spend much of their time with adults may feel this to be an overgeneralization. Many of the adult clients seen for speech and language diagnoses are understandably overwhelmed by their speech, language, and often more pervasive problems. Some have suddenly undergone significant alterations in their life-styles. One day they are active and the next day because of a cerebrovascular accident they have been reduced to an invalid and a haltingly communicative, partial person. Others have just undergone surgery as a lifesaving procedure and are flooded with concern over their health and disgust, sadness, and anger over their loss. Some come from families that are themselves fearful; others have no families or supportive persons. These adults have lost more than speech and language. All of these clients may be overwhelmed by their problems and their concomitant effects on their personal, social, and vocational pursuits.

For many of these clients the diagnostician may represent the one professional who has time and interest, who allows them to talk about their concerns, and who has the ability to help them do something about their problems. It is imperative that the diagnostician be sensitive to these needs and adapt his diagnostic design accordingly. In many instances it may be important to acknowledge how concerned the client is over his health or how hard it must be for him to cope with the new problems. The client may well need to express his fears and frustrations; he may need to be depressed or simply cry. He may need to voice his feelings before he can undertake testing. While the diagnostician must be able to offer support and concern, he also must show the client that his purpose is to help as best he can, to do something about the problem. With these clients it is particularly important to explain what the tools are intended to do and why the information gained is important. Letting the client know what is happening helps him feel more in control. At all times, however, the diagnostician must not be swept away by compassion, offering more than is warranted. He must remain realistic in his comments, as nothing in the long run is more shattering than unfulfilled hope.

In addition to attending to the adult clients' feelings about themselves and their problems, the diagnostician may have to modify the presentation of tools to facilitate their ability to respond. Distraught or disoriented clients must be given time to respond. At times the instructions may be given too fast, and when a response does not come immediately, the diagnostician may think the client does not understand and proceed to another item. Adults can be frustrated by this; their responses worsen, and yet they may not be able or willing to tell you that you are doing something wrong. For example, latency of response is common in the aphasic and must be accounted for when testing with a formal tool or in conversation. Too much stimulation, too fast, can result in an emotional reaction—the only means by which the aphasic can handle the situation. These clients are adults; the diagnostician is an adult—a common ground for an interpersonal interaction.

This interpersonal aspect of data collection is far more difficult to learn than the skill of administering a specific diagnostic tool. The information that provides the data base for assisting the diagnostician comes from many sources. Information about communicative interaction is essential, as discussed in Chapter 2. The diagnostician also uses his broad base of knowledge in child rearing and management, management of the ill and handicapped, child growth and development, human personality, psychological growth and development, learning theory, and many other areas. One of the most important areas of knowledge he needs is self-knowledge—what he is as a person.

Ours is a "talking profession." Our concern is with a person's ability to use speech and language. If diagnosticians are not skilled in relating through communication, how can they be skilled in solving speech and language problems?

Interpersonal-professional relationship. From the moment the client and the diagnostician meet they enter into an interpersonal-professional relationship—a contract is formed between the parties. The perceptions the client has of the diagnostician and vice versa will have an important bearing on the diagnostic process.

The diagnostician may assume that the client comes in order to achieve greater homeostasis in his daily functioning, greater integration among all the aspects of his life: cognitive, sensorimotor, and interpersonal. He is attempting to achieve a better "gestalt." Since diagnosis is an active and not a passive process, the diagnostician enters into the client's existence just as the client enters into the diagnostician's existence. The diagnostician must be aware of the client's reactions to his "help." As well, he must be aware of his own needs to help. The diagnostician must discover the client; the client must teach the diagnostician. Both must respect each other, be authentic in what they feel, and be ready to "weather the storms" that may occur; they must arrive at some degree of commitment to each other.

These interpersonal interactions are vital; many clients are "lost" because something goes amiss in this aspect of the process, even when appropriate test information has been obtained. A good diagnosis relies on the feelings that have resulted as much as on the tools that were administered.

There are many important ideas that can be borrowed from Gestalt psychology for an understanding of the interpersonal interactions that occur in the diagnostic process. A good introduction to this material can be found in Polster and Polster (1973). Schultz (1972) and Schultz and Carpenter (1973) present useful information about clinical interactions.

The interaction or relationship between the diagnostician and the client is often blithely called "establishing rapport" and somehow is supposed to magically occur. We all know that rapport is essential to the diagnostic process, but we do not always know how to achieve it. Somehow the diagnostician is expected to be "on" with each client he sees, no matter what his own day or personal life may be like.

Discovering the primary ingredients for successful interpersonal interactions is difficult. We sometimes hear remarks like "You have to be born with it" or "He really knows how to plan a diagnosis, but he can't relate to the client." Much work needs to be done in this area before we understand why one diagnostician seldom has difficulty relating to all types of clients; whereas another always seems to have screaming children. Shriberg (1971) conducted a study to determine the effect of the examiner's social behavior on children's articulation test performance. During their interactions with the children, the examiners assumed various social behaviors that were judged to represent real behaviors. Even though Shriberg's main variable of the examiner's social behavior was not significant, further studies like his can be important for discovering interpersonal factors affecting client performance. Perhaps, instead of assuming "artificial" behaviors, real diagnosticians with real behaviors should be studied.

Probably most difficult for the diagnostician is understanding himself in the relationship. It is much easier to look toward others as the problem and pretend that whatever we contribute to the relationship is optimal. However, relationships are a two-way street: diagnosticians have no fewer difficulties than do their clients. The diagnostician needs to know what his anxieties and needs are in the situation, his manner of relating, and the life experiences that have made him respond to people as he does.

Even with considerable self-insight and self-change, there will probably always be some personal characteristics in a diagnostician that are going to be reacted to negatively by some of the clients he sees. He cannot be all things to all clients. Furthermore, some characteristics negatively reacted to cannot be changed. For example, the diagnostician may be young rather than old, white rather than black, or male rather than female. Our skills as diagnosticians must counteract these reactions and impressions, the ultimate basis by which we hope to be judged by our clients. Age, however, is often a problem with student diagnosticians who may be perceived as both young and without experience. How can clients respect their skill and opinions? If student diagnosticians demonstrate good skills and maturity, they usually are accepted. At other times the issue needs to be confronted, quite appropriately allowing that in fact the student is in training and is being supervised by a professional, who has final responsibility for any decisions made.

We have so little information about the client-examiner interaction during the diagnostic process. The diagnostician often assumes that the client will do what is expected, and if they reinforce him appropriately, expected behavior will be forthcoming. Students in training need to understand that some failures in diagnostic procedures may stem from clients who, because they do not perform in expected ways, do not provide the student with reinforcement. In diagnosis both the client and diagnostician may be reinforcing and punishing one another. What factors did Stech et al. (1973) report as being reinforcing and punishing to the clinician?

In relating to clients the diagnostician must develop an understanding and acceptance of the client as well as an understanding and acceptance of himself. The diagnostician must regard his client as the result of a particular set of life experiences and demonstrate to the client that his aim is to help him with any information gained. In some cases, clients may be reluctant to give information as they fear the information will be used against them. For example, all parents do not necessarily have equal levels of concern about their children. In truth, some do not care for their children at all, and the fact that the child demonstrates a speech or language disorder only heightens their dislike for the child. Is this something they could reveal to the diagnostician? Parents view their children as extensions of themselves—as their child is judged, so they may be. If the diagnostician can develop and project the attitude that individuals do the best they can with whatever life has presented them, this attitude will contribute to a feeling of appreciation, understanding, and acceptance by the client.

Schein's model (1969), presented in Fig. 2-5, is a helpful way to view interpersonal contacts between the diagnostician and the client. Can all communications be open? No client is ready to flood the diagnostician with the truths of his life during this initial diagnostic contact. Presumably most clients are ready to give some information but not all information. Many clients have unknown, blind, and concealed selves, as do the diagnosticians. Clients do not and should not share everything. They may give more information than is usual for them simply because the diagnostician is a professional, and they have come to him for some type of help. The more supportive and accepting the professional, the more likely is the client to offer whatever may be pertinent to an understanding of the problem. There are, however, instances when a client reveals too much, using the diagnostician for relief of many anxieties and concerns about his life. Such outpourings may produce tremendous guilt, and the client may not be able to return to the setting. The diagnostician must therefore be careful of how much he lets the client reveal.

At the same time the diagnostician must be careful of how much he reveals about himself. For example, should a diagnostician, who has his own stuttering under control, reveal that he is a stutterer to a client being seen for stuttering? Or should a diagnostician talking to a mother whose child has a significant behavioral problem reveal that his child, too, has a behavior problem? How much does a diagnostician use his personal life experience as a way of relating to the concerns of the client being seen? There may be no answers to these questions, but there are cautions to exercise. Suppose, for instance, that the diagnostician with controlled stuttering revealed his experiences with stuttering, including the information that he is now experiencing little or no difficulty with his speech. Will the client feel he can do the same thing? Will this external motivation bring him to therapy? Or will his lack of success be expressed as hostility toward the diagnostician who has been too successful. Using someone else as a model for motivation at times may create more harm than good. The client may have only perceived the diagnostician's success at controlling his behavior but not the effort, anxieties, and hard work that went into controlling the behavior.

Work setting. Different work settings require that the diagnostician acquire somewhat different information for developing the skill of interpersonal interaction. The diagnostician in an acute care hospital needs more information about interacting with sick people than does the public school diagnostician; whereas the public school diagnostician needs to know more about interacting with active, healthy children at various age levels. The diagnostician in a children's hospital may concentrate on skills used in working with the sick child, while a diagnostician in a nursing home will concentrate on the special needs of the elderly, invalid population. In each of these settings the diagnostician will need to refine his interpersonal skills with the client, other professionals, and the client complex if he is to solve the special speech and language problems that exist in each setting. Whatever the setting, the diagnostician must try to gear himself to the particular requirements and personalities of the client rather than expecting the client simply to adapt to his personality and his need to collect information.

Pat DiCioccio is employed in an extended care facility where she frequently works with patients who are dying. She contributes the following about the special interpersonal characteristics in this circumstance.

The patient population in an extended care facility not only includes the invalid geriatric patient, but also the patient with progressive neurological disease who can no longer be managed at home. This patient is usually a young to middle-aged adult who is in the severe stages of his disease process. There are diagnostic and therapeutic services that one may offer such a patient; however, it is ultimately important that the diagnostician/clinician first have the necessary interpersonal skills that are essential for interacting with this type of patient. The professional in this setting must develop his own understanding of the disease process and the dying patient. He must evaluate his own thoughts and reactions to the dying patient and the magnitude of the patient's problems, and the impact of his situation must be felt by the clinician. He must be able to deal with his own feelings as well as those of the patient as the diagnostic/therapeutic relationship begins to grow, and he must truly understand what he as a professional can offer. These interpersonal skills one develops in this situation are most important in helping the professional provide appropriate diagnostic and therapeutic services. Interacting honestly, compassionately, and professionally with the dying patient, all three somehow equally balanced, must be the underlying framework for any diagnostic or therapeutic service that is provided.*

Interview

Most diagnoses include an interview as one of the tools of diagnosis selected for data collection. It is usually formalized into a distinct task of data collection, and therefore, because of its separateness, we will present information about it as a tool to be administered apart from the remainder of the information on tool administration.

The topic of interviewing often is treated in awe by the student trying to learn it and, perhaps to some extent, by the person trying to teach it. If the student approaches the subject in a practical way, he will discover he "interviews" every day of his life. People interview each other daily; they ask questions for information; they discuss areas of concern; they ask questions of each other about problems they are having; and they ask questions about feelings, health, attitudes, etc. This is done using all the methods of interviewing: the direct question, the multiple-choice response,

*From DiCioccio, P., Personal communication. Cleveland: Sunny Acres Hospital (1975).

etc. under all types of conditions: friendly, hostile, angry, open, closed, and dozens of others. Thus our daily personal interactions can serve as the bases for learning to conduct interviews in our job setting. The diagnostician moves from this area of personal general knowledge to the specific interview knowledge needed for diagnosis of speech and language disorders.

Interviewing is a complex skill used by many professionals, each having a special purpose and use for the techniques. But overriding all the special uses of the interview is the basic purpose, to obtain information. There is one basic way of obtaining this information—by asking "questions." Each person develops his interviewing style from this basic method of interviewing and from his own personal characteristics during interpersonal interaction.

The student should become familiar with the various orientations to interviewing. Each has something to offer the diagnostician of speech and language disorders. As a project, develop an outline of the common principles of interviewing revealed in the following: Bingham and Moore (1941), Emerick and Hatten (1974), Garrett (1972), Rogers (1942), Stevenson (1971), Sullivan (1954).

In the previous chapter we discussed how the diagnostician plans his interview, considering the areas of information in which he is interested, and how he may frame certain questions to obtain this information. He now approaches the interview as a coalition between himself and the informant; a coalition developed for the purpose of understanding the speech and language problem, what caused it, what can be done about it, who is concerned about it, and who can do something about it. It is important to help the informant see his active role in helping to solve the problem. An interpersonal-professional relationship must be established.

We believe in making it clear to the informant that both of us are in this process together, and that our findings and solutions are dependent on his involvement. Approaching the interview as a team usually has an energizing effect, particularly on family members. It helps to eliminate parental expectations of easy cures in which they have nothing to do and removes the professional from an authoritarian position. We like to tell parents that they have the information about their child as they live with him 24 hours a day, and we have the training to help put the pieces of information together.

The skill of interviewing is concerned with the how-to aspects: how to obtain the most pertinent information without creating undue anxiety, stress, frustration, helplessness, or other unpleasant feelings in the person being interviewed. The diagnostician must develop skills for interviewing the hostile mother, the defensive father, the denying adult, the unsophisticated child—each client as himself. Any diagnostician can develop and ask pertinent questions at some level—this is questioning—but the skill of interviewing comes when he knows how to do this in various ways, with different people, with different ideas and concerns. Most of the time the diagnostician is fortunate; the client and his family come with a problem they want solved. They usually want to cooperate the best they can during the interview. Thus the diagnostician gets answers to his questions. However, even with willing clients, difficulties can be encountered, for example, a parent who wants to know why his child has not begun to talk but who is denying slow development or mental retardation as a possible explanation. This parent may give all kinds of accurate information about the child's development, but does not dare to offer one ounce of information about what he thinks caused it. Parents like this are not simply being hostile or defensive; they are sometimes being protective of themselves and of their child.

As well as the questions he designs, the diagnostician should consider the use of tools that have been specially designed as interview techniques. These are available as commercial tools and are also present in the research literature. What specific information would the following provide: *Parents Attitudes Scale* by Wiley (1955), *Verbal Language Development Scale* by Mecham (1959), the *Vineland Social Maturity Scale* by Doll (1965), and the *Receptive-Expressive Emergent Language Scale (REEL)* by Bzoch and League (1971)?

The diagnostician must decide how he will record the information offered in the interview. Choices range from tape recording the entire interview to making no notations during the interview. Tape recording the session may inhibit the informant's responses, particularly when the information is emotional or highly personal in nature or if the informant questions the diagnostician's motives in using the information. On the other hand, relying on recall of all the detailed information following the interview is a skill achieved by few diagnosticians. Most diagnosticians choose a method somewhere in between these two alternatives, developing their own system for recording pertinent information. The diagnostician must be sure, however, that his note taking does not impede the information flow, slow down the discussion, or create a barrier between himself and the client.

The diagnostician can set the tone for note taking by asking for or being sure that all identification information and certain other factual information are accurately recorded. Usually recording such information in the presence of the informant creates no difficulty, for he knows what is being written down and expects it to be written down. Having set the tone for note taking, the diagnostician, as he proceeds in the interview, can jot down abbreviated notes in the form of key items that will serve as memory jogs at a later time. Letting the informant know enough times early in the interview what was written down (for example, "I just wrote down that Jonathan was easy to toilet train") can assure the informant that the diagnostician is recording what they say, not judging it. This procedure also assists in developing the coalition between the diagnostician and the informant.

Another approach used by diagnosticians is to take a few minutes immediately following the interview to write down the salient aspects of the interview information. Some professionals, social workers in particular, are trained to make detailed "process recordings" following the termination of the interview. Early in his training the student should learn a method of recording during the interview in which he can become highly skilled.

We have found that when the interview is presented as a problem-solving effort between the diagnostician and the informant, permission is generally obtained for use of the tape recorder. The informant can be instructed to have the recorder stopped if information is being discussed that he prefers not be recorded. Having used this technique over a number of years, we have not noticed any particular difference between interviews using a recorder and those that do not. Our clinical experience is that the informant quickly disregards the presence of the recorder, particularly if placement of the recorder and microphone are inconspicuous. This approach to recording information is invaluable in teaching the interview process or for experienced diagnosticians to check on their own interviewing skills.

Tool administration

To administer the tools he has selected, the diagnostician must have general knowledge about tool presentation as well as the specific knowledge about each tool he is planning to use. As a part of tool administration, the diagnostician also concerns himself with accurate recording procedures.

Tool presentation. The diagnostician must know each tool and its specific administrative procedures. He must understand all the stimulus-response variables that exist in any given tool. Many tools specify the basic stimulus-response modalities being tested but make little or no mention of other modalities necessary to complete the task. For example, the *Northwestern Syntax Screening Test* (Lee, 1969) aims to test auditorally presented syntactic "reception and expression"; however, successful completion of this tool also requires rather astute visual perception. Many tools for measuring comprehension of language are of this type, requiring both auditory and visual processing of information. Some tools provide an auditory stimulus for presentation that is only incidental for facilitating a response. The *Templin-Darley Tests of Articulation* (Templin and Darley, 1969) provide a stimulus frame to elicit the name of the item pictured: "We fasten the _____," where the expected response is *zipper*. However, if the client can understand that he is to name the picture, the auditory stimulus can be abandoned in testing. Many tests require visual interpretation of a picture in order for the client to respond, which has always created a certain amount of consternation among diagnosticians. Tests are frequently criticized for lack of adequate pictorial representation—"No wonder he can't name cat, the picture looks more like a dog."

There are some tools that provide for alternate modes of stimulation and response. *Examining for Aphasia* by Eisenson (1954) exemplifies this. In many of his subtests, if the aphasic does not or cannot respond to one mode of stimulation, an alternate will be provided. Presumably the data obtained with the alternate methods is equally adequate, although this is not stated in the test manual. Reseach evidence provides some information that, at least for naming tasks from visual stimulation, the examiner could use pictures, objects, photographs, line drawings, etc. to elicit equally appropriate naming responses from aphasics (Corlew and Nation, 1975).

As well as stimulus-response modality variables, the diagnostician should be completely aware of all the speech and language levels represented in the stimulus items. Again, many tools specify their primary purpose as testing for a certain linguistic level; whereas the test items require processing of more than one level. For example, the *Auditory Discrimination Test* by Wepman (1958) requires auditory presentation of pairs of words that are either the same or different. The question that arises is how the completion of the task is to be interpreted—on the basis of discrimination of speech sounds or on the basis of semantic comprehension since the stimuli are words. The same is true of any "discrimination" test based on word pairs. Any tool designed for syntactic comprehension would most likely also require semantic comprehension. Because of this, the *Assessment of Children's Language Comprehension* (Foster et al., 1972) first determines if the child comprehends all the test words (semantic level) before putting them into combinations called critical elements, interpreted as syntactic word orders.

There are few tools that are relatively "pure" in terms of stimulus-response modalities and levels of language being tested. The diagnostician must rely on his analysis of the test items, remaining alert to the fact that there will be variables incidental to the test designer's basic concern.

We (Aram and Nation, 1975) developed a test battery for viewing language patterns in language-disordered children. We were confronted with specifying tools for isolating levels of language products and processes. How successful were we in developing our test battery?

Tools are essential to the diagnostician. They provide detailed ordering of the stimuli to be presented and ways for observing specified response levels. Required in all these tools are administration procedures that the diagnostician uses if at all possible or if they are applicable to his client. Most tools come with manuals or instructions for administration—how to present the items, what order they come in, establishing basal levels and ceiling levels of performance, alternate stimulations, number of stimulations, score forms for recording responses, response scoring systems, etc.

It should go without saying that before using a test instrument for its explicit purposes, the diagnostician should be well grounded in its administrative procedures, particularly with methods of recording and scoring the responses. Without question, students in training should obtain good groundwork in tests and measurements that will give them the background and respect for the careful use of instruments of measurement—background that can be utilized for learning each new tool that is developed in their profession.

In speech pathology we are being introduced to a practice that has been common in psychology: "certification" in the use of specific tests such as the *Porch Index of Communicative Ability* (1967) and the *Porch Index of Communicative Ability in Children* (1974). This practice seems to be waning for some in clinical psychology (Palmer, 1970); however, we wonder if speech pathology is now going to go through this phase. Our hope is that it will not!

"Auditory discrimination" has always been difficult to conceptualize and measure. How have the following test designers gone about this task: *Templin Picture Sound Discrimination Test* (Templin, 1957), *Goldman-Fristoe-Woodcock Test of Auditory Discrimination* (Goldman et al., 1970), the *Test of Listening Accuracy in Children* (Mecham et al., 1969), and Wepman's *Auditory Discrimination Test* (1958)? How have they provided for administering the auditory stimuli, what type of stimuli have they chosen, and how do they record and score the responses? Would all of these tools give you the same information about "auditory discrimination"?

Some additional remarks are necessary about changing the standard instructions that accompany testing tools. If possible, the diagnostician using structured objective tests should present them according to their standard instructions. However, varying the stimulus presentation sometimes allows a client to respond better. For example, young children at times have difficulty responding to the phrase "Show me" or "Point to _____"—the recommended stimulus presentation for the *Peabody Picture Vocabulary Test* (Dunn, 1965). By making a slight alteration in directions and saying "Touch _____," "Put your finger on _____," or "Put the penny on _____," the child will respond. Stimulus phrases such as "Make ducky sit on _____" also motivate a child, who has long since become disinterested in "showing me" or "pointing to" the said picture. We mentioned earlier that Eisenson's *Examining for Aphasia* (1954) presents alternate modes of stimulation, a practice few tools provide, but a practice we feel should be reintroduced into test design. At times there may be undue concern with the standardization of the stimulus presentation when it is the response that is more important.

When presented initially with standardized items from a test, some clients may not grasp what they are to do. At this point it may be very appropriate to alter the task considerably. Clients should not be penalized for lack of understanding the task. For example, in the *Language Modalities Test for Aphasia* (Wepman and Jones, 1961a, b) the first item in the structured section is the presentation of a visual stimulus. The examiner says, "What is this?" as he points to the picture. If the client does not respond, the question can be repeated, and if he still does not respond, it is recorded as an NR (no response). This seems to be a simple, clear instruction that would need no alteration. However, clinical experience tells us that many aphasics cannot respond initially to such simple instructions and may require more guidance

before they understand a testing task. In this instance the examiner might want to offer other stimulation: "You say the name of this"; "This is not a chicken, it is a _____"; "This is a fish; you say the name"; or any other number of alterations until the client understands he is to name the picture or whatever the task item is. Then subsequent items can be presented in the standardized way.

Review the administration procedures for several tests of phonetic structure. What differences are evident in administrative procedures? Could the procedures from one test be used with a second test without affecting the reliability or validity of the results? Start your review with a comparison of the *Arizona Articulation Proficiency Scale* (Fudala, 1972), the *Laradon Articulation Scale* (Edmonston, 1963), and the *Goldman-Fristoe Test of Articulation* (Goldman and Fristoe, 1969).

When altering the standard presentation, the diagnostician must be aware of the possible invalidation of the tool and be cautious of using the normative data that has been gathered under the standard presentation. While it is unlikely that "Touch *boat*" or "Put your finger on *boat*" substantially changes a child's level of vocabulary comprehension, other presentation modification may. For example, if the child is asked to "point to what grandma and grandpa have on their lake," the child is responding to the visual representation of boat rather than the spoken word, boat. These two tasks are not equivalent.

The *Vocabulary Usage Test* (Nation, 1972) is first administered using a cloze procedure. A stimulus is presented with an inflection that signals the child to fill in the slot with the word. What if the diagnostician alters this procedure and simply asks the client, "What is this?" Does this change of procedure alter the vocabulary usage score? Would naming on command be the same as a cloze procedure?

Most tools are designed to obtain as typical a response as possible from the client.

However, when a client cannot or will not respond to the stimulus, the diagnostician may resort to repetition as an alteration of the stimulus-response mode. Repetition of stimuli has often been used as a major testing method even though its use has been heavily criticized. This issue was frequently raised in regard to testing for phonetic structure. Statements were made that imitated word productions will not be representative of the client's ability to produce speech sounds; that is, he will usually perform better on the repeated task. However, one of the major standardized tools for phonetic structure, the *Templin-Darley Tests of Articulation* (Templin and Darley, 1969), rests somewhat on a repetition foundation. The issue is still being debated as seen in the article by Kresheck and Socolofsky (1972). They presented evidence that 4-year-old children performed significantly better on an imitative articulation test than on the same test when spontaneous responses were elicited. They concluded that if an accurate sample of articulation behavior is wanted, then imitation in any form cannot be used for assessing articulation.

On the other hand, repetition as a method for discovering information about language usage gained greater respectability with the advent of the work of Fraser et al. (1963). Menyuk and Looney (1972) presented evidence that repetition of sentences, varying in length and structure, can differentiate between normal and language-disordered children. Even under a repetition task, children demonstrated errors that were comparable to errors they made in spontaneous speech. The errors made were related to difficulties the language-disordered children were having in understanding the transformational structure of the sentences and reflected the rule systems they had for generating sentences.

The criticisms raised about using repetition to sample speech and language behavior seem somewhat overstated. True, repeated speech and language is not necessarily representative of spontaneous speech and language use; however, it is representative of repeated speech and language and can be interpreted as such. The relevant point is, What does repeated speech and language behavior reveal to the diagnostician about the client's ability to process speech and language? If in testing for phonetic structure repeated responses are better than spontaneous responses, this may tell the diagnostician about the client's potential capabilities or his progress in mastery of the task. Actually this is just how repeated responses have frequently been used; they form the basis of much of the stimulability testing the diagnostician will do to make some estimate of prognosis. Van Riper and Erickson (1968) have developed the *Predictive Screening Test of Articulation* based on this premise.

To us, imitated or repeated responses tell the diagnostician something about underlying language processes. Repetition may be different than spontaneous responses, but repetition cannot be accomplished without certain internal processes being intact. If repetition is the only way a test can be used with a client, alter the test format; repeated responses are far better than no responses. On the positive side, if the client matches the model, it is demonstrable evidence that he can produce the response, which may be evidence that his speech and language disorder can be changed. Given certain cautions about using repetition as a mode of eliciting responses, it can be used efficiently as a method of data collection.

Berry-Luterman and Bar (1971) have presented an interesting repetition task that they feel has diagnostic significance for language-impaired children. Syntactic structures that were incorrectly produced in the child's own spontaneous speech were used as items for repetition, followed by repetition of the sentence correctly constructed, and then followed by repetition of the correct sentence produced in reverse order. What implications did Berry-Luterman and Bar draw from their study? Do you feel this would be a productive area to continue developing as a clinical tool?

If the diagnostician keeps in mind that his goal is to collect information about the client's speech and language problem, he can adapt standard procedures to facilitate the client's ability to respond. The aim is not to make clients into statistics, rather the interest is in understanding their disorder. However, once the diagnostician modifies presentation and response procedures, he must interpret the data he has gained in light of those modifications.

Different tools have been designed to measure similar behaviors. What do the following tools offer for measuring formulation of various aspects of syntax (grammar): the expressive portion of the *Northwestern Syntax Screening Test* (Lee, 1969), the *Berry-Talbott Tests of Language* (Berry, 1966), Lee's *Developmental Sentence Scoring* and her *Developmental Sentence Type* analysis, (1974) the expression portion of the *Michigan Picture Language Inventory* (Wolski, 1962), and the *Carrow Elicited Language Inventory* (Carrow, 1974)? How many different types of stimuli are used for these tasks? Do they represent what might be considered as stimulus alterations?

Every other source of speech and language stimulation that occurs in the diagnostic session (the immediate speech and language environment) must be structured just as carefully as the items from selected tools. Frequently, diagnosticians forget that their spontaneous remarks may be too complex to be comprehended by the client. If the diagnostician expects the client to respond, he must monitor all the verbal stimulation he provides. For example, a 3-year-old child with a language disorder may respond marginally to questions formed in the present tense but not to questions formed in the future tense, or he may not be able to give responses that require the use of the past or the future tense. Using graded verbal stimuli, the diagnostician can discover, through conversation, the general level at which a child with a language disorder may be able to comprehend and formulate responses and the point at which he no longer can respond.

As well as controlling the complexity of language stimulation, the diagnostician must take care not to overstimulate. Overstimulation sometimes occurs with young children who are not talking or giving any indication of comprehension. It is also seen with aphasics who have comparable language difficulties. The diagnostician may resort to an overinflected, loud, sing-song speech pattern—a truly dreadful type of overstimulation. When observing this behavior, we sometimes think that the diagnostician hopes the client will talk because he talks this way. Overstimulation is also seen by the use of extensive questioning: "What is this? What is your name? What is that? Did you come with mommy?"— endless questions that the client may not be able to answer, does not want to answer, or is not given time to answer.

Leach (1972), in an interesting article, explores parents' use of the interrogative in interaction with their children. One of his major interests was the relationship between environmental events, the language input of the parent, and the characteristics of the language responses of the child. This article holds important implications for controlling the stimulation diagnosticians provide in the immediate diagnostic setting. How might you develop data collection procedures for children with language disorders following the model developed by Leach?

Observation and recording. How to observe and record the client's responses is fundamental to data collection. Everything the diagnostician needs to learn about the client may well be right before his eyes and ears; however, if he is not able to see, hear, and keep track of what is there, he may lose the very information he needs.

The diagnostician should maintain close scrutiny of all the behaviors exhibited by the client. No behavior should be thought of as simply incidental; it should be observed, recorded, and considered in terms of its relationship to the clinical hypothesis. Frequently, significant responses emerge from unplanned or unorthodox stimulus presentation. For example, a diagnostician was testing Joe whose causal hypothesis was a significant hearing loss. In the test room Joe was not responding to any auditory stimulations. He did not turn his head toward any sound source, differentiate between sound toys—nothing. An observer was behind the two-way observation mirror and tapped lightly on the glass. Joe turned toward this sound source. To check this response, the examiner in the room engrossed the child in play, the observer repeatedly tapped and the child repeatedly turned. The diagnosticians had observed a response to sound. Information was obtained for their clinical hypothesis from an unplanned stimulus.

Planned or unplanned, every behavior may offer a source of information to the observant diagnostician. Even crying behavior, while it might impede other data collection, is useful. For example, 2-year-old Bonnie whose causal hypothesis was inadequate velopharyngeal closure secondary to a repaired cleft palate was being seen. She seemed terrified of any procedures that might mean discomfort for her and cried excessively at the onset of the session. The diagnostician here could be both comforting and observing. Is the crying behavior nasal? How nasal? Does it vary with the intensity of the crying?

The diagnostician's planned use of the SLPM as a framework for observation makes it possible for him to organize the many variables under study. He can plug in the various behaviors as they occur. Each relevant behavior can be recorded as a product, a behavioral correlate, or as associated behavior. The diagnostician can record the details he obtains from his observations until he builds up enough information to signal that the diagnosis can be concluded. Observing all behaviors from this framework prevents the diagnostician from unwarranted interpretations of isolated responses.

While the diagnostician has the SLPM framework for observing his client's responses, he must know how to record the details he observes. He needs some means

of capturing what the client is doing so he may analyze, refer to, and report that data at a later time. He must know how to use notational systems for recording his data. He can use test forms, behavioral observation forms, and systems of his own making as long as the recording of the data reflects the reality of the data collection session. It is the rare circumstance when the diagnostician does not have to make constant, on-the-spot records of his client's responses. When recording his measurements, he immediately interposes himself between the actual response and his recording of that response. At the moment of response the diagnostician usually records his impression of the correctness of the response and the quality of the response, particularly if he has judged the response as incorrect. He does this by comparing the response to some internal criteria for adequacy.

Recording in its limited sense would be description or getting down what the client said, any other type of recording requiring judgment of the correctness and quality of the response is scoring. Thus recording and scoring of responses are intimately bound together; seldom is all scoring done after all responses are made. The diagnostician generally must record and score each item as it occurs for later use.

The diagnostician has basically three procedures available to him for recording and scoring the response, and most scoring protocols accompanying tests use one or more of these.

1. He can determine if the response is correct or incorrect.
2. He can judge the quality of the response along some scale.
3. He can describe the response, that is, record what the client did.

For example, when the diagnostician records that Bertheva made a /b/v/ substitution error, he has used both the descriptive and correctness procedures—noting the type of error is automatically making a statement of correctness. The recording procedures of most tools greatly depends on the complexity inherent in the response required and on the information the diagnostician wants to obtain from the response. Where categorical responses of the yes/no type are required, the diagnostician can score them as right or wrong at the time the response is elicited. Where more complex responses are elicited, the choice is often to describe: to record what the client did for later use in multidimensional scoring.

At first glance it would seem easy to at least differentiate a correct response from an incorrect one. However, we know this is hardly true. Our experience indicates that the range of variability for judging correctness of certain types of responses may be broad, particularly considering responses in context; that is, a sound produced in isolation is usually easier to judge than a sound produced in conversational speech.

There are no absolute criteria for perceptual measurements; experimenters obtaining intra- and interjudge reliability will attest to this. Shriberg (1972) confirms this impression in his study conducted to determine the perceptual judgments made on the /s/ and /r/ phonemes. And yet, the diagnostician must develop internal criteria for making accurate perceptual measurements on the responses made by the individual client. Unlike the experimenter, he usually cannot obtain interjudge reliability of his response recording. Instead, he relies on his own established reliability for each tool he uses. Tools such as Wepman's *Auditory Discrimination Test* (1958) and the *Full-Range Picture Vocabulary Test* (Ammons and Ammons, 1948) rely basically on categorical scoring; the primary interest of these tools is the correctness of the response, not the type of error made. A major test for aphasia, the *Minnesota Test for Differential Diagnosis of Aphasia* (Schuell, 1965), uses a correctness scoring procedure and because of this draws some criticism.

Many of the measures taken of speech and language responses cannot be scored as right or wrong. Instead, responses are qualitatively recorded. Rating scales are frequently used as qualitative recording devices, particularly for disorders such as voice and stuttering. As well, rating scales are used to provide estimates of severity and intelligibility. As he listens to the response, the diagnostician judges the kind, amount, and degree of variation that occurs. Thus the ability to plot responses on these psychological scaling procedures is dependent on the diagnostician's knowledge of the range of variation that can occur.

The most common scales are those that ask for three judgments, for example, mild-moderate-severe, low-average-high, or poor-average-good. Others, however, may require the listener to rate behavior on a scale from 1 to 5 or 1 to 7. The presumption made is that the intervals on these scales are equal and can be converted to numerical quantities. The diagnostician must be trained to judgmental criteria if he is to use these scales appropriately. If not, he will not know if the pitch is high-appropriate-low; if the distortion is mild-moderate-severe; or if the amount of nasality is absent-mild-moderately severe-severe-extreme.

What did Berry and Silverman (1972) discover about the Lewis-Sherman (1951) scale of stuttering severity?

We have often asked classes of students in training to rate a client's speech responses on various scales. The variability of ratings is always amazing. It becomes readily apparent that interjudge and intrajudge reliability is crucial to accurate recording of client responses. Our profession is in great need of training tools to assist students in developing perceptual criteria for various speech and language behaviors they will be asked to rate. In training programs and research settings the use of audio- and videotape recorders is advocated. Recording all or part of the diagnostic session has unquestionable advantages in training programs and allows for later interobserver reliability and more studied analysis.

Many tools use some form of rating scale for recording responses, either for the entire test or for selected subtests. For example, in the *Boston Diagnostic Aphasia Examination* (Goodglass and Kaplan, 1972) "articulation" is rated throughout a number of subtests. Their scale rates "articulation" on a normal-stiff-distorted-fail continuum.

Because the diagnostician is generally interested in the type of error made by the client, he also employs descriptive recording procedures. In this procedure the diagnostician puts down on paper the "exact" response made by the client. He will then categorize the response into a "type of error" category and may at the same time record a correctness judgment. If Fred was asked to name pictures and was shown a fish and he said "bird," the diagnostician would record the word, "bird," score it as incorrect, and categorize it as a type of error; perhaps in this case an in-class semantic error. In the *Language Modalities Test for Aphasia* (Wepman and Jones, 1961a, b) each response is scored according to a six-point category, each number representing a type of response that might be made to the standardized stimuli. Or in another example, when Diane points to the incorrect picture on the *Peabody Picture Vocabulary Test* (Dunn, 1965) and the diagnostician records the number of the picture to which she pointed, he then has obtained

some information about the types of vocabulary comprehension errors Diane is making. Or yet another diverse example: listening to Jill's voice the diagnostician records that it is breathy and hoarse. In this instance the diagnostician bypasses recording what Jill says and instead describes categorically the dimensions of voice quality he has heard. Testing tools available abound with various examples of the use of the descriptive recording-scoring procedure.

Many tools utilize all three recording-scoring procedures. Since speech and language behavior is not unidimensional, tools are designed to obtain several dimensions of behavior from a single response or from a series of responses. Tools like this require multidimensional scoring, isolating as many dimensions as can be observed and recorded simultaneously. Experimental and clinical studies have been instrumental in isolating important dimensions of speech and language disorders. For example, Prins and Lohr (1972) studied 46 visible-audible variables of stuttering behavior. From their analysis of the data they identified 10 factors that, to them, identified the dimensions of stuttering behavior. For the diagnostician, studies such as these assist in determining which behaviors to observe and which provide the most differential information, rather than observing a set of variables that all give similar types of information.

When using standardized and objective tools, the diagnostician is obliged to record and score the response accordingly if he wants to use the standardization data available. However, at times he may find that using only the recommended procedures limits the information he might obtain. Therefore he may choose to amplify on the recording-scoring procedures to gain additional information. This is particularly true in tools like the *Minnesota Test for Differential Diagnosis of Aphasia* (Schuell, 1965), which uses primarily correctness scoring procedures. The diagnostician would probably amplify his recording, adding descriptive procedures to gain data about the type and quality of the responses made to the test items. The diagnostician must always remember that he learns more from knowing what the error is than from knowing an error occurs.

In test construction for aphasia, Porch (1967) and Wepman and Jones (1961a,b) have been instrumental in developing multidimensional scoring procedures, whereas Schuell (1965) maintained a plus-minus scoring procedure. Review the scoring procedures of these tests. Which would provide the most information about responses that aphasics make? Which would be the easiest to use in a clinical setting? Read Porch's article (1971) about multidimensional scoring for assistance in this review. What do Davis and Leach (1972) add to scaling procedures for aphasic errors?

Diagnostician's tasks

Many questions occur to the diagnostician about the realities of the diagnostic session. Foremost among them is, Will the client cooperate with my plan, will we be able to interact in a positive manner to achieve what we both want—a solution? And he should be asking, How much like my preplanning will this diagnosis be? What circumstances may arise that require alterations in my plan?

To complete this fourth step we have specified three tasks the diagnostician must accomplish.

1. He prepares for the diagnostic session, arranging the physical space and materials and then meets the client.
2. He collects his data through the use of interviewing and testing.

3. He closes the diagnostic session, determining when he has sufficient information to provide for appropriate management plans.

Prepares for the diagnostic session

In preparing for the diagnosis, the diagnostician must attend to the physical arrangements for the session and to the inital contact with the client.

Physical arrangements. The diagnostician should select and arrange his room, materials, and forms to be ready for the session. The furniture should be appropriate to the age of the client; doors should be wide enough for wheelchairs; materials should be arranged in order of use and hidden from view if necessary; all equipment being used should be in working order; simple things like ashtray availability, opening windows on hot days, and turning on the lights should all be thought about. There are innumerable details about the physical arrangements that could be discussed. Many are specific to the work setting—what is available in terms of rooms, furniture, and materials. However, there is one major consideration regardless of the circumstances. The diagnostician should prepare and arrange the physical environment to be as conducive as possible for eliciting cooperation and responsiveness. Being concerned about interpersonal interactions generally overcomes any limitations imposed by a poor physical environment, and we have yet to see carpeting on the floor and expensive furniture substituting for professional skill in personal interaction and systematic observation. Thus, when the client arrives in the diagnostician's room, his physical comfort should be attended to; taking off coats, arranging seating, commenting on the conditions of the physical setting if needed, pointing out toilet facilities, etc.

Initial client contact. The diagnostician must decide how he is going to introduce himself to the client complex. This initial contact is essential for the further establishment of interpersonal-professional relations. Depending on the setting, the client may be sent to the diagnostician's office or the diagnostician will go to the waiting room to meet the client. With adult clients the usual introductions are sufficient, providing information about who you are, where you will be taking them, and some information about what you will be doing and how long it may take. Giving information about the general features of the diagnostic session allows the client to develop a grasp of what it all may mean and what part he may be playing.

Children are quite another matter. If the child has already established separation from his parents, he may go readily with the diagnostician. A procedure that is helpful is to allow the child to approach the diagnostician. While talking to the parent, glance at the child, winking at him, smiling at him, and letting him see that his parent thinks you are safe. This often arouses his natural curiosity and he may approach you. When this seems likely, the diagnostician can say, "You must be Donald, I'm Jim." From this point, conversation can ensue; the diagnostician can begin to inform the child of what is going to happen, thereby getting him interested in the upcoming proceedings. Moving to the diagnostic room then may be accomplished with ease. Learning how to interact with young children is the key ingredient.

At other times child-parent separation can be quite problematic. It must be handled with care. How does the diagnostician get a child to come with him to the testing room? Along with the procedures just suggested, the diagnostician should let the parent help. Often the parent is the best solver of a potential separation problem. Take cues from the parent-child interaction; go slow and do not force yourself on the child. The parents often know if the child will go with you, or they will know the things to say to the child so he is willing to go with you.

The parent's and child's advice and consent are essential to the diagnostic contract. Should the child go alone or should the parent accompany him? Different professionals take very different approaches to this issue. While some practice routine separation of children from their parents, we feel this practice is ill advised for many preschoolers. Children between the ages of 2 and 4 are in a period of working out their feelings of separateness from their parents, and at this age separation may be a particularly difficult situation for them. Even when some children separate with no problem, there is no assurance that they have not experienced some separation anxiety.

We feel the issue of child-parent separation rests with our purpose—to provide the best help we can for the client. If a parent can assist in this, then it is appropriate to have the parent present. When a child feels secure about "mommy," he is more likely to perform optimally. Likewise, whenever the parent is present, an opportunity for parent-child interaction is available to the diagnostician. Often an interacting bond must first be established among parent-diagnostician-child until the parent bond can be faded. However, there are times when the parent will not allow the child to perform on his own, continually interjecting advice, correction, and help or becoming distraught by the child's performance. In these interfering instances the parent must be "separated." When the child is engaged with the diagnostician and appears to have developed confidence in him, the parent can be politely asked to leave. Once the child and the diagnostician are interacting well, this separation is not too difficult for the child, but there may be some concern over how difficult it was for the parent.

Palmer (1970) provides some important viewpoints about the initial client contact with children.

Collects the data

The interview and the tools to be used are now administered in as structured, objective, systematic, and efficient a manner as possible, given the many variables that make up the diagnostic session. The diagnostician needs many skills to control variables in the immediate clinical testing situation: the client variables, the setting variables, the tools variables, and the diagnostician variables.

Actually, data collection begins the moment the diagnostician first observes or introduces himself to the client. As a matter of fact, this initial interaction may provide enough data for the diagnostician to verify that he is on the right track. On the other hand, he may discover he was on the wrong track and immediately must put into effect new plans. For example, if a language disorder was hypothesized for Norma and at the moment she responded to the diagnostician's greeting she blocked on every word she uttered, an obvious change in plans is required. It does not mean that language may not be disordered, only that Norma may both stutter and have a significant language disorder. Probably the diagnostician would study these two products in interaction: Does the stuttering behavior increase as expected language responses increase in complexity?

Throughout the diagnostic session the diagnostician remains alert to all variables that signal needed changes in plans. We do not wish to impart the idea that collection of data is simply the carrying out of the plans arrived at previously. In many instances the diagnostician will discover that a tool previously selected is inappropriate for the client; thus he must have the ability to switch procedures. Alterations in planning also can occur as a result of information obtained in the interview. Wherever and whenever they occur, the diagnostician must recycle his diagnostic design. The new information is now a part of a new constituent analysis, leading to a reformulation or adjustment of the clinical hypothesis and requiring a redesigning of tools to collect his clinical data.

Interviewing. From his design the diagnostician has delineated the information he hopes to obtain in the interview and has given thought to how best to frame questions to get that information. Now he needs to execute his planned questions. The interpersonal nature of the interview comprises the new element to which the diagnostician must adjust his diagnostic design. The characteristics and needs of both the informant and diagnostician will interact to mold and modify what has been planned to this point.

In approaching interviewing, the diagnostician will need to attend to three aspects of the "live" interview. He first will need to structure his interview as a part of the total diagnostic session. He then will launch into the interview with the informant. Finally, he will enter the heart of the interview, collecting and recording pertinent information.

STRUCTURING THE INTERVIEW. Interviews are often difficult to conduct within the confines of the time limitations of the diagnostic session. With adults this can be accomplished by incorporating the interview as part of the clinical testing. The questions asked can be used to obtain more information about the problem, and serve as samples of speech and language behavior as well: how well the client can comprehend what is said to him, how well he can hear, how he formulates language, and how well he produces it through the speech-producing mechanism. Communicative interaction with adult clients often becomes the basis for obtaining interview and clinical data simultaneously; at times no further specific clinical tools are needed.

With children clients, however, interviewing becomes more problematic. Generally the diagnostician wants to interview the parent or whoever brings the child prior to testing the child. The question immediately arises as to what to do with the child. If the interview is conducted in the presence of the child, how will this affect what the diagnostician asks or how the parent may respond? Will the child feel ignored if he is not attended to during this time? In many situations there may be no satisfactory answers to these questions; but since the major purpose of the diagnosis is to see the child, the interview must not take up all the time available.

Interviewing the child's parents takes on a different structure dependent on the work setting, the diagnostician's philosophy about interviewing, and separation plans. Some professionals advocate seeing the parent for a separately scheduled interview session, followed by a second testing session with the child. If the setting and parents are such that multiple diagnostic visits are possible, this method of seeing the parents and child on different visits often is ideal. When the child arrives, all the attention is his, and the problem of what to do with him during the interview is circumvented. In addition, seeing the parents prior to the child's visit allows the parents to prepare themselves as well as the child for what to expect when the child is tested. Other professionals advocate using a team approach: one interviewing the parent while another sees the child. Such an approach is often used in multidiscipline settings as well as in training centers. In yet other settings a playroom may be provided for the child staffed by a student, an aide, or someone who attends to and possibly makes observations of the child.

These latter two approaches, however, necessitate separation. If separation is not accomplished and the child remains in the interview room, some diagnosticians set up a play corner for the child that distracts him while the interview is being conducted. There are instances, however, when the child stays on his mother's lap and is present throughout the interview. In such situations the diagnostician must guide the interview so that questions and answers are limited to what can appropriately be said in the child's presence. The diagnostician can indicate this directly to the parent, for example, "Let's try to discuss Darwin's problem in such a way that he does not feel uncomfortable about what we say." Similarly, the diagnostician needs to let the child know what they are talking

about. He may say, for example, "Your mother is going to be telling me what things you have been doing, so that I know more about you. We will be talking for a short while, and then you and I will have a chance to talk together." At other times the diagnostician is confronted with a child who cannot be separated and who dominates the interview by his behavior. Probably every diagnostician at some time in his career has had a child dismantle his office or shriek throughout an attempted interview. At such times the only alternative may be a telephone conversation with the parent following the diagnosis or a conference scheduled for a later day.

■ In the following example situations decide how you would structure the interview within the total diagnostic session. What modifications might be necessary? How can the interview be arranged to gain the best data possible? What impact will the interview have on all persons involved, including the informant and others who may be present?

1. Three-year-old Reagan arrives with both his mother and father at a university speech and hearing center. The interview and testing are planned to be conducted simultaneously, although Reagan indicates he does not want to leave his parents. How should the diagnostic team proceed?

2. Mrs. Lewis comes with her husband who is very depressed over his recent stroke and resulting physical and language problems. With whom does the diagnostician, Mrs. Sekeley, hold the interview? Will the interview and testing sessions be distinct or integrated? If integrated, what is Mrs. Lewis' role?

3. Fourteen-year-old Norris is brought by his very anxious mother, Mrs. Leonard, for help with his stuttering problem. Who is interviewed? What is Norris told about the interview? What is Mrs. Leonard told?

4. Four-year-old Kim is brought to a setting in which one diagnostician is to hold both the interview and testing sessions on the same day. No provisions are available for another person to care for Kim during the interview. Since Kim is a very active and at times out-of-control child, the mother is

not able to attend well to the questions she is asked. Indeed, Kim is quite disruptive and very little interviewing is possible. What should the diagnostician do to obtain the interview information he wants?

LAUNCHING THE INTERVIEW. After the diagnostician has dealt with the structure of the interview as part of the total diagnostic context, he must begin the actual interview. Earlier in this chapter we stressed approaching the interview as a coalition between the informant and the diagnostician. We therefore suggest the diagnostician launch the interview by explaining the purpose of the interview and the importance of the informant in this process. For example, the diagnostician may want to begin in the following manner: "Mrs. Blatt, we are glad that you were able to come with Pam today. Before we test her, I'd like to spend a little time talking with you so that I can better understand her problem as you see it. Since I will see Pam for such a relatively short time and cannot observe everything about her, I will have to rely on you to tell me the things that I cannot observe. You will be very important in helping me understand many aspects of Pamela's problem, why she is having the problem, and what we can do about it." Such an introduction explains the purpose of the diagnosis and also includes the informant as an integral part of the process.

■ Plan how you would introduce the purpose of the diagnosis and explain the informant's role to the following informants. How would the diagnostician explain the purpose of the interview to the following people? What language would he choose to do this?

1. Mrs. Reidel, a social worker with the department of child welfare, has brought 10-year-old Darren to the community hearing and speech agency. Darren lives at home with his mother and seven other siblings.
2. The diagnostician, Dr. Lipkowitz, is to begin an interview with Dr. Whitney a well-known pediatrician in the community, whose 7-year-old son is hypothesized to have a minor articulation problem.
3. Miss Mayfield, a black diagnostician, is to interview Mrs. Lund, a working-class white mother of 4-year-old Sandra.
4. Mr. Sugarman, a public school diagnostician, has scheduled an interview appointment with Mrs. Becker, the fifth grade teacher of Kathy who has a stuttering problem.

After introducing the purpose of the diagnosis, we suggest the diagnostician acknowledge the information he has received about the client prior to the interview. For example, he might say, "I appreciate your taking the time to fill out the questionnaire we sent you. I was wondering if Bethany's speech has changed any since you returned the form?" Or in another instance, the diagnostician might say to the wife of the client, "Dr. Kronenberg said your husband had a stroke 2 months ago. Tell me what changes you have seen in his speech? Mentioning the information he has received lets the informant know the scope of information that the diagnostician possesses and serves as a starting point to talk about the problem. If the informant has submitted information, it lets the informant know that the diagnostician has read what he has written and that its content need not be repeated. If reports have been sent from persons other than the informant, we also feel the diagnostician should mention these, unless explicitly asked not to by the one who sent the report. Letting the informant know what information has been received allows for more open, direct communication.

We want to point out, however, that acknowledging the receipt of information from other sources is quite a different matter than sharing the contents of that information. For example, while a diagnostician may say, "We have received reports from Dr. Nordell [the school psychologist] and Mrs. Elson [the child's teacher]," we do not feel the diagnostician should report another person's findings. Usually reports from other professionals will indicate what information has been given to the client or parents. If not, and the informant asks about the other professionals' findings, the diagnostician may simply say, "I suggest that you ask Dr. Nordell these questions as he was the one who tested your child, and he will be better able to explain his results."

■ Acknowledge receipt of information in the following situations.

1. A parent, Mrs. Weiss, has returned a children's speech and language history form with most of the items left blank.
2. The diagnostician has received a report from the neurologist in charge of Mr. Zeitz during his recent hospitalization following his stroke. Mr. Zeitz claims he does not know what happened to his speech.
3. Mr. Kronenberg has completed a history form in exacting detail. He has also mentioned that he is seeing a psychiatrist, from whom he has requested a report be sent to the hearing and speech center. The psychiatrist's report has not been received at the time of the interview.
4. The diagnostician has received no information other than basic identifying information about Ray Harold, a 20-year-old man with a voice problem.
5. A parent, after learning that the psychologist who tested her 5-year-old son Bart has sent a report, asks what IQ her son received.

COLLECTING THE INTERVIEW DATA. Having explained the purpose of the diagnosis and acknowledged the available information, the diagnostician is ready to begin asking the questions he has planned in order to get the information he wants. It is generally a good idea to begin the question-answer process in a nonthreatening manner. The diagnostician will want to be sure the informant can feel successful in responding to the initial question. With some clients the diagnostician may begin by asking a general question first such as, "Have you seen any changes in John's speech since you filled out the history questionnaire?" Or if the informant has not provided any previous information, perhaps the diagnostician would begin by saying, "How would you describe Larry's speech and language problem?" or "What con-

cerns you about Larry's speech and language problem?" Such a general circumscribed amplification question allows the diagnostician to assess the informant's level of understanding of the problem and also focus the interview immediately on the client's speech and language. Emerick (1969) has suggested that the diagnostician listen before he talks, thus allowing the informant to let you know where he is. From this the diagnostician can better determine how to employ his preplanning strategy. Such an approach also subjects the clinical hypothesis to test without first limiting the range of possible topics or biasing the focus of the interview.

If the diagnostician senses that the informant may not initially feel comfortable in providing a relatively lengthy and unstructured response, he may alternatively choose to begin the questioning by asking for some very specific, readily obtainable information such as identifying information or clarification of some item on the history form. For example, "Is your address still 2897 Berkshire?" or "You mentioned on the phone that you saw Dr. Warner at the psychology clinic. When did you see Dr. Warner?"

Having started with a general question, the diagnostician can continue by picking up a point in the informant's response and asking for further information about that point. For example, if Mrs. Ledowsky says that 4-year-old Amy stutters and has a hard time getting her words out, the diagnostician might then ask Mrs. Ledowsky to describe further what it is that Amy does when she stutters, what situations make her stuttering more or less severe, or if she has noticed any letters or words that Amy has particular difficulty with. If the diagnostician has framed specific questions about Amy's speech and language, he will then want to insert those questions here.

In proceeding through the interview, we find it helpful to approach the questioning by general topic areas. The topic headings of the speech and language history questionnaire can serve this purpose. These topics include identification; statement of the problem; speech, language, and hearing history; general development, including pregnancy and birth history as well as developmental history; medical history; behavior; educational history; and home and family information.

The extent to which each topic is explored will depend on the information available prior to the interview, the design of the interview, and the informant's ability to provide the requested information. If detailed information was available, the diagnostician may only need to address a few topic areas. If little information was available, the diagnostician may need to initiate each new topic area with a general, circumscribed amplification question, followed by more structured questions to gain the specific information needed. In this manner the diagnostician can balance open and closed questions, gaining the kind of information both has to offer. Approaching the interview by general topic areas helps the diagnostician remember what information he planned to obtain without being bound to notes, and thus leads to more thorough and smooth data collection in the interview. A topic approach to interviewing helps guard against simple rotelike presentation of a series of nonrelated, preplanned questions. Finally, approaching the interview from topic areas also allows the informant to see the continuity of the interview and helps him understand why certain questions are being asked.

As mentioned previously, we suggest the interview begin or at least very early focus on the client's speech and language. The client's speech and language problem is what brought the client, and therefore it is a logical point to begin from both the informant's and the diagnostician's perspectives. The informant undoubtedly expects to talk about the problem, and thus discussing the speech and language problem provides an initial common ground between the informant and the diagnostician. After the informant has been able to say

what he wants to about the speech and language behavior, and the diagnostician has been able to ask the questions he has framed, the diagnostician will then want to move the interview to other topics.

Many of the remaining topics will help the diagnostician understand causal factors, although the purpose of some of these topic areas may not be obvious to the informant. We suggest that in moving on to these other topics the diagnostician may want to introduce the new area by explaining why he is interested in such information. For example, in addressing medical history, the diagnostician may say, "I would now like to discuss your child's medical history as sometimes we can identify illnesses or accidents that may be related to his speech and language problem. How has Arick's health been?" Or if considerable information is available, the diagnostician may say, "You mentioned on the history questionnaire that Arick has had several earaches. For what period of time did he have these, and how were they treated?" Or in entering questions in the area of general behavior, the diagnostician might say, "I'm interested in getting a picture of Jimmy's other behavior so that I can put his speech and language into broader perspective. Let's start by telling me how he spends a typical day from the time he gets up in the morning until the time he goes to bed at night."

Along with gaining the information he wants, the diagnostician will have to execute the recording procedures he has decided on if these are to be done within the interview session. If he has planned to tape-record the interview, he will need to explain his purposes in recording the session and gain the informant's consent. If the diagnostician has decided to write information down only after the session, he will need to pay close attention to the specifics given. If identification data has not appeared in written form, most diagnosticians will want to make sure this information is recorded accurately at the time it is given. Whatever method of recording the diagnostician chooses, he will need to let the informant know what he is doing and keep check so that his recording does not interfere with the interpersonal interaction. Often the context makes it obvious what he is writing down. For example, if the parent is giving names or dates, it is generally understood that this information is written down. The diagnostician, however, may want to make this explicit; for example, he may say, "I am going to jot down the dates you mention so that I am sure that I remember them exactly as you give them to me."

The real skill involved in interviewing is being able to adapt the questions and recording of information to the individual characteristics of the informant. The diagnostician may well approach the interview via topic areas and have settled on a recording method; however, the specifics that evolve are very much dependent on the interpersonal dynamics that take place between the diagnostician and the informant.

■ This project is designed as a role play between one person designated as a student diagnostician and a second person who will serve as the informant. The diagnostician plans to gain the following information as a part of the interview.

1. The student diagnostician wants to tape-record the session. He must explain his purpose in wanting to record the session and ask for the informant's consent.
2. The diagnostician wants to get a more detailed description of a 5-year-old child's language comprehension. Information available prior to the interview simply stated, "He doesn't seem to understand everything said to him."
3. The diagnostician has no information pertaining to developmental milestones.
4. The child has been described by the referring pediatrician as "irritable," "difficult to manage," and "prefers to play alone."

The diagnostician is to gain this same information from the following three informants role played by the second person. How will he modify his approach and interactions to gain this information?

1. Mrs. Robbins is a middle-class housewife who is concerned about her adequacy as a mother. Her husband tends to blame her for Raymond's unmanageable behavior, claiming that if she knew how to manage him, Raymond would not have all of his current problems. She fears that Raymond may be retarded and is very concerned about the cause of his language and behavior problems; however, she attempts to present him in the most favorable light and to minimize his difficulties.
2. Mrs. Watkins is a lower-class mother who communicates her information and impressions about her son through a "restricted code." While she knows Arnold is not "stupid," she has little knowledge of other factors contributing to speech and language functioning. While her understanding of Arnold's problem is limited, she very much wants to do whatever is best for him.
3. Mrs. Roth is a social worker in the residential treatment program where Joshua has been living for the past 8 months. She is young and only recently out of school. She has been trained in process recording and tells the diagnostician that she feels use of the tape recorder for interviews is inappropriate. Mrs. Roth has relatively little information about Joshua since she just recently was assigned his case. In addition, she has had little experience with children with speech and language problems. She is, however, very interested in learning about speech and language in general as well as learning specifically about Joshua's problem.

Following the role play with each informant, the participants and observers may want to discuss the following points.

1. Interpersonal interactions: How did each participant behave toward the other one? What was each participant feeling during the interview?
2. Information flow: Did the informant give and get the information he wanted? Did the diagnostician give and get the information he wanted? Was all the relevant information exchanged?

After the diagnostician has gained the information he wants in the interview and the informant has been given ample oppor-

Table 15. Interview with Mrs. Compardo

Diagnostician's aim	Diagnostician's and Mrs. Compardo's statements (D = Diagnostician, C = Compardo)
Explain the purpose of the interview.	D: Mrs. Compardo, before working with Katherine I'd like to spend some time talking with you about her speech and language. Your information will be most useful in helping understand her problem and in giving us a broader picture of her. We'll be working together in determining Katherine's problem and in doing something about it.
	C: I'm glad to finally be here today. I really don't know why Katherine is having trouble talking, and I hope that we'll be able to do something about it.
Acknowledge the information received prior to the interview.	D: I appreciate your taking the time and thought to have filled out the history questionnaire so completely. I have gone over it carefully and it has helped me plan what I will be doing with Katherine today. It also has helped me think of a few other things I'd like to ask you.
	C: On some of the questions, I just wasn't sure what to say.
	D: I know that sometimes it's hard to know just what is intended by some of the questions. We'll be discussing some of those here.
Inform parent of recording method chosen.	D: From time to time, you may see me jotting notes down. Some of the things you say I will want to write down exactly as you have said them so that I will be sure to have the correct information.
Begin interview proper with a general, circumscribed amplification question that addresses the speech and language problem.	D: Since you completed the history form, have you noticed anything else that you might like to add about Katherine's speech and language?
	C: Not too much has changed, although I think she is starting to call the cat "nana"—our cat's name is Nerja. She also has really been involved in picture books. She's always trying to get me to read to her. One other thing I've been noticing lately is that compared to my other children, she is really a messy eater. She uses both hands and really makes a mess.
Follow up open question with a more structured question based on earlier response.	D: By messy eater, what do you mean? Does she play with her food, or does she seem to be have trouble keeping food in her mouth?
	C: She's a good eater; that is, she likes to eat and doesn't really play with her food. Rather, she's just sloppy in the way she eats. Her milk is always running out of the corners of her mouth or bits of food fall out of her mouth. She also doesn't chew her food very well, swallows huge bites, and sometimes gags. As a baby she accepted solid foods much later than my other children did and had problems moving the food around in her mouth to chew it and swallow it. I didn't think we'd ever get her off baby food. I wish we would have owned stock in Gerber's.
Follow up point made by parent to get further information having to do with Katherine's understanding.	D: One thing you said a little earlier I'd like to discuss a little more. You said Katherine is always trying to get you to read to her. What kinds of books does she like? Does she seem to like the stories, or is she mostly involved in looking at the pictures?
	C: Katherine used to favor books like the ABC's and simple picture books, but now she seems to be bored by those. She likes books that have more of a story to them. She loves the *Three Little Pigs* and some of the Dr. Seuss books.

Continued.

Table 15. Interview with Mrs. Compardo—cont'd

Diagnostician's aim	Diagnostician's and Mrs. Compardo's statements (D = Diagnostician, C = Compardo)
Insert planned question relevant to topic area under discussion.	D: Can you give me other examples of situations in which Katherine understands the language used?
	C: Well, since she loved the *Three Little Pigs* so much, I bought her the record at the grocery store—you know one of those 49¢ records that she later can play herself. Now she wants me to play that over, and over, and over. She laughs when the pigs say "not by the hair of my chinny, chin chin," and sometimes blows when the wolf says "then I'll huff and I'll puff and I'll blow your house down."
	D: Can you think of any other situations. Sometimes it's tricky to know if a child understands the words we say to them or gets the message through our gestures or other clues. Can you think of any situations in which it was quite clear that Katherine understood what you said rather than what she saw?
	C: Let's see . . . oh, the other day I was busy cooking in the kitchen and I wanted a magazine that I had left on the nightstand next to our bed. I asked Katherine to go upstairs and get it, and she did. Sometimes she won't do what I want her to, but I think that's more a matter of stubbornness than not understanding.
Continue role playing the remainder of the interview.	

tunity to offer what he wants, the diagnostician will need to close the interview. He can do this by thanking the informant for his cooperation and the information he has provided. He then will need to specify what is to happen next and when and how he will get back to the informant. For example, he might say, "You have been very helpful in giving me a lot of information about Perry. While we could probably continue to talk for some time, I would like to begin testing Perry before he gets too restless. You may remain in the waiting room while I am with Perry. After we are finished, I will again meet with you to discuss my findings and to plan our next steps."

■ We now return to our client, Katherine Compardo, to conduct an interview with Mrs. Compardo. The interview has been structured so that Katherine is playing quietly in a sandbox in another corner of a large room. Mrs. Compardo and the diagnostician can thus interact without distraction as Katherine is actively involved in her play. Table 15 sketches part of this interview. The student is encouraged to com-

plete the interview through role play. He will want to refer back to Chapter 13 where further information needed about Katherine has been delineated and where questions have been framed. He will also need to refer to the children's speech, language, and hearing history questionnaire that Mrs. Compardo has completed (Appendix II).

Clinical testing. As previously discussed, a major ingredient of clinical testing is the interpersonal interaction that takes place. Cooperation from the client is necessary to obtain the data needed. With adults this is seldom problematic. Even with adults with major physical and psychological problems cooperation can be obtained if the diagnostician keeps in mind that he will have to work with and through certain behaviors. Usually within the session he can obtain enough cooperation from the adult to do his clinical testing.

With children this is not the case. Much attention must be paid to getting cooperation from the child, not only initially but throughout the diagnostic session. A child may start out well but be unable to maintain this behavior throughout the entire session.

ORIENTING PROCEDURES. At the outset of clinical testing clients must be given information that orients them to the diagnostic session. Structure is provided that lets a client know what is expected. A balance must be maintained between formality of testing and informality of interaction. Natural interests and spontaneous responses to the setting and the materials, including getting off the subject, must be allowed for if interest in the procedures is to be maintained throughout the session. Fatigue, boredom, restlessness, negativism, frustration, anger, etc. must be combated. The initial contract should specify in some sense the rules each will play—this is what I do, and this is what you do. Within this framework the client is given decisions to make.

For the child it may be well to establish more rules at the onset of the testing session. First, we are going to sit down; then we are going to look at some pictures; then you will have to say some words—various ways of putting structure into the session so the child knows what he is doing, why he is doing it, and what may be coming next. After the ground rules are laid, the child can then be made an integral part of the decision making. He can be given choices of things to do, which task to do first, which chair to sit in, what to do next, how long to do it, when to take a break, etc. The child can be made an assistant to the diagnostician. He can help get out the materials, put them away, turn pages, and arrange the tables and chairs; he can assist in any number of activities that turns him into an active participant in his session rather than simply a passive recipient of test stimuli to which he responds. Being a part of the decision-making process keeps a child interested, motivated, curious, and in some control over what happens to him.

The choices offered can be structured in such a way that each alternative is acceptable to the diagnostician. For example, if in the testing room two chairs are placed, one red and one blue, the child can be asked, "Which chair would you like, the red one or the blue one?" He is given a choice; but the choices are limited, and both chairs should be appropriate for the child. Giving assent to a child's wishes gives him a feeling that he has a part to play in decisions that will affect him in some way.

Fremon (1972) has presented an interesting article directed to parents about using yes responses as often as possible with children. A side effect of this approach to discipline has been the positive effects on the parents about their children. How might the ideas discussed by Fremon be applied to the diagnostic session?

CARRYING OUT THE TESTING STRATEGY. The diagnostician has a plan for testing the client and the necessary materials ready for doing so, including backup procedures that may be necessary for testing alternate hypotheses. The plan is made up of a series of "puzzle pieces," some more detailed than others. Gathering all the pieces is now essential for filling in the plan. It was suggested in the last chapter that the diagnostician develop a flowchart representing how he might move from one procedure to the next, indicating alterations of procedures that would not affect the accumulation of data.

Hannah and Sheeley (1975) have presented a seven-stage sequence flowchart for audiologic evaluation. Their overall concern is how audiologists might select testing procedures to arrive at a diagnostic profile. Compare their model of test selection to the framework being developed in this book for the diagnostic process, particularly as it relates to the selection of tools and collection of data steps of the process.

The general flowchart of most help is that which first proposes a tool to obtain baseline data about the behaviors of interest, followed by tools that provide more specific detail. Establishing baseline data about the cause-effect relationship gives immediate information, and in the case when the client cannot or will not continue, the diagnostician has some information to use.

A common tool used to establish early baselines is conversational speech, a basic tool for any speech and language disorder and sometimes considered a routine procedure. For an adult client this could be incorporated in the interview, providing the diagnostician specific data about speech and language while providing the client an opportunity to discuss his problem. For children, however, conversation is not easy and a conversational situation will generally have to be structured. Probably the least successful structure for young children is the question-asking approach. Children meeting strangers do not respond well to direct questions—even of the most innocuous types like "What is your name?" Children, on their first contact with an adult, must be drawn into verbal interaction. They must understand that they can respond in their own time, in their own manner, and with all their adequacies and inadequacies.

The use of parallel talking with children is often effective. The diagnostician can select an activity that initially requires no speech; for example, while playing together with some toys of interest at a stand-up sandbox, the diagnostician can comment on what he is doing and what the child is doing, slowly adding to his comments instructions for the child to follow. "Let's take our cars to the garage." Does the child proceed to do so; be sure to wait to see.

Children tend to be inquisitive; their curiosity often "gets the best of them," and it can be used to advantage by the diagnostician. Let children look into things, discover things, be surprised by things, laugh at things, and enjoy their surroundings. A technique for stimulating conversation that takes advantage of children's curiosity is the old hiding trick. The diagnostician can have a flannel board set up and a big bag of carefully selected pictures that is his se-

cret. The child can be intrigued by the examiner's interest in the bag until he wants to get into the bag. Once the "stage is set," the child can be instructed to close his eyes, reach in, take one picture, and put it on the flannel board. The flannel board could have sections: the city, the farm, the house, the department store, etc. The pictures in the bag can relate to these sections. When the child pulls out a picture the examiner can say, "Oh, you found a cat; I think that goes in the house. Let's put it in the house." Natural spontaneity is required of the diagnostician. Verbal overreaction on his part can set off overreaction in the child.

Does the child follow the instructions? Further questions can be asked, "Where did you put the cat? In the house? In this way the diagnostician can model various speech and language structures for the child to use when it is the diagnostician's turn to close his eyes, reach in the bag, take one picture, and put it on the flannel board. Depending on the child's disorder, the diagnostician can structure this technique to get at any aspect of speech and language: reception, comprehension, formulation, repetition, and production. He should know at what age levels the tasks he designs can be performed by children; that is, he selects his activity and his verbal stimuli according to normative information. A carefully structured activity such as the preceding usually gets a child to interact verbally through which the diagnostician obtains baseline data, a spontaneous language sample, and, as well, sets up a comfortable interpersonal relationship. Since talking and listening are the mainstays of diagnosis, this procedure may provide enough data to understand the effect component of the cause-effect hypothesis.

Develop a procedure similar to the one described that is structured to obtain specific information about (1) the ability to use the articulatory mechanism, (2) the child's ability to hear, (3) pitch, quality, and loudness, (4) the complexity of syntax, and (5) the ability to produce phonemes.

There are many general suggestions that could be offered for working with children. Among them we list the following that the diagnostician may find helpful.

1. Remember, that most children are easy to test. They go through the paces in a remarkably matter-of-fact manner. Take a hint from this. Make your manner likewise. Assume that "here is something we are going to do." It may be enjoyable but that is really secondary. In most cases, time is saved and the actual creation of emotional reactions is avoided if the diagnostician does not approach the testing as a thrilling, exciting game that the child is going to "just love." Any extremes of emotion by the diagnostician may create problems in the child. There is no need or justification for building up an atmosphere of excitement in anticipation of a fascinating game. The older the child, the more apparent this statement becomes. You are securing a representative sample of the child's speech. The more simply and efficiently this can be done, the less wear on the diagnostician and child.

2. Administer the tools quickly and efficiently. For most children the process must move along at a reasonably good rate in order to hold their attention and to prevent prolonging the testing beyond its maximum usefulness. But do not push the child too fast. You do not need rapid-fire responses. If he appears interested in looking at a test picture or talking about it, let him. Rapidity of administration varies greatly from child to child. Do not expect a response on every item—let some of them go and pick them up later. Struggling to get a response from the child on every item by asking again and again or saying, "You know that" can build up a condition of nonresponding.

3. Allow children to have temporary diversions during the testing. They should be able to make comments, ask seemingly irrelevant questions, and get up and move around without being made to feel guilty. On the other hand, too much freedom or too prolonged distractive activities may be disastrous. The diagnostician should maintain control of the testing situation. This control can be gentle though insistent. In most cases it is sufficient to direct attention to the testing materials after brief diversion. At other times it may be necessary to say or imply, "We have played a while, now let's go back to this."

4. Be careful of asking the child if he wants to do something. This often sets off negativism, and what if the child says "no" to a task you had every intention of doing. The diagnostician then runs the risk of the child discovering that his wishes may be ignored. So guard against requests that you suspect may be met with refusal. Negativism cannot usually be reduced by prodding to respond and certainly not by displaying disapproval of his "uncooperative" behavior. When a child is thrust into a potentially threatening (to his way of feeling) situation, he has a right to be negative until such time as he can evaluate the situation. Negativism is often acceptable behavior that does not need to call forth any particular emotional reaction on the part of the diagnostician.

5. The use of reinforcement must be considered carefully for maintaining continued participation. Verbal reinforcement usually works, but in some instances other primary and secondary reinforcers will be needed. But the reinforcing device should not impede the flow of testing. A device that helps to keep young children moving to completion is the use of a timing device. A nonworking clock can be set, and the examiner can point out where the big hand must go before the child can stop. "In 10 minutes we will be done with this." Children often have vague time concepts and 10 minutes will not be too meaningful. The diagnostician and child can move the hand on the clock to show the passing of time, making the hand arrive at the designated place at the time the testing is over.

6. There is also one rather specific suggestion we would like to offer. When doing speech mechanism examinations with children, never assume that you will get to look in their mouths as often as you would like. Make every observation count. If the

child cooperates the first time, do as much as you can, look for everything you can, do one task immediately after another as there may be no second chance.

Once the interaction pattern has been established and some baselines of information obtained, the diagnostician can move into his more detailed and specific clinical testing. Each tool is introduced matter-of-factly. "Now we are going to look at some pictures, and I want you to tell me the name of each one. I'll help you if you don't know the name. You turn the pages." Or "Mrs. Valtille, I have a test to give you to help us understand your problem better."

Knowing when to discontinue using a tool is as important as knowing when to use a certain tool. It requires knowing when enough details about the behaviors under study have been obtained or when a client no longer is performing adequately or with interest. There is no rule to follow other than knowing what information is being obtained and how useful it will be in discovering the essentials of the clinical problem. For example, one of our favorite observations was of a child who was asked to repeat sounds in sequences. The sequences were created by the child who threw a set of dice (wooden blocks) on which the sounds were printed. Dice were added or removed to change the length of the sound sequences to be repeated. This procedure continued, to our way of thinking, beyond its meaningfulness, and after a time the child confirmed this by saying: "When are we going to stop playing with these stupid blocks?" The student was spending too much time getting details at the risk of losing the child's interest and cooperation.

When using standardized tools, the intent is to complete the test if at all possible or else the normative data will not be usable. Some tools are designed to establish basal and ceiling levels of performance such as the *Peabody Picture Vocabulary Test* (Dunn, 1965). Others require completion in their entirety, for example, Wepman's *Auditory Discrimination Test* (1958). Still others supply a screening portion to help make decisions about going on to the remainder of the test for added details such as the *Language Modalities Test for Aphasia* (Wepman and Jones, 1961a, b). However, even with such tools, testing should be discontinued if the client is evidencing significant difficulties in performance or attention that could hinder any remaining testing. When tools are designed to present items graded for difficulty level, they are easier to use than those that are not.

Another situation that occurs is with the client who manifests immediate behavior indicative of his clinical problem, for example, the adult stutterer who stutters significantly from the moment the diagnostic session begins. The diagnostician knows he has a prosody disorder. Can testing be discontinued? If the diagnostician's intent was only to discover this fact, then testing could be discontinued. However, diagnosis is designed to obtain more than an obvious sample of manifest behavior. He will go on to obtain as many details about the disordered prosody in as many situations as possible, exploring the full range of cause-effect relationships. He works toward gaining as much information as possible to answer any number of clinical questions for making management decisions.

At other times the client does not readily manifest the behavior reported by the referring source. This is seen to occur quite frequently in young children reported to be stutterers. If anxiety-provoking situations create greater nonfluencies, we should expect that a child coming into the strange diagnostic setting, meeting strange people, and being separated from his parents would be anxious and would demonstrate the nonfluencies that concern his parent. However, we have seen many instances where the child performed with little or no hesitation in verbal interaction, nor did he reveal any disfluencies.

The diagnostician should question the

situations under which the child was asked to perform. Was their enough immediate situational stress present to elicit disfluent speech? How could the diagnostician introduce communicative situations that might elicit the stuttering behavior for which the child was referred? Various techniques have been developed based on environmental stress as a causal factor in stuttering. We also have seen instances when the child seemed to be very happy, relaxed, and highly verbal but began to present disfluencies when "stress" was introduced into the interpersonal interaction. One technique found to elicit these nonfluencies has been to ask the child questions rather rapidly, without giving him the opportunity to answer or express himself fully. These instances seem to bring out the nonfluencies. But it does not appear to create any particular anxiety in the child or emotional stress. What we see is often in line with what parents report; he is excited and wants his turn to talk, but it is not an easy talking situation. We like to have the parents observe in these situations to confirm the behaviors we hear or do not hear as the case may be.

Some experimentation has been done to determine under what conditions disfluencies appear in the speech of children. What does the work of Martin et al. (1972a-c) offer the diagnostician gathering data on children suspected of stuttering?

We will now proceed to a series of diagnostic situations reflecting different aspects of data collection. Only the schematics of the client background and tools selected will be given. The student is encouraged to fill in the many missing details that may have led to these data collection circumstances.

■ Mr. Robert Chester saw the following three clients.
  1. Edward James, a 4-year-old boy, diagnosed as severely hypernasal because of inadequate velopharyngeal closure
  2. Mr. Donald George, 47 years of age, diagnosed as having a severe articulation problem due to paresis of the speech musculature
  3. Carl Richards, 5 years old, medically diagnosed as having spastic cerebral palsy

For each of these clients, Mr. Chester performed a speech mechanism examination. For Edward James, he concentrated his procedures on evaluating the extent of velopharyngeal closure. For Mr. George, he concentrated on the articulatory musculature. For Carl Richards, he concentrated on the phonatory, articulatory, and resonatory mechanisms. Considering his procedural concentration, what speech and nonspeech activities would Mr. Chester use for each of these clients? As a general guide to speech mechanism examinations, Appendix IV presents a speech mechanism examination form. This form is designed primarily as an overview speech mechanism examination; it does not provide many of the details that may be necessary to proceed with the examinations of the preceding clients. To assist the student in designing their specific procedures and observing the responses, the following references are offered: Darley (1964), Darley et al. (1969a, b, 1975), Hixon and Hardy (1964), Mason and Grandstaff (1970, 1971), McWilliams et al. (1968), and Mysak (1971). A quote from Darley can serve as a further procedural guide in planning your examination:

... speech is no slow-motion summation of the movements of dissociated though adjacent structures; a static view in the course of somewhat artificial activities will not truly tell us about the dynamics of the speech mechanism *in speech.* ...

We must discover malfunctioning of the speech apparatus during utterance. Observation of the deviation in speech may unveil the deviation in structure or function. Lifting of the tongue outside the mouth may not be duplicated within it; the tongue may rise in silence and during breath holding but not in speech or during exhalation. The smooth function of a single part may break down when built into a complex pattern of overlapping movements requiring efficient coordination. A compensatory movement used to overcome an anatomical or physiological deficiency may serve well in isolation, but it may create more problems than it solves when it is fitted awkwardly into a sequence. It is manifest, then, that we must supplement tests of function of individual parts with a thorough appraisal of the structures operating simultaneously *in speech.*[*]

[*]From Darley, F. L., *Diagnosis and Appraisal of Communication Disorders.* Englewood Cliffs, N.J.: Prentice-Hall, Inc., pp. 103-104 (1964).

■ Each of the following clients has been hypothesized as having a voice disorder. No causal factor has been hypothesized.

1. John Herbert, 7 years of age, in the second grade
2. Fred Josephs, a high school athletic instructor, aged 29 years
3. Margaret Josephina, aged 16 years, and lead cheerleader of her high school
4. John Pardio, aged 72 years, a retired farmer

Mr. Julius Weiss, the diagnostician has planned the following general procedures, not necessarily in this order, for these four clients:

1. General conversational speech
2. Procedures for habitual and optimal use of the voice
3. Controlled measures of voice use: words, isolated vowels, phrases, sentences, situational roles

From these general procedures, develop a specifically outlined plan adapting these procedures for each of the preceding clients. Consider how the following "rules" may apply to your procedures.

1. Listen to one component of the voice at a time.
2. Listen only for disordered characteristics.
3. Describe the voice characteristics in perceptual (product) terminology.
4. Do not use causal terminology for a description of the voice characteristics.

The following references will be helpful for determining the procedures you might use: Boone (1971), Moore (1971), Perkins, (1971a, b), and Wilson (1972).

■ Mr. William Cross will be seeing the following two aphasic clients.

1. Mr. Jack Metz was referred by Dr. Tom Harris for diagnosis and therapy. Dr. Harris diagnosed him as aphasic with accompanying visual problems. What procedure might Mr. Cross introduce into his testing to determine the type of visual problem and if the problem interferes with Mr. Metz's language functions?
2. Mr. James Grogan, aged 41 years, was referred to determine the appropriateness of language therapy. Mr. Grogan's family doctor, Dr. Ken Maras (general practitioner), felt he might not benefit from therapy because of his "emotional lability, extreme depression, disorientation, and loss of intellectual function." Mr. Grogan has been diagnosed by Dr. Bill Burcham (neurosurgeon) as aphasic after removal of a tumor of the left temporal lobe.

There are many factors about these two clients affecting the selection of tools and data collection. Assume that Mr. Grogan is aphasic; concentrate on how you would make your observations of the factors mentioned by Dr. Maras. What tests for aphasia and other tools might you select? How would you interpret Dr. Maras' remarks about Mr. Grogan's emotional and mental status in light of associated factors often seen in aphasic clients? How do neurologists examine the functions presented in Mr. Metz's and Mr. Grogan's referral? Look into general neurologic examinations, visual field testing, mental status, orientation, etc. The following references will assist you: Brookshire (1973), Chusid (1970), and Mayo Clinic (1971).

■ The following clients were found to have speech sound errors with no disruptions of the speech-producing mechanism. Adapt the stimulability (integral stimulation) procedures suggested by Milisen et al. (1954) to each of these clients. Consider how you would stimulate for each of the sound errors.

1. Brian, 3 years of age, made errors of omission and substitution on all fricatives and affricates.
2. Sheila, 7 years of age, made distortion errors on the /θ, s, z, tʃ, and dʒ/.
3. Mr. Danny Nichols, 23 years of age, made distortions on all productions of the /r and ɝ/ phonemes.

Consider the following in planning your stimulability procedures.

1. Gaining and maintaining attention
2. Examiner-client physical proximity
3. Teaching the stimulability technique
4. Number of stimulations to apply
5. Signaling the client to respond without intervening verbalization
6. Amount of auditory, visual, and phonetic placement information to provide
7. Use of phonemes the client can produce
8. Use of stimulation in isolation, nonsense syllables, and words

■ Mr. Jack Russo will be screening four groups of individuals suspected of having errors of sound production. He is given 10 minutes with each person. He plans on using word productions for obtaining his information. When he is finished, he wants to know:

Table 16. Initial client contact and clinical testing with Katherine Compardo

Diagnostician's tasks	Information obtained
Room	
The room selected was a large nursery with a stand-up sandbox and several well-demarcated areas. In one corner was a kitchen setting with children's furniture; the sandbox was in another area; a chalk board and cabinets with toys behind closed doors were in the room. In a separate area was a child's table and chairs. Each area was set up with materials for use with Katherine.	
Initial client contact	
Katherine and her mother were met in the lobby of the agency. The diagnostician sat and talked with both of them. Katherine was seated next to her mother, and the examiner pulled up a chair to face them.	Katherine responded to "Hi Katherine" by smiling. The examiner reached out to hold her hand and she took it. They held hands while the conversation took place. Katherine made no verbalizations.
Separation	
Initially, all three went to the nursery. But it seemed to the examiner, and the mother confirmed it, that Katherine would have gone with him.	Katherine became engrossed in the sandbox while an interview with the mother proceeded. The interview lasted a short time, since so much information had already been obtained. After the interview, Katherine was asked if it was all right for her mother to leave the room; she shook her head "yes" and only momentarily followed her mother with her eyes. Still no verbalization had occurred.
Orienting procedures	
The diagnostician went to the sandbox with Katherine, commented on what she was doing, and joined in the activity.	She responded appropriately to the following instructions as well as to others of a similar type: "Put some sand in the bucket," "Put the dog in the house," "Where's the cat?", "Put the cat by the dog," and "Put some sand under the house."
	During this task she made several unintelligible "screeching" sounds. When asked to name the dog and cat, her responses were /ɔˀɪ/ and /æˀ/.
Tools	
Katherine was asked to come to the table to do some looking at pictures, listening, and talking.	She moved immediately to the table and sat in a chair.
Peabody Picture Vocabulary Test and *Vocabulary Usage Test* were used for a combined comprehension, formulation, and repetition task.	
Form B of the *Peabody Picture Vocabulary Test* was used for comprehension as it is used in the *Vocabulary Usage Test;* after the *Vocabulary Usage Test* item was given, Katherine was asked to repeat it.	Example plates: she pointed correctly but did not respond to the vocabulary usage items, nor would she attempt imitation of the words.
	Comprehension was tested through plate 15, at which time Katherine got up from her chair, shook her head "no," and ran back to the sandbox.
Took her to the kitchen area to explore the area.	Again, she demonstrated ability to follow directions and seemed to know the relationships among the various pieces of furniture in the area.
Asked her if she would do some talking for me, since I need to know how well she can do.	She shook her head "yes," reached out for my hand, and started toward the table.
Asked her to imitate a new way of getting to the table. We jumped in place, hopped, stood on one leg, ran several steps, and several other motor tasks.	She attempted all tasks and performed them with some awkwardness.

Continued.

Table 16. Initial client contact and clinical testing with Katherine Compardo—cont'd

Diagnostician's tasks	Information obtained

Tools—cont'd

Direct repetitions of sounds and words were attempted. The diagnostician held Katherine on his lap so they were face-to-face, emphasizing to her how much he wanted to hear how well she talked.		

	ITEMS STIMULATED	RESPONSE
Vowels	/a,i,æ,o,u/	All repeated
Consonants	/b/	/b/
	/p/	/b/
	/d/	/di/
	/t/	/d/
	/k/	/d/
	/g/	/d/
	/m/	/b/
Words	Shoe	/d/
	Button	/bʌfə/

She would attempt no more imitation of speech.

Diagnostician's tasks	Information obtained
Imitation of speech musculature movements.	Tongue protrusion: seemed to be trying but could not protrude it Tongue lateralization: moved it to the left but not to the right Lip protrusion: again, seemed to try but did not accomplish. Other observations: tongue appeared to be held flat in the mouth; saw little tongue tip activity; rather constant drooling with little effort to swallow the saliva; she tended to wipe it off with her hand. Gave cereal to eat, she chewed and swallowed; she drank water from a cup.
One last chance to elicit names. Had her open the toy chests and explore the toys, but she was not given any until she said the name. Stimulus: "What is it?"	She understood, produced /i/ for doll, dog, cup, and /hɪʔʌ/ for shoe, cat, and spoon.
Guided observations throughout the session.	See previous comments. She appeared to have an awkward gait with some toeing in, no facial asymmetry, licked a lollipop that was given at the end of the session.
Interpersonal interaction.	She responded well to the tasks, although she made it clear when she was finished. She seemed to enjoy doing things with the diagnostician and did go along with some tasks, that she might not have enjoyed.

1. Are errors present that are outside expected norms?
2. How many errors are present?
3. What is the type of error?
4. What position in the word does it occur?
5. Are there any patterns of consistency?

For his test words, Mr. Russo will go to objective standardized articulation tests, and select 20 words for each population. He will develop a recording-scoring form for each screening. How will he do this for the following groups?

1. Four-year-old children in a large nursery school

2. Nine-year-old children in a Catholic elementary school
3. Fifteen- to seventeen-year-old mentally retarded adolescents in a vocational workshop for the retarded
4. Adult male prisoners in the state penal institution

■ Information is now provided about Katherine Compardo, our ongoing client example. Table 16 schematizes the initial client contact and clinical testing done with Katherine based on the tools that were selected in the previous chapter. Not all the tools and observations are discussed but enough to provide an example of how the diagnostician proceeded with his testing strategy and recorded his observations of the responses that were made.

Closes the testing session

As well as knowing how to open his clinical testing session, the diagnostician must do some planning for closing the session. Children who have been separated from their parents now must be separated from the diagnostician. We have seen instances of children who have screamed because it was time to go home. No matter how the session started, the client usually comes to realize that the diagnostician is working with them to solve a problem. Even very young children have an awareness that this event is meaningful, that just playing games did not occur. Therefore separation from "this person who has been helping me" is important. Abrupt separations can lead to negativism when the next appointment comes. Clients who leave with good feelings return for therapy with good feelings.

Closing the session is actually initiated at the beginning of testing. Clients can be informed how long the session may be and periodically informed that there is only so much time left. Closing the session, then, is task oriented; each tool completion leads to final completion.

For children, it is especially important that the last task be one designed to give him as much praise for success as possible and one that places little demand on him. As an aside, we want to emphasize that throughout testing, where possible, a tool should be ended with successful performance by the client. For example, using the *Peabody Picture Vocabulary Test* (Dunn, 1965), we will continue "testing" after the ceiling has been reached, making up names for two or three successive plates that we know the child can point to successfully. Praise at this time for his success also assists in gaining cooperation to move on to the next task.

At times when the client knows he is doing the final task, his performance is affected. Generally, being glad the session is coming to an end, his responses may become perfunctory and careless. Nontypical responses may occur. Thus it is wise to use final procedures that are either very different from others used or those that may be less essential to the diagnostician's findings. Some diagnosticians use a period of free play with children to close the session. With adults general conversation is appropriate. When the end of the session has come, it should be stated as such, and the client given the opportunity to respond about his feelings of what took place and what is going to happen next.

Muma (1973) has presented a discussion of seven underlying assumptions that diagnosticians should consider in language assessment. The assumptions discussed are (1) quantitative and descriptive approaches, (2) language knowledge and usage, (3) language structure and function, (4) formal and informal approaches, (5) sampling, (6) data handling, and (7) validity. Apply these assumptions to the selection of tools and the collection of data steps of the diagnostic process presented in this chapter.

SUMMARY

In this fourth step of the diagnostic process the diagnostician implements his clinical design; he collects his clinical data. Here he applies the information studied and organized in the previous steps. He also calls on his knowledge and professional skill in tool presentation, response observation and recording, and interpersonal interactions. These sources of information allow him to adapt his design to new data and to the individual needs of the clients he sees.

Three tasks are involved in collection of the clinical data.

1. The diagnostician first *prepares for the diagnostic session.* He must ready the room and his materials, ensuring that his physical props are in order.

He also will establish his initial contact with the client complex. In doing this he prepares the client for what they may expect to take place, and he himself samples what he may expect from them.

2. The diagnostician then proceeds with *collecting his data*. Usually this includes both an interview with the client and the actual clinical testing. These may or may not occur on the same day. Both the interview and testing will include tool presentation, adaptation of the session to new information and the interpersonal context, and recording systematic observations.

3. Finally, the diagnostician will need to *close the testing session*. Here he will want to let the client complex know how things stand and what next steps will be taken.

Having concluded the data collection the diagnostician will next analyze that data.

CLIENT PROJECTS
Michael T. Durall

Michael T. Durall has been referred to the Eastern Speech and Hearing Clinic as a part of the vocational services offered by the Bureau of Vocational Rehabilitation. Currently Mr. Durall is unemployed. According to the referral, Mr. Durall is a stutterer and he confirms this in the client history form. The material available on Mr. Durall is reproduced in Appendix II. Complete a constituent analysis and all other steps through collection of data. What are the advantages of approaching causal factors from a contemporary versus a historical view? Consider the value of the following tools with Dr. Durall: Riley's *Stuttering Severity Instrument* (1972) and the *Southern Illinois University Speech Situations Check List* (Brutten and Shoemaker, 1974). In Johnson et al. (1963) there are also a number of measures that can be taken regarding rate of speaking and oral reading. They use one particular speaking procedure that might be quite interesting

in this referral. It is referred to as the *Job Task*. What information do adaptation procedures add to your data collection (Peins, 1961; Williams et al., 1968; Wingate, 1966).

Some diagnosticians working with clients who stutter may spend little time collecting detailed information about the behaviors manifested. Instead, their concern is with the personal motivations, level of interests, and attitudes the client has about changing his stuttering behavior. These diagnosticians save data collection of the specifics of the stuttering pattern until therapy begins if they feel they are even necessary to do. What would be your reaction to this type of diagnosis—a diagnosis that concentrates on management concerns rather than on an analysis of a behavior that is readily evidenced in most adult stutterers?

Previous clients: William Gafford, Isadore Alexander, and Derek Park

Return to the clients you have been studying. Now consider how you would collect the data using the tools you have selected for these clients. Keep in mind the settings in which you are working for each of the clients. You will have to project the data you obtain. You should do this precisely, using appropriate recording forms where available, so you will have this information for use in later steps.

REFERENCES

Ammons, R. B., and Ammons, H. S., *Full-Range Picture Vocabulary Test*. Missoula, Mont.: Psychological Test Specialists (1948).

Aram, D. M., and Nation, J. E., Patterns of language behavior in children with developmental language disorders. *J. Speech Hearing Res.*, **18**, 229-241 (1975).

Berry, M., *Berry-Talbott Tests of Language: I. Comprehension of Grammar*. Rockford, Ill.: 4322 Pinecrest Road (1966).

Berry, R. C., and Silverman, F. H., Equality of intervals on the Lewis-Sherman scale of stuttering severity. *J. Speech Hearing Res.*, **15**, 185-188 (1972).

Berry-Luterman, L., and Bar, A., The diagnostic significance of sentence repetition for language-impaired children. *J. Speech Hearing Dis.*, **36**, 29-39 (1971).

Bingham, W. V., and Moore, B. V., *How To Interview.* New York: Harper & Row, Publishers (1941).

Boone, D. R., *The Voice and Voice Therapy.* Englewood Cliffs, N.J.: Prentice-Hall, Inc. (1971).

Brookshire, R. H., *An Introduction to Aphasia.* Minneapolis: BRK Publishers (1973).

Brutten, G. J., and Shoemaker, D. J., *Southern Illinois University Speech Situations Check List.* Carbondale, Ill.: Southern Illinois University Press (1974).

Bzoch, K., and League, R., *Assessing Language Skills in Infancy.* Gainesville, Fla.: Tree of Life Press (1971).

Carney, P. J., and Sherman, D., Severity of nasality in three selected speech tasks. *J. Speech Hearing Res.,* **14,** 396-407 (1971).

Carrow, E., *Carrow Elicited Language Inventory.* Austin, Tex.: Learning Concepts (1974).

Chusid, J. G., *Correlative Neuroanatomy and Functional Neurology.* (14th ed.) Los Altos, Calif.: Lange Medical Publications (1970).

Corlew, M. M., and Nation, J. E., Characteristics of visual stimuli and naming performance in aphasic adults. *Cortex,* **11,** 186-191 (1975).

Darley, F. L., *Diagnosis and Appraisal of Communication Disorders.* Englewood Cliffs, N.J.: Prentice-Hall, Inc. (1964).

Darley, F. L., Aronson, A. E., and Brown, J. R., Differential diagnostic patterns of dysarthria. *J. Speech Hearing Res.,* **12,** 246-269 (1969a).

Darley, F. L., Aronson, A. E., and Brown, J. R., Clusters of deviant speech dimensions in the dysarthrias. *J. Speech Hearing Res.,* **12,** 462-496 (1969b).

Darley, F. L., Aronson, A. E., and Brown, J. R., *Motor Speech Disorders.* Philadelphia: W. B. Saunders Co. (1975).

Davis, N., and Leach, E., Scaling aphasics' error responses. *J. Speech Hearing Dis.,* **37,** 305-313 (1972).

Doll, D. A., *Vineland Social Maturity Scale.* Circle Pines, Minn.: American Guidance Service, Inc. (1965).

Dunn, L. M., *Peabody Picture Vocabulary Test.* Circle Pines, Minn.: American Guidance Service, Inc. (1965).

Edmonston, W., *Laradon Articulation Scale.* Los Angeles: Western Psychological Services (1963).

Eisenson, J., *Examining for Aphasia.* New York: The Psychological Corporation (1954).

Emerick, L., *The Parent Interview: Guidelines for Student and Practicing Speech Clinicians.* Danville, Ill.: The Interstate Printers & Publishers, Inc. (1969).

Emerick, L. L., and Hatten, J. T., *Diagnosis and Evaluation in Speech Pathology.* Englewood Cliffs, N.J.: Prentice-Hall, Inc. (1974).

Foster, R., Giddan, J. J., and Stark, J., *Assessment of Children's Language Comprehension.* Palo Alto, Calif.: Consulting Psychologists Press (1972).

Fraser, C., Bellugi, U., and Brown, R., Control of grammar in imitation, comprehension, and production. *J. verb. Learning verb. Behav.,* **2,** 121-135 (1963).

Fremon, S. S., Creative discipline that works. *Parent's Magazine,* **47,** 50-51, 84-86 (1972).

Fudala, J. B., *Arizona Articulation Proficiency Scale.* Los Angeles: Western Psychological Services (1972).

Garrett, A., *Interviewing: Its Principles and Methods.* (2nd ed.; Revised by E. P. Zaki and M. M. Mangold) New York: Family Service Association of America (1972).

Goldman, R., and Fristoe, M., *Goldman-Fristoe Test of Articulation.* Circle Pines, Minn.: American Guidance Service, Inc. (1969).

Goldman, R., Fristoe, M., and Woodcock, R. W., *Goldman-Fristoe-Woodcock Test of Auditory Discrimination.* Circle Pines, Minn.: American Guidance Service, Inc. (1970).

Goodglass, J., and Kaplan, E., *The Assessment of Aphasia and Related Disorders.* Philadelphia: Lea & Febiger (1972).

Hannah, J. E., and Sheeley, E. C., The audiologist's model for test selection. *Asha,* **17,** 83-89 (1975).

Hixon, T. J., and Hardy, J. C., Restricted motility of the speech articulators in cerebral palsy. *J. Speech Hearing Dis.,* **29,** 293-306 (1964).

Johnson, W., Darley, F., and Spriestersbach, D. C., *Diagnostic Methods in Speech Pathology.* New York: Harper & Row, Publishers (1963).

Kresheck, J. D., and Socolofsky, G., Imitative and spontaneous articulatory assessment of four-year-old children. *J. Speech Hearing Res.,* **15,** 729-733 (1972).

Leach, E., Interrogation: A model and some implications. *J. Speech Hearing Dis.,* **37,** 33-46 (1972).

Lee, L. L., *Northwestern Syntax Screening Test.* Evanston, Ill.: Northwestern University Press (1969).

Lee, L. L., *Developmental Sentence Analysis.* Evanston, Ill.: Northwestern University Press (1974).

Lewis, D., and Sherman, D., Measuring the severity of stuttering. *J. Speech Hearing Dis.,* **16,** 320-326 (1951).

Martin, R. R., Haroldson, S. K., and Kuhl, P., Disfluencies in child-child and child-mother speaking situations. *J. Speech Hearing Res.,* **15,** 753-756 (1972a).

Martin, R. R., Haroldson, S. K., and Kuhl, P., Disfluencies of young children in two speaking situations, *J. Speech Hearing Res.,* **15,** 831-836 (1972b).

Martin, R. R., Kuhl, P., and Haroldson, S., An experimental treatment with two preschool stuttering children. *J. Speech Hearing Res.,* **15,** 743-752 (1972c).

Mason, R. M., and Grandstaff, H. L., Evaluating the velopharyngeal mechanism in hypernasal speakers. *Ohio J. Speech Hearing,* **4,** 23-28 (1970). (Reprinted in *Language, Speech, Hearing Services in Schools,* **4,** 53-61 [1971].)

Mayo Clinic, *Clinical Examinations in Neurology.* (3rd ed.) Philadelphia: W. B. Saunders Co. (1971).

McWilliams, B. J., Musgrave, R., and Crozier, P., The influence of head position upon velopharyngeal closure. *Cleft Palate J.,* **5,** 117-124 (1968).

Mecham, M. J., *Verbal Language Development Scale.* Circle Pines, Minn.: American Guidance Service, Inc. (1959).

Mecham, M., Jex, J., and Jones, J., *Test of Listening Accuracy in Children.* Provo, Utah: Brigham Young University Press (1969).

Menyuk, P., and Looney, P. L., A problem of language disorder: Length versus structure. *J. Speech Hearing Res.,* **15,** 264-279 (1972).

Milisen, R., et al., The disorder of articulation: A systematic clinical and experimental approach. *J. Speech Hearing Dis. Monogr. Suppl.* 4 (1954).

Moore, G. P., *Organic Voice Disorders.* Englewood Cliffs, N.J.: Prentice-Hall, Inc. (1971).

Muma, J. R., Language assessment: Some underlying assumptions. *Asha,* **15,** 331-338 (1973).

Mysak, E. D., Cerebral palsy speech habilitation. In L. Travis (Ed.), *Handbook of Speech Pathology and Audiology.* New York: Appleton-Century-Crofts (1971).

Nation, J. E., A vocabulary usage test. *J. Psycholing. Res.,* **1,** 221-231 (1972).

Palmer, J. O., *The Psychological Assessment of Children.* New York: John Wiley & Sons, Inc. (1970).

Peins, M., Adaptation effect and spontaneous recovery in stuttering expectancy. *J. Speech Hearing Res.,* **4,** 91-99 (1961).

Perkins, W. H., Vocal function: A behavioral analysis. In L. Travis (Ed.), *Handbook of Speech Pathology and Audiology.* New York: Appleton-Century-Crofts (1971a).

Perkins, W. H., Vocal function: Assessment and therapy. In L. Travis (Ed.), *Handbook of Speech Pathology and Audiology.* New York: Appleton-Century-Crofts (1971b).

Polster, E., and Polster, M., *Gestalt Therapy Integrated.* New York: Brunner/Mazel, Inc. (1973).

Porch, B. E., *Porch Index of Communicative Ability.* Palo Alto, Calif.: Consulting Psychologists Press (1967).

Porch, B. E., Multidimensional scoring in aphasia testing. *J. Speech Hearing Res.,* **14,** 776-792 (1971).

Porch, B. E., *Porch Index of Communicative Ability in Children.* Palo Alto, Calif.: Consulting Psychologists Press (1974).

Prins, D., and Lohr, F., Behavioral dimensions of stuttered speech. *J. Speech Hearing Res.,* **15,** 61-71 (1972).

Riley, G. D., A stuttering severity instrument for children and adults. *J. Speech Hearing Dis.,* **37,** 314-321 (1972).

Rogers, C. R., *Counseling and Psychotherapy.* Boston: Houghton Mifflin Co. (1942).

Schein, E. H., *Process Consultation: Its Role in Organization Development.* Reading, Mass.: Addison-Wesley Publishing Co., Inc. (1969).

Schuell, H., *Minnesota Test for Differential Diagnosis of Aphasia.* Minneapolis: University of Minnesota Press (1965).

Schultz, M. C., The bases of speech pathology and audiology: What are appropriate models? *J. Speech Hearing Dis.,* **37,** 118-122 (1972).

Schultz, M. C., and Carpenter, M. A., The bases of speech pathology and audiology: Selecting a therapy model. *J. Speech Hearing Dis.,* **38,** 395-404 (1973).

Shriberg, L. D., The effect of examiner social behavior on children's articulation test performance. *J. Speech Hearing Res.,* **14,** 659-672 (1971).

Shriberg, L. D., Articulation judgments: Some perceptual considerations. *J. Speech Hearing Res.,* **15,** 876-882 (1972).

Stech, E. L., Curtiss, J. W., Troesch, P. J., and Binnie, C., Clients' reinforcement of speech clinicians: A factor-analytic study. *Asha,* **15,** 287-289 (1973).

Stevenson, I., *The Diagnostic Interview.* (2nd ed.) New York: Harper & Row, Publishers (1971).

Sullivan, J. S., *The Psychiatric Interview.* New York: W. W. Norton & Co., Inc. (1954).

Templin, M. C., *Templin Picture Sound Discrimination Test.* In M. C. Templin, *Certain Language Skills in Children.* Minneapolis: University of Minnesota Press (1957).

Templin, M. C., and Darley, F. L., *Templin-Darley Tests of Articulation.* (2nd ed.) Iowa City: University of Iowa Press (1969).

Van Riper, C., and Erickson, R., *Predictive Screening Test of Articulation.* Kalamazoo, Mich.: Western Michigan University Press (1968).

Wepman, J. M., *Auditory Discrimination Test.* Chicago: Language Research Associates (1958).

Wepman, J. M., and Jones, L. V., *Language Modalities Test for Aphasia.* Chicago: Education-Industry Service (1961a).

Wepman, J. M., and Jones, L. V., *Studies in Aphasia: An Approach to Testing.* Chicago: Education-Industry Service (1961b).

Wiley, J. H., A scale to measure parental attitudes. *J. Speech Hearing Dis.,* **20,** 284-290 (1955).

Williams, D. E., Silverman, F. H., and Kools, J. A., Disfluency behavior of elementary school stutterers and non-stutterers: The adaptation effect. *J. Speech Hearing Res.,* **11,** 622-630 (1968).

Wilson, D. K., *Voice Problems of Children.* Baltimore: The Williams & Wilkins Co. (1972).

Wingate, M., Prosody in stuttering adaptation. *J. Speech Hearing Res.,* **9,** 550-556 (1966).

Wolski, W., *Michigan Picture Language Inventory.* Ann Arbor, Mich.: The University of Michigan Press (1962).

Chapter 15

Analysis of the clinical data

Analysis of the clinical data is the fifth step of the diagnostic process. All of the data available about the client is now ready for analysis—determining what significance the data may have for solving the clinical problem. Analysis of the clinical data is only an epilogue to collecting the clinical data and a prologue to interpretation of the data.

At the outset it is important to realize that this step of the diagnostic process is somewhat artificial, since data analysis is seldom separate from either its collection or interpretation. The diagnostician cannot wait until all testing is completed before beginning some analysis and interpretation. For example, he may alter his test procedures during the session because of preliminary analysis of the data being obtained. Similarly, when the diagnostician scores and analyzes the data for significance, he cannot always keep separate interpretive evaluations.

However, we consider analysis of the data to be an important step to consider separately, particularly for the diagnostician in training. It is designated as a separate step primarily to illuminate the mental processes that occur when the data is analyzed for significance. Unlike the researcher who may lay out all his data and determine its significance through a series of statistical analyses, the diagnostician must do an ongoing analysis—he cannot wait until all his data is in before he determines if it is significant. But the diagnostician must develop the mental operations of this step, thought of as the nonjudgmental organization of the "facts" that have been obtained throughout the diagnosis. The diagnostician needs to develop the skill of scoring the data, objectifying the data, comparing the data to normative data, and organizing the data in relationship to the hypotheses—all without interpreting its meaning. It is a phase of data analyses, not data interpretation.

Developing this step assists the diagnostician in keeping bias out of the diagnosis; it forces him to stay with the "facts" before entering the interpretive stage. This step is therefore analogous to the stage in research where the results are reported after the data is in prior to any interpretation of their meaning.

To accomplish the clinical analysis the diagnostician engages in four tasks. First, he scores his new data, objectifying it quantitatively and descriptively and comparing it against standard information. He also determines how reliable and valid the data may be—the overall quality of the data. Second, he lists and categorizes the new data in terms of his cause-effect hypothesis from the SLPM framework. Third, he adds the data from his constituent analysis to this listing and categorization, revising the constituents as indicated by the new data. Fourth, he determines the significance of the data for providing a solution to the clinical problem—what support can be offered, what negates a clinical problem, and what is still missing. Following these tasks, the diagnostician will have analyzed his data and can then enter into his clinical interpretation.

CLINICAL ANALYSIS: HOW IT IS DONE

The diagnostician arrives at the analysis step fully prepared. He now has all the information, complete or incomplete, that will go into making his clinical diagnosis. The analysis of data step of the diagnostic process is quite similar to, or perhaps just a continuation of, the constituent analysis step. Just as the constituent analysis prepared the available information for the development of the clinical hypothesis, so also does the clinical analysis ready the accumulated data for the next step—the clinical evaluation. Thus whatever the diagnostician does at this stage will be reflected in his subsequent clinical evaluation. The objectivity and security with which he proceeds here will determine the quality of his eventual diagnosis.

Information bases

The information bases the diagnostician uses at this fifth step of the diagnostic process have been specified in all the previous steps. The only "new" information he draws on here would be the *emphasis* placed on analysis. He must now concentrate on any information that teaches him how to score and analyze the tools he has used, how to develop summary analysis forms for categorizing the detailed information obtained, and how to draw comparative analyses, that is, comparing his client to normative data and to other clients having a similar disorder.

Sources of data for clinical analysis

To analyze his data the diagnostician uses the data available from both the constituent analysis and collection of data steps of the diagnostic process, including all the intermediate processes that went into getting the data collected. From the constituent analysis the diagnostician has available all the historical data he has analyzed to develop his clinical hypothesis and its alternates. Emphasis was placed in that step on the source, amount, type, reliability, and validity of the information obtained prior to testing. Because the mental processes that are necessary for the analysis of the clinical data are so similar to those for doing the constituent analysis, it is suggested that the student return to that step for review.

From the data collection step just completed, the diagnostician has available all the contemporary data he was able to obtain. Tool administration, interviewing, observing, and recording-scoring were emphasized as a part of data collection. All this previous information becomes relevant to the diagnostician as a source of information for clinical analysis. Again, we suggest review of this information.

Nature of clinical analysis

What new data the diagnostician collected was dependent on how well the diagnosis was designed as well as the diagnostician's observation, measurement, and recording skills. Whatever the diagnostician was able to systematically observe, measure, and keep track of becomes the raw material for clinical analysis. At times some of this data becomes useless; too much of one kind was collected and not enough of another. But the analysis must be done with the data collected; it is too late to wish for something else. The data obtained must be "objectified" and compared to standard criteria for completion of the analysis prior to interpretation.

"Objectifying" the data. As a major part of data analysis, the diagnostician objectifies the data obtained. How did the client perform with the different tools that were used? The diagnostician objectively scores the response to each tool, test, subtest, and item, all the relevant stimulus-response situations that occurred during the diagnostic session.

The diagnostician objectifies the client's performance on the tools by whatever method of scoring he has available—numbers, descriptions, and qualitative judgments as discussed in the previous chapter. He describes what the client said and did, rates the performance according to perceptual criteria, determines pass-fail responses, judges the correctness of the response, describes the type of errors made, counts the number of errors made, and records the consistency of the errors. He notes the situations that resulted in error responses, in better or normal responses, and in response variability, and he judges the extent of the errors—how many errors were made out of how many responses. The diagnostician goes through many general and specific procedures to objectify the client's response to the tools that were presented.

All these analysis procedures are attempts to specify the degree and extent of the variation and not, at this time, to judge the presence or absence of a speech and language disorder. For example, if the diagnostician used a phonetic structure test to determine the errors 4-year-old Donald makes and discovered that he made 43 errors out of 50 possible responses, he would know how many errors Donald made. He might then ask, What are the characteristics of the errors? Were the errors primarily omissions, substitutions, or distortions? What sounds were used in place of other sounds? What sound features were characteristically in error? Were early developing sounds used in place of later developing sounds? Was manner of articulation affected more than place of articulation? Were voiced sounds used for voiceless sounds? And what was the rule system Donald used to generate phonologic strings? These and other details of Donald's errors could be "scored" and analyzed by the diagnostician. All these provide much greater information for interpretation than just knowing he made 43 errors out of 50.

Seldom do diagnosticians use a physical analysis for specifying the details of speech and language variations. Physical analysis is most often used in basic research. How have Faircloth and Faircloth (1970) used graphic level recordings and spectrographic information to support their findings that making diagnostic judgments about speech sound errors in isolated word production is not as valid as making them from connected speech testing?

From his objective analysis the diagnostician also provides summary descriptions that characterize the details of the variation, noting any variables that may interfere with the reliability and validity of the data—the reliance he places on the data as being "good" data. Objectification, then, is the analysis procedure by which the details of the client's disorder are specified. This results in data of basically two types, quantitative (numerical) and descriptive.

Most objective standardized tools provide for some quantification of the results obtained, usually for comparative purposes. For example, the test form that accompanies the *Templin-Darley Tests of Articulation* (Templin and Darley, 1969) derives a series of numerical scores concerned with the number of errors the client makes in relation to the total number of responses, sound categories, positions of the sound, etc. The *Peabody Picture Vocabulary Test* (Dunn, 1965) provides a basal score and a ceiling score from which a raw score is derived. The *Assessment of Children's Language Comprehension* (Foster et al., 1972) for Part A of the test scores number correct and for Parts B, C, and D scores percentage correct. The student is encouraged to review Chapters 13 and 14 and Appendix III for discussion of the tools and to study the scoring protocols for each tool they consider using.

Diagnosticians often use a spontaneous speech and language sample to gain information about the level and structure of speech and language development. Because of its importance in obtaining information about the typical use of speech and language, its validity, reliability, and form of analysis is crucial. The spontaneous speech sample seems to be one of the most frequently studied tools. Beyond the methods used to elicit the sample and the considerations given to its reliability and validity (Minifie et al., 1963), the diagnostician must also be able to record, transcribe, and analyze (score) the responses accurately. There are a number of quantitative and descriptive forms of analyses derived from a spontaneous speech and language sample—mean length of utterance (Brown, 1973), mean length of response (Johnson et al., 1963; Shriner, 1969), number of different words and structural complexity score (Johnson et al., 1963), length complexity index (Miner, 1969; Shriner, 1967); developmental sentence types (Lee, 1966, 1974), and developmental sentence scoring (Lee, 1974).

Sharf (1972) presented information that compares some of the measures taken and used for analysis of children's speech and language development. What suggestions does he offer that might assist the diagnostician? How would you reconcile his concerns about the use of age comparisons and the need to sample over time? What further information do the following articles offer for use of the spontaneous speech and language sample (Johnson and Tomblin, 1975; Shriner and Sherman, 1967; Shriner et al., 1969; Wilson, 1969)?

Many tools and procedures used for diagnosis are not amenable to numerical reduction, nor is it desirable to do so. For example, there is still no number that describes a hoarse voice. Metric analysis is only one way of scoring data. Data is also objectified through the use of clear descriptions of the behaviors observed. Generally it is not enough simply to get a score that reflects performance; the diagnostician will want to provide more descriptive information, describing the patterns of behavior of his client. Some of the objective and standardized tools provide for analysis of behavioral patterns. Again, using the test form

that accompanies the *Templin-Darley Tests of Articulation* (Templin and Darley, 1969) as an example, we see that it provides for an analysis of the patterns of misarticulations with some emphasis on the differences in production between phonemes as singles and phonemes in blends.

Since so many tools used in diagnosis do not provide for detailed pattern analysis, the diagnostician must develop his own system for scoring and analyzing the information he has obtained. The diagnostician does not have to be bound to the test designer's analysis recommendations or limitations. He can expand his analysis in any way suggested by his funds of knowledge about speech and language and its measurement. As an example, many phonetic structure tests score the response only by type of error—substitution, omission, distortion, or addition. The diagnostician can analyze the results beyond this. He could do a distinctive feature analysis (McReynolds and Huston, 1971), a kinetic or acoustic analysis (Van Riper and Irwin, 1958), etc. Rather than just analyzing the type of error that was made, he can analyze how the error was made in relationship to how the sound should have been made (Table 4). Was the error sound close to the target sound, or was it far from the target sound in terms of manner and place of articulation or in terms of distinctive features.

How does Weber (1970) suggest we approach "patterning of articulation"?

Information from these analyses is important for management decisions. If a diagnostician analyzed the results of testing with Mrs. Wicker, an aphasic, only in terms of correct or incorrect responses, he would miss data of importance for interpretation of the results. If Mrs. Wicker misnamed 90% of the pictures requested, the diagnostician would be fairly certain that she has a "naming" problem. However, if he knows what type of responses she made, he has more information about her problem. Are low frequency of occurrence nouns (hammock) replaced by high frequency of occurrence nouns (bed), or by a statement of usage (you lay on it), or by a descriptive qualification (it's canvas—you know, for outside, for the breeze)? From this analysis the diagnostician can say much more about the type of naming problem as opposed to saying only that a naming problem exists.

Van Demark and Tharp (1973) report that much information is lost in articulation testing because of concern with and ease of counting correct responses versus analyzing the nature of the responses made. They have developed a computer program for data reduction of the results of articulation testing with cleft palate individuals. Can this coding system be adapted for clinical use when no computer is available for reduction and analysis of the data?

More formalized descriptive analysis methods are needed and do seem to be forthcoming, as seen by the emphasis placed on using analyses of spontaneous speech and language samples. The influence of linguistic science on clinical analysis of language behavior has been significant. Often, however, some of the analysis systems offered are far too complex or beyond the diagnostician's knowledge. He may not be expert and facile in all the theories and techniques offered by linguistic science. What he needs are more practical, facilitative analysis techniques. In the future we hope to see more clinical adaptations of these analysis systems.

Engler et al. (1973) have provided what they consider to be a practical guide for linguistic analysis of language samples. What approach have they taken that makes their system practical? How does it compare to other systems of analysis, for example, Lee's (1966, 1974) developmental sentence types?

Descriptive objectification focuses on behavior in context, on describing patterns of behavior. From this pattern analysis the diagnostician attempts to discover the principle by which a specific client may be generating his speech and language behavior—a principle that puts the diagnostician in a better position for interpretation and management.

Objectifying the data sets it up for the next task, a comparative analysis. The details from which the diagnostician objectifies the data provide greater reliability and validity to his observations. He has viewed the data from more than one perspective, objectifying it in order to gain greater security for his comparative analysis—to prevent impressionistic comparisons.

■ In the last chapter (p. 285) we suggested a project for gathering data on several clients using the speech mechanism examination. Now that you have examined this tool (Appendix IV) and considered what data you might collect with it, determine how you would objectify your findings. Consider both quantitative and descriptive procedures.

Comparative analysis. All of the objectified data are compared in some way to standard information (normative data from standardized tests and from the diagnostician's fund of knowledge), or the data are compared to intradisorder information (to other clients who have similar speech and language disorders).

The purpose of this comparative analysis is to plot the client's performance and behavior against the standard behavior of the comparison group. Is he above, at, or below the mean? Is he at the 25th, 50th, or 75th percentile? Is his variation mild, moderate, or severe? Does he fall into group I, II, or III? Ultimately these comparative analyses lead to clinical interpretations that conclude whether a speech and language disorder exists.

In order to perform his comparative analyses the diagnostician must have standard information to use for comparison. The standardized tests have such normative information for ready use (Chapter 13). The diagnostician quantifies his client's responses and compares them to the scores of the standardization group, but as discussed in Chapter 13, standardized tools are not always applicable to a clinical population. At times the standardization group is not comparable to the clients seen in a particular setting, as in the case of a setting that sees a large population of black children. Or the procedures by which the standardization data were gathered cannot be duplicated with a client with a speech and language disorder or within the time constraints imposed by the diagnostic session. Seldom in diagnosis can we duplicate the sampling procedures recommended by the experimental literature. At other times the standardization data may not extend to the age levels of the clients being seen. This is so often the case for diagnosticians seeing many young children between the ages of 2 and 4 years. Few tools have been developed for measuring speech and language skills at this age level, and the reliability of the measures is frequently not stable. Finally, the standardization data may not reflect the theoretical orientation of the diagnostician and thus may not be suitable to him. Some of these difficulties are illustrated in the following two paragraphs.

Hollien and Shipp (1972) have presented normative data on the fundamental frequency of the male voice between the ages of 20 and 89 at decade intervals. This data was obtained through a sophisticated instrumental analysis in their laboratory, using the "fundamental frequency indicator" described by them as a "digital readout f_0 tracking device." The information made available by them can be important for the diagnostician, but how can he use the same measuring device to arrive at his client's fundamental frequency for comparative purposes? Most likely, he cannot. Instead, the diagnostician will have to rely on his clinical perceptual measures to determine his client's fundamental frequency. He will have to use measures different from those by which the normative information was gathered and yet make a comparison to that normative information.

Many clients seen for diagnosis have disorders of phonetic structure or phonology.

The normative data available regarding the development of "articulation" came from studies done some time ago and from a different theoretical orientation than is currently used (Poole, 1934; Templin, 1957; Wellman et al., 1931). There is question about the current applicability of this information, a question addressed somewhat by Sander (1972). Using the data from Wellman et al. (1931) and Templin (1957), Sander demonstrated that the acquisition of phonemes is best viewed from an age range rather than as age norms. Further work along similar lines has been completed by Prather et al. (1975) in studying the development of articulation in children between the ages of 2 and 4 years. The work by Sander (1972) and Prather et al. (1975) indicates that the normative data that were heavily used may no longer be appropriate, and it assists in drawing more contemporary comparative analyses (Chapter 6).

The primary basis for comparative analysis resides in the diagnostician's funds of knowledge about normal and disordered speech and language, the subject of Chapters 3 through 8. The diagnostician throughout his training and professional life builds in standards for comparison; this building-in process is called "clinical experience." By way of illustration, many clients do not respond to direct, objective procedures for testing a specific speech and language behavior. Attempts to get young children to name specific words on a phonetic structure test are limited by the child's vocabulary ability, willingness to participate in a naming task, attention span, motivation, and other factors. Instead, the diagnostician may have to rely on some spontaneous speech, repetition, and a little naming to obtain a sample of the child's use of phonemes. He must, however, compare this nonstandard sample to the normative data available if he is to make decisions regarding the child's abilities.

■ Brian, aged 3 years, 5 months, made errors on the following phonemes during spontaneous speech production: /f, t, s, ʃ, k, and g/. Using the chart (Fig. 6-3) from Prather et al. (1975), analyze and interpret these errors. Would your analysis vary depending on whose information you used (Prather et al., 1975, or Sander, 1972)?

Of particular relevance to diagnosticians for comparative analyses are the data that characterize a disordered population (intradisorder comparison). Much information is available about groups of people with speech and language disorders, grouped behaviorally or causally, for example, stutterers, aphasics, voice disorders, mentally retarded. (See Chapters 7 and 8 for a detailed discussion of speech and language disorders.) This intradisorder information is crucial to the diagnostician. For example, if the diagnostician is to see 7-year-old Danny who is classified as educably mentally retarded, he will want to know how Danny compares to normal children his age and younger as well as to other educable retarded children (Chapman and Nation, 1974). In a sense standards for disordered behavior are established, and a new client is compared with these standards to determine if he fits, that is, if he is typical of the general description of the disordered population.

It is easy to see why the diagnostician must be careful when drawing comparisons such as these. Just as normative data can be faulty and misused so can the data gathered on disordered populations. There have been many studies done with the intent of describing the typical speech and language behavior of a special group of individuals; however, there is often little commonality among the studies, particularly in the way the data have been gathered and described.

■ You have just completed the diagnosis of Sheila, a 12-year-old girl with a mental age of 7 years. You have taken a spontaneous language sample that you feel was quite adequate under the diagnostic circumstances. How helpful would the information provided by Naremore and Dever (1975) be to you in your analysis of the language sample? What would you expect of Sheila's speech and language performance?

Because of new information that accrues and changes that occur in theories about speech and language behavior, the diagnostician must continue to renew his theoretical perspectives on the analysis of the behaviors that signal a speech and language disorder. The experimental and clinical literature provide much of the current information needed for data analysis. The student in training must develop and maintain an awareness of and an appreciation for the insights the literature provides for data analysis and interpretation.

What does the following literature offer to the diagnostician for data analysis and interpretation: Silverman (1973), differentiation between normal disfluencies and stuttering in young children; Ramer and Rees (1973), comparisons between standard American English and black English; Wiig and Semel (1973), comprehension differences between children with learning disabilities and normally achieving children; Morehead and Ingram (1973), early language acquisition of normal and linguistically deviant children; Yoss and Darley (1974), differentiating developmental apraxia from other articulation disorders; De Hirsch (1967), differentiating the speech and language behavior of the aphasic and schizophrenic child; Menyuk and Looney (1972), language performance differences between normal and language-disordered children?

Diagnostician's tasks

Now that we have discussed the information bases needed by the diagnostician for clinical analysis, we turn to the four tasks performed by him on all the information gathered.

1. He scores his new data and objectifies it, getting it ready for the second task.
2. He lists and categorizes the data in relationship to his clinical hypothesis.
3. He adds the information from the constituent analysis, revising it as called for by his new findings.
4. He determines the significance of all the data, readying it for the next step of the diagnostic process, clinical interpretation.

The tasks the diagnostician performs at this fifth step of the diagnostic process are similar to the tasks done during the constituent analysis and will not be amplified to a great extent here. In a general sense, at this step, the diagnostician wants to know what data he has and how good it is for interpreting the specific characteristics of the client's speech and language disorder and its causes.

When these four tasks are done on the same day as the diagnostic session to prepare for an immediate clinical interpretation, many quick mental operations are necessary. In those settings where interpretation does not occur on the same day, the diagnostician would complete these tasks in greater detail before calling the client back for final interpretation. But even in those settings where the analysis and subsequent interpretations are done immediately following testing, the diagnostician then returns again to this step for more detailed analysis and specification than was first possible.

Scores the new data

The diagnostician sits down with all his tools, scoring protocols, manuals, notes, tape recordings, and his memory and scores all his new information. He wants to find out what he has and how good it is. Actually much of the objectification and comparative analyses of the data occurred while they were being collected. Responses and descriptive statements were recorded, how the client performed, and what he did. The conditions under which the data were obtained were notated, particularly those that would be reflected in the reliability and validity of the information. Thus in this first clinical analysis task all the data that has not yet been scored will now be objectified, and the data recorded and scored during the collection step will be reviewed for accuracy and completeness. Greater detail and specification are added.

■ Table 16, detailing the information obtained on Katherine Compardo, demonstrates the initial step in objectifying the new data that were

obtained. Because of Katherine's level of performance, the data are primarily descriptive objectification—what Katherine did under what circumstances. Return to Table 16 and continue to score and do comparative analyses of the information presented. On what basis will you make comparisons of her data: norms from standardized tests, norms from your funds of knowledge about normal and disordered speech and language and/or your knowledge about children with similar types of speech and language disorders—intradisorder comparisons? Katherine completed the *Peabody Picture Vocabulary Test* up to plate 15; what information does this provide regarding comprehension of single words? What comparative analysis would you draw from her responses to comprehension stimuli throughout the testing session? For example, she responded appropriately to directions that had the following prepositions embedded in them: in, by, and under. What normative data would you apply for comparison to her formulated language? Are specific normative data needed? Continue asking yourself comparative questions for application to Katherine's clinical data.

Data analysis is colored by the methods used in collection and by cooperation from the client. The diagnostician must understand all the variables that entered into the diagnostic session and that may have affected the quality of the information obtained. He will have to separate the information that is considered nonusable from that he can rely on; he can note the strength of each bit of data or note generally the overall quality of the data. These general notations often are seen at the beginning of the testing section of clinical reports: "Buddy entered the testing room willingly, interacted appropriately with the diagnostician, and performed all tests required of him. His performance is considered to be a valid and reliable estimate of his abilities."

■ In Table 16 the diagnostician recorded a number of the circumstances under which Katherine Compardo's data were obtained. Reading his remarks, do you get a clear feeling of how well Katherine performed on the tasks required? Would you be able to make a general statement about the reliability and validity of her performance? Do you think the diagnostician obtained typical performance, or are there indications that Katherine was withholding speech and language? One way of checking on validity is to compare the behavior obtained with behavior reported by others—in Katherine's case, the mother.

We will now proceed to a series of client examples for you to score. For each of them you will want to objectify the data presented and make comparative analyses.

■ Chloe Paxton, aged 5 years, 5 months, was given the *Templin-Darley Screening Test of Articulation*. She correctly produced 22 out of the 50 responses required. The errors made on this test were as follows:

Substitutions

INITIAL	MEDIAL	FINAL
s/θ	f/θ	f/θ
d/ð	s/ʃ	v/ð
s/ʃ	s/ʒ	s/ʃ
l/j	s/tʃ	s/tʃ

Distortions: The /r/, /r/ blends, and the /ɝ/ were consistently distorted.

Compare these findings to the normative information provided for this test and its recommended analysis procedures. Also do a kinetic and acoustic analysis as recommended by Van Riper and Irwin (1958). What additional information would a distinctive feature analysis provide (McReynolds and Engmann, 1975; McReynolds and Houston, 1971)?

■ The following are a series of observations made on Jack Butts, aged 3 years, 8 months.

Jack was first observed in the reception room by the diagnostician. He was building a block tower with his father. He verbalized /m: ba:/ and /ba ba/ repeatedly during this task. He built a six-block tower, and when it fell he said, "aw aw." The diagnostician pounded on the filing cabinet; Jack did not turn to the sound the first time but did the second time. The diagnostician said "Hi" and Jack repeated "Hi." Jack entered the testing room quietly, and at the request of the examiner took his seat. When given a graduated color cone, he worked by trial and error for some time before working out the size relationships—finally he did, and he placed the pieces on the cone in order. He followed commands such as "turn on the radio, throw the ball, and put the ball in the basket." When he dropped objects, he would stand, screech, and quiver while he pointed to the object on the floor. He responded to a toy that made a noise when he picked it up by jumping up from his chair and running to the waiting room. He returned with the examiner, and after explanation and demonstration of the toy he played with it, repeatedly getting the toy to make the noise. While playing with colored plastic eggs he said /mo hɛg/—more eggs. He became engrossed in this activity, taking the eggs apart and putting them together. While doing this, he usually matched the colored halves correctly. When he made an error he said, "oh oh" and corrected the color match. During this activity he made no direct communicative interactions with the examiner. When the examiner again obtained his attention with a new task, Jack immediately became interested. Throughout the observation period he could be easily distracted, changing from one activity to the next even when quite engrossed in his current activity. He frequently left his chair and went to the door but each time could be brought back to the table by being shown a new item.

Analyze these observations into a set of comparative "scores." Where will your information come from for this analysis? What information do you have that might be causal, that might be effect? If you had to select testing procedures for this child, what might you use?

■ The following are examples of the language formulation skills of Gretchen Warner, aged 3 years, 7 months. A total of 40 responses were recorded during the course of the diagnostic session.

Gretchen used primarily three-word phrases; however, in the language sample the range was from one- to four-word responses. Phrases used were typically verb phrases; for example, "hear mommie," "ride car," and "eat cookie" and simple subject-verb combinations—"baby broke," "car gone," and "Gretchen jump." For questions and negatives the following types of responses were heard: "you pen, huh?" "mommie no sit," and "me no cookie." Other examples of her language responses were "me bite snake," "there barber," "no you turn," and "ride on a car."

How would you score these responses? What systems of analysis would you use? Diagnosticians often rely heavily on an objective analysis of spontaneous speech and language responses obtained during a single diagnostic session. Many questions have arisen about the reliability and validity of such language sampling. Recommendations have been made that speech and language behavior should be sampled over two or more sessions and at different times during the day. This, of course, is not a likely practice in diagnosis unless diagnosticians extend their sessions over days or weeks. Can diagnosticians, then, ever obtain a reliable, valid, typical sample of a child's speech and language behavior? Are samples of behavior of language-disordered children the same as language samples of normal children? If diagnosticians are to compare their disordered clients to the various systems of language analysis, which index of development will be best to use? How can these indices be used along with other data collected to assure the diagnostician that he is making appropriate analyses? See the previous discussions and references to the use of a spontaneous speech and language sample.

Lists and categorizes the new data

In this second clinical analysis task the new data the diagnostician has objectified and compared are now listed and categorized in relationship to the clinical hypothesis within the SLPM framework. He now has many bits of new data that need to be inventoried; just as in the constituent analysis he inventoried the bits of information for deriving a hypothesis, he now inventories the new data for deriving his clinical diagnosis. The student is referred back to Chapter 11 for the details and concepts presented about listing and categorizing. These same tasks are used in the clinical analysis and thus will not be reiterated here.

However, we want to point out once again the importance of the SLPM as an organizing principle for the diagnostician in clinical analysis. Gearing his analysis to the SLPM, the diagnostician would order his data within the components of the model, not just the hypotheses that were formulated. Using the model at this stage keeps bias to a minimum. He should order the new data that falls into all the components of the model, even if his hypothesis did not include all the components. For example, the diagnostician might not have been focusing on input stimulation factors; however, if data were accumulated that fits into this component, he should consider it in his clinical analysis.

Using the SLPM in his clinical analysis, the diagnostician can go beyond the data that was obtained. Just as he did when formulating his clinical hypothesis, the diagnostician can list and categorize (or-

der) the data in terms of both the factual data and the inferences he makes. For example, measures of structure and function of the speech mechanism may be objectified and provide direct evidence for associated causal factors. On the other hand, information about causal factors within the speech mechanism may come inferentially from behavioral (product) data. If the diagnostician heard excessive nasality (product), he might infer inadequate velopharyngeal closure as a potential causal factor within the speech mechanism. The SLPM demonstrates how these relationships can be drawn, giving the diagnostician support for some of the later interpretations he may derive from the data. If the diagnostician derives his hypotheses from the SLPM, it follows that his clinical analysis can rely on the same model. This listing and categorizing task provides the diagnostician with a pattern analysis—what data fits each part of the hypothesis—the distribution of details that specify causal factors and effects.

In Chapter 11 we provided a constituent analysis form in some detail (Form 9), specifying the components of the SLPM, cause-effect categorization, statements of the problem, purposes of the referral, management considerations, behavioral considerations, and incidental information. This form is again useful at this step; however, the diagnostician can adapt its format for clinical analysis adapted more to each specific clinical hypothesis. This adapted format serves as a specific summary form to list and categorize the data obtained about each client.

■ A clinical analysis form adapted from Katherine Compardo's clinical hypotheses might look like Table 17. On this form we have not categorized the specific response items from Table 16. Instead, we only point out generally some of the information that applies to the listing and categorization—emphasis is on the inferences that might be drawn from the data. The new data from the interview will be incorporated into the next diagnostic task rather than here. The student is encouraged to specify

Table 17. Clinical analysis form for listing and categorizing data obtained on Katherine Compardo in relationship to her cause-effect hypothesis

CNS disruption	Physical processes	Behavioral correlates	Products	Other information
Central language segment	Language represen- tation Speech programming	Formulation Sequencing	All language levels "Aphasia" "Apraxia"	This would be speci- fied as in Form 9 or specifically re: Katherine Compar- do's hypothesis
See overall motor abilities See overall use of speech mecha- nism See overall abili- ties on tasks of language, inter- personal reac- tions, and cog- nitive perfor- mance	Same Use of speech mus- culature	Same See items related to speech and lan- guage product Stimulability testing	See all information about the speech and language produced under all conditions (stimulability testing seems important here) Naming are the only responses from which to work	*Referral* Overall motor abilities Limited speech and language leads to several causal questions *Comprehension* See all responses to directions and *Pea- body Picture Vo- cabulary Test* re- sponses

the items for analysis and to add those we have not included.

Adds the data from the constituent analysis

The information from the constituent analysis must now be listed and catego- rized along with the new data. As previ- ously stated, the clinical analysis is pri- marily a continuation of the constituent analysis with newly collected data added.

The data from the constituent analysis are "brought down" intact to the clinical analysis, unless the newly acquired data collected during the diagnostic session warrant revision of any of the constituents. The interview data often require the diag- nostician to revise certain constituents. In the interview he has amplified, clarified,

and verified the questionable constituents; now he can add these revised constituents to the clinical analysis form in the appro- priate cause-effect and other categories.

■ For Katherine Compardo it is suggested that the student return to her constituent analysis and bring down those constituents that are ap- propriate for clinical analysis. What has the interview information with Katherine's mother (Table 15) added to your interpretation of the constituents? Do any of the major constituents need revision? What new information was of- fered in regard to her eating habits, and where might you add this information to the clinical analysis?

Often, referral is a part of the manage- ment considerations planned for clients. As previously discussed, referrals should be made based on specific information obtained and specific information needed to interpret cause-effect relationships. As a part of listing and categorizing, the diagnostician will want to carefully specify which data may lead him to referral considerations.

■ The very nature of Katherine Compardo's clinical hypothesis should lead the diagnostician to consider a referral. The causal factors hypothesized cannot be tested directly by the diagnostician. What information is now available on Katherine that would be categorized under "need for referral"? For example, what information might lead to a neurologic referral, a psychological referral, a general medical referral, etc.?

Determines the significance of all the data

In this fourth task of clinical analysis all of the data now listed and categorized must be examined for significance, for its relevance to the clinical hypothesis, alternate hypotheses, or new hypotheses. The questions the diagnostician asks himself in this task are how can the data be used, how can it assist me in making my clinical interpretations, and is it relevant for deriving my clinical diagnosis? Again, the student should return to Chapter 11 for a full discussion of the diagnostician's task, determining the significance of his constituents. The same process applies to determining the significance of his data in the clinical analysis. He is basically ruling in and ruling out data that provides him with support for interpretation.

The diagnostician continues to compare the data obtained with his funds of knowledge, with some emphasis on intradisorder comparisons. He uses his funds of knowledge to determine what data are supportive of causal factors, what data specify effects, and what data support a cause-effect relationship. He wants to know how confident he can be using the data to draw his interpretations. Does the data offer him a potential solution to the clinical problem, or does he start again?

As was done in Chapter 11, the diagnostician can develop a significance table to systematically view the data that are now listed and categorized. The diagnostician is now engaged in "differential diagnosis"—a process applicable to all clients.

Myklebust (1954) has developed a table as a type of summary analysis. His information is what we refer to as both intradisorder and interdisorder comparisons and provides the basis for determining the significance of constituents and collected data. Compare Myklebust's concept of "differential diagnosis" of auditory disorders to our concept that all diagnoses are differential.

■ The student should now complete Table 18 for our example client, Katherine Compardo.

Table 18. Determination of significance of all the data on our example client, Katherine Compardo

Data	Significance
Summary statement of information collected about language product, for example:	What does this tell about language formulation?
The mother's reports are accurate; Katherine responds only occasionally in single-word responses that are often unintelligible.	Can she formulate language, but does not produce it? Is the speech programming process affecting the output; that is, could she formulate the message but not program it for production?

SUMMARY

This fifth step in the diagnostic process scores, orders, and determines the significance of all the data available on the client; the new data collected during the interview and clinical testing sessions, and the prior data used in the constituent analysis. While, typically, this step runs imperceptibly from the previous step (collection of the clinical data) and into the following step (clinical interpretation), we feel it is important for teaching purposes to discuss analysis as a separate step, thereby underscoring the objectivity that is its essential characteristic. To guard against bias, it is advantageous to develop this practice of nonjudgmental consideration of the data before it is interpreted.

The diagnostician is encouraged here to objectify his data both quantitatively and descriptively, using standard criteria from information available in his fund of knowledge, from his internalized perceptual norms, from intradisorder comparisons with clinical populations, and from standardized test norms. Descriptive analyses provide broader specification of the data and are particularly useful in planning client management.

Four tasks comprise the clinical analysis step.

1. The diagnostician first *scores his new data.* He objectifies the data through quantitative and descriptive comparative analyses that provide the context and the pattern to the behavior.

2. He *lists and categorizes the new data.* This task is similar to the same task in the constituent analysis. He plots his data in accordance with his clinical hypothesis within the SLPM perspective. He inventories his data to determine what he has available to use for interpretation of the clinical problem.

3. He *adds the data from the constituent analysis.* The clinical analysis has been discussed as a continuation of the constituent analysis. In this task the diagnostician "brings down" the relevant constituents needed for in-terpretation of the clinical problem. He adds them to the previous listing and categorization.

4. The diagnostician *determines the significance of all the data.* Again, this task is similar to that performed in the constituent analysis. Here the diagnostician is attempting to discover how relevant all his data are, how they can be used for clinical interpretation.

Once the clinical analysis is completed, the diagnostician is now ready to enter the clinical interpretation stage of the diagnostic process.

CLIENT PROJECTS
Marie Abadie

Ms. Marie Abadie was admitted to the rehabilitation unit of Kankakee General Hospital 3 weeks following the onset of her condition. She was brought over from 6 West, the neurology-neurosurgical ward. In Appendix II her discharge summary report as dictated by Dr. Denise Aronson is reproduced. Also included in Appendix II are the results of Dr. Sandy Mayfield, speech pathologist, who has used selected items from various tests of aphasia following a processing schema. Analyze the results of the testing. What significance do her findings have to a classification of processing deficits in aphasia? Whose schema is basically being followed in this format of testing and analysis?

Previous clients: William Gafford, Isadore Alexander, Derek Park, and Michael Durall

Now that you have collected the data on the above clients, do a clinical analysis of your data, following the procedures suggested in this chapter.

REFERENCES

Brown, R., *A First Language: The Early Stages.* Cambridge, Mass.: Harvard University Press (1973).

Chapman, D., and Nation, J. E., Language patterns of certain primary level educable mentally retarded children. Paper presented at the Annual Convention of the American Speech and Hearing Association, Las Vegas (1974).

De Hirsch, K., Differential diagnosis between aphasic and schizophrenic language in children. *J. Speech Hearing Dis.*, **32**, 3-10 (1967).

Dunn, L. M., *Expanded Manual for the Peabody Picture Vocabulary Test*. Circle Pines, Minn.: American Guidance Service, Inc. (1965).

Engler, L. F., Hannah, P., and Longhurst, T. M., Linguistic analysis of speech samples: A practical guide for clinicians. *J. Speech Hearing Dis.*, **38**, 192-204 (1973).

Faircloth, M. A., and Faircloth, S. R., An analysis of the articulatory behavior of a speech-defective child in connected speech and in isolated-word responses. *J. Speech Hearing Dis.*, **35**, 51-61 (1970).

Foster, R., Giddan, J. J., and Stark, J., *Manual for the Assessment of Children's Language Comprehension*. Palo Alto, Calif.: Consulting Psychologists Press (1972).

Hollien, H., and Shipp, T., Speaking fundamental frequency and chronologic age in males. *J. Speech Hearing Res.*, **15**, 155-159 (1972).

Johnson, M. R., and Tomblin, J. B., The reliability of developmental sentence scoring as a function of sample size. *J. Speech Hearing Res.*, **18**, 372-380 (1975).

Johnson, W., Darley, F. L., and Spriestersbach, D. C., *Diagnostic Methods in Speech Pathology*. New York: Harper & Row, Publishers (1963).

Lee, L. L., Developmental sentence types: A method for comparing normal and deviant syntactic development. *J. Speech Hearing Dis.*, **31**, 311-330 (1966).

Lee, L. L., *Developmental Sentence Analysis*. Evanston, Ill.: Northwestern University Press (1974).

McReynolds, L. V., and Huston, K., A distinctive feature analysis of children's misarticulations. *J. Speech Hearing Dis.*, **36**, 155-166 (1971).

McReynolds, L. V., and Engmann, D. L., *Distinctive Feature Analysis of Misarticulations*. Baltimore: University Park Press (1975).

Menyuk, P., and Looney, P. L., A problem of language disorder: Length versus structure. *J. Speech Hearing Res.*, **15**, 264-279 (1972).

Miner, L. E., Scoring procedures for the length-complexity index: A preliminary report. *J. Commun. Dis.*, **2**, 224-240 (1969).

Minifie, F. D., Darley, F. L., and Sherman, D., Temporal reliability of seven language measures. *J. Speech Hearing Res.*, **6**, 139-148 (1963).

Morehead, D. M., and Ingram, D., The development of base syntax in normal and linguistically deviant children. *J. Speech Hearing Res.*, **16**, 330-352 (1973).

Myklebust, H. R., *Auditory Disorders in Children*. New York: Grune & Stratton, Inc. (1954).

Naremore, R. C., and Dever, R. B., Language performance of educable mentally retarded and normal children at five age levels. *J. Speech Hearing Res.*, **18**, 82-95 (1975).

Poole, I., Genetic development of articulation of consonant sounds in speech. *Elem. Eng. Rev.*, **11**, 159-161 (1934).

Prather, E. M., Hedrick, D. L., and Kern, C. A., Articulation development in children aged two to four years. *J. Speech Hearing Dis.*, **40**, 179-191 (1975).

Ramer, A. L. H., and Rees, N. S., Selected aspects of the development of English morphology in black American children of low socioeconomic background. *J. Speech Hearing Res.*, **16**, 569-577 (1973).

Sander, E. K., When are speech sounds learned? *J. Speech Hearing Dis.*, **37**, 55-63 (1972).

Sharf, D. J., Some relationships between measures of early language development. *J. Speech Hearing Dis.*, **37**, 64-74 (1972).

Shriner, T. H., A comparison of selected measures with psychological scale values of language development. *J. Speech Hearing Res.*, **10**, 828-835 (1967).

Shriner, T. H., A review of mean length of response as a measure of expressive language development in children. *J. Speech Language Dis.*, **34**, 61-68 (1969).

Shriner, T., and Sherman, D., An equation for assessing language development. *J. Speech Hearing Res.*, **10**, 41-48 (1967).

Shriner, T., Holloway, M., and Daniloff, R., The relationship between articulatory deficits and syntax in speech defective children. *J. Speech Hearing Res.*, **12**, 319-325 (1969).

Silverman, E.-M., Clustering: A characteristic of preschoolers' speech disfluency. *J. Speech Hearing Res.*, **16**, 578-583 (1973).

Templin, M. C., *Certain Language Skills in Children: Their Development and Interrelationships*. Institute of Child Welfare Monograph Series, No. 26, Minneapolis: University of Minnesota Press (1957).

Templin, M. C., and Darley, F. L., *The Templin-Darley Tests of Articulation*. (2nd ed.) Iowa City, Iowa: University of Iowa Press (1969).

Van Demark, D. R., and Tharp, R., A computer program for articulation tests. *Cleft Palate J.*, **10**, 378-389 (1973).

Van Riper, C., and Irwin, J. V., *Voice and Articulation*. Englewood Cliffs, N.J.: Prentice-Hall, Inc. (1958).

Weber, J. L., Patterning of deviant articulation behavior. *J. Speech Hearing Dis.*, **35**, 135-141 (1970).

Wellman, B., Case, I., Mengert, I., and Bradbury, D., Speech sounds of young children. *University of Iowa Studies in Child Welfare*, **5**, 1-82 (1931).

Wiig, E. H., and Semel, E. M., Comprehension of linguistic concepts requiring logical operations by learning-disabled children. *J. Speech Hearing Res.*, **16**, 627-636 (1973).

Wilson, M. E., A standardized method for obtaining a spoken language sample. *J. Speech Hearing Res.*, **12**, 95-102 (1969).

Yoss, K. A., and Darley, F. L., Developmental apraxia of speech in children with defective articulation. *J. Speech Hearing Res.*, **17**, 399-416 (1974).

Chapter 16

Interpretation of the clinical data: clinical evaluation

After the data has been scored, categorized, and its significance considered in relationship to the clinical hypothesis, the diagnostician is then ready to interpret his data, the sixth step of the diagnostic process. This step is a synthesis and integration of all the preceding steps. It is the culmination of the diagnostic process, where the aim is to come to decisions about the nature and extent of the speech and language disorder and its causes. This phase of the diagnostic process particularly tests the diagnostician's problem-solving skills, as it is here that he must put all the pieces together into their most logical order.

Interpretation, clinical evaluation, has at its core client concern; it lays the groundwork for management proposals. How he interprets the clinical data underlies the conclusions the diagnostician will draw from it, how he will communicate his understanding with others, and what management proposals he will choose. The clinical evaluation is, in a sense, the answer to the clinical questions that have been posed.

As the clinical analysis parallels the constituent analysis, the clinical evaluation parallels the clinical hypothesis. The constituent analysis sets up the information for the derivation of the clinical hypothesis; likewise the clinical analysis sets up the data for the clinical evaluation. In many ways the clinical evaluation step represents a continuation of hypothesis formulation. Only now the diagnostician has firsthand data and is better able to judge the strengths and weaknesses of the interpretation he offers. Probably many clinical evaluations are more accurately still clinical hypotheses with greater degrees of probability. The diagnostician hopes his interpretation has a high level of certainty.

Three tasks make up the clinical evaluation step. The first task, interpreting the results of the clinical analysis, draws heavily on the diagnostician's problem-solving abilities. Here the diagnostician figures out how the data best fits together to explain the problem, to explain the most likely cause-effect relationship. In essence, this task is the thinking process that allows the diagnostician to formulate his diagnosis.

After the diagnostician has completed his interpretation, he undertakes the second task, stating the diagnosis. This task is a formal, succinct statement of his diagnosis. The "statement" may be a mental solidification or may be written explicitly. It expresses the most likely cause-effect relationship, addressing both the speech and language disorder and the probable contributing causes.

The third task, supporting the diagnosis, is a formal support paper for the diagnostic statement, again paralleling the similar task performed in the development of the clinical hypothesis. As a formal support paper, this task draws from literature support, the constituent analysis, and the analysis of the clinical data. The clinical evaluation tasks set the stage for the next and final step in the diagnostic process, drawing conclusions and proposing management considerations.

CLINICAL EVALUATION: HOW IT IS DONE
Information bases: culmination of problem-solving skill

As the culmination of the diagnostician's problem-solving skills, the clinical evaluation is based on information from all the previous steps and on all information used by the diagnostician as a "solver" of speech and language problems. All the information gained and examined in the earlier steps is brought together to contribute to the final diagnosis. If there were any uncorrected "errors" in the previous steps, they will most likely be reflected in the clinical interpretation. As mentioned previously, this step closely parallels step two of the diagnostic process, the derivation of the clinical hypothesis. The reader is directed to Chapter 12 for review of the information presented there, which is entirely applicable to the current step being discussed.

Since the decisions made about the management of the client's speech and language problem rest on the diagnostician's clinical interpretation, this step of the diagnostic process may be the most crucial. If the diagnostician does not exercise extreme care in this final problem-solving stage of diagnosis, inappropriate management decisions may easily result.

The diagnostician must consider the strengths and weaknesses of all his information. He must remember that some of the tools used may not have provided a typical sample of the client's behavior. He must be careful not to overemphasize some pieces of data that may support his interpretation in favor of other information that may weaken his interpretive position. He must state a case, but unlike a trial attorney he must also present evidence that may weaken his case. The diagnostician is not trying to "win his hypothesis"; he is offering his best reasoning to solve the problem, proposing alternate interpretations if they seem warranted for understanding and treating the client's problem.

At this step the diagnostician is not primarily supporting or rejecting his hypothesis in a manner similar to the experimenter. Instead, he is adding to and subtracting from his original hypothesis that acted as a clinical guide for the diagnostic process. When the process ends, the diagnostician cannot simply say his hypothesis was not supported. Rather, he must come up with a new hypothesis (solution) that better explains the data. Thus while he makes his clinical evaluation in terms of his clinical hypothesis, he is not solely bound to supporting or rejecting his most likely hypothesis, a major reason for proposing alternate hypotheses.

Client concern, as the highest priority of diagnosis, requires the diagnostician to remain free of the "bias trap." All along the diagnostic process he should have maintained an objective attitude toward the nature of the client's problem. If he has done this, then his interpretation of the information will be appropriate to the client and not just an interpretation that reflects his bias. The diagnostician's interpretations must bear a supportable relationship to the known information; they must be clearly reasoned and appropriately limited.

In practice, it generally is not as difficult to arrive at an interpretation of the disordered speech and language behavior as it is the probable causal factors contributing to the problem. This is generally true because the speech and language behavior is more accessible to direct observation, while causal factors are often understood only through inferences from secondary behavior. The diagnostician's fund of knowledge about speech and language disorders, as represented in Chapters 3 to 8 becomes as crucial to his clinical evaluation as it was in deriving his clinical hypothesis.

Diagnostician's tasks

The diagnostician now engages in the tasks that will fulfill two of his primary job functions: to determine the nature and extent of the speech and language disorder and to understand the causal factors associated with it. Therefore his major function at this step is to draw reasonable relationships among the cause-effect data to arrive at a diagnostic statement. He asks himself if his interpretation bears a reasonable relationship to what is known in the field of speech and language disorders, if the causal factors used to explain the speech and language disorder bear a reasonable relationship to known facts, if he has enough facts and careful inferences to support his interpretation, if his interpretation verifies the interpretations of other workers in the profession, if his interpretations provide new insights into speech and language disorders, and if his interpretations provide for appropriate management decisions to be made.

To do this, we have proposed three tasks to be performed by the diagnostician at this seventh step of the diagnostic process.

1. He interprets the data from the clinical analysis, examining cause-effect relationships and formulating the basis for his diagnostic statement.
2. He formalizes his interpretation by stating his diagnosis, specifying his cause-effect relationship.
3. He supports his diagnositc statement through a formal support paper, a clinical evaluation, that considers his position on the clinical problem, offering his reasons why his diagnosis is more appropriate than other conclusions might be.

Interprets the results of the clinical analysis

From the clinical analysis the diagnostician developed a clear perspective on the significant results of the diagnostic process. He now focuses on his professional interpretation of the meaning of these results. Does the client have a problem? If so, what is the disorder and what may have caused it? His clinical hypothesis pointed the direction; now the diagnostician determines if he was on course. In the same way that the clinical hypothesis offered the diagnostician a potential solution to the problem, the clinical interpretation has a forward reference; it becomes the diagnostician's "solution" to the problem from which the proposed course of management comes.

Some diagnosticians often resort to overuse of test results for interpretation, particularly in those settings that use or require the use of certain tests routinely. Instead of integrating all the data accumulated on the client, they make interpretations based entirely on test scores. Some

FUNKY WINKERBEAN   By Tom Batiuk

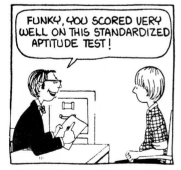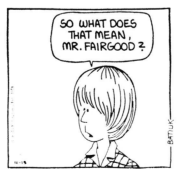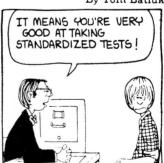

Fig. 16-1. A very careful interpretation of test scores. (FUNKY WINKERBEAN by Tom Batiuk. Courtesy Field Newspaper Syndicate.)

tests gain greater use this way than others (Chapters 13 and 14). Each diagnostician must guard against replacing clinical evaluation with reporting test results. The use of test results (the clinical analysis) is only a part of the overall clinical evaluation. The diagnostician must differentiate between reporting test scores and interpreting clinical data (Fig. 16-1). Overreliance on test scores can lead to faulty management decisions to say nothing of faulty diagnoses. If the diagnostician only uses a given tool, the only inferences and conclusions that can be drawn are dependent on the findings from that tool.

What do Vellutino et al. (1972) have to say about the use of Wepman's *Auditory Discrimination Test* (1958)?

In his clinical analysis the diagnostician systematically viewed all information that specified what the disorder might be and any information that reflected potential causes of the disorder. His emphasis in interpretation is drawing the probable relationships among these sets of data. At times the relationship is easy to see: "Mr. Grogan has aphasia due to a stroke," "Mr. Catlow has no vocal tone due to a recent laryngectomy," and "Ms. Wicker's hoarse voice quality is currently due to the presence of large vocal nodules." At other times, as discussed in some detail in Chapter 8, the relationships are difficult to impossible to draw. Cause-effect relationships are complex interactions; diagnosticians often do not see a direct cause of the speech and language disorder, particularly in young children with developmental disorders. Thus the diagnostician's use of his inferential measurement strategy is vitally essential if he is to support his cause-effect relationship.

Interpreting the nature of the speech and language disorder requires knowing the characteristic patterns seen in the various disorders. The interpretation is two pronged. First, the diagnostician must differentiate the client's disorder from other types of disorders, for example, a prosody disorder from a semantic disorder, a language disorder from a phonetic structure disorder, etc. Second, he must go on to differentiate the client's individual disorder pattern from characteristics of clients with similar problem types, that is, stuttering$_1$ from stuttering$_2$ from stuttering$_3$, etc. The individual patterns of behavior presented by clients with similar disorders vary significantly. The clinical analysis should provide the diagnostician with needed information for making these differentiations, that is, if he has been able to observe enough speech and language behavior.

Interpreting the nature of the speech and language disorder is often easier than determining the causal background for the disorders or for the individual behavioral patterns seen. Again, if the diagnostician has gathered his causal data carefully, he will arrive at a more likely probable causal basis for the disorder than arriving at a least likely probability. As was discussed, the diagnostician has three ways of relating causal factors. First, he can view the causal basis for a speech and language disorder from a purely historical perspective: what happened in the past that might account for the disorder. Second, he can view the contemporary basis for the disorder: what is currently operating that may account for the behaviors manifested—a processing viewpoint. Of course, the diagnostician has a third option—interrelating these two viewpoints about causal factors. In most instances he should attempt the latter.

■ The following are a set of findings on 4-year-old Adeline Eichelberger.
1. Language comprehension-formulation is delayed 1 year.
2. Intelligibility is severely limited.
3. Medically diagnosed at 1 year of age as having mild cerebral palsy.
4. Discovered moderate sensorineural hearing loss at 3 years of age. Bilateral hearing aids recommended and used since that time.
5. Intelligence tested within normal limits within the past month.

Interpret the causal factors operative in Adeline's problem from the three options for viewing causation: historical, contemporary, and combined.

How does the diagnostician go about drawing and interpreting the most likely cause-effect relationship? For example, how does the diagnostician know that Amy's history of significant ear infections and hearing problems are related to her current errors of phonology? This assumed relationship would mean that at some point Amy was unable to hear the sounds of speech or to discriminate the phonologic cues in the speech of her environment, and that in some way this has resulted in her inability to generate appropriate phonemes and phoneme sequences. Hearing loss, of either short- or long-term duration in young children, is often cited as a causal factor for speech and language disorders. However, there is little direct evidence that indicates what type and degree of hearing disorders disrupt the learning and use of the phonologic level of language.

Is the article by Owens et al. (1972) helpful in interpreting cause-effect relationships that may exist between hearing loss and phonemic errors?

The diagnostician's interpetation of cause-effect relationships relates somewhat to the concept of the normal distribution curve, a device heavily used in the method of science. In order to infer a cause that is more than chance, the diagnostician relies on his knowledge of widely held correlations between causal factors and patterns of disordered behavior (intradisorder comparisons). For example, the diagnostician might interpret that Alex's lack of language development is related to a severe bilateral sensorineural hearing loss that was due to the reported maternal rubella because he knows that in a significant percentage of cases of maternal rubella, severe hearing losses result. By relating his client information to the expected probability he is closer to a more likely cause-effect rela-

tionship. However, the diagnostician must keep in mind that when using intragroup disorder comparisons, as with any population-sample comparisons, there is some degree of error. Therefore he must always be parsimonious in drawing his clinical interpretation. The lower the correlations reported (that is, the discrepancies or lack of cause-effect relationships reported in the literature), the more cautious the diagnostician must become. The concept of error due to chance is extremely applicable and indeed necessary in clinical interpretation. It reminds the diagnostician of the limitations of his results, the tentative nature of his diagnosis.

What cause-effect relationships seem to be the most difficult to interpret? All reported literature that is directed toward discovering patterns of speech and language behavior related to specific causal factors is relevant. As well, what do the following articles offer for helping professionals interpret cause-effect relationships: Bankson and Byrne, 1962; Carrow, 1957; Davis and Blasdell, 1975; De Hirsch et al., 1964; Farmakides and Boone, 1960; Greene, 1960; Pitzner and Morris, 1966; Raph, 1967; Rosenberg, 1966?

Intradisorder comparisons do form a major framework by which diagnosticians interpret their cause-effect relationships, and the use of the SLPM framework is partially designed to specify more validly and reliably these relationships. A precise and theoretically sound attempt to draw cause-effect relationships for interpretation is the type of work done by Darley et al. (1969a, b, 1975). From their work, the diagnostician knowing the client's neurologic disease could predict the disordered behaviors, or on the other hand, seeing a client with certain speech behaviors could allow the diagnostician to infer a potential neurologic disease. Of equal importance in their work is the emphasis on interacting, overlapping processing systems responsible for the clusters of speech behaviors seen. That is, because the speech-producing processes have certain neurologic controls in common (see discussion of speech and language product), speech behaviors tend to cluster. Thus a particular disease or a particular lesion may lead to a fairly predictable set of disordered speech patterns.

■ The following is adapted from the clinical report written on Mr. Isadore Alexander, one of the example clients used throughout this book. From these findings interpret the probable causal factor responsible for this speech disorder.

Mr. Alexander was accompanied by his wife but taken alone for the evaluation. His spontaneous speech did not evidence any symbolic comprehension-formulation disturbances (aphasia) but was severely unintelligible and bizarre. [NOTE: Intelligibility and bizarreness are two of the dimensions of dysarthria investigated by Darley et al. (1969a, b). Their articles form the basis for the dimensions observed and evaluated in Mr. Alexander and the conclusions drawn from the evaluation.]

These two dimensions are overall judgments of the speech. Intelligibility relates to how well the listener is able to understand the speech of the patient, and bizarreness relates to the degree to which the speech calls attention to itself. It was possible to understand what Mr. Alexander was saying because in most cases the context of his responses was known and also because a manner of "speechreading" was employed. The examiner visually noted the direction of movement of the articulators and to some extent assumed the speech product because it was distorted by extremely weak articulatory contact and slow rate.

In evaluating the speech/voice variation more specifically, the following component dimensions of intelligibility and bizarreness were rated: pitch, loudness, vocal quality, breathing for speech, prosody, and phonetic structure.

Mr. Alexander's pitch level, overall, was somewhat low and monotonous (monopitch). When asked to follow the examiner up and/or down the scale on /a/, he demonstrated inability to vary pitch to any great extent.

A significant aspect of loudness was monoloudness; a consistent level of loudness was maintained that was somewhat louder than normal. Significant aspects of vocal quality were severe vocal harshness (a rough, raspy quality), strained-strangled voice, voice stoppages, and hypernasality.

The most prominent feature of breathing for speech was audible inspiration. The prosodic variations were slow rate, short phrases, reduced stress, intervals prolonged, inappropriate silences, and excess and equal stress.

A spontaneous speech sample indicates the prosody variations listed above. "What's the trouble [pause for inspiration] I can't [pause] say [pause] anything [pause] to [pause] her [pause] and she [pause] don't [pause] see." Each pause represents a brief, audible breath intake. Each word is spoken with excessive and equal stress and at the same pitch and loudness level.

Mr. Alexander's phonetic structure variations were characterized primarily by imprecise consonants. That is, the consonant sounds showed slurring, inadequate sharpness, distortions, and lack of crispness. There is clumsiness going from one sound to another. To some extent phonemes were prolonged, especially vowels, which had the effect of distorting the vowels. Specific testing of diadochokinetic rate showed slower than normal rate for all alternating movements of the articulators and repetition of monosyllables such as /kakaka/ and /lalala/. The most markedly slow rate was in production of /kalakala/, which involves moving from a back to a front phoneme. Phoneme substitutions did not involve inappropriate place or direction of articulation, but reduction of force and range, which had the effect of distortion of the phoneme. Voicing of unvoiced phonemes, /b/p/ and /g/k/, tended to occur. Voiceless fricatives either were not produced or were replaced by a plosive, /p/f/. The factor that seemed to underlly these phonetic structure variations was that insufficient closure of the velopharyngeal port prevented impounding of air for plosive and fricative production. Indeed, observation of palatal function both in production of sustained /a/ and short, rapid productions of /a/ indicated very little palatal movement. This would also account for the hypernasality.

As the evaluation progressed, Mr. Alexander's speech became slower in rate even than the initial slow rate, and there were more frequent pauses, inappropriate silences, and voice stoppages. Phonation simply ceased and the voice was "squeezed" into a whisper. Even this examiner was exhausted, a seeming reflection of what appeared to be the tremendous effort it increasingly required for Mr. Alexander to communicate.[*]

Intradisorder comparisons are quite useful when the information is available; however, there is still much to be discovered about cause-effect relationships. The variability in patterns of behavior is great; certain causal factors seem to result in any number of behavioral differences. We are just beginning to isolate some of the basic language disorders seen in young children and have hardly tapped their causal bases (Aram and Nation, 1975; Hardy, 1965). As we learn more about how speech and lan-

[*]Our thanks are extended to Ms. Janet Whitney, speech pathologist, formerly at the Cleveland Hearing and Speech Center, Cleveland, Ohio, for permission to use this portion of her clinical report.

guage are processed by the human being, we will learn more about how causal factors disrupt these processes, resulting in characteristic patterns of speech and language behaviors. Until all the data is in, the diagnostician must use his skills as a problem solver to arrive at the most likely solution to the clinical problem (Chapter 9).

Establishing cause-effect relationships is not easy. Diagnosis is not easy, but the diagnostician must strive to understand, to make the best interpretations possible, and to report them with caution. He has an obligation to the profession to continue to seek for reasonable explanations for why speech and language disorders exist, no matter how tentative they may be. Often the findings and interpretations of the diagnostician can point the way for further experimental research. The diagnostician may have arrived at a fairly unique explanation for the disorder he is seeing. He may arrive at an insight about the nature and cause of speech and language disorders that the researcher may use to develop experimental studies: studies that then feed back into the diagnostician's fund of knowledge. For example, a diagnostician may interpret certain phonetic structure errors on the basis of a neurologic disruption of the tongue. However, further study will be required to place this inference by the diagnostician into better perspective. It may be the anatomist, physiologist, neurologist, or speech scientist who provides the necessary data to turn this interpretation-inference into data that may truly demonstrate the relationship and become usable for future diagnoses.

Case studies reported in the literature often are presentations of rare diagnostic circumstances. These studies, however, provide insights for use in more general diagnostic situations—they often present information related to processing disruptions. What do the following example clinical reports offer for diagnostic use: Aronson, 1971; Fisher and Logemann, 1970; Garstecki et al., 1972; Kent and Netsell, 1975; Stein and Curry, 1968; Weinberg et al., 1975?

Because of the lack of factual and theoretical security for many potential cause-effect interpretations, the diagnostician must exercise care in his explanations. He must carefully consider all the information in order to offer the client his most reasonable interpretation. And, we should not be misled; clients with speech and language disorders want to know: "What caused me to talk this way?" The diagnostician should be prepared to respond to the question. Client's are not always satisfied with an explanation that a disorder is present; they often already know that. Nor are they always satisfied that something will be done about it. Client's have a natural desire to know, and often a high level of anxiety about what caused their disordered behavior. Our clinical interpretations should allow us to respond with a reasonable explanation within our professional boundaries.

Parsimonious interpretations are called for. The diagnostician should stick to the best set of data about each client, information at low levels of abstraction rather than highly theoretical explanations. He must try to interpret on the basis of the factual rather than inferential if at all possible. The diagnostician's intent is to synthesize his information to present the interpretation that fits the data best. What evidence does he have to support his interpretation that Anthony's hypernasality is due to inadequate velopharyngeal closure, that Deli's phonetic errors are due to her short lingual frenum, that Mr. Van Meter's hoarse voice is due to vocal abuse, or that LaVerne's distorted speech sounds are related to his high-frequency hearing loss. At this point the information in Chapters 8 and 12 will be of most use to the student in interpreting the clinical data.

States the diagnosis

The diagnostician formalizes his diagnosis and states it as carefully and succinctly as possible. The formal diagnostic statement is often used in interprofessional communication and at times may be used directly with the client complex. Therefore the diagnostician should work out several ways of stating his diagnosis at various levels of abstraction to suit his communication purposes. Everything that was discussed regarding the statement of the clinical hypothesis in Chapter 12 is relevant to the statement of the diagnosis and should be reviewed.

■ The following serve as examples of various ways a diagnostic statement could be framed for communication with different individuals concerned with Robert's problem. With whom might these statements be used?

1. Robert has a severe phonologic formulation problem. He has not learned the phonologic rule system for producing appropriate phonemes of his language. The causal factors relating to this mislearning are unclear at this time but may have some relationship to long-standing middle ear infections during critical language-learning periods.

2. Robert has great difficulty making sounds. He has not learned how to do this yet.

3. Robert has a severe problem using the sounds of his language. We think he has not learned how to use them because of his significant hearing problems.

4. Robert has a severe language formulation problem on the phonologic level. His phonologic rule system is very rudimentary for his age. We suspect his difficulties are due to his early history of significant middle ear problems that reduced the amount of phonemic information he received at very critical ages. Even though he demonstrates no current auditory processing difficulties, we infer that they existed and resulted in his current language processing difficulty.

We are reminded by Johnson et al. (1963) that our diagnosis may only be tentative. The clinical hypothesis from which the diagnostician worked may never be fully verified. Therefore, although the diagnostician must express his findings in a diagnostic statement, this statement does not necessarily imply that the final conclusion has been reached. As the clinical hypothesis is predictive and explanatory, so is the diagnostic statement. Since our

major interest is client concern, our diagnostic statement should reflect the projections the diagnostician will make regarding management proposals. He utilizes his conclusions, his diagnostic statement, to inform the client, to plan therapeutic objectives, and to make appropriate referrals.

As an additional guide to clinical interpretation and stating his diagnosis; the diagnostician will find the general semantics information presented by Korzybski (1941, 1948) and adapted by Ptacek (1970) to the diagnostic process helpful. Darley (1964) also presents a set of guiding principles that would be useful to review.

Supports the diagnosis: clinical evaluation

The clinical evaluation task, supporting the diagnosis by developing a formal support paper, basically presents the diagnostician's reasoning processes for arriving at his diagnostic conclusion. He "argues" for his position, incorporating, as well, any points that may detract from his position. Rarely will all of the diagnostician's findings relate positively to his diagnosis. Therefore he must make effective use of the negative results; that is, the data that tend to systematically weaken rather than support his position. If the diagnosis is both logically sound and empirically based, then negative results that weaken rather than confirm the diagnosis are valuable for focusing the diagnostician's attention on potential alternative problems.

This task of supporting the diagnosis is taught as a formal presentation of the interpretation of the findings with documentation from the literature. The support paper synthesizes all the information that bears on the client's problem. The diagnostician offers his best possible explanation, an explanation that may be based as much on inference as it is on fact. The interpretation reflected in the support paper should allow for the logical proposal of management plans. This support paper can then serve as the basis for the clinical evaluation section of the clinical report.

This last task of clinical evaluation is similar to the final task performed in deriving the clinical hypothesis, that is, evaluating the quality of the clinical hypothesis and presenting a formal support paper. It is recommended that the student review that information. Three examples are now presented to demonstrate the task of supporting the diagnosis.

For our first example we offer a clinical *hypothesis* support paper adapted from one developed by Mrs. Karen Wolf on Michael Durall, a client project first presented in Chapter 14.

For the diagnostician the behavioral manifestations of prosody disorders in adults are relatively easy to observe. Therefore many diagnosticians spend their time obtaining many details of the stuttering pattern, the circumstances under which it occurs, the stutterer's attitude toward his disorder, and the effect it has had on his life. The emphasis in the diagnosis is often contemporary; what is happening now when the stutterer attempts to speak. Histories are taken with some interest in how the condition started and developed, but often little use is made of this information for deriving a causal hypothesis from a historical viewpoint or for developing and selecting tools for causal observation. Conflicting theories exist about the causes of stuttering, and this seems to have led to a behaviorally oriented view of stuttering at the expense of understanding causal factors.

In keeping with the theme developed in this book, we see a need for diagnosticians to strive to uncover the potential cause of the stuttering in each client they see. These clinical attempts may lead to better views of causation for stuttering.

Presentation of this *hypothesis* derivation is not necessarily meant to represent our position on causation of stuttering, but rather represents the task of supporting a cause-effect relationship from the literature. Even though this work is not a clinical evaluation, we are presenting it as an example of the reasoning process that occurs similarly in clinical interpretation.

Clinical hypothesis

Michael Durall has a disfluency disorder (characterized by repetitions, prolongations, and blocks) due to a constitutional deficiency in motor coordination of the speech production processes that is still present. In addition, verbal and nonverbal speech modifiers, various covert reactions (situation/word fears), and a self-concept centering around the disfluency disorder may be present due to conditioning processes throughout his life.

Clinical hypothesis support

As could be seen in the constituent analysis, the number of substantial constituents from which to make causal inferences about Michael Durall's stuttering are limited. Therefore the hypothesis I have formulated is primarily based on my funds of knowledge with respect to the disorder of stuttering.

The primary causal factor to which I attribute Michael's disfluency is that of a constitutional deficiency in motor coordination of the speech production processes. By the term constitutional I mean the physical makeup of the individual that contributes to the person he is or will become. All of us have constitutional differences in the many abilities we possess. Some of us are less adept at certain activities than others. I hypothesize that Michael's constitutional makeup has not allowed him to develop the intricate, precise motor coordinations necessary for normally fluent speech.

It has been found that substantially more males than females stutter. Van Riper (1971) reviewed the literature on the subject and concluded that in general the ratio of male stutterers to female stutterers was from three or four to one. Many attempts have been made to explain this difference with little definitive results except that the difference definitely occurs in all cultures. Van Riper (1971) suggests that the difference reflects a less stable "neuromuscular control system for speech in the male" in the early years that may mature over time. Dr. Charlotte Avila, a pediatric neurologist at Metro, states that males are constitutionally inferior in many respects to females and cites the more frequent occurrences of childhood illnesses, speech and language problems, and higher mortality rates in males as examples of this belief. It would appear that just by virtue of being a male Michael stood a greater chance of having a disfluency disorder.

Another fact that substantiates the notion of a constitutional basis to stuttering is that stuttering tends to occur through successive generations in families. Studies supporting this view include that of Andrews and Harris (1964), Nelson et al. (1945), and Wepman (1939). Even though Michael did not report any familial incidence of stuttering, these findings tend to support a constitutional factor involved in stuttering.

It has long been observed in the literature that most stuttering begins in early childhood. Andrews and Harris (1964) and Morley (1957) report that more of their subjects had an onset at 4 years of age than at any other age. This coincides with Michael's report of stuttering for as long as he could remember. In posing a constitutional deficiency in Michael's motor coordination for speech, however, it is necessary to assume that his disfluencies were present from the onset of speech. It has been found by Berry (1938) that of 500 stutterers, 72% began to stutter within the first year after speech began. In Aron's 1958 study, reported by Van Riper (1971), 9 out of 16 parents reported that stuttering began at speech onset. Perkins (1977) states that judgments of sound and syllable disfluencies are usually made when language has context. This statement would tend to explain why age of onset is often reported between 3 and 4 years of age, for this is the time when sentence length and structure is expanding rapidly.

Of further interest is the fact that spontaneous recovery occurs in so many of these children. The exact percentage of children cited as recovering varies with individual studies. Andrews and Harris (1964) report that out of 27 children in a large population of children followed from birth to 15 years of age who had stuttered at least 6 months or more 80% had recovered. Sheehan and Martyn (1970) interviewed a large sample of college students during the course of several years and found 147 who had stuttered at some point in time. The authors reported that spontaneous recovery had taken place in 80% of these subjects. Dickson (1971) studied an elementary and junior high school population, 9% of which had been reported to have stuttered at some time. Approximately 55% of these children had recovered spontaneously. Wingate (1964) also looked at a population of college students who had reportedly stuttered at some point and found that 73% of them recovered in adolescence. I interpret these findings as support for a constitutional deficiency in stutterers. For example, it is possible that motor coordination of the speech processes reaches its peak at different ages in all of us. While the majority of us acquire this ability during early childhood, it may be that many of these stutterers reached their peak coordination at later points of maturation. Quite some time ago Steer (1937) commented on this point. He felt that stuttering might well be a function of maturation of the speech mechanism used in speaking, and adults who stuttered were arrested in development of the speech mechanism.

Evidence that stuttering may come from motor incoordination of certain of the speech production processes comes from several sources. The first notable effect that is relevant to this hypothesis is the rhythm effect. Bloodstein (1950) conducted a questionnaire study of the events that would or would not facilitate fluency and found that speaking in time to various rhythmic activities was often cited as creating a significant reduction in stuttering. Fransella and Beech (1965) conducted a study in which stutterers were asked to say each word or syllable of a word list in time with a rhythmic metronome (the authors ruled out distraction as a cause by having the subjects listen carefully to an arrhythmic beat while reading material similar to the above). The rhythmic condition significantly reduced stuttering, and since there was no effect from the arrhythmic listening condition, it was felt that distraction did not account for the effect. Brady (1969), however, found that speaking in time to an arrhythmic metronome was nearly as effective in eliminating stuttering as speaking in time with a rhythmic metronome when one syllable per beat was produced. Bloodstein (1972) explains the rhythm effect in terms of syllabification and rhythm combined. He states that in reducing speech into syllabic units there is in turn a simplification in motor planning. Bloodstein (1972) further suggests that substantial decreases in stuttering while on delayed auditory feedback can be explained in terms of the simplification of motor planning due to a slower rate of speech. Wingate (1969) attributes this effect to the fact that the individual must emphasize intentional vocalization to produce stress patterns centering on the syllable. This same explanation is given by Wingate (1969) to explain the effects of singing and choral speaking on stuttering. Bloodstein (1950), among others, has reported stutterers to become fluent when singing and also when speaking in unison with one or more persons on either the same or different material (choral speaking). One last condition that reduces stuttering significantly is shadowing (Cherry and Sayers, 1956). In all of these conditions Wingate (1969) emphasizes the point that continuity of speech production is present.

Wingate (1969) states that support for his hypothesis comes from studies on phonation and articulation in stutterers. It has been found that initial sounds in words or syllables are stuttered on more than later sounds, and that final sounds are never stuttered (Froeschels, 1961). In addition, the first words of sentences tend to be stuttered on more frequently than later words in nearly all studies on the subject (Van Riper, 1971). Wingate (1969) attributes these points to the fact that "soundmaking" has been initiated after these first sounds and thus induces continuity of phonation. Recently, Adams and Reis (1971) tested 14 stutterers on their phonation abilities. They had the subjects read two passages, one composed of all-voiced sounds and the other of a combination of voiced and voiceless sounds. They found significantly less stuttering and more rapid adaptation of the all-voiced passage. The authors say this supports the hypothesis of a positive relationship between frequency of stuttering and the frequency with which phonatory adjustments must be made. The authors infer that the repetitions and prolongations exhibited by their subjects were a reflection of their difficulty in initiating, maintaining, and coordinating phonation with articulation in order to make fluent phonetic transitions. Stromstra's spectrographic findings, reported by Perkins (1977), showed repetitions and prolongations of stuttering children were often associated with abnormal, abrupt termination of phonation and that in those children exhibiting this trait, stuttering still existed 10 years later.

A study by Brenner et al. (1972) looked at stutterers' ability to recite 10-syllable sentences from memory after conditions of silent rehearsal, aloud rehearsal, lip rehearsal, whispered rehearsal, and no rehearsal. Aloud rehearsal yielded significantly fewer stutterings than any other condition. The authors state that vocalization is the only distinguishing feature between these conditions and therefore stutterers must have trouble coordinating phonation and articulation. They suggest that aloud rehearsal facilitates coordination of these functions, and they attribute the adaptation phenomenon to this fact. Finally, Wingate (1967), in explaining the stutterer's increased difficulty with longer and more unfamiliar words (Soderberg, 1966), suggests that these words are more diffiult because of their difficult or unfamiliar motor plan.

Early studies dealing with breathing irregularities fit well with the incoordination of speech production processes hypothesis. It is interesting to note that one study (Starbuck and Steer, 1953) found that the irregularities in the respiration of stutterers during speech decreased with adaptation in successive readings. As Brenner et al. (1972) explained adaptation as being due to rehearsal of articulatory and phonatory coordinations, so can this adaptation be explained as rehearsal of the coordination of the breathing for speech subprocess with the other subprocesses of speech production.

While I advocate the hypothesis that Michael's disfluencies per se are the result of an inherent constitutional weakness, there is reason to believe that operant conditioning may play a considerable role in the secondary (verbal and nonverbal speech modifiers) mannerisms so often associated with the disorder of stuttering. Brutten and Shoemaker (1967) recognize the application of instrumental conditioning principles to the secondary mannerisms found in stuttering. When an operant (a nonverbal speech modifier) is emitted and followed by reinforcement (a chance termination of a block), there is a greater likelihood of that response occurring again. Wischner (1952) talks about the operation of instrumental avoidance behaviors to avoid stuttering (although he states reinforcement is through the attendant anxiety reduction). Most of the research on the role of operant conditioning deals with the involuntary disfluencies per se and not the secondary mannerisms. However, as reported by Van Riper (1971), Webster did find that in one of his two subjects the word "wrong" used as contingent reinforcement during stuttering moments served to decrease "voluntary" stuttering behaviors (verbal/nonverbal speech modifiers).

In addition to the preceding, it has been found that many stutterers have fears of certain situations, certain words, etc. Van Riper (1971) reviews the literature and concludes that stuttering will increase in situations containing high communicative importance. Some studies have shown that stutterers will stutter less when alone than when in groups of two or more and that listeners evaluated as difficult to speak to elicit more stuttering (Porter, 1939). Also, several investigators have found significant relationships between the degree of expectancy to stutter on certain words and the stuttering on them (Knott et al., 1937; Johnson and Ainsworth, 1938). These effects can be accounted for in terms of learning theory—the more these situations or words are paired with stuttering, the more the stutterer will fear them.

Finally, it has been found by Rahman (reported by Van Riper, 1971) that the only real difference between a group of stutterers and their controls in his study was in the real self-concept relating to social interaction. The ideal self-concepts were the same in general. As reported by Van Riper (1971), Nelson found that stutterers tended to perceive themselves primarily in terms of their speech. These findings are in close agreement with Michael's statements concerning the effects stuttering has had on his social and personal life. These are difficult to find support for in the literature other than in statements of common sense. It is quite understandable that the stutterer's self-concept would be affected by his disorder, and therefore it is necessary to include this as an important aspect of the total problem.[*]

The preceding example demonstrated extensively the use of the literature to derive a clinical hypothesis.

The second example presents a clinical evaluation of test results in a manner that might appear in a clinical report. Test results are presented first. The constituent analysis from which the hypothesis was derived is not presented.

Testing and observation

Evelyn was seen on June 16 and June 30, 1969. On the first date, the *Peabody Picture Vocabulary Test* (PPVT), the *Templin-Darley Screening Test of Articulation,* a speech mechanism examination, and an audiometric test were administered. It was requested that Evelyn return for a dual speech and hearing

[*] Our appreciation is extended to Mrs. Karen Wolf for permission to include this material. Mrs. Wolf developed this support paper while a graduate student in the Department of Speech Communication, Case Western Reserve University, for a course in diagnosis-evaluation of communication disorders.

evaluation on June 30. On this date, further audiometric testing was done. Evelyn's speech and language abilities were also further investigated with pictures to elicit spontaneous speech and six subtests of the *Illinois Test of Psycholinguistic Abilities* (ITPA).

On the *Peabody Picture Vocabulary Test* (Form B) that was given to test vocabulary comprehension, Evelyn achieved a vocabulary age of 2 years, 8 months as compared to her chronological age of 5 years, 8 months.

On the 50-item screening test of the *Templin-Darley Screening Test of Articulation,* Evelyn produced five correct responses. The mean number of correct responses for 5-year-old girls is 40.6, and the cutoff point of inadequate performance is 31 correct items. Analysis of whole-word responses on the test showed the following basic pattern.

1. All stops were correctly produced in initial and medial positions but were sometimes omitted in a final position.
2. Substitutions or omissions of fricatives always occurred—the most frequent substitutions were /p/f, t/s/, and /t/ʃ/.
3. The two affricates, /tʃ/ and /dʒ/, were not produced but were substituted for by various sounds.
4. Of the four sounds, /l/, /w/, /j/, and /r/, the first two were usually produced, the third always had a substitute, and the fourth was produced correctly in the initial position only.
5. Nasal sounds were produced in appropriate positions, with /n/ and /ŋ/ usually omitted in a final position.
6. The "r-colored" vowel had no coloring.
7. In consonant clusters, blends of /s/ plus one or more consonants always had the /s/ omitted; blends of a consonant plus /r/ were usually produced as the consonant plus /w/; and a consonant followed by /l/ was usually produced correctly.

Attempts to modify the phonetic production using Milisen stimulability techniques resulted in some change from /p/ to /f/; /v/ was not produced; /θ/, could be approximated; and /ʃ/ and /s/ were not produced even with strong stimulation.

Little spontaneous speech (consisting mainly of naming) was elicited with situational pictures. During the administration of the *Illinois Test of Psycholinguistic Abilities,* a few spontaneous comments were produced; those that were longer than one word consisted mainly of vowels with many of the consonants omitted.

On the six subtests of the *Illinois Test of Psycholinguistic Abilities* that were given, the following age level scores were obtained: auditory reception, 3.3; visual reception, 4.1; visual sequential memory, 6.2; auditory sequential memory, 4.2; visual association, 2.4; verbal expression, 3.10.

A speech mechanism examination revealed no difficulty in producing movements with the articulators. Diadochokinetic rate was difficult to assess since Evelyn would not produce the syllables more than a few times.

The first audiometric testing found a pure tone air conduction threshold of 43 dB in both ears when the average was taken of 500, 1,000, and 2,000 Hz. Pure tone bone conduction thresholds with masking ranged from 5 to 15 dB in both ears. The second audiometric test found a pure tone air conduction average of 28 dB in the right and 27 dB in the left ear, with a masked bone conduction average of 8 dB in both ears. The speech reception threshold for the right ear was 20 dB and for the left it was 15 dB, with 100% discrimination at 50 dB. The examiners noticed that it was necessary to raise the loudness of their voices more on the first day Evelyn was seen than on the second.

Evelyn's responses to test stimuli were very softly spoken when she was first seen. She was a shy, quiet, well-behaved child who attended to the examiners but made no attempts to speak spontaneously. The second time she was seen, Evelyn was still highly cooperative but offered only a few spontaneous remarks toward the end of the testing session.

Clinical evaluation

Evelyn is a child with a language disorder that is severe and is complicated by visual, hearing, and environmental problems. The omission and substitution of consonants and the mixing of Spanish and English made Evelyn difficult to understand in what little speech she produced that was more than a one-word response.

Tests of comprehension and formulation of language (utilizing both visual and auditory channels) indicated language performance on an age level much lower than Evelyn's chronologic age. However, all of these scores may not be completely indicative of Evelyn's ability. When the *Peabody Picture Vocabulary Test* was administered, the examiner had to say the stimuli very loudly and more than once to elicit any response. Also, on the *Illinois Test of Psycholinguistic Abilities,* the examiner felt that Evelyn did not always understand the task in spite of repeated instructions; this was particularly true of the visual association subtest. On the one subtest—visual sequential memory—where Evelyn quickly understood what was expected of her and eagerly performed, the score was more commensurate with her chronologic age.

Even though the test results may not be a maximal reflection of Evelyn's ability, the language scores are so much lower than the norms for children of her age that it is doubtful that she will be able to achieve much success in verbal tasks when she enters the first grade in September.

Whether the lack of normal development in language was caused or merely complicated by respiratory infections and ear infections with resultant conductive hearing loss is difficult to determine. The bilingual home-school environment also is probably not aiding Evelyn's acquisition of either language.

As a third example we now present an abbreviated, somewhat abstract clinical evaluation on our demonstration client, Katherine Compardo.

Katherine Compardo demonstrates a severe language formulation disorder on all levels of language. The characteristics of her disorder would lead us to call it childhood aphasia, and in her case the concept of accompanying apraxia seems warranted. If this diagnosis is on target, the potential cause would reside in cerebral dysfunction that has significantly affected the language processing areas needed for formulating language.

Interestingly, Katherine exhibits a less comprehensive childhood aphasia than typically seen in that her comprehension skills seem relatively intact. Her understanding of language as reported by the mother and as observed during testing appear to be appropriate for her age. However, because it was difficult to maintain Katherine's attention to comprehension tasks, definitive test results are not available. More testing will be needed to gain greater security regarding the level of her comprehension skills.

It is Katherine's language formulation skills that are obviously quite limited for her age. This, of course, was the mother's report and was verified in the diagnosis. She has only a few words that are intelligible, the remainder of her speech output consists of certain stereotyped sound combinations. Other than this, she uses "gestures" to communicate. She uses nothing we would call a sentence, and children of her age should be talking in relatively complex sentence structures.

In Katherine's case we feel that her limited output cannot be explained just by calling it aphasia. She is having significant difficulty using the speech musculature. There may be some question about a concomitant dysarthria indicated by drooling and difficulty keeping food in her mouth, but there is little other evidence for this type of motor speech disorder. If dysarthria were the basis for her problem, we would expect more speech production output than we are seeing. Instead, we find it more useful to consider that Katherine has an accompanying apraxia, that is, difficulty with voluntary control of the speech musculature for speech production. She has little ability to control the use of the speech mechanism on command or in imitation even though we see similar behaviors performed involuntarily, for example, tongue protrusion. When she is asked to repeat speech sounds and words, there is some minimal modification but during testing it was negligible. If this "additional" component to the aphasia is present, it would better explain the severe limitations she demonstrates. Thus beyond her limitations of creating messages, she seems unable to program the motoric sequences needed to put speech sounds together.

Conditions such as Katherine's are characteristic of children who have been described as expressive aphasics and/or apraxics—a condition associated with cerebral dysfunction. In Katherine's case the suspected cerebral dysfunction is apparently congenital since no evidence is present to indicate any brain damage after birth. The only evidence currently available to support cerebral dysfunction as a causal factor is Katherine's history of language development, her current disorder of language, and the observations made of the use of the speech mechanism. Other than this, she demonstrates only mild behavioral signs that are sometimes used as indicative of cerebral dysfunction—the slight general incoordination and slow motor development, the distractibility, and the inability to attend to a directed task for a long period of time. These characteristics, however, all must be viewed in relationship to Katherine's age.

Even though additional information is needed we feel it is important at this time to consider Katherine as severely deviant in language formulation on all linguistic levels as a concomitant of childhood aphasia and apraxia.

SUMMARY

At this step of the diagnostic process the diagnostician offers his clinical evaluation, his diagnosis of the speech and language disorder and its probable causes. It is here that the diagnostician must pull together all that has gone before, using his funds of knowledge and problem-solving skill to arrive at his diagnosis. He achieves his clinical evaluation through interpretation of the clinical data in a process very similar to the development of the hypothesis. He uses all the information available prior to the contact with the client as well as the new information collected during the interview and diagnostic sessions. This step marks the culmination of the diagnostician's application of his professional skills.

At this step the diagnostician performs three tasks.

1. He *interprets the results of the clinical analysis.* This is the thinking process behind his diagnostic statement in which he synthesizes the information available and arrives at the most likely delimitation of the speech and language disorder and its probable causes.

2. After thinking through his interpretation, the diagnostician *states the di-*

agnosis. This becomes a succinct, formal statement of the client's disorder and the causes.

3. He finally *offers a clinical evaluation supporting the diagnosis*. Here the diagnostician offers his support or position for the diagnosis. He documents how he arrived at the diagnosis.

Having interpreted the clinical data and formulated the diagnosis, the diagnostician now will draw conclusions based on that diagnosis. This problem-solving road to diagnosis should lead to the best management of the problem. If the diagnostician has been unsuccessful in finding a best answer, he must begin again, adjusting his procedures and using his mistakes to discover a better answer to the problem.

CLIENT PROJECTS
Katherine Compardo

The information presented on Katherine Compardo throughout the steps of the diagnostic process plus the additional information developed by the student can now serve as a project for the clinical evaluation tasks. Interpret the findings from the clinical analysis, state the diagnosis, and develop a support paper that argues your position.

Previous clients

For each of the previous clients used throughout the steps of the diagnostic process we will now present the diagnosis arrived at. The student is to use the previous information they have gathered on these clients, match it to the diagnosis presented here, and develop an interpretation and support paper for each client that leads into these diagnostic statements.

William Gafford

Reverend Gafford has a severe voice problem characterized by low pitch, hoarseness, pitch breaks, and limited pitch range. The vocal characteristics are related in part to his current bilateral contact ulcers, but more importantly they are related to the vocal abuse that brought on the ulcers. The vocal abuse is characteristic of his habitual forceful use of the phonatory mechanism, using too low a habitual pitch, achieving loudness by tightening the muscles of the laryngeal area, and using hard glottal attacks. The condition is aggravated by constant throat clearing.

Isadore Alexander

Mr. Alexander presents a severe dysarthrophonia that has its basis in impaired neurologic functioning affecting all speech production processes. Strong evidence from the characteristic speech pattern suggests amyotrophic lateral sclerosis as the basis for the dysarthrophonia.

Derek Park

Derek Park has an articulation-resonation processing disorder resulting in deviant phonetic structure. His phoneme production is characterized primarily by hypernasality and nasal emission along with numerous other phoneme distortions. This disorder results rather directly from inadequate velopharyngeal closure and deviant dentition secondary to a repaired cleft of the primary and secondary palates.

Michael Durall

Mr. Durall manifests a prosody disorder characterized currently by prolongations, circumlocutions, and word modifiers. He also presents associated secondary mannerisms that assist him in maintaining the flow of speech, and he evidenced extreme tension in the speech musculature during his difficult speech periods. The onset of this disorder was in early childhood and has developed to its current status.

Marie Abadie

Marie Abadie demonstrates a nonfluent (Broca's) aphasia characterized by slow labored speech, lack of inflection, and lack of many functor words, particularly auxiliary verbs, word endings, and tense markers. This aphasia resulted from a cerebrovascular accident subsequent to the ligation of a left internal carotid artery aneurysm.

REFERENCES

Adams, M., and Reis, R., The influence of the onset of phonation on the frequency of stuttering. *J. Speech Hearing Res.,* **14,** 639-644 (1971).

Andrews, G., and Harris, M., *The Syndrome of Stuttering.* London: William Heineman, Ltd. (1964).

Aram, D. M., and Nation, J. E., Patterns of language behavior in children with developmental language disorders. *J. Speech Hearing Res.,* **18,** 229-241 (1975).

Aronson, A. E., Early motor unit disease masquerading as psychogenic breathy dysphonia: A clinical case presentation. *J. Speech Hearing Dis.,* **36,** 115-124 (1971).

Bankson, N. W., and Byrne, M. C., The relationship between missing teeth and selected consonant sounds. *J. Speech Hearing Dis.,* **27,** 341-348 (1962).

Berry, M. F., Developmental history of stuttering children. *J. Pediat.,* **12,** 209-217 (1938).

Bloodstein, O., A rating scale of conditions under which stuttering is reduced or absent. *J. Speech Hearing Dis.,* **15,** 29-36 (1950).

Bloodstein, O., The anticipatory struggle hypothesis: Implications of research on the variability of stuttering. *J. Speech Hearing Res.,* **15,** 487-499 (1972).

Brady, J. P., Studies on the metronome effect on stuttering. *Behav. Res. Ther.,* **7,** 197-204 (1969).

Brenner, N. C., Perkins, W. H., and Soderberg, G. A., The effect of rehearsal on frequency of stuttering. *J. Speech Hearing Res.,* **15,** 483-486 (1972).

Brutten, E. J., and Shoemaker, D. J., *The Modification of Stuttering.* Englewood Cliffs, N.J.: Prentice-Hall, Inc. (1967).

Carrow, M. A., Linguistic functioning of bilingual and monolingual children. *J. Speech Hearing Dis.,* **22,** 371-380 (1957).

Cherry, E. C., and Sayers, B. M., Experiments upon the total inhibition of stammering by external control, and some clinical results. *J. psychosom. Res.,* **1,** 233-246 (1956).

Darley, F. L., *Diagnosis and Appraisal of Communication Disorders.* Englewood Cliffs, N.J.: Prentice-Hall, Inc. (1964).

Darley, F. L., Aronson, A. E., and Brown, J. R., Clusters of deviant speech dimensions in the dysarthrias. *J. Speech Hearing Res.,* **12,** 462-496 (1969a).

Darley, F. L., Aronson, A. E., and Brown, J. R., Differential diagnostic patterns of dysarthria. *J. Speech Hearing Res.,* **12,** 246-269 (1969b).

Darley, F. L., Aronson, A. E., and Brown, J. R., *Motor Speech Disorders.* Philadelphia: W. B. Saunders Co. (1975).

Davis, J., and Blasdell, R., Perceptual strategies employed by normal-hearing and hearing-impaired children in the comprehension of sentences containing relative clauses. *J. Speech Hearing Res.,* **18,** 281-295 (1975).

De Hirsch, K., Jansky, J. J., and Langford, W. S., The oral language performance of premature children and controls. *J. Speech Hearing Dis.,* **29,** 60-69 (1964).

Dickson, S., Incipient stuttering and spontaneous remission of stuttered speech. *J. Commun. Dis.,* **4,** 99-110 (1971).

Farmakides, M. N., and Boone, D., Speech problems of patients with multiple sclerosis. *J. Speech Hearing Dis.,* **25,** 385-390 (1960).

Fisher, H. B., and Logemann, J. A., Objective evaluation of therapy for vocal nodules: A case report. *J. Speech Hearing Dis.,* **35,** 277-285 (1970).

Fransella, F., and Beech, H. R., An experimental analysis of the effect of rhythm on the speech of stutterers. *Behav. Res. Ther.,* **3,** 195-201 (1965).

Froeschels, E., New viewpoints on stuttering. *Folia Phoniatrica,* **13,** 187-201 (1961).

Garstecki, D. C., Borton, T. E., Stark, E. W., and Kennedy, B. T., Speech, language, and hearing problems in the Laurence-Moon-Biedl syndrome. *J. Speech Hearing Dis.,* **37,** 407-413 (1972).

Greene, M. C. L., Speech analysis of 263 cleft palate cases. *J. Speech Hearing Dis.,* **25,** 43-48 (1960).

Hardy, W., On language disorders in young children: A reorganization of thinking. *J. Speech Hearing Dis.,* **30,** 3-16 (1965).

Johnson, W., and Ainsworth, S., Studies in the psychology of stuttering: X, Constancy of loci of expectancy of stuttering. *J. Speech Dis.,* **3,** 101-104 (1938).

Johnson, W., Darley, F. L., and Spriestersbach, D. C., *Diagnostic Methods in Speech Pathology.* New York: Harper & Row, Publishers (1963).

Kent, R., and Netsell, R., A case study of an ataxic dysarthric: Cineradiographic and spectrographic observations. *J. Speech Hearing Dis.,* **40,** 115-134 (1975).

Knott, J. R., Johnson, W., and Webster, M., Studies in the psychology of stuttering: I, A quantitative evaluation of expectation of stuttering in relation to the occurence of stuttering. *J. Speech Dis.,* **2,** 20-22 (1937).

Korzybski, A., *Science and Sanity: An Introduction to Non-Aristotelian Systems and General Semantics.* (2nd ed.) Lancaster, Penn.: Science Press Printing Co. (1941).

Korzybski, A., *Selections from Science and Sanity.* Lakeville, Conn.: Institute of General Semantics (1948).

Morley, M. E., *Development and Disorders of Speech in Childhood.* Edinburgh: Churchill Livingstone (1957).

Nelson, E. E., Hunter, N., and Walter, M., Stuttering in twin types. *J. Speech Dis.,* **10,** 335-343 (1945).

Owens, E., Benedict, M., and Schubert, E. D., Consonant phonemic errors associated with pure-tone configurations and certain kinds of hearing impairment. *J. Speech Hearing Res.,* **15,** 308-322 (1972).

Perkins, W. H., *Speech Pathology.* (2nd ed.) St. Louis: The C. V. Mosby Co. (1977).

Pitzner, J. C., and Morris, H. L., Articulation skills and adequacy of breath pressure ratios of children with cleft palate. *J. Speech Hearing Dis.,* **31,** 26-40 (1966).

Porter, H. V. K., Studies in the psychology of stuttering: XIV, Stuttering phenomena in relation to size and personnel of audience. *J. Speech Dis.,* **4,** 323-333 (1939).

Ptacek, P. H., The evaluative process in speech pathology. In J. Akin, A. Goldberg, G. Meyer, and J. Stewart (Eds.), *Language Behavior: A Book of Readings in Communication.* The Hague: Mouton Publishers (1970).

Raph, J. B., Language and speech deficits in culturally disadvantaged children: Implications for the speech clinician. *J. Speech Hearing Dis.,* **32,** 203-214 (1967).

Rosenberg, P., Misdiagnosis of children with auditory problems. *J. Speech Hearing Dis.,* **31,** 279-282 (1966).

Sheehan, J. G., and Martyn, M. M., Stuttering and its disappearance. *J. Speech Hearing Res.,* **13,** 279-289 (1970).

Soderberg, G. A., The relations of stuttering to word length and word frequency. *J. Speech Hearing Res.,* **9,** 584-589 (1966).

Starbuck, H., and Steer, M. D., The adaptation effect in stuttering speech behavior and normal speech. *J. Speech Hearing Dis.,* **18,** 252-255 (1953).

Steer, M. D., Symptomatologies of young stutterers. *J. Speech Dis.,* **2,** 3-16 (1937).

Stein, L. K., and Curry, F. K. W., Childhood auditory agnosia. *J. Speech Hearing Dis.,* **33,** 361-370 (1968).

Van Riper, C., *The Nature of Stuttering.* Englewood Cliffs, N.J.: Prentice-Hall, Inc. (1971).

Vellutino, F. R., DeSetto, L., and Steger, J. A., Categorical judgment and the Wepman test of auditory discrimination. *J. Speech Hearing Dis.,* **37,** 252-257 (1972).

Weinberg, B., Dexter, R., and Horii, Y., Selected speech and fundamental frequency characteristics of patients with acromegaly. *J. Speech Hearing Dis.,* **40,** 253-259 (1975).

Wepman, J. M., Familial incidence in stammering. *J. Speech Dis.,* **4,** 199-204 (1939).

Wepman, J. M., *Auditory Discrimination Test, Manual of Directions.* Chicago: Language Research Associates (1958).

Wingate, M., Recovery from stuttering. *J. Speech Hearing Dis.,* **29,** 312-321 (1964).

Wingate, M., Sound and pattern in "artificial" fluency. *J. Speech Hearing Res.,* **12,** 677-686 (1969).

Wingate, M. E., Stuttering and word length. *J. Speech Hearing Res.,* **10,** 146-152 (1967).

Wischner, G. J., An experimental approach to expectancy and anxiety in stuttering behavior. *J. Speech Hearing Dis.,* **17,** 139-154 (1952).

Zisk, P. K., and Bialer, I., Speech and language problems in mongolism: A review of the literature. *J. Speech Hearing Dis.,* **32,** 228-241 (1967).

Chapter 17

Conclusions: management considerations, interpretive conference, and follow-up

This seventh step of the diagnostic process brings us full circle and returns us to Chapter 1. It is now the job of the diagnostician to fulfill the diagnostic purposes for the client complex. Since his ultimate concern is the client, the diagnostician must now present his conclusions about the speech and language disorder, its causes, and what he would propose be done about it to the client. The diagnostician must offer his solution to the problem. This step is the logical end result of all the diagnostician has done. The diagnostic process is not concluded until the diagnosis formulated in the previous step is translated into a management plan for the client.

This last step of the diagnostic process incorporates four tasks the diagnostician must perform: first, he determines the management plan; second, he holds an interpretive conference to discuss his diagnostic findings and management plans; third, he writes his reports; and fourth, he completes administrative follow-up.

CONCLUSIONS: HOW THEY ARE DONE
Information bases

In drawing his diagnostic conclusions, the diagnostician will need information from three sources: (1) the previous steps in the diagnostic process, (2) knowledge of management of speech and language disorders, and (3) knowledge and skill in communicating information.

Previous steps

In arriving at a management plan and imparting this information to the client and other professionals, the diagnostician is obviously dependent on the information gained in the previous steps. Management considerations follow from the clinical evaluation formulated in the previous step, which was possible, of course, only because of the steps that led up to it. From all these steps the diagnostician also gathers clues about the best way to present his diagnostic findings. For example, he uses what he has learned from the interview about the level of sophistication, insight, and concern of those with whom he will confer.

Management of speech and language disorders

As an information base for formulating management proposals, the diagnostician draws information from his general knowledge of disordered speech and language, his own expertise in treating various disorders, and his experience with health-related services available in the community. Management of clients with speech and language disorders and associated problems is the subject of a large body of literature, information the diagnostician must have but most of which is beyond the scope of this book.

Our focus here is on three general topics:

323

(1) therapeutic intervention, (2) prognosis, and (3) referrals. The diagnostician needs information in these areas to make management decisions.

Therapeutic intervention. Therapy information can be found in many books currently in use in our field either as general books in speech and language disorders (Berry and Eisenson, 1956; Dickson, 1974; Van Riper, 1972) or books specific to a single speech or language disorder (Boone, 1971; Eisenson, 1972; Van Riper, 1973; Winitz, 1969). Currently, our profession is gaining greater sophistication in the treatment of speech and language disorders. Diagnosticians must continually keep abreast of new information about therapeutic success to determine how and if the disorder they have diagnosed can be treated.

Approaches to therapy have been proposed, both of a general nature (applicable to many types of disorders) and of a specific nature (therapeutic techniques for a specific set of symptoms). For example, the disorder of stuttering seems to have lent itself to a wide range of treatment considerations, ranging from strict operant conditioning approaches for modifying specific bits of behavior to the psychiatric approach intended to help the stutterer understand the psychosexual and interpersonal basis for his stuttering behavior. The diagnostician must weigh these various alternatives to therapeutic intervention against what he knows about the effectiveness of each approach as well as what he knows about his client as a total person (Fig. 17-1). The diagnostician must also have knowledge of the specific procedures and techniques that could be recommended for any given problem he has diagnosed.

The personal characteristics of the client will temper the general approaches recommended. The diagnostician may have to offer specific modifications for the individual client. So the diagnostician must know what the literature reports about the use of a therapeutic approach with clients of different types. An example of this could be the specification of a therapy approach for a phonetic structure disorder with a 4-year-old child versus an 8-year-old child. Therefore a major area of knowledge needed by the diagnostician is a consideration of the general and specific therapeutic approaches that have been used for speech and language disorders.

Prognosis. Prognostic information is fundamental in choosing among the various management possibilities and planning their sequence. The diagnostician needs to know what procedures are required to *effect a change* in the client. No recommendations, no matter how assiduously carried out, will be of any value if the client cannot or will not change. Just because a problem exists does not always mean that something can be done about it.

THE WIZARD OF ID   By Parker and Hart

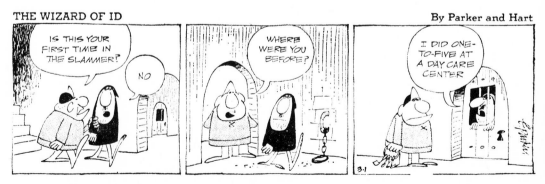

Fig. 17-1. Alternate management. (Courtesy John Hart and Field Enterprises, Inc.)

Twenty-eight-year-old Paxton, with an estimated IQ of 30, may very well be severely limited in his use of speech and language, but how likely is it that a change will result from direct therapy? Even if some improvement in communication (possibly through using a nonverbal system) may be brought about, does the amount of change justify the time and expense invested? Would a management plan other than therapy be more appropriate to the client's total needs and possibly bring about as much improvement as direct speech therapy? Few speech pathologists work in settings that can make therapy available to everyone, regardless of the probable prognosis. The diagnostician must determine who can benefit the most from therapy. At times prognostic decisions eliminate some clients from therapy considerations; those who have a low probability of change may be excluded from consideration if the degree of change would not offset time and money considerations. At the other extreme, some clients with a very favorable prognosis may not need special intervention.

What suggestions do Flower et al. (1967) offer regarding case selection for the mentally retarded?

Prognosis for better speech and language behavior is dependent on many factors, but one of the most important is the cause of the speech and language disorder. If the diagnostician is to predict changes in speech and language behavior, he has to view disorders in reference to their causal factors and not just the behavioral manifestations. Based on causal factors, the diagnostician knows that certain speech and language disorders are more amenable to change than others. For example, with children having developmental speech and language disorders the diagnostician may be on safe ground in prognosticating considerable improvement and even for some completely normal speech and language behavior. Maturation in these children con-

tributes considerably to the changes seen in speech and language. However, if the child is deaf or severely retarded, the prognosis will be far different.

Likewise, we know that adult aphasics can make changes in their speech and language, but they seldom achieve complete recovery of their premorbid skill level. Rather, recovery is dependent to a great extent on the site and extent of the cerebral lesion and the resulting pattern of language deficits and concomitant physical, psychological, and emotional problems. Physical processing causal factors relevant to prognosis are many, including the localization and extent of the lesion, status of the disease (static or progressive), and associated pathologies.

Even though they did not include the site and extent of brain injury in their variables, Keenan and Brassell (1974) provide clinical information about recovery from aphasia based on initial diagnostic statements of prognosis. How did they retroactively go about determining the effectiveness of their prognostications? What would you add to the factors that they felt were important influences on the judgments made about potential recovery?

Prognosis also depends on variables not related to disease that affect either the speech and language input or internal processing. For example, the age, intelligence, education, general health, emotional status, and motivation of the client as well as the attitude and resources of the family all affect the degree of improvement that can be expected.

The student should return to Chapters 7 and 8 and review causal factors associated with speech and language disorders. Which factors would you predict might allow for the best prognosis, which for the worst?

As more and more questions are asked about accountability for health services, the diagnostician must develop greater predictive measures. He must know what disorders are amenable to treatment and what a particular therapy plan will do for the client. Speech pathology has long been concerned with prognosis, but little has been done to develop measures that are predictive of change in speech and language behavior as a result of therapeutic intervention. The diagnostician needs to be able to predict what management plan will best facilitate change, that is, bring about the best prognosis. Is therapy the best plan alone or in conjunction with other treatment plans? For example, while the resonance and phonetic structure characteristics of a child with velopharyngeal insufficiency may be anticipated to improve, the diagnostician must decide which therapeutic plan will allow for maximal improvement. How much can be accomplished with speech therapy alone? At what point should surgical intervention intercede?

Develop a list of variables that have been considered as important prognostic indicators for the following speech and language disorders: stuttering in adults, phonologic/phonetic structure problems in elementary schoolchildren, adult aphasics, laryngectomees, "aphasic" children, and adults with voice disorders not associated with pathologic conditions. The following resources will be helpful: Cooper, 1973; Eisenson, 1972, 1973; Kleffner, 1973; Snidecor et al., 1962; Van Riper, 1972, 1973; Wilson, 1972.

Referrals. As a part of management planning the diagnostician must consider referrals to other professionals who will be helpful in the diagnosis and treatment of the client. Referrals for adjunct services are pursued for two basic reasons. First, referrals are often considered when the diagnostician needs more definitive information about causal factors. For example, if the diagnostician feels the speech and language disorder may be related to neurologic disease, he would refer the client for neurologic testing. Second, referrals are made if other professionals are needed in the treatment program. For example, a client may benefit from psychotherapy in addition to, or instead of, speech therapy. Referrals and interprofessional liasons are important considerations for proposing a management plan.

Referrals are made for psychological, neurologic, social work, educational, and other specialized medical services. Within these broad categories of services are embedded many specialists to whom referrals can be made. Because of these multidisciplinary needs, the diagnostician must have a broad knowledge of what specialties and agencies can assist in the management of a speech and language disorder. He must have access to the facilities in his community that can provide these services as either adjuncts to his own treatment or as primary treatment services. For example, the diagnostician has seen Kenneth who has a severe language disorder related to suspected mental retardation. The problem is exacerbated by parents who do not understand why Kenneth behaves as he does, and they feel guilty about his condition. To confirm his suspicions of mental retardation, the diagnostician referred the child to a psychologist for intelligence testing. Together with the psychologist, a management plan was formulated that included seeing Kenneth for language therapy, placing him in a special preschool for retarded children, and providing counseling for the parents by the psychologist. Many management plans involve joint rather than unilateral decisions. When several professionals are involved, the management plan needs to specify who does what and when. Only then can the treatment program be efficiently coordinated.

The diagnostician must make intelligent, informed referrals for these needed services. He must be well trained in recognizing what makes a specific referral the logical and correct thing to do. A referral should never be based on "it seems like a good idea." It should be made on the basis of positive, objective, and logical information. Therefore the diagnostician must know (1) when to refer for services, (2) to whom to refer, (3) what to expect from the referral, and (4) how to interpret the results obtained.

The following topics should be developed in detail for each potential referral service used by the diagnostician.

1. Referral for type of service: For example, the neurologic examination.

2. Criteria for referral—when to refer: This section should include the various types of behaviors observed, tests used, and any results of the diagnosis that indicate the need for the referral. For example, (a) the level of speech and language development could be indicative of mental retardation; (b) drooling a sign of a more generalized motor dysfunction; and (c) oververbalization a sign of emotional disturbance.

3. To whom referral should be made: From the preceding criteria this may be self-evident, but not always. For example, (a) for mental retardation, signs of emotional disturbance, or school failure, you may choose among the psychologist, the psychiatrist, or the educational specialist; or (b) for a child suspected of learning disabilities or minimal cerebral dysfunction, you may opt to refer to a pediatrician, a neurologist, a pediatric-neurologist, etc. Generally, in each community you will discover who works best with the various problems you see.

4. What to expect: Generally a report or telephone call is forthcoming, depending on the reporting practices of the referral. You should work toward obtaining the tests and observations made and how they were interpreted by the referral source. For example, what is done to determine intelligence?

5. Interpretation of results obtained: The interpretation for the referred problem will be done by the professional referred to; that is, if the referral was to determine intellectual abilities, this interpretation will be done. At times the referral person may relate his findings to the speech and language disorder. However, it is the task of the diagnostician to determine how the findings assist him in understanding the speech and language disorder and planning appropriate management.

• • •

In summary, the diagnostician must have in his repertoire an understanding of the total aspects of management of any given speech and language disorder or the means to obtain this information. He must be able to determine if therapeutic intervention is warranted, what effect therapy would have in modification of the disorder, and what other services may be indicated for resolution of the problem. In order to achieve his purpose of "solving" the speech and language problem, the diagnostician must have in his fund of knowledge information pertinent to the management alternatives for any given speech and language disorder.

Communication of information

As part of concluding the diagnostic process, the diagnostician will need information and skills that allow him to communicate his findings effectively. He must be able to transmit his information to the client complex in an interpersonal interaction, the interpretive conference, and also must share his findings in written form.

Interpretive conference. Communication of the diagnostic findings to the client is important. None of us, for example, like to leave a physician's office without an explanation of our illness or disease, its cause, and a plan for treatment. Client understanding of the problem fosters cooperation and trust. There is little likelihood that persons will act on advice if they do not understand and accept the information given them. The importance of communicating the diagnostic information to the client cannot be stressed too strongly.

Emerick (1969) and Marshall and Goldstein (1969, 1970) are among the few who have written about the actual imparting of diagnostic information. Most of the literature in our area concentrates on parental counseling (Derman and Mana-ster, 1967; Sander, 1959; Webster, 1966, 1968; Wood, 1948) and is directed toward helping parents understand the speech and language problems presented by their child while the child is undergoing therapy. For example, Webster (1966, 1968) discusses various counseling techniques for parents of children with speech and language disorders. Her emphasis is on helping parents work through their communication problems with the child to prevent interpersonal difficulties from occurring because the significance of the disorder is not understood. A resource book helpful for understanding the counseling process with parents of the ill and handicapped has been compiled by Noland (1971).

Conferencing shares with counseling the goal of helping clients define and cope with the facts of their problem. However, we see a distinction between the two processes. Counseling, for us, implies a process in which the person is helped to verbalize, explore, and alleviate his feelings regarding the communication problem, the emphasis here being the feelings of the person counseled. Thus, for us, counseling is a longer, more introspective process requiring considerable interpersonal commitment by all parties involved. Very little counseling, in this sense, can be achieved on a one-shot basis with a virtual stranger.

The interpretive conference, in contrast, emphasizes the transmission of information from the diagnostician to the client for the purpose of jointly arriving at a management plan. The interpretive conference is an interpersonal interaction; thus all that has been said regarding interpersonal relations during the interview applies equally here. As well, many counseling techniques are useful during the interpretive conference just as they were during the interview. As the interview was used to gather information about the problem, its causes, and what has been done about it, so the interpretive conference is used to impart information about the diag-

nostician's findings: the nature of the problem, its potential causes, and his proposed solution for it.

Of particular importance in the interpretive conference is how the diagnostician imparts information. The client, family members, or others came to the diagnostician in order to gain understanding and help with the speech and language problem. They are entitled not only to an evaluation, but also a clear, concise explanation of the diagnostic findings. The amount of information given during the interpretive conference varies depending on many variables, particularly the personal characteristics of the client complex. The information may vary from specific test findings to only a general impression of the problem. Whatever is presented must be presented clearly and concisely—the client must not be overwhelmed with information he cannot or does not want to handle at this time. The information of prime importance to impart is who is going to do what, when, and where.

It is often said that "comprehension precedes expression" in the acquisition of language. The same holds true for the diagnostician in the conference. Diagnostic information cannot be imparted to the parent in a comprehensible manner until it is thoroughly understood by the diagnostician. Too frequently, professional jargon replaces understanding. Everyday the diagnostician uses terms such as phonologic, motor programming, disinhibition, and minimal brain dysfunction. What he must understand is that most clients do not understand what these words mean. The diagnostician needs a clear, down-to-earth means of expressing these concepts. In a sense, he must be a "walking thesaurus" capable of clarifying and interpreting processes, products, and causal factors that may not be readily understood by others. The following example illustrates the significance of the diagnostician's use of terminology in regard to parental understanding of diagnostic information.

During a particular conference session, a

diagnostician related his findings to the mother of the child he had just tested. The diagnostician was quite thorough in his description of the child's problem, and his diagnosis seemed quite accurate: "Devin has a severe language formulation problem that is particularly evident on the phonologic level. His problem seems to represent a verbal apraxia that is probably part of the more general minimal brain damage that has been reported by the neurologist, Dr. Ecklemann." After giving this diagnosis, the diagnostician asked the mother if she had any questions; the mother responded that she did not. Fortunately, the diagnostician then added, "Now tell me what you will tell your husband about your child's problem when you go home." The mother's reply was quite inadequate, and after stumbling over a few sentences, she said, "I don't know." The diagnostician in this situation may have a clear understanding of the problem but did not use words that transmitted information to the mother.

The diagnostician must keep in mind how much of the information the client can absorb, how technical his terminology can be. He must develop a way of talking to clients that allows them to understand and act. Clients will want to know if the diagnostician saw the problem they saw, if it is a significant problem, if it can be changed, why it is there, and what they can do about it. The diagnostician must have some knowledge of the attitudes and beliefs of the client and his family if he is to present information they will use—an advantage gained by holding an interview prior to this time. For example, a mother who believes her son stutters because he was in a car accident—"he began to stutter after that"—may not be ready to accept any other explanation, especially one that includes an interpretation of her attitudes toward the child following the auto accident. The diagnostician may have discovered that her interactions with the child seemed based on guilt (she was responsible for the auto accident), and he may consider these interactions as the more significant variables. In his interpretive conference with this mother, the diagnostician may have to deal with causal factors on one level in the interpretive conference, using later counseling sessions to explore the mother's attitudes and feelings about her son's stuttering and the role she may be playing in its development.

Therefore the information base needed by the diagnostician should provide him with knowledge about holding interpretive conferences: what information to impart and the manner of imparting the information.

Report writing. Other than the interpretive conference the diagnostician's major form of communication is a written report. The written report serves as a "permanent" record to be used by various individuals involved with the client including the client and his family. These written reports take many forms from short summary letters to elaborate clinical reports containing much detailed information.

The style and format of the report may vary depending on the person to whom it is written. The professional's *clinical report,* as a part of the agency records, will be used by the professional who sees the client for services. This clinical report is usually quite detailed, specifying all components of the diagnosis that occurred and the recommendations made. This same report may be sent, as well, to certain of the referral sources, generally another professional involved with the client. At other times separate reports, usually much shorter, are sent to the referral source or other professionals. Abbreviated reports or short letters often become the primary means of reporting between experienced professionals who have knowledge of each other's work and rely on one another to be informed and objective.

Other types of written reports are also used. Sometimes a summary report is given to the parents of the child seen. This summary report may be completed at the time of the interpretive conference, giving the parent present the information to share with the absent parent, or they may use the report in further contacts they make with teachers, their physician, etc. At times, letters are written to the parents following the diagnostic session summarizing the findings and emphasizing the management plan that was worked out. This type of follow-up communication again serves as a record for them and gives them assurance that the diagnostician is still involved with them. Thus there are many ways to write reports, each facilitating communication in different ways. What is written on a medical chart in a hospital may vary significantly from the comprehensive clinical report written in a community speech and hearing agency. Many factors go into the decisions regarding the style and format of reports; however, there is one overriding concern; that is, the report must communicate the diagnostician's findings clearly.

The diagnostician can be taught and can teach by the reports he writes. In providing detailed information, the diagnostician can teach other interested professionals something about speech and language beyond the specific client's problem. Other professionals cannot evaluate the importance or validity of the diagnostician's findings if they know little or nothing about his area of expertise. To illustrate the teaching function of a clinical report, we can draw a reverse example. If a diagnostician receives a report from a physician who says that the EEG findings were abnormal and stops there, the diagnostician learns little. He would have to find out the meaning of these findings. If the physician had included information about how abnormality is determined and what abnormal findings may mean in terms of brain function, brain injury, etc., he then has taught the diagnostician something useful about his own profession. The diagnostician can do the same thing. When he says that speech is deviant, he says little. When he says speech behavior varies from normal in the following way . . . , he says much more and

provides the physician with a broader view of abnormal speech. Many examples could be provided about the teaching role of clinical reports.

We have found professional report writing to be among one of the most difficult skills to teach. It seems as if some students have the knack and others do not. However, writing reports helps to develop problem-solving discipline. By having to commit himself on paper, the student is forced to think through his interpretations carefully. Even if report writing will later become abbreviated, we feel it is important for students to first develop the skill of writing detailed clinical reports. If he initially learns to write thorough, exacting reports, he can always reduce their length when he becomes accomplished in the diagnostic process and has established himself as a diagnostician.

Clinical report writing should follow, quite naturally, the steps of the diagnostic process. As the researcher must communicate his findings through a well-reasoned research report, so the diagnostician must develop a well-reasoned clinical report. To this end, we believe that report writing can best be taught by learning how scientific papers are written; an article in a professional journal serves a parallel purpose to a clinical report. The report should indicate clearly the process the diagnostician has gone through to arrive at the diagnosis he is reporting. If the diagnostic process has been well thought out, the report will also be. If the diagnostician has developed a clear perspective about his client, it will be reflected in his report. We have presented many examples, projects, and demonstrations of what goes on in the diagnostic process, designed first to give the diagnostician a clear perspective on the client and his problems; however, they were also designed to give initial practice with some of the elements of report writing.

If report writing is difficult, it may stem from one of two reasons. First, and often the case, is that the diagnostician has not yet developed a clear perspective on the client and, second, that he truly has difficulty writing. In the first instance we would suggest going back over the information and clarifying it until the perspective develops and can be conveyed in written form. In the second instance the only recommendation that can be made is hard work, self-criticism, and write, write, write.

We do offer the following resources as assistance. We mentioned previously that learning how research articles are constructed and written is an important guide to clinical report writing. The article by Forscher and Wertz (1970) can serve as a useful guide. Several other sources are helpful. Hammond and Allen (1953) give extensive information about report writing geared for psychologists. Their ideas and suggestions are equally relevant to the speech pathologist. A comforting thought they discuss is the reality of the tediousness of report writing, and how it can be combatted. Chapter 16 suggested general semantics concepts as useful adjuncts for interpreting data and stating diagnoses. These concepts are especially pertinent to report writing. Science and semantics go hand in hand and assist the diagnostician in maintaining control over his reasoning processes, his use of observation, and control over his use of language. These ideas have been expressed by Ptacek (1970) as related to the diagnostic process and English and Lillywhite (1963) as related to report writing. Most recently a report writing handbook for students and clinicians has appeared (Knepflar, 1976).

Two other articles, besides being interesting and humorous, provide specific information on report-writing style. Moore (1969) and Jerger (1962) demonstrate via specific examples the poor writing seen in research literature and clinical reports with general rules for correcting these examples. Their emphasis is on clarity and brevity—two aspects of style everyone should hold on to. Because these two articles express similar ideas from different perspectives, because this coincides with our view that clinical and research reporting are comparable, and because we feel they express report writing ideas better than we could, these articles are reproduced in Appendix V.

Pannbacker (1975) draws on the articles by Jerger (1962) and Moore (1969) in her discussion of diagnostic report writing. What further insights does she offer?

Whenever a writer presents information about writing skills, he immediately runs the risk of having the reader say, "Why didn't you use these ideas more assiduously in your own work?" We are running the risk and own up to many instances of poor, unclear, complicated writing.

Diagnostician's tasks

In this last step the diagnostician must determine what to do about the disorder. When this step is finished, it is hoped that everyone will go home knowing what was done, what was said, and what is going to happen later.

To conclude the diagnosis the diagnostician performs four basic tasks. First, he determines the management plan that he will propose to the client. Second, he holds an interpretive conference with the client complex to present his findings and potential management plan and works out the details with the client. Third, he writes his reports for those who are to receive them. Fourth, he completes any administrative follow-up necessary to assure that action is taken and completed. When all these tasks are completed, the diagnostician can consider the diagnosis finished. Sometimes this closure is achieved within a few days; at other times it may take some months before the plans for management have been carried out.

Determines the management plan

After the diagnostician has completed his clinical evaluation, he determines his major management needs. The diagnostician must consider whether the speech and language variation/disorder truly constitutes a problem for either the client or someone else. If a problem is specified, a solution must be offered to the client, his family, or whoever referred him. Management alternatives must be considered by the diagnostician, not only the best management of the problem but also alternatives that consider the effect on the client and the practicality of the management plan.

The diagnostician asks himself four interrelated yes/no questions. Can the client change his disordered behavior? Is therapeutic intervention necessary to do so? Are referrals necessary? Is service available? Depending on his answers to these questions, he proceeds to think through the various management alternatives appropriate to the disorder, its causes, and the personal characteristics of the client. He develops a definitive plan of action to offer to the client during the interpretive conference.

Can the client change? Can the aphasic client alter his speech and language performance? Can the hypernasal child develop nonnasal speech production? Can the adolescent stutterer become fluent? Will the young child "outgrow" his phonologic errors? The diagnostician must know from his interpretation of the data what the prognosis for change in behavior might be. At times this prognostic information can be based specifically on his test results; the client was able to modify his behavior. At other times he will have to make prognostic judgments based on prior experience with clients who have demonstrated similar disorders or on the basis of what the literature tells him can be done with problems of this type. From this information the diagnostician should be able to answer the question: "Can the client change his speech and language disorder?"

If he answers yes to this prognosis question, he must organize the information that indicates the client can change for discussion with the client complex and for later use in writing his clinical report. If he answers no to the prognosis question, he must be prepared to discuss with the client complex why a speech and language therapy plan is not offered when a known disorder exists.

Are there any speech and language disorders you would not expect the client to change? What are the many variables that have to be considered to answer this prognosis question, such as the effects of maturation, length of time the problem has existed, and the severity of the disorder?

Of special significance to the diagnostician are the specific prognostic tools he has available that give direct evidence about a client's ability to change. He has a most valuable tool at his command, his own professional expertise. Work such as that by Van Demark et al. (1975) illustrates this point. They studied the ability of three measures of velopharyngeal competency to predict the need for further surgical management of the palate. Their interest was to reduce the instance of unnecessary speech therapy and indecision regarding the form of management needed. As a single measure, the best predictor of need for secondary palatal surgery of the three clinical tools studied was the articulation score as elicited by the examiner using the *Iowa Pressure Articulation Test* (Morris et al., 1961; Templin and Darley, 1969). The best overall predictor was the articulation score in combination with the lateral x-ray rating.

The student should return to the discussion about tools and procedures that provides information about "prognosis for change." What, actually, do these tools tell us? Do they predict overall change in the disorder? Do they predict success in amount of change? Are they related to recovery curves for specific speech and language tasks? How much can we predict from these tools about the overall ability of a client to alter his disorder? How much do the tools tell us, and how much does our knowledge about the disorder and its causes tell us?

The diagnostician's attitude about treatment for different types of speech and language disorders is crucial to the prognosis question. Since the diagnostician makes the recommendations, clients may receive treatment based only on his particular beliefs. For example, if a certain diagnostician does not believe that aphasics benefit from language therapy, will he recommend it? Treatment recommendations based on prognostic data, however, should make this diagnostician assume an attitude other than his own. Even if he does not believe aphasics improve significantly enough to warrant treatment, he should realize that other professionals do and make his recommendations based on other information rather than just his own bias. Client concern should be his interest.

■ Mr. Carl Baldwin, 45 years of age, has been a severe stutterer since childhood. Between the ages of 22 and 37 years, he has attempted therapy four different times with four different therapists using various methods for changing his stuttering. You have just seen him for diagnosis and now must decide if he is a candidate for therapy. Answer this first yes/no question: "Can the client change?" On what would you base your answer?

Insight into the client's personal characteristics and general attitude about changing his disorder is also vital in determining if the client can change.

Dr. Darrell Cook, speech pathologist at the Cleveland Hearing and Speech Center, offers the following remarks regarding his assessment of prognostic variables for clients who stutter.

Three variables that I believe I can begin to assess during the first interview have to do with the following matters: (1) acceptance of responsibility for change, (2) willingness to take risks in therapy interactions, and (3) awareness of patterns of avoidance and escape behaviors.

In regard to the first variable, I look for statements such as "I understand that there's a machine that will make me stop stuttering," or "My boss says I can't get ahead in the company unless I stop talking this way," or "She/he [referring to wife/mother, brother/boss, etc.] makes me stutter." Although there may be a grain of truth in each of these statements, I think that the person who is perceptive enough to see how he fits into the picture, in terms of what he does, how he feels, and how he must alter his behavior in order to modify the speech pattern, is the person who will probably be better able to accept clinical suggestions designed to alter his way of speaking.

In regard to risk taking, I usually have a more positive feeling about the client who will readily go along with an attempt at trying "three-bounce" or "easy prolongation" techniques with a minimum of overt resistance (that is, saying, "I don't see what good *that* will do!"), my assumption being that the client who does this has already put himself "into the hands" of a therapist and already perceives that the unlearning of the escape/avoidance behaviors entails a certain amount of openness, willingness to experiment, etc.

In regard to the third variable, self-awareness, I sometimes find that clients come to the first interview already sensitized to how they stutter. To be sure, where this level of understanding has not been reached, it must be taught. But where it is in evidence in a client not previously experienced in therapy, I believe it represents some level of ability at looking at the self objectively. If so, it would be a significant contributor to change.[*]

What are your reactions to these variables? Are they variables that can be measured directly? Could they be quantified?

Is therapy needed for change? If the diagnostician answers yes to this therapeutic intervention question, he must be prepared to tell the client complex that therapy is needed, why it is needed, what the client can expect from it, how often it may be needed, the length of the sessions, and even perhaps some of the tasks the client may be required to do. The objectives of the therapy should be proposed. If the client is a child, the parent's role in the therapeutic process should be made explicit, especially if parental counseling is to be incorporated into the therapeutic plan.

If the diagnostician answers no to the therapeutic intervention question when a problem is present, he will have to tell the client why therapy may not be warranted. Perhaps his evaluation of the prognostic question or the referral question provides his answers; that is, prognosis is too poor, or service is required elsewhere.

---

[*] From Cook, D., Personal communication. Cleveland: Cleveland Hearing and Speech Center (1975).

Knowing that the client can change his behavior and that therapy is needed, the diagnostician must work out his proposed therapy plan before offering it to the client. He must be well versed in alternate plans appropriate for any given speech and language disorder at any age. For example, not all problems of phonetic structure, phonology, stuttering, etc. are treated alike. He must be able to propose and recommend the best treatment plan for the specific client, suggesting an effective approach to the disorder. His plan may consider such factors as when to start, individual or group therapy, the number of times and length of sessions per week, the sequence of events needed including referrals, and the involvement of any members of the client complex. He may suggest a "wait-and-see" approach in cases where he feels maturation may be effective, putting the client in a "holding pattern" and recommending periodic reevaluations to assess again whether direct therapy is needed. This wait-and-see question arises quite frequently over certain problems seen in young children, frequently over the young child whose parents feel he stutters. For example, there is evidence that children do "outgrow" their stuttering or nonfluent speech patterns (Sheehan and Martyn, 1970; Young, 1975).

At times, at the conclusion of the initial diagnostic session, the diagnostician has little definitive information on which to base a diagnosis. He may be left with an alternate hypothesis, little information due to problems in carrying out his diagnostic plan, or a series of suspicions, hunches, and guesses. Therefore before instituting a particular intervention plan, he may recommend regular sessions designed primarily to uncover more information about the cause-effect relationship rather than as a treatment program. He must plan clearly what the intent of these sessions will be, what procedures he would like to follow to obtain the information of interest. These procedures can be therapeutic as well as diagnostic and have been referred to as "diagnostic therapy."

How did Hegrenes et al. (1970) devise therapeutic measures that assisted them in determining the causal basis for the client they discuss?

The diagnostician should plan the objectives of therapy and what changes might be expected if the therapeutic recommendations are carried out, another level of prognostication. He must make the client complex aware of their commitment for achieving the objectives of the proposed therapeutic plans. What is the outcome to be? Will it be complete eradication of the speech and language disorder; will it be movement toward more acceptable speech production; will it be movement toward increased interpersonal communicative abilities; will it allow the client to achieve his social and vocational objectives? How realistic are the recommendations made by the diagnostician in relationship to the personal goals of the client and his family? Are the hopes and expectations of the family the same as the diagnostician's view of what can be done about the disorder? Will they be ready to pursue the plans of action that are needed?

Therapy recommendations go far beyond the statement that therapy is needed. If an appropriate contract is to be established for therapeutic intervention, the diagnostician must develop the beginnings of the contract as realistically as possible. The client must not develop unrealistic expectations on the basis of recommendations made by the diagnostician. A contract entered into unrealistically is bound to result in failure, the diagnostician cannot deliver or the client cannot succeed. Thus the diagnostician must specify in his recommendations what is likely to be achieved and what cannot be accomplished. For example, he may be able to improve the intelligibility of a child with inadequate velopharyngeal closure, but he may not be able to decrease the amount of hypernasality.

Are referrals needed? If the diagnostician answers yes to the referral question, he and the client will want to know to whom to refer, how to refer, and what to expect from the referral source. He will have to explain the referral to the client complex in a way that they will be willing and able to follow through. If the referral is essential to understanding the problem and its cause, the referral should be stressed as needed before therapy begins or as soon after as possible. If the referral is to another specialty thought more suitable for the client's problem, then again, immediate referral is essential since the client may not be seen in speech and language therapy.

At certain times immediate referrals may not be too helpful and, in fact, may be premature. When some causal factors are obscure, quite historical, and no longer operating, and the diagnostician is assured that therapy can proceed without confirmation from another speciality, he may delay a referral until he feels more certain about its need. For example, if minimal cerebral dysfunction is suspected, even though little evidence has accrued, this might not be the best time to suggest a referral. It might be better to wait until the client responds to a therapy program—often a suspected brain-injured client is a rambunctious child who can be settled down during the therapy sessions. Or if the diagnostician feels the client complex is not ready to pursue a referral, he may not make an immediate referral. For example, the parents of a child just diagnosed as severely deviant in language development may not be ready to accept the diagnostician's suspicions of mental retardation. Therefore he may not make an immediate recommendation for psychological referral to the parents. He can pursue the referral once the child enters therapy for the language disorder and he has established a better relationship with the parents.

If the diagnostician answers "no" to the referral question, there is no referral planning necessary following the diagnosis unless the client asks for a "second-opinion" referral. In this case the diagnostician is obligated to assist the client in finding another diagnostician.

■ The following clients were seen for diagnosis in a community speech and hearing agency. A basic diagnostic statement is provided. From this statement consider an overall management plan including any referral needs.

1. Mrs. Silverman has severe aphasia (group IV on the *Minnesota Test for Differential Diagnosis of Aphasia*), resulting from a cerebrovascular accident 3 months ago.
2. Four-year-old David Hayes has severely unintelligible speech related to an extremely short lingual frenum.
3. Five-year-old August Hatten has a severe phonologic disorder possibly precipitated by temporary hearing losses associated with chronic middle ear infections since an early age. Habit strength and association with an older brother who also has a phonologic disorder are both considered as maintaining factors.
4. Karen Weiss has a severe speech production problem. There is little ability to initiate phonation or control the speech production mechanism. This disorder is directly due to the brain injury she sustained in an automobile accident.
5. Geoffrey, aged 4 years, 3 months, has a severe articulation problem accompanied by moderate to severe hypernasality and nasal emission resulting from inadequate velopharyngeal closure subsequent to a repaired cleft lip and palate.
6. James Catlow, aged 23 years, has an excessively high-pitched voice due to failure of the voice to change during puberty, at times referred to as "mutational falsetto."

Is service available? Many agencies providing speech and language services are unable to schedule immediate therapy for all clients who need it. There may be extensive waiting lists; in some school systems many children in the lower grades are automatically, by policy, excluded from service; in a rehabilitation unit priority may be given to the client with the more complicated problems.

When the demands exceed the supply, the agency must formulate ways of assisting the client whose problem has been diagnosed until such time as the therapeutic plan can be implemented. The sensitivity and policies of the agency become extremely important during this time, keeping in touch with the clients who are on waiting lists, giving them approximate times when service may be implemented, and finding ways to assist them while they are waiting for direct services. At times home programs or group programs can be of some assistance in the interim.

Besides the service availability of his own agency, the diagnostician must know the nitty-gritty of obtaining other needed community services. There are many practical interagency "in's and out's" he will need to learn with each specialty and agency. He must know what services and personnel are available and the quality, flexibility, location, and expense of the specific service. He must be able to mesh the requirements of the specific service agency with the client. Can the client afford the service? Can he get there at the times the service is offered—usually between 9:00 A.M. and 5:00 P.M.?

Unfortunately, adjunct professional services are sometimes limited within the community in which the diagnostician works. If the community has a wide range of health and educational services available, it is fortunate, and the client can probably get the management alternatives needed. However, in many instances the diagnostician is functioning in a limited-resource community. In these cases the recommended management alternatives may not exist, and the choices made by the diagnostician will need alteration. For example, there may be no special classes for the child with a significant learning disability accompanying his speech and language disorder. Therefore the diagnostician cannot refer to a special class unless the family is willing and able to send the child to a special school away from home or they are willing and able to move to a location where the services are available. When services considered important are not available, the diagnostician must work out management alternatives best suited to the circumstances of his community. There may be options available, although some of these may not be optimal.

One of the first things diagnosticians should do when they arrive in a new community, on a new job, is to develop a resource book on available community services including the exact name, address, and telephone number of the agency; the type of services generally and specifically provided; and the personnel of major contact. As a project, do this for your local hospital. What departments exist in the hospital that may provide you with services or that may refer clients to you for services?

■ From Katherine Compardo's clinical evaluation presented in Chapter 16 plus your own analysis and evaluation, develop a mangement plan for Katherine. Does she need therapy to change her level of language abilities? Are referrals necessary to help with overall diagnosis and management of Katherine? If so, to whom would you refer, and what would you expect from the referral?

Holds an interpretive conference

During the interpretive conference the diagnostician will want to accomplish at least two purposes. First, he aims to provide the client complex with a clear understanding of the speech and language problem and its probable causes. Second, he will want to explore the available management alternatives with them so that together they can decide on a management plan. In the interpretive conference the diagnostician and the client become a team, working toward understanding the nature and cause of the speech and language problem in order to effect an appropriate management plan—one with which everyone concerned can work comfortably with the knowledge that if it is put into effect, the client can make modifications in his speech and language behavior.

At the outset the diagnostician has to determine when to hold the interpretive conference. Is he to do it immediately following the diagnostic session, or will he schedule a separate appointment for the conference? There is no rule to apply to this situation. It depends solely on the complexity of the problem and the diagnostician's need for time. When the conference can be held at the end of the session, do so; when it cannot, inform the client complex that you need time to go over the results and if possible make an immediate appointment for the interpretive conference.

The diagnostician must have a plan of action. In imparting his diagnostic findings he can begin by summarizing the areas that were evaluated in a very general sense. "During the time we tested Don, we were looking at how well he understands and uses words and sentences." Then the diagnostician can mention the client's strengths, perhaps areas of relatively high performance, or if appropriate, behavior that facilitated testing. In any event, try to relate something positive about the testing session. "Our tests showed that Mary hears well. She is able to use her tongue, lips, and jaw very well to make speech sounds." Or "Don really worked hard during the session, even though some of the things I asked him to do were frustrating for him."

Following this general picture of strengths and weaknesses, continue into a description of the speech and language disorder, giving specific examples and possibly explaining specific test results. For example, "You remember the test on which Mary named pictures. That test showed us that Mary is not able to make all of the speech sounds that most 5-year-old girls make." After the detailed description of the disorder, the diagnostician will then want to resummarize the major points.

After describing the speech and language disorder, the diagnostician can then proceed to address the probable causes. Clients and their families usually seek a statement of cause. They may feel that a specific cause will relieve them of the responsibility for the problem or that a discovery of cause will indicate an immediate method of treatment to correct the defect. In the discussion of causation the diagnostician can encourage the client to review

his own attempts to account for the speech and language problem. While the diagnostician's statements surrounding the topic of cause and effect must be as accurate as possible, attitudes and comments should be directed more toward allowing the client complex an opportunity to bring out into the open their own thoughts on the subject, rather than simply presenting them with detailed causal information (Rheingold, 1945).

If the explanation offered by the client seems reasonable and constructive, the diagnostician should encourage exploration, leading to an accurate representation of causal factors. If the client's explanation is so divergent as to suggest misconception of the cause, then the diagnostician must discourage their belief and develop another approach to causation.

Oftentimes, implicating causal factors is a very sensitive subject in that it tends to precipitate more stress for the family. Revealing that the child's speech and language problem may be due to mental retardation, brain damage, or emotional disturbance may serve only to create anxiety and needless fears and adverse home reactions. Of course, if the child has not been examined or assessed by a psychologist, neurologist, or other medical personnel previous to the speech and language diagnosis and the diagnostician suspects causation that may require referrals or additional testing, then he has to work through the needs for a referral with the client complex. "We would like Don to be seen by the Mental Development Center for further testing so that we can get a better idea of his abilities in areas other than speech and language." "We would like to make an appointment for Mary to see a neurologist so that we can obtain additional information about some of the difficulties Mary is having moving her tongue. Once we have this information, it will help us in planning a therapy program for her." If the parent asks, for example, "Is Don mentally retarded?" then it is necessary to give the parent an honest and direct answer. "Most of Don's skills and behavior seem to be around the 2- to 3-year age level." If a previous diagnosis of mental retardation has been made and has been interpreted to the family, then refer to these findings. However, in discussing causal factors it is important to be aware of the parent's conception of the terms used. Frequently parents' knowledge about similarly diagnosed persons is the basis for their reactions to and acceptance of certain labels. For example, one mother, because of her severely retarded brother, considered all retarded children incapable of attaining any social or intellectual maturity. Her experience had lead her to consider "retarded" to be synonymous with "vegetable."

■ You have just seen Arthur, the son of Mr. and Mrs. Gregory Schwartz. Arthur is now 5 years old, but in all the testing and observation you did he performed at about the 3-year level. You also know, as reported by the psychologist, that Arthur is mentally retarded, a reliable reported IQ of 60. The parents do not yet know this, and the psychologist has recommended they not be told at this time. Apart from how you might handle that information, consider how you would discuss your findings with the parents. How will you discuss causal factors in response to their questions?

Many times it is not possible to report definitive causal factors. In such instances we find the concept of historical and contemporary causation a particularly useful way in which to approach a discussion of causal factors. For example, the diagnostician might say, "Mary does not produce many of her sounds clearly because she is having difficulty making her tongue move as she would like it to"—contemporary causation. Or "We are not sure exactly why Mary is having this difficulty with her tongue"—historical causation. Also, in interpreting causation, the diagnostician must keep in mind the multiple nature of causation, serial causation, direct and indirect interactions, and the other perspectives on causation discussed in Chapter 8. Translated into layman's terms, such perspectives are useful for the interpretive conference.

In describing the speech and language disorder and reporting probable causal factors, some diagnosticians find the use of a summary or profile form to be a useful device for making the information clear. A written summary for the parents aids in transmitting information and also provides the client with basic information for future reference. For example, a mother who goes home from the diagnosis and is asked by her husband, "What did they tell you?" will then have the summary available for discussion with her husband. A summary form can aid the diagnostician in conveying the whole picture and also can aid the person receiving the information in retaining the whole picture.

Bangs (1968) recommends the use of summary analysis charts in parent conferencing. The profile charts she discusses with the parents cover the specific areas of testing given the children before and during placement in their treatment program. Can a procedure similar to this be established for routine use in diagnosis of different types of speech and language disorders? How would you do this for children who stutter, have voice problems, or have phonologic disorders?

Beyond imparting diagnostic findings, the major purpose of the interpretive conference is to arrive at a management plan. The diagnostician enters the interpretive conference with a proposal for future steps to be taken, having considered prognostic factors, management alternatives, and practical considerations. The diagnostician, as the professional, brings with him his recommendations as to what he thinks would be the best plan and why. He offers a tentative solution to the problem. However, he tries to do this from the perspective of the client's total concerns and problems. For example, one client may be primarily concerned about his medical and physical treatments and consider speech a very low priority. Another client may have a strong desire to improve his speech despite the fact that the speech disorder is very minimal.

The diagnostician comes only with a proposal. During his interpretive conference any number of alterations in the plan may take place, depending on the reactions of the client complex to the plan or their ability to carry out the proposed plans. Thus the diagnostician must get used to having his optimal plans altered by the practicalities inserted by the client complex. They must be allowed to influence and contribute to the decision. If they are involved in the decision, they will be more likely to follow through and feel the plan is appropriate for them. At times the points that need to be reconciled are minor. Perhaps the timing for initiating therapy does not fit in exactly with their other plans or the client would prefer to try to find a therapist closer to his home than those suggested. At other times there may be considerable discrepancy between what the client complex believes or is ready to hear and what the diagnostician recommends. An example would be a child referred by his teacher because his speech is unintelligible to her, but the parents feel the child will "outgrow" the problem. The diagnostic findings, however, reveal a significant problem. In this case the diagnostician must help the parents understand the degree of the problem before they will be able to accept therapy as a needed solution. The diagnostician must know how to work this through in his interpretive conference.

In another instance the diagnostician may purposely recommend an alternate plan, paving the way to a more appropriate management solution. For example, Mrs. Eckelmann seemed to fear the possibility that her daughter Dorathy was retarded. However, she denied such feelings and rejected such a possibility. The diagnostician, however, also suspected retardation. Because he felt the parents would not follow through with a referral for psychological testing, he recommended immediate language therapy and parental counseling to help the parents understand Dorathy's problem. From this management plan hopefully would evolve a more appropriate treatment plan for Dorathy—a combination of professionals trained to work with all aspects of the retardation.

In still other instances, the diagnostician may alter his original plan for direct therapy during the interpretive conference. Early during the conference he may hold his recommendation for direct therapy while he assesses the family's understanding of the problem, what they may be able to carry out, and on this basis alter his original plan—an on-the-spot alteration that may serve the needs of all concerned better than direct therapy. This type of alteration is frequently considered when the problem seen has a strong maturational component—the child may well grow out of many of the speech and language behaviors given appropriate amounts and types of stimulation at home.

For example, Judi, 4 years of age, was seen for a stuttering problem. Her parents had been concerned since she was 2 years of age and had been advised to ignore it. However, the speech difficulty persisted and they brought Judi for diagnosis. Judi exhibited significant disfluencies in the form of rapid repetitions of sounds, words, and phrases, usually occurring at the beginning of an utterance. She became increasingly disfluent if asked to answer questions quickly or when not given a chance to respond. If the diagnostician ignored her, her verbal attempts to attract his attention were filled with nonfluencies. During the conference the diagnostician worked to help the parents understand Judi's specific difficulties, assessing their sensitivity to the problem and judging their ability to follow through with suggestions for creating easier communicative situations for Judi. Because of the parent's responses, the diagnostician made the decision to help them develop a program at home with periodic conferences to check on the progress being made. With other parents less able to understand and provide the desired environment, the diagnostician would have recommended a different management strategy, probably direct therapy accompanied by parent counseling. The point is that in the interpretive conference the diagnostician must make judgments about parents, their understanding of the problem, and their ability to follow through with general and specific management proposals. This requires finely tuned insight into clients and their families.

Dreher and Baltes (1973) recommend the use of bibliotherapy as an adjunct to treatment of speech and language disorders. They provide an annotated list of materials they feel will be useful. Can reading materials be developed and distributed to clients and their families as part of the recommendations given for management of the speech and language problem? Review the material presented by Dreher and Baltes as an initial source of such information.

■ The following dialogue is an example of an interpretive conference with Mrs. Russo, whose 5½-year-old son Jack has just been seen for a speech and language diagnosis. Evaluate the diagnostician's comments and approach in terms of the information reported, the appropriateness of the language used, and the sensitivity to the mother. What aspects would you emulate? What would you change? Keep in mind that many of the points discussed are related to a number of questions and comments posed by the mother in the history form and the interview.

D: We want to share with you what we did with Jack and to try to help you understand what kinds of problems he is having with speech and language. What I would like to do now is give you the findings of our testing with Jack, and then we can discuss the next steps we want to take.

Please stop me at any time if you do not understand what I am saying or if you have additional questions.

My first purpose is to help you understand Jack's problem as we see it. This will be our first step in working together on his problems. Roughly, what we did was give him a number of tests that helped us to find out how he is understanding and using language. What we generally found was that Jack's understanding and use of language is at about the 2- or 3-year level.

Sometimes we see children whose understanding is at one level and their expression is at another level. This was not particularly true for Jack. Both his understanding and his expression were at about the same level. We also gave him some other tests to see how well he can produce different kinds of sounds—the types of sounds that we use in words. He had a minor problem with making the different sounds correctly, but for the most part, he is able to produce the correct sounds in easy situations.

Mrs. R: Well then, why do I have trouble understanding him?

D: Sometimes in conversational speech his ability to produce sounds is not as good as his use in single words. The test we gave him used single words, but he does not maintain his level of intelligibility when the words are together in everyday conversational speech. Although in conversation his speech is difficult to understand, in comparison to his other language skills, his ability to produce all the different sounds in single words was really relatively good. But we will also be concerned about working to improve his ability to make sounds correctly in connected speech. The nice thing we know is that he is very, what we call, stimulable. That is, I say a sound and he can sometimes imitate it back to me. If I say /p/ and he says /p/ after me, that is a favorable sign meaning that he can change the way he makes his sounds and with some help will be able to produce them all by himself.

We did attempt to look at how Jack lifted his tongue and produced the motor movements for speech, but as you know Jack just had a tooth out and was not too anxious to have us looking in his mouth.

But the fact that he can produce so many sounds, that is, his articulation is relatively good, indicates to us that he is probably able to use his tongue correctly and is having no problems lifting it or moving it. For example, he can make the t, d, n, and l sounds that require him to put his tongue tip to the top of his mouth like this [demonstration].

So, essentially, what we see is that Jack's ability to understand and use both single words and connected speech is what we would expect from a child of about 2 to 3 years of age.

I thought you might be interested in looking at some of the language tests that we gave Jack to show you briefly the kinds of things we did and the kinds of tasks Jack had problems with.

In terms of his understanding of language, the first thing we looked at was his ability to understand single words, like a vocabulary test. We would say one word and he would have to point to it [Mrs. Russo shown the *Peabody Picture Vocabulary Test*]. For instance on this page we would say ball and he would point to it. Here we presented him with one single word—usually this kind of task is easier for children to do than to understand longer sentences. On this test he scored at about the 2½-year age level. Then we gave Jack a second test where the language becomes longer and he has to listen to connected speech and choose the correct picture [Mrs. Russo shown the *Assessment of Children's Language Comprehension*]. For example, the phrase "horse standing," requires Jack to listen to both parts—if he listens to just the last word, he might point to "bird standing." The speech continues to get longer and longer. All through this test he was at about the 2- to 3-year level.

In terms of his use of speech, we had him name pictures to see what level his expressive vocabulary was [Mrs. Russo shown the *Vocabulary Usage Test*]. For example, he would see a picture like this, and we would say "This is a _____." Jack would have to fill in the right words from what he saw in the picture. Here we were looking at his expressive vocabulary and on this test he scored at the 2½-year age level.

Then we listened to his conversational use of speech. Here we found that he used two words together and occasionally three words. This is not what we would expect of a 5-year-old child. Again, it is more like a 2- or 3-year-old child.

Do you have any questions so far?

Mrs. R: Jack does seem quite slow for his age, but will he ever catch up or will he always be slow.

D: We can never really predict when a child is as young as Jack how much progress he will make. We do know that he is going to change, that he is going to learn more. How much we cannot be sure. I would expect his ability to produce sounds is going to show quite a bit of improvement since we know that he is able to produce them correctly with help. Now in terms of the level of his understanding and use of language we are really not sure how far he may go. Most children by 5 years of age have acquired most of their basic sentence structure. So since Jack has been slow all along, he may continue to put more words together. It will not be like catching up with children who do not have problems, but he will be able to understand and say more than he is now.

Mrs. R: I knew Jack was slow but never wanted to find out why. I was afraid he was retarded.

D: I did want to talk with you about the reasons for Jack's slow use of speech and language. There are a number of factors to consider. One of these factors is a possible hearing problem. But you have never noticed a problem with hearing, and we did not suspect any when we were working with Jack.

You just mentioned another major factor why children are slow, like Jack, in developing speech and language. You indicated that you were afraid Jack was retarded. That is a factor we will want to look at carefully with Jack—his general level of mental growth. Here are some things we may want to look for. Are all of his skills at one level, or are speech and language skills reduced more than his other skills? In other words, we are interested in whether Jack is having more problems with language than with other nonlanguage areas—for example, his ability to put puzzle pieces together, his ability to color, his ability to do self-help activities such as dressing and undressing—things that do not require speech and language. What we will want to assess are the other areas of mental growth; language is only one area. Sometimes we find children where this is the only problem; sometimes there are children who have problems in a number of areas. So this is an additional area where we would like to do some more testing. We would like to schedule Jack for a more thorough psychological evaluation—to see if just his speech and language are reduced or if other areas are also at a lower level.

NOTE: At this point the diagnostician and Mrs. Russo have information about some of Jack's overall abilities and skills beyond speech and language. A decision here could be made to work through with Mrs. Russo some of that information, depending on how Mrs. Russo is reacting and how much she might need or want to know at this time rather than waiting for a referral. In interpretive conferencing the diagnostician has to decide how much to reinforce a possible causal factor.

Mrs. R: Will you do this, or will I go somewhere else?

D: It could be handled either way. We have a clinical psychologist here to do psychological testing, or we could refer you elsewhere. What would you prefer?

Mrs. R: Either way.

D: I think it would be best then for us to do it. We have all the information here, and after testing is completed it would be easier for all of us to get together.

Mrs. R: Will you be placing Jack in speech therapy now?

D: I think we will wait to decide that. There are a number of things we might do, but first we should have the results from the psychologist. After testing is finished, you, the psychologist, and I will work out the best plan for Jack. I know that you are anxious to get started, so let's go down to the scheduling office and work out a time that you can bring Jack for the psychological testing. If possible, it would be a good idea for your husband to come.

■ The following is a partial set of diagnostic findings on Lee Newton, aged 5 years, 5 months. Two hypothetical Mrs. Newtons are described. From this information consider what might be the major differences in your approach to the interpretive conference with these two mothers.

Mrs. Newton I

Mrs. Newton is a middle-class housewife who is concerned about her adequacy as a mother. Mr. Newton tends to blame his wife for Lee's impulsive, occasionally unmanageable behavior, claiming that if she knew how to manage him, Lee would not have all of his current problems. She fears that Lee may be retarded and is very concerned about the "cause" of his behavior and language problems; however, she attempts to present Lee in the most favorable light and to minimize his difficulties. Although Mr. Newton makes an adequate salary to support his family, the family has felt the effects of inflation and has not had much money for nonessentials. While willing to do whatever is necessary for Lee, Mrs. Newton is worried about the cost of the evaluation and possible therapy, about which she has no information.

Mrs. Newton II

Mrs. Newton is a lower-class mother who communicates her information and impressions about Lee through a "restricted language code." While she knows Lee is not "stupid," she has little knowledge of other factors contributing to speech and language functioning. While her understanding of Lee's problem is limited, she very much wants to do whatever is best for him.

Partial diagnostic findings

Templin-Darley Screening Test of Articulation: raw score—25 correct; norm—34.7; cutoff—31

ERRORS: /w/r and d/ð/ initially and medially; /w/l, b/v, f/θ/ initially; /f/θ/ in the final position; /w/ substituted for /r/ and /l/ in /spr, br, tr, kr, gr, fr, θr, skr, ʃr, pl, kl, fl, and spl/

ADDITIONAL ERRORS: noted in spontaneous speech—/s/t and t/s/ inconsistently in the initial position; /d/l/ in medial positions

STIMULABILITY: /d, t, and θ/ produced correctly in nonsense syllables but not words; /v, l, and r/ not produced correctly

Peabody Picture Vocabulary Test: 2-year, 9-month age level (chronologic age is 5 years, 5 months)

Preschool language profile: pointed to four body parts (24 months); obeyed five of seven simple commands (24+ months); correctly identified eight pictures (21 months); comprehended three of five prepositions (32 months); comprehended two of five questions (39 to 42 months); pointed to two of four pictures that answered questions (less than 36 months); expressively named four of four objects (30 months); named six of ten picture objects and pointed to two others (30 months); responded to pictures with one or two words; on the action agent test answered eight of twenty questions (3-year-old answers 60% to 70% correctly); told sex (30 to 36 months); named one of four colors (norm for all four is 5 years of age)

Hearing testing: audiometric sweep test attempted at 15 dB from 250 to 8,000 Hz; ring-drop toy used as a conditioning device, but responses obtained in this manner were erratic; thresholds varied as much as 50 dB; however, Lee did respond to several low-intensity tones at most frequencies, when became restless after 15 to 20 minutes, testing discontinued

Recommendations

1. Additional nonverbal psychological testing
2. Social service referral to learn more about management factors at home
3. Additional hearing testing

■ Now, plan your interpretive conference about Katherine with Mrs. Compardo. A referral to a pediatric neurologist should be included in the plan. How will you explain Katherine's disorder and its causes? How much information do you feel Mrs. Compardo will be able to handle? Could you just describe the language behavior and make a referral? Does she not already have a clear understanding of how well

Katherine uses language? Will you schedule language therapy without the results of the referral? Consider two approaches for your conference: first, an approach where you describe speech and language of aphasic children; second, an approach where you want causal information to come from the referral.

At this time you may be interested in what such a referral might tell you. We are including here an example of a report that might have been received from the pediatric neurologist. What additional information did this referral give you? What additional information will it give Mrs. Compardo? Will the causal factor be clarified for her? This information is provided now for your understanding of what to expect from a referral; the information cannot be used during your interpretive conference with Mrs. Compardo, since it would not yet be available to you.

I saw Katherine Compardo on November 4, 1974. This 2-year, 8-month-old girl has a major problem with delayed speech and a secondary problem of poor gait. According to Mrs. Compardo, her language development is significantly delayed. She still does not talk in more than a few single words or two-word phrases, and the only one she uses consistently is "Here, Ma." Most of the rest of her speech is an occasional portion of a word, and the mother can name maybe six or eight such words and that is the sum extent of expressive language. Mother states she understands everything including two-stage commands. And yet, she does not seem to understand too well in conversation, though one cannot be absolutely sure about this. However, single objects are fairly well understood. She knows more than four body parts, recognized many objects in excess of 50 by name, but still does not point to objects in books. She has poor concentration and does not play for long. She sits close when watching TV and seems to enjoy it.

She was born following a full-term pregnancy. The mother was in labor 3½ hours and had a normal delivery under spinal anesthesia. Birth weight was 8 pounds. Sucking and swallowing were normal, and she was nursed for 3 months. She walked at 14 months. Mother keeps going back to the fact that the child did not cry right from the beginning, that she babbled and cooed little, and that at 3 to 4 months her laugh was most peculiar and unusual. There is no other significant language disability in this family.

Physical examination showed a pleasant-looking youngster with head circumference of 47 cm. The child was irritable and would not concentrate on anything for long. I did not hear any language except a few noises. During periods when she was more friendly, she would look at me, copy all my gestures, mimic facial grimacing, and copy my examination. It is quite clear that this child understands a good deal more by the visual route than any other. With language, she was able to comprehend a fair amount, carry out one-stage commands, and point to some objects, but she soon lost concentration. Her play was repetitive with little concentration and not much imagination. She would carry the doll around and throw it about without any apparent awareness of what she was doing with it.

The eye movements are full, and funduscopic examination was normal. The discs and maculae are unremarkable. Hearing is grossly normal and was not tested further. There is no facial asymmetry. She has no difficulty protruding her tongue and licks a lollipop without much problem. Her motor strength seems unimpaired, the reflexes are symmetric, and plantar flexion is normal.

The mother had a question about an additional problem, namely, poor gait for which she has seen an orthopedic surgeon. I noticed some toeing-in but no serious difficulty here.

This child has a very definite and significant expressive and probably receptive language disorder. I think she would fall into the category of what I would call "moderate developmental language delay" (receptive and expressive aphasia being less good terms for this). There is nothing evident in the neurologic examination that accounts for this. We will schedule an EEG and look into it. Speech therapy plus nursery school are going to be very important for this young lady. The speech pathologist indicated to me in a conversation that comprehension is apparently age level. There is a question on their part about apraxia, but I think that most of what she is showing now represents the expressive language difficulty. There is no doubt that the observation of possible apraxia could be relevant, because as the years go by, we do find that many of these children do show other disorders of learning including significant sensory disorders and perceptual disorders as well as some motor difficulties that are easier to examine at that time. I will let you know the result of the EEG and will also be discussing the management further with the speech pathologist. I thank you for the referral.

Writes his reports

The diagnostician must now record his diagnosis in some written form or in a number of written forms depending on where the information is to go. At the very least, he must record his diagnosis on the clinical report that stays with his agency. Because of the many purposes for writing reports, the diversity of settings in which diagnosticians work, the many different referral sources, and the policies and practices about report writing dictated by agencies, specification of how to construct reports is difficult if at all possible. However, guidelines can be offered. Generally, regardless of the format of the report or to whom it is written, it will include information about the statement of the problem, what was done in the diagnostic session, an interpretation of the findings, and what is to be done about the problem. Following these general guidelines, a number of formats for structuring clinical reports have been offered (Emerick and Hatten, 1974; Johnson et al., 1963; Knepflar, 1976; Sanders, 1972).

Reports must be organized and written for the reader, whoever he may be. The diagnostician must develop a report-writing style that allows each reader to find what he wants quickly. But there may be many readers for each report or the need to write a number of different reports for each client. There is a point of practicality that must be entertained; that is, how many reports can a diagnostician be expected to write for any given client seen for services? Therefore we advocate the use of a single, rather comprehensive clinical report that can be readily adapted for sending to various involved individuals but that has as its primary function use within the diagnostician's agency. This comprehensive clinical report serves as a resource document about the client at the time he was initially seen. We believe it essential that students in training be taught this method of report writing before moving on to others.

The format that we are presenting is not unlike other formats; however, we are tying the sections of the report to the steps of the diagnostic process, indicating the general nature of the information to be included within each section. The sections should stand relatively independent from each other; that is, each section can be read as a separate unit. The most vital component of this report is the clinical evaluation section. This section should provide a relatively complete summary of the diagnostician's interpretation of the problem and his reasons for his diagnosis. It can be written in a deductive fashion, stating the diagnosis and then how and why it was arrived at. Once it is clearly written, it serves as a practical device in that it can be sent as it is to certain individuals or easily adapted for others.

The following is a suggested format for constructing a clinical report. The heading titles are suggestive, and exactly how information is ordered and discussed in each section is dependent on the client and the type of problem. Some sections could be collapsed into larger units if needed. At the left are indicated the steps of the diagnostic process from which information is applicable to each of the sections of the report.

Following this format a clinical report becomes similar to a research article. If presented this way, the report allows the reader to make judgments about the nature and quality of the diagnosis that took place. The reader can review the information presented, make his own interpretations, accept or reject the diagnostician's conclusions, ask for more information, etc. A report written this way does not demand that the reader be accepting of the diagnostician's findings, only that he give careful consideration to how the diagnostician went about the diagnosis and how he arrived at his interpretation of the data. A clinical report of this type is an open communication rather than a closed communication. It is open to other interpretations; it does not unequivocally state this is the disorder, and this is what should be done about it. The clinical report should invite other considerations; it should open doors for clinical interpretation and new insights, rather than close the avenues of further communication. Our interest is client concern, not unchallenged diagnoses.

We have included an appendix (Appendix VI) that amplifies report writing by presenting examples of information that might be included in each of the sections of the format. As well, Appendix VI includes samples of reports written to parents, adapted from the clinical report. Keep in mind that these examples are out of context with the remainder of the report.

One additional general comment about

Steps of the diagnostic process	Sections of the clinical report
CONSTITUENT ANALYSIS	*Section I: Identification information* This is usually prescribed in standard form by the agency and includes such items as name, address, and agency number.
CONSTITUENT ANALYSIS	*Section II: Statement of the problem* This is the client's, not the diagnostician's, statement of the problem as well as any that have come from the referral sources. The information here gives the reader a clear idea of how people involved with the client have viewed the problem and the sequence of events that led to the referral. Keep in mind that the reason for referral and the statement of the problem may not be the same, and different sources report them differently. What is wanted in this section is a clear statement of how the problem is seen and how the client came to you.
CONSTITUENT ANALYSIS CLINICAL HYPOTHESIS	*Section III: Background history* This section can become quite lengthy depending on what information is included. What is used comes from information available prior to the diagnosis as well as certain information gathered during the interview. Basically, the history information that is most directly relevant to the problem should be included. The information should be ordered by topic and sequence—it is time-dimension reporting. It can be structured according to such topics as presented on the children's case history questionnaire or any topics suitable to the client. A guideline for inclusion is to use that information that will be needed for the clinical evaluation. Remember that this information has been used to derive the clinical hypothesis, which included a determination of the significance of the information. Thus information in this section can be presented in light of its relevance to the overall clinical problem as long as *all* relevant information is presented. This comment is not meant as a license for including only that which supports your conclusions; it is a license for pertinency. Generally, the diagnostician's hypothesis is not included in a report as we have previously discussed. But a case could be made for including it in some instances, and if so, it would most logically appear at the end of the history section, perhaps as stated in the following example: "This history led us to believe that Mr. Goldstein was exhibiting a severe dysarthria related to his diagnosed neurologic disease, multiple sclerosis."
CLINICAL TOOLS DATA COLLECTION DATA ANALYSIS	*Section IV: Testing and observation* This section would include all the procedures that were used, the results of the procedures, and the analysis of the data—the objectification of what took place during the diagnostic session. This, too, could become quite a lengthy section depending on how much was included and how it is structured. We recommend basic information be provided in the report and not all the details of the analysis. The emphasis should be summary analyses rather than reporting all the raw data, again depending on the nature of the problem. This section could be ordered test by test in the sequence in which they were given; however, this would be a test-oriented report rather than a client-oriented report. Instead, we suggest ordering the testing under umbrella headings and reporting appropriate information within these headings regardless of the sequence in which they occurred unless, of course, sequential reporting is indicated. We would recommend using a processing system for ordering the results. The broad headings of reception, comprehension, formulation, and production could be used as needed. Within each, the tools that are appropriate could be discussed, reporting the results in product and behavioral correlate terms. In this section a general statement of the client's reactions to the diagnostic session could be included. It can be placed at the beginning of the section so the reader gets immediate knowledge about the effects of the client's behavior on the test results.

Continued.

Steps of the diagnostic process	Sections of the clinical report

CLINICAL
EVALUATION
	Section V: Clinical evaluation
	   In this section the diagnostician draws together all the information into a summary interpretation. He presents his diagnostic interpretation and offers his support from the history and his testing. This can be done in a deductive manner, starting out with a diagnostic statement and then providing the evidence for the diagnosis. The criteria for this section is: can it stand alone and be read as a "report"? We consider this section to be the most vital of all the sections; it requires considerable writing skill.
	
	Section VI: Diagnostic statement
	   This section is included only for the convenience of the reader. It can be located quickly to obtain an immediate statement of the diagnostician's findings.

CONCLUSIONS	*Section VII: Recommendation* This section states as succinctly as possible the management proposal for the client, including any practical considerations for carrying out the management plan. It should not be just a statement of what the diagnostician recommends but rather it should let the reader know who is to do what, when, and where.

report writing seems unavoidable. The diagnostician must be sure to edit and proofread the final copy once it is typed. This last step, although tedious, serves as a fresh look at what has been written and corrects any number of errors that may occur in the typing process.

■ Now that all the information has been considered for Katherine Compardo, the student should plan and write a clinical report. Since a referral has been recommended for Katherine, we would suggest that a parental letter (report) also be written. These we have found to be especially useful when follow-up beyond therapy scheduling is indicated.

Completes administrative follow-up

In Chapter 10 the administrative aspects of the diagnostic process including follow-up were discussed. The diagnostician basically has two roles to play in follow-up. First, he must make sure that all management decisions are carried out or, if not, why they will not be followed through. Second, he will have some function to play in record keeping, of which his clinical reports are one part.

The diagnostician's job is not completed until he knows the final disposition of his client. This means careful and consistent follow-up. Once again, setting demands often dictate the nature of follow-up responsibilities. If the therapy recommended is done in the same setting as the diagnosis and by the staff member who has done the diagnosis, then it is a matter of scheduling the client for therapy as soon as the professional has an opening in his schedule. If there is a long waiting list, the diagnostician should feel obligated to refer the client elsewhere if other services are available. If this is not feasible nor desired by the client, the diagnostician must make the client aware of how long he may have to wait for therapy services. In the meantime the diagnostician might put the client on a once-a-month visit to do a quick check of progress, offering suggestions for things to do while waiting. A periodic telephone call to the client may also help him during this waiting period. Many clients are lost because contact by the agency is not forthcoming.

The diagnostician should keep a logbook on each client seen and the disposition of that client. Even if scheduling in the agency is done by the administrative support personnel, the diagnostician must be the one who keeps in professional contact until the client is scheduled. If the client is scheduled with other staff members in the agency, the diagnostician must be available for consultation and assistance in the scheduling and interpretation of the management plan he has proposed.

More follow-up difficulty is encountered when referrals to other agencies are required. If it is a referral to another agency for therapy, the diagnostician may have to convince the agency to accept the client without undergoing a second diagnostic process. In communities where the professionals have developed a working relationship based on mutual respect for one another's work this is readily accomplished. Unfortunately, however, many agencies refuse to start the therapy process with a client diagnosed at an outside agency. In any case, if the diagnostician refers outside for therapy, he must follow through with his recommendation. He may want to talk directly with the personnel of the outside agency to arrange a time if possible. He should, at least, alert the agency that the client may be calling for an appointment. He should have obtained permission from the client to forward the diagnostic information along with his letter of referral. It is the obligation of the agency to which the client is referred to let the diagnostician know they have accepted and scheduled a client; however, this is not always done. We feel the diagnostician who has not received such a confirmation should check with the agency referred to so he can know and record in his clinical records the final disposition of the client.

If therapeutic recommendations are being withheld until an examination is made by another professional to whom the client has been referred, it is important for the diagnostician to keep on top of the progress made in completing these rec-ommendations. Besides making the purpose of the referral clear to the client, the diagnostician must make sure that the agency or professional he refers to understands his purpose in making the referral. As with all referrals, the diagnostician should make direct contact with the professional via telephone, referral letter, and reports. He must let the client know how to go about getting seen by the professional to whom he has been referred. Again, many clients are lost to therapy because of long delays that occur in this process. They may lose patience with the process and give it up as not being worth it.

Record-keeping systems vary significantly in different settings, ranging from basic notations on charts about the predominant symptoms and causes to complex data-retrieval systems maintained over the time period the client is seen. In general practice the records kept on a client are the clinical report followed by a series of log notes recording the day-to-day therapy activities and progress made. This system fulfills the professional's first responsibility, getting the information down accurately for later use by himself or other professionals.

Record keeping, however, forms the basis of much needed research about clinical problems. Therefore we recommend that each setting in which the diagnostician works develop and maintain a standard, and yet flexible, record-keeping system devised for easy recording and retrieval of information for both clinical and research purposes. The data accumulated during the diagnostic process and the clinical report can serve as the basis for recording data in master data files to facilitate retrieval.

An extensive discussion of data-retrieval systems is beyond the scope of this book, but we want to point out some information of interest to the reader. We have moved full blast into the computer age, and as computers are adapted to clinical functions, most of us will become involved in some way with retrieval systems based on computer technology. Several systems of data recording have been reported (1) for general clinical use (Elliott and Vegely, 1971; Elliott et al., 1971), (2) specific to a type of causal disorder, for example, cleft lip and palate (McCabe, 1966), and (3) directed to recording details from a specific test (Van Demark and Tharp, 1973).

Time, personnel, and costs currently prohibit the extensive use of highly complex computerized systems for most settings. But computers are not the only means to record adequate information for retrieval. The intent to keep such information is the primary ingredient for any record-keeping system. Data summary sheets can be utilized to transfer the information collected during the diagnostic process.

In developing the system the diagnostician must begin with a set of objectives that guide his creation of the system. His objectives for the system lead him to consider the amount and type of information to include. Rees et al. (1969) presented a standardized data-recording system to meet the needs of public school clinicians working in the Los Angeles area. The descriptions they provide for setting up their system, although not complex, are similar to systems set up for computers. Regardless of the method of storage and retrieval, the system must have a set of objectives, a system for reducing and recording the data, and a system for facilitating use by the various people who will be using it—either as recorders, storers, transmitters, receivers, or interpreters.

What are the basic objectives stated by Rees et al. (1969)? Could you develop a data collection and retrieval system for the diagnostic process discussed in this book?

SUMMARY

The diagnostician concludes the diagnostic process by fulfilling the diagnostic purposes for the client—client concern. All that has gone on before this point has allowed him to delineate the speech and language disorder and to achieve some level of understanding of the causal factors involved. Now he must translate his diagnosis into feedback and payoff for the client. In determining a management proposal, he must draw from the information he has gathered during the diagnostic process as well as what he knows about changing speech and language behavior. Having developed a management plan, he will then need to communicate his diagnostic findings as well as his recommendations for management to the client complex and involved professionals. Thus he needs knowledge and skill in interpersonal information giving as well as in report writing. Finally, he must apply his administrative talents to ensure that what has been planned actually takes place and that the needed paperwork gets done.

In summary, the final step of the diagnostic process involves four tasks.

1. The diagnostician will *determine a management plan*. In doing this he needs to know if the client can change his speech and language disorder with or without direct speech and language therapy. He plans for any referrals that are needed to fulfill the management plan, considering what services are available throughout the community in which he works.

2. Armed with a management plan, the diagnostician then *holds an interpretive conference* with the client complex, during which he discusses his diagnostic findings and works out the management plan with them, including any practical alterations that are needed.

3. The diagnostician then *writes his reports*, the number and type varying with his work setting and special needs for communicating his concerns about the client. At the very least he will write a clinical report for the agency in which he works, for

self-recall or later use by other professionals.

4. Finally, the diagnostician will need to *complete his administrative follow-up,* seeing to it that all management plans are worked out and appropriate paperwork and record keeping completed.

CLIENT PROJECTS

Each of the clients presented as examples throughout this book represented different disorders and management needs. For each of them, consider your management plan, your approach to the interpretive conference, write your clinical reports, and determine how you would work through any necessary follow-up.

REFERENCES

Bangs, T. E., *Language and Learning Disorders of the Pre-Academic Child.* New York: Appleton-Century-Crofts (1968).

Berry, M. F., and Eisenson, J., *Speech Disorders: Principles and Practices of Therapy.* New York: Appleton-Century-Crofts (1956).

Boone, D. R., *The Voice and Voice Therapy.* Englewood Cliffs, N.J.: Prentice-Hall, Inc. (1971).

Cooper, M., *Modern Techniques of Vocal Rehabilitation.* Springfield, Ill.: Charles C Thomas, Publisher (1973).

Derman, S., and Manaster, A., Family counseling with relatives of aphasic patients at Schwab Rehabilitation Hospital. *Asha, 9,* 175-177 (1967).

Dickson, S. (Ed.), *Communication Disorders: Remedial Principles and Practices.* Glenview, Ill.: Scott, Foresman & Co. (1974).

Dreher, B. B., and Baltes, L., Bibliotherapy for the communication disordered: Rationale and materials. *Asha, 15,* 528-534 (1973).

Eisenson, J., *Aphasia in Children.* New York: Harper & Row, Publishers (1972).

Eisenson, J., *Adult Aphasia: Assessment and Treatment.* New York: Appleton-Century-Crofts (1973).

Elliott, L. L., and Vegely, A. B., Notes on clinical record-keeping systems. *Asha, 13,* 444-446 (1971).

Elliott, L. L., Vegely, A. B., and Falvey, N. J., Description of a computer-oriented record-keeping system. *Asha, 13,* 435-443 (1971).

Emerick, L. L., *The Parent Interview.* Danville, Ill.: The Interstate Printers & Publishers, Inc. (1969).

Emerick, L. L., and Hatten, J. T., *Diagnosis and Evaluation in Speech Pathology.* Englewood Cliffs, N.J.: Prentice-Hall, Inc. (1974).

English, B. H., and Lillywhite, H. S., A semantic approach to clinical reporting in speech pathology. *Asha, 5,* 647-650 (1963).

Flower, R. M., Leach, E., Stone, C. R., and Yoder, D. E., Case selection. *J. Speech Hearing Dis., 32,* 65-70 (1967).

Forscher, B. K., and Wertz, R., Organizing the scientific paper. *Asha, 12,* 494-497 (1970).

Hammond, K. R., and Allen, J. M., *Writing Clinical Reports.* New York: Prentice-Hall, Inc. (1953).

Hegrenes, J. R., Marshall, N. R., and Armas, J. A., Treatment as an extension of diagnostic function: A case study. *J. Speech Hearing Dis., 35,* 182-187 (1970).

Jerger, J., Scientific writing can be readable. *Asha, 4,* 101-104 (1962).

Johnson, W., Darley, F. L., and Spriestersbach, D. C., *Diagnostic Methods in Speech Pathology.* New York: Harper & Row, Publishers (1963).

Keenan, J. S., and Brassell, E. G., A study of factors related to prognosis for individual aphasic patients. *J. Speech Hearing Dis., 39,* 257-269 (1974).

Kleffner, F. R., *Language Disorders in Children.* New York: The Bobbs-Merrill Co., Inc. (1973).

Knepflar, K. J., *Report Writing in the Field of Communication Disorders.* Danville, Ill.: The Interstate Printers & Publishers, Inc. (1976).

Marshall, N. R., and Goldstein, S. G., Imparting diagnostic information to mothers: A comparison of methodologies. *J. Speech Hearing Res., 12,* 65-72 (1969).

Marshall, N. R., and Goldstein, S. G., The maintenance of diagnostic information imparted by three methods: One year later. *J. Speech Hearing Res., 13,* 447-448 (1970).

McCabe, P. A., A coding procedure for classification of cleft lip and cleft palate. *Cleft Palate J., 3,* 383-391 (1966).

Moore, M. V., Pathological writing. *Asha, 11,* 535-538 (1969).

Morris, H. D., Spriestersbach, D. C., and Darley, F. L., An articulation test for assessing competency of velopharyngeal closure. *J. Speech Hearing Res., 1,* 48-55 (1961).

Noland, R. L. (Ed.), *Counseling Parents of the Ill and the Handicapped.* Springfield, Ill.: Charles C Thomas, Publisher (1971).

Pannbacker, M., Diagnostic report writing. *J. Speech Hearing Dis., 40,* 367-379 (1975).

Ptacek, P. H., The evaluative process in speech pathology. In J. Akin, A. Goldberg, G. Myer, and J. Stewart (Eds.), *Language Behavior: A Book of Readings in Communication.* The Hague: Mouton Publishers (1970).

Rees, M., Herbert, E. L., and Coates, N. H., Development of a standard case record form. *J. Speech Hearing Dis., 34,* 68-81 (1969).

Rheingold, H. L., Interpreting mental retardation to parents. *J. Consult. Psychol., 9,* 142-148 (1945).

Sander, E. K., Counseling parents of stuttering children. *J. Speech Hearing Dis., 24,* 262-271 (1959).

Sanders, L. J., *Procedure Guides for Evaluation of Speech and Language Disorders in Children.* (3rd ed.) Danville, Ill.: The Interstate Printers & Publishers, Inc. (1972).

Sheehan, J. G., and Martyn, M. M., Stuttering and its disappearance. *J. Speech Hearing Res., 17,* 121-135 (1970).

Snidecor, J. C., et al., *Speech Rehabilitation of the Laryngectomized.* Springfield, Ill.: Charles C Thomas, Publisher (1962).

Templin, M. C., and Darley, F. L., *The Templin-Darley Tests of Articulation.* (2nd ed.) Iowa City, Iowa: University of Iowa Press (1969).

Van Demark, D. R., and Tharp, R., A computer program for articulation tests. *Cleft Palate J., 10,* 378-389 (1973).

Van Demark, D. R., Kuehn, D. P., and Tharp, R. F, Prediction of velopharyngeal competency. *Cleft Palate J., 12,* 5-11 (1975).

Van Riper, C., *Speech Correction: Principles and Methods.* (5th ed.) Englewood Cliffs, N.J.: Prentice-Hall, Inc. (1972).

Van Riper, C., *The Treatment of Stuttering.* Englewood Cliffs, N.J.: Prentice-Hall, Inc. (1973).

Webster, E. J., Parent counseling by speech pathologists and audiologists. *J. Speech Hearing Dis., 31,* 331-340 (1966).

Webster, E. J., Procedures for group parent counseling in speech pathology and audiology. *J. Speech Hearing Dis., 33,* 127-131 (1968).

Wilson, D. K., *Voice Problems of Children.* Baltimore: The Williams & Wilkins Co. (1972).

Winitz, H., *Articulatory Acquisition and Behavior.* New York: Appleton-Century-Crofts (1969).

Wood, K. S., The parent's role in the clinical program. *J. Speech Hearing Dis., 13,* 209-210 (1948).

Young, M. A., Onset, prevalence, and recovery from stuttering. *J. Speech Hearing Dis., 40,* 49-58 (1975).

Administrative forms

REQUEST FOR SERVICE

Date _____

Service requested for _____ Birth date _____

Address _____ Phone _____
           (Street)   (City)   (State)   (Zip)

Requested by (referral) _____ Relationship _____

Address of referral source _____ Phone _____

Responsible relative: Name _____

                 Address _____

Address for appointment _____

What seems to be the problem? (Remarks) _____

_____

_____

Any previous evaluations or therapy at (agency name)?   Yes _____   No _____

Recorded by _____

- -

Correspondence record (Please initial each entry.)

                                                  Date sent   *Date returned*

Acknowledgment, client history, release forms   _____ _____

Follow-up acknowledgment letter   _____ _____

Letters to other sources (name and address)

_____ _____ _____

_____ _____ _____

_____ _____ _____

_____ _____ _____

Scheduled for diagnosis: Date _____ Time _____ Diagnostician _____

Appointment letter sent: Date _____

ACKNOWLEDGMENT OF REQUEST FOR SERVICE

Date _____

To _____

_____

_____

Dear _____ :

We have received a request for an appointment for _____ at the Hearing and Speech Center.

In order for our evaluation to be most effective, past history information is needed. We are enclosing a client history form. Please fill it out carefully to the best of your knowledge. The enclosed release forms, which allow us to obtain information from appropriate professional people or agencies (doctors, hospitals, etc.), also need to be signed.

Since we can schedule only a limited number of people, a prompt return of the client history and release forms will allow us to give you an earlier appointment. Please use the enclosed self-addressed envelope for your completed forms.

Sincerely,

_____

FOLLOW-UP ACKNOWLEDGMENT LETTER

Date _____

To _____

_____

_____

Re _____

_____

Dear _____ :

On _____ we received a request for a diagnosis for _____ . On _____ a client history and release forms were sent. These forms need to be completed and returned to our agency before we can schedule an appointment.

If you still desire an appointment, complete the forms and return them to the Hearing and Speech Center by _____ . If we do not receive the forms by this date, we will assume that you do not wish to have an appointment at this time. Enclosed please find an extra set of forms for your use.

Sincerely,

_____

PATIENT HISTORY: APHASIA

Our evaluation of your speech and language difficulties will depend on information about your past history. Fill out the form as completely as possible and return in the enclosed envelope. No appointment is given until the form has been returned and evaluated.

NOTE: *All information given is kept confidential.*

Date _____

Person completing this form _____

Relationship to patient _____

I. IDENTIFICATION

Name _____ Sex _____ Age _____

Address _____ Phone _____
        (Street)   (City)   (State)   (Zip)

Birth date _____ Birthplace _____
        (Month)   (Day)   (Year)

Referred by _____

Address _____ Phone _____
        (Street)   (City)   (State)   (Zip)

II. PERSONAL AND FAMILY HISTORY

Marital status: Single __ Married __ Separated __ Divorced __ Widowed __ Remarried __

Spouse's name _____ Address _____
                                        (Street)   (City)   (State)

Spouse's occupation _____

Children:

Name	Age	Living Yes	Living No	Address
1.				
2.				
3.				
4.				
5.				

Do you have brothers and sisters? Number _____ List ages _____

III. MEDICAL HISTORY

When did the illness or accident occur? Date _____

Describe the illness or accident: _____

_____

Were you unconscious? _____ Paralyzed? _____ Did you have convulsions? _____

If yes, describe. _____

How soon were you seen by a physician? _____

Physician's name _____ Address _____

Continued.

PATIENT HISTORY: APHASIA—cont'd

III. MEDICAL HISTORY—cont'd

Were you hospitalized? _____ If yes, how long? _____

Name of hospital _____ Address _____

If not hospitalized, describe how you were cared for. _____
_____

Are you now under a physician's care? _____ If yes, for what reason? _____
_____

Physician's name _____ Address _____

Are you now taking medication? _____ Name and dosage _____
_____ Are you responsible for taking your medication? _____

Your health before this illness or accident was: Excellent __ Average __ Fair __ Poor __

Before this illness or accident have you ever had a: Heart condition? _____ High blood pressure? _____ Previous strokes? _____ Seizures? _____ Fainting spells? _____

Describe any other serious illnesses, accidents, and operations you have had.

When	Problem	Where hospitalized	Attending physician
1.			
2.			
3.			
4.			
5.			

Describe any visual problems you have. _____
_____ Glasses? Yes _____ No _____

Describe any hearing problems you have. _____
_____ Hearing Aid? Yes _____ No _____

Please give information below about any of the following services you have had.

	Date or dates	Person/agency	Address
Speech/language examination			
Speech/language therapy			
Hearing examination			
Psychological testing/ counseling			
Vocational counseling			
Physical therapy			
Occupational therapy			

PATIENT HISTORY: APHASIA—cont'd

IV. EDUCATIONAL HISTORY

University

Circle highest grade completed: 1 2 3 4 5 6 7 8 9 10 11 12   1 2 3 4

Graduate school degree? Yes _____ No _____ Area of university study or specialization.

_____

Describe any other education or special training. _____

_____

_____

V. EMPLOYMENT HISTORY

Last occupation _____ How long? _____

Employer _____

Address _____
       (Street)   (City)   (State)   (Zip)

Are you still employed? _____ What present employment arrangement do you have with your employer? _____

_____

Describe briefly the type of work you were doing in your past occupations. _____

_____

Check here if you are a housewife. _____ What are your primary sources of income? (Check all the appropriate blanks.) Salary _____ Hourly wages _____ Commission _____ Savings and investments _____ Profits and fees _____ Public welfare _____ Other (Please give details). _____

_____

_____

_____

VI. SPEECH AND LANGUAGE HISTORY

In what country have you lived most of your life? _____ What is your native language? _____ What other languages do you speak, understand, read, or write? _____ What languages other than English do you speak at home? _____ When did the present speech difficulty begin? _____ What was your speech like at that time? _____

How has it changed? _____

_____

Describe any speech problems you had before this illness or accident. _____

_____

_____

_____

_____

_____

_____

Continued.

PATIENT HISTORY: APHASIA—cont'd

VI. SPEECH AND LANGUAGE HISTORY—cont'd

The following items are very important for helping us plan our test procedures so as to keep the time spent in evaluation at a minimum. Please check as carefully as possible those items you can and cannot do.

I CAN I CANNOT

Speech

I CAN	I CANNOT	
____	____	Indicate meaning by pointing or gesture
____	____	Say a word if I write it first
____	____	Repeat words spoken by others
____	____	Articulate sounds
____	____	Say words
____	____	Say short phrases
____	____	Say short sentences
____	____	Talk without using "roundabout" way of getting meaning across
____	____	Speak with relative fluency
____	____	Be easily understood
____	____	Relate a story read or seen on television
____	____	Carry on a telephone conversation

Comprehension

I CAN	I CANNOT	
____	____	Understand single spoken words
____	____	Understand simple spoken sentences
____	____	Understand conversational speech with one person
____	____	Understand conversational speech with several persons
____	____	Follow radio or television speech
____	____	Understand spoken directions
____	____	Recognize objects
____	____	Understand the use of these objects
____	____	Understand everything I listen to

Reading

I CAN	I CANNOT	
____	____	Read signs with understanding
____	____	Read numbers with understanding
____	____	Read single words with understanding
____	____	Read newspaper headlines with understanding
____	____	Read magazine articles with understanding
____	____	Read books with understanding
____	____	Tell time

Writing

I CAN	I CANNOT	
____	____	Copy numbers, letters, or words
____	____	Write my name by myself
____	____	Write single words by myself
____	____	Write short sentences by myself
____	____	Write personal letters by myself
____	____	Write creatively by myself

PATIENT HISTORY: APHASIA—cont'd

VII. DAILY BEHAVIOR

I CAN   I CANNOT

Orientation

I CAN	I CANNOT	
____	____	Remember past events
____	____	Remember events relative to my accident or illness
____	____	Remember recent events
____	____	Find my way about my home town
____	____	Find my way about a strange town

Daily living

____	____	Do simple arithmetic
____	____	Dress myself
____	____	Tie shoes
____	____	Tie necktie
____	____	Handle all bathroom needs by myself
____	____	Shower myself
____	____	Shave myself
____	____	Handle money
____	____	Plan my own activities
____	____	Go shopping alone
____	____	Answer the telephone

Walking

____	____	Walk unaided by myself
____	____	Walk with leg brace
____	____	Walk with cane
____	____	Rise to a standing position from a seated position without assistance
____	____	Seat myself from a standing position

Eating

____	____	Eat unassisted
____	____	Eat with special eating utensils

Using hands

____	____	Use both hands easily for all tasks
____	____	Use right hand easily for all tasks
____	____	Use left hand easily for all tasks
____	____	Open doors easily by myself

Were you right- or left-handed before the present illness or accident? Right ____ Left ____
Check those hobbies and interests that apply to you.

Reading

____ Books
____ Magazines
____ Newspapers

Music

____ Play instrument
____ Listening
____ Going to concerts
____ Other _____
        (Specify)

Sports

____ Baseball
____ Football
____ Basketball
____ Hockey
____ Golf

Writing

____ Letters
____ Other _____
        (Specify)

Interests

____ Gardening
____ Cooking
____ Sewing
____ Fishing
____ Boating
____ Traveling, Sights
____ Painting
____ Other _____
        (Specify)

How many hours per day do you watch television? _____

Continued.

PATIENT HISTORY: APHASIA—cont'd

VIII. HOME

Housing (Please check.): House _____ Apartment building _____ Apartment over a business _____ Other (Please describe.) _____

_____

How many rooms? _____ Members of household other than family? _____

_____

Neighborhood (Check all that best describe your neighborhood.): Residential _____ Business _____ Poor _____ Rural _____ Above average _____ Crowded _____ Average _____ Run-down _____ Excellent _____ Suburban _____ Tenement _____ Housing development _____

Please date and sign these release forms that allow the Hearing and Speech Center to obtain appropriate information from other professional persons or agencies.

Authorization to obtain information

I hereby authorize _____
(Source from whom information is to be obtained)

to release information regarding _____ to the Hearing
(Name of client)

and Speech Center.

Signed _____ Date _____
(By the client or by responsible relative)

Authorization to obtain information

I hereby authorize _____

to release information regarding _____ to the Hearing
and Speech Center.

Signed _____ Date _____

Authorization to obtain information

I hereby authorize _____

to release information regarding _____ to the Hearing
and Speech Center.

Signed _____ Date _____

Authorization to obtain information

I hereby authorize _____

to release information regarding _____ to the Hearing
and Speech Center.

Signed _____ Date _____

Authorization to obtain information

I hereby authorize _____

to release information regarding _____ to the Hearing
and Speech Center.

Signed _____ Date _____

REQUEST FOR INFORMATION

Date _____

To _____

  _____

  _____

Dear _____:

_____ has requested an evaluation at the Hearing and Speech Center for _____ . In order for our evaluation to be complete, no appointments are given until pertinent history has been obtained. It has been suggested that you would be able to give us helpful information. Please provide us with information in the areas checked below:

____ Birth history	____ School adjustment
____ General development	____ Behavioral problems
____ Health history	____ Physical therapy
____ Operations	____ Emotional adjustment
____ Physical defects	____ Psychological evaluation
____ Occupational therapy	____ Psychometrics
____ Vision	____ Speech and hearing problems
____ ENT examination	____ Vocational guidance
____ Neurologic examination	____ Other _____

Enclosed please find a signed authorization allowing you to send us the desired information.

Sincerely,

_____

APPOINTMENT LETTER: INFORMATION FOR CHILDREN

Date _____

To _____

_____

_____

Dear _____:

_____ has been scheduled for an evaluation at the Hearing and Speech Center on _____. This appointment time has been set aside for you alone; however, if for any reason you are unable to keep the appointment, please let us know a day or so in advance so we can use the time for someone else. On the day of your appointment please arrive on time since we have a lot to do in the 1½ hour evaluation. Although we try to complete our evaluation in one appointment, there are times when we have to ask that you return for a second visit.

Oftentimes children and their parents do not know what to expect from their visit here. While here, a Speech Pathologist will be testing your child's speech and language abilities. The tests used require the child to name pictures; to repeat words, sounds, and sentences; to talk about pictures, etc. He will also be asked to listen carefully to instructions so we can find out how well he understands speech and language. We sometimes will do an examination of your child's mouth. Here we are interested in how the tongue, jaw, lips, etc. are used in speech. This examination is in no way painful for the child. If indicated, we often give your child a hearing test using an audiometer and earphones. This is an easy task for most children requiring them to listen carefully to different tones and then let us know if he hears them. Sometimes this testing is done in a special soundproof room.

Like most of us, children are afraid of the unknown. They are more relaxed and cooperative when they know ahead of time where they are going and what they will be doing. This is where part of the parent's work comes in. The following are general guidelines of what some parents have found helpful, although preparation should fit your particular child.

1. Tell him he is coming to the center.
2. Tell him that most children have fun.
3. Tell him it is a place very much like school. This is especially helpful for children under 5 years of age who have older brothers and sisters in school; however, a suggestion like this would not be helpful for a child who hates school.
4. Tell him about our special rooms for testing and our tests.
5. Be sure he understands there is nothing in our evaluation that will hurt in anyway.

If we can be of further assistance in helping you prepare your child or answer any questions, please call me at the center. We are looking forward to meeting you and your child.

Sincerely,

_____

SCHEDULING FORM

Name _____ Birth date _____ Age ____ Center No. ____
         (Last)   (First)

Address _____ Phone _____ Agency No. _____

_____ CBR No. _____

Assignment by _____ Date _____

Suggested schedule

Problem _____

_____

Staff, group, or program _____

_____

Days _____ Times _____ Reeval: Month _____
Year _____ Notations _____
_____
_____
_____

Management decision (check)

Add _____
Reevaluation _____
Change _____
Transfer-reschedule _____
Drop-reschedule _____
Drop-closure _____
Drop-close-reeval _____

Routing (date and initial)

Dept. office (A-R) _____
Scheduling _____
Dept. office (T-D) _____
Scheduling (DCR) _____

Current schedule

	Staff	Days	Times	I	G
1.	_____	_____	_____	___	___
2.	_____	_____	_____	___	___
3.	_____	_____	_____	___	___
4.	_____	_____	_____	___	___
5.	_____	_____	_____	___	___

New schedule

	Staff accepting	Days	Times	I	G	Beg. date
1.	_____	_____	_____	___	___	_____
2.	_____	_____	_____	___	___	_____
3.	_____	_____	_____	___	___	_____
4.	_____	_____	_____	___	___	_____
5.	_____	_____	_____	___	___	_____

RELEASE FORM

Authorization is given to the Hearing and Speech Center to release information concerning

Name _____ Date _____

Address _____ Birth date _____

_____

to the following persons or agencies:

1. Name _____

   Address _____

   _____

2. Name _____

   Address _____

   _____

3. Name _____

   Address _____

   _____

Signed _____

Relationship to client _____

NOTE: Reports may be sent *only* to the sources listed above. Requests for reports made by other sources must be accompanied by a separate release form.

Client projects

REQUEST FOR SERVICE: Katherine Compardo

Springfield Speech and Hearing Center
2661 Euclid Heights Boulevard   Area code 217
Springfield, Illinois 82233   624-5521

Date _May 15, 1974_

Service requested for _Katherine Compardo_   Birth date _3-2-1972_

Address _One St. Mary's Court   Springfield, Illinois   82233_   Phone _644-5454_
(Street)   (City)   (State)   (Zip)

Requested by (referral) _Dr. D. Wasser_   Relationship _Pediatrician_

Address of referral source _McGee Medical Building_   Phone _624-2233_

Responsible relative: Name _Mrs. Lois Compardo—Mother_

Address _Same_

Address for appointment _Same_

What seems to be the problem? (Remarks) _Katherine doesn't talk much; she only speaks a few words. Her pediatrician suggested we call you to have an evaluation. We know she is young but we're very concerned. She should be talking much more by now._

Any previous evaluations or therapy at SSHC?   Yes_____   No ✔_____

Recorded by _Wolpaw_

- -

Correspondence record (Please initial each entry.)

	Date sent	Date returned
Acknowledgment, client history, release forms	_5-16-74_	_6-3-74_
Follow-up acknowledgment letter	_____	_____
Letters to other sources (name and address)		
No other information requested at this time	_____	_____
_____	_____	_____
_____	_____	_____

Scheduled for diagnosis: Date _6-10-74_ Time _9:00_   Diagnostician _Bobkoff_

Appointment letter sent: Date _6-4-74; following telephone appointment_

CHILDREN'S SPEECH, LANGUAGE, AND HEARING HISTORY: Katherine Compardo

Our evaluation of your child's speech, language, and hearing problems will depend on information about his past history. Fill out the form as completely as possible and return in the enclosed envelope. If there are any items you do not fully understand, put a check mark in the left margin and we can discuss them when you come for your appointment.

Date *June 1, 1974*

Person completing this form *Lois Compardo* Relationship to child *Mother*

I. IDENTIFICATION

Name *Katherine Compardo* Birth date *March 2, 1972* Sex *F* Age *27 mo.*

Address *One St. Mary's Court* Phone *644-5454*

Mother's name *Lois* Address *Same* Age *38*

Father's name *Frank* Address *Same* Age *42*

Referred by *Dr. Wasser* Address *McGee Medical Building*

Family doctor *None* Address

Child's pediatrician *Dr. Wasser* Address *McGee Med. Bldg.*

II. STATEMENT OF THE PROBLEM

Describe as completely as possible the speech, language, and hearing problem. *Only speaks a few words. Can say ma but won't call me unless I'm there. Points to Daddy and says it. Understands everything she is told. She won't say anything else.*

When was the problem first noticed? *Quiet as an infant*

How has the problem changed since you first noticed it? *She just isn't talking.*

What has been done about it? Has this helped? *Nothing*

What do you think caused the problem? *No idea*

Are there any family members or relatives who have or had speech, language, or hearing problems? *My nephew didn't start talking till he was 29 months.*

III. SPEECH, LANGUAGE, AND HEARING HISTORY

How much did your child babble and coo during the first 6 months? *not much*

When did he speak his first words? *2 yrs.* What were the child's first few words?
Here — Daddy — Hi

How many words did the child have at 1½ years? *none* When did he begin to use two-word sentences? *none*

Does he use speech? Frequently _____ Occasionally *✔* Never _____

Continued.

CHILDREN'S SPEECH, LANGUAGE, AND HEARING HISTORY—cont'd

III. SPEECH, LANGUAGE, AND HEARING HISTORY—cont'd

Does he use many gestures? (Give examples if possible.) *gestures—knocks on me for my attention, then pulls me*

Which does the child prefer to use? Complete sentences _____ Phrases _____

One or two words ___✔___ Sounds _____ Gestures _____

Does he make sounds incorrectly? *yes* If so, which ones? *most of them*

Does he hesitate, "get stuck," repeat, or stutter on sounds or words? _____
If so, describe. _____

How does his voice sound? Normal ___ Too high ___ Too low ___ Hoarse ___ Nasal ___

How well can he be understood? By his parents *everything* By his brothers and sisters and playmates *everything* By relatives and strangers *everything*

Did your child ever acquire speech and then slow down or stop talking? *no*

Does he imitate speech but not use it? *no*

How well does he understand what is said to him? *understands everything*

Does your child hear adequately? *yes* Does his hearing appear to be constant or does it vary? _____ Is his hearing poorer when he has a cold? *I don't think so.*

Has your child ever worn a hearing aid? *no* Which ear? _____ How long? _____

Hours per day? _____ Does it seem to help him? _____

NOTE: If the child has a hearing aid, please bring it and the earmold along with you when you come in for your appointment.

IV. GENERAL DEVELOPMENT
A. Pregnancy and birth history

Total number of pregnancies __5__ How many miscarriages, stillbirths? *None*
Explain. _____

Which pregnancy was this child? *Last* Length of pregnancy? *9 mo.* Was it difficult? *No*

What illnesses, diseases, and accidents occurred during pregnancy? *None*

Was there a blood incompatibility between the mother and father? *No*

Age of mother at child's birth __36__ Age of father at child's birth __40__

What was the length of labor? *5 hrs.* Were there any unusual problems at birth (breech birth, caesarean birth, others)? If so, describe. *No*

What drugs were used? *None* High or low forceps? *No* Weight of child at birth _____

Were there any bruises, scars, or abnormalities of the child's head? *No*

CHILDREN'S SPEECH, LANGUAGE, AND HEARING HISTORY—cont'd

IV. GENERAL DEVELOPMENT—cont'd

Any other abnormalities? *No*

Did infant require oxygen? *No*   Was child "blue" or jaundiced at birth? *No*

Was a blood transfusion required at birth? *No*

Were there any problems immediately following birth or during the first 2 weeks of the infant's life (health, swallowing, sucking, feeding, sleeping, others)? If so, describe.

None

At what age did infant regain birth weight?

B. Developmental

At what age did the following occur? Held head erect while lying on stomach *2 or 3 wk.*
Rolled over alone ___ Sat alone unsupported *3 mo.* Crawled *10 mo.* Stood alone *15 mo.*
Walked unaided *15 mo.* Fed self with spoon *1½ yr.* Had first tooth ____ Bladder trained
_____ Bowel trained _____ Completely toilet trained: Waking_____ Sleeping _____ Dressed
and undressed himself ___ What hand does he prefer? *Both* Has handedness ever been
changed? _____ If so, at what age? _____ How would you describe your child's current physical development? *She seems much slower than my other children.*

Check these as they apply to your child.

	Yes	No	Explain: give ages if possible.
Cried less than normal amount		✔	
Laughed less than normal amount		✔	
Yelled and screeched to attract attention or express annoyance	✔		*all along*
Head banging and foot stamping			
Extremely sensitive to vibration			
Very alert to gesture, facial expression, or movement	✔		*since she was a baby*
Shuffled feet while walking			
Generally indifferent to sound		✔	
Did not respond when spoken to		✔	
Responded to noises (car horns, telephones) but not to speech		✔	
Difficulty using tongue	✔		*when she talks*

Continued.

CHILDREN'S SPEECH, LANGUAGE, AND HEARING HISTORY—cont'd

IV. GENERAL DEVELOPMENT—cont'd

	Yes	*No*	*Explain: give ages if possible.*
Difficulty swallowing		✔	
Talked through nose		✔	
Mouth breather		✔	
Tongue-tied		✔	
Difficulty chewing		✔	
Drooled a lot		✔	
Food came out nose		✔	
Constant throat clearing		✔	
Difficulty breathing		✔	
Large tongue		✔	
Difficulty moving mouth	✔		*when she talks*

V. MEDICAL HISTORY

Is your child now under the care of a doctor? *Yes* Why? *general check-ups*

Is he taking medication? *No* Type? _____ Why? _____

At what ages did any of the following illnesses, problems, or operations occur? Please indicate how serious they were.

	Age	Mild	Mod.	Severe		Age	Mild	Mod.	Severe
Adenoidectomy					Earaches				
Allergies					Ear infections				
Asthma					Encephalitis				
Blood disease					Headaches				
Cataracts					Head injuries				
Chickenpox	1½	✔			Heart problems				
Chronic colds					High fevers				
Convulsions					Influenza				
Cross-eyed					Mastoidectomy				
Croup					Measles				
Dental problems					Meningitis				
Diphtheria					Mumps				

CHILDREN'S SPEECH, LANGUAGE, AND HEARING HISTORY—cont'd

V. MEDICAL HISTORY—cont'd

	Age	Mild	Mod.	Severe		Age	Mild	Mod.	Severe
Muscle disorder					Rheumatic fever				
Nerve disorder					Scarlet fever				
Orthodontia					Tonsillectomy				
Pneumonia					Tonsillitis				
Polio					Whooping cough				

Has the child ever fallen or had a severe blow to the head? ___*no*___ If so, did he lose consciousness? _____ Did it cause a concussion? _____ Did it cause: Nausea _____ Vomiting _____ Drowsiness _____ Describe any other serious illnesses, injuries, operations, or physical problems not mentioned above. _____

_____

What illnesses have been accompanied by an extremely long, high fever? _____

Temperature _____ How long did the fever last? _____

Which of the above required hospitalization? ___*none*_____

Where was the child hospitalized? _____ For how long? _____

Who was the attending physician? _____

VI. BEHAVIOR

Check these as they apply to your child.

	Yes	No	Explain: give ages if possible.
Eating problems		✔	
Sleeping problems		✔	
Toilet training problems		✔	
Difficulty concentrating	✔		*she runs around a lot*
Needed a lot of discipline		✔	
Underactive		✔	
Excitable			
Laughs easily			
Cried a lot		✔	
Difficult to manage		✔	
Overactive	✔		*runs around a lot*
Sensitive			

Continued.

CHILDREN'S SPEECH, LANGUAGE, AND HEARING HISTORY—cont'd

VI. BEHAVIOR—cont'd

	Yes	No	*Explain: give ages if possible.*
Personality problem		✔	*she just won't talk*
Gets along with children	✔		
Gets along with adults	✔		
Emotional			
Stays with an activity			
Makes friends easily	✔		
Happy			
Irritable			
Prefers to play alone		✔	*plays alone and with other children*

How do you discipline your child? _____

_____

What are the child's favorite play activities?   *picture books — bike — outdoors*

_____

VII. EDUCATIONAL HISTORY

Did child attend day care or nursery school? _____ Where? _____ Ages _____

Kindergarten? _____ Where? _____ Ages _____

School now attending _____ Address _____

Grade he is now in _____ Grades skipped _____ Grades failed _____

What are his average grades? _____ Best subjects _____ Poorest _____

Is the child frequently absent from school? _____ If so, why? _____

How does child feel about school and about his teacher? _____

_____

What is your impression of your child's learning abilities? _____

_____

Has anyone ever thought he was a slow child? _____

_____

Describe any speech, language, hearing, psychological, and special education services that have been performed including where this was done. How often was your child seen in this service? _____

_____

_____

CHILDREN'S SPEECH, LANGUAGE, AND HEARING HISTORY—cont'd

VIII. HOME AND FAMILY INFORMATION

Father's occupation *Senior Lieutenant*   Last grade completed in school   *12*

Mother's occupation *Housewife*   Last grade completed in school   *12*

Brothers and sisters:

Name	Age	Sex	Grade in school	Speech, hearing, or medical problem
1. *Jennifer*	6	F	1	
2. *Nancy*	5	F		
3. *Diane*	18	F	12	
4. *Frank*	20	M	College	
5.				
6.				
7.				
8.				

Are there any other languages spoken in the home? *No* If so, by whom and how often?

_____

Home and neighborhood (check all that apply): Residential ✔ Business area _____

House ✔ Rural ___ Above average ___ Housing development ___ Excellent condition ___

Apartment area ____ Average ✔ Crowded ___ Suburban ✔ Number of rooms? 6

Members of household other than family? *None* _____

Primary source of income (check the appropriate blanks): Salary ✔ Hourly wages ____

Commission _____ Welfare _____ Profits and fees _____ Savings and investments _____
Other _____

Please add any additional information you feel will help us in understanding your child and his problem: *I am calling you because my doctor suggested it. When baby was infant, I questioned her hearing because she was so quiet. Now I am sure she can hear. I have just convinced myself there was nothing wrong; now I have to start thinking otherwise.*

REQUEST FOR SERVICE: William Gafford

Speech and Hearing Clinic
2897 Berkshire Road
Chile, Ohio 12142

Area code 216
321-3981

Date *October 17, 1975*

Service requested for *Reverend William G. Gafford*   Birth date *2-18-1929*

Address *173 E. 86th St.   Chile,   Ohio   12142*   Phone *321-0214*
      (Street)   (City)   (State)   (Zip)

Requested by (referral) *Drs. G. Gershon and L. Lefkoff*

Relationship *Ear, Nose, and Throat Specialists*

Address of referral source *Parkway Medical Center*   Phone *368-2381*

Responsible relative: Name *Mrs. Tillie Gafford*

             Address *Same*

Address for appointment *Same*

What seems to be the problem? (Remarks) *Hoarse voice from ulcers on my vocal cords.*
When I was young, my voice never changed until my professor told me to lower it. Two
years ago my throat started to bother me and I got hoarse. I had an operation and it was
better, but now it feels like something is in my throat all the time.

Any previous evaluations or therapy at SHC?   Yes _____   No ✔

                        Recorded by *Aversano*

- -

Correspondence record (Please initial each entry.)

	Date sent	Date returned
Acknowledgment, client history, release forms		
Follow-up acknowledgment letter		
Letters to other sources (name and address)		
Called Gershon and Lefkoff following call	*10-17-75*	*10-19-75*
from Rev. Gafford. They will send a referral		
letter.		

Scheduled for diagnosis: Date *10-19-75* Time *9:00* Diagnostician *Seligman*

Appointment letter sent: Date _____

REFERRAL LETTER: William Gafford

October 19, 1975

Dorothy M. Aram, Ph.D.
Speech and Hearing Clinic
2897 Berkshire Road
Chile, Ohio 12142

Dear Dr. Aram:

We have seen Rev. William Gafford on several occasions for complaints of hoarseness, aphonia, and laryngeal pain. Rev. Gafford is plagued with recurring hoarseness that we feel is secondary to vocal abuse. After prolonged speaking, he has developed contact ulcerations on the posterior aspect of the vocal cords. We have treated these ulcerations with vocal rest and they do improve. However, we are referring him for voice therapy in the hope that recurrence of the contact ulcers can be prevented by removing the cause and establishing better speaking habits.

We would appreciate a report of your evaluation. Should you need more information, please feel free to contact us.

Sincerely yours,

Gerald Gershon, M.D.
Lewis Lefkoff, M.D.

GG/LL:val

CONSULT NOTES: Isadore Alexander

Department of Otolaryngology
University Hospitals
923 Spaight Road
Loami, Illinois 82233

Identification information   Date: September 20, 1974

Name: Isadore Alexander
Address: 147 Orton Court
   Loami, Illinois 82233
Birth date: August 4, 1906
Age: 68

Consult notes

I saw Mr. Alexander today on referral from Dr. William Fowles who saw him on recommendation from Dr. Lee Uransky. Mr. Alexander's chief complaint was hoarseness. Findings were negative.

IMPRESSION: Functional dysarthria
COMMENT: I advise speech therapy for Mr. Alexander.

Jarius Lambert, M.D.

LETTER OF INFORMATION: Isadore Alexander

William Fowles, M.D.
Practice Limited to Otolaryngology
Loami Medical Building
1532 West Monroe Street
Loami, Illinois 82233

September 25, 1974

Dear Dr. Eichelberger:

My only contact with Mr. Alexander was very brief. I saw him on June 15, 1974, on referral from Dr. Uransky. Mr. Alexander complained of hoarseness and blurred speech. I could find no laryngeal pathology, although I did hear the hoarseness and the blurred speech. I did a hearing test that was essentially negative, a slight loss in the high frequencies. I did not feel equipped to handle this man's complaint, so I referred him to Dr. Lambert at University Hospitals.

Sincerely,

William Fowles, M.D.

LETTER OF INFORMATION: Isadore Alexander

Lee Uransky, M.D.
Practice Limited to Neurology and Neurosurgery
Loami Medical Building
1532 West Monroe Street
Loami, Illinois 82233

September 25, 1974

Dear Dr. Eichelberger:

I am pleased to hear that Mr. Alexander is being seen for speech services. I had recommended that to him when I saw him on May 20, 1974, but did not feel he would follow through. When I saw him, his voice was hoarse and he exhibited a bizarre speech pattern. His speech was slow with little affect. My neurologic examination was negative, and I felt this man was demonstrating a functional speech disorder perhaps secondary to some organic mental changes. His personality and anxiety about his condition led me to suspect some possible psychiatric implications. I referred him to Dr. Fowles for further consultation.

Sincerely,

Lee Uransky, M. D.

LETTER OF INFORMATION: Derek Park

September 22, 1975

Mr. Maurice Posch, M.A.
Iles Elementary School
1818 So. 14th Street
Springfield, Illinois 82233

Dear Mr. Posch:

Derek Park was born June 10, 1970, with a left complete cleft lip and palate following a full-term pregnancy. The repair of the lip was performed on July 12, 1970.

On July 12, 1971, a bone graft was performed to the anterior cleft area. On November 2, 1971, the cleft palate was repaired.

He was last seen in my office on November 7, 1974. It was my feeling that there was a fair amount of nasal escape.

I would appreciate a report from you after completion of your evaluation.

Very truly yours,

M. Sugarman, M.D.

MS:val

LETTER OF INFORMATION: Derek Park

September 21, 1975

Mr. Maurice Posch, M.A.
Iles Elementary School
1818 So. 14th Street
Springfield, Illinois 82233

Dear Mr. Posch:

When Derek Park last came to the Cleft Palate Clinic, there was an evaluation of his speech. It was generally immature with articulation defects related to this immaturity. His problems with weak and nasally emitted fricatives, however, seem to be the effect of poor velopharyngeal pressure. It is felt that better articulation may be stimulated by intensive speech therapy when Derek starts school.

Although Mr. and Mrs. Park have agreed with our recommendation, it should be noted that in the past we have found Mrs. Park to be somewhat evasive and passively resistive. She does follow through but seems to "hold back."

Please send your report to our Cleft Palate Clinic.

Sincerely yours,

Lois Fry, Ph.D.
Speech Pathologist

LF:val

REQUEST FOR SERVICE: Michael Durall

Eastern Speech and Hearing Clinic
2661 Coventry Road
Cleveland, Ohio 44106

Area code 216
444-8223

Date *September 15, 1974*

Service requested for *Michael T. Durall*   Birth date *7-17-51*

Address *432 E. 96th Street   Cleveland, Ohio   44105*   Phone *822-1933*
          (Street)   (City)   (State)   (Zip)

Requested by (referral) *Al Butts—BVR*   Relationship *Vocational Counselor*

Address of referral source *Room 104—Eastern Speech and Hearing Clinic*

Phone *444-8223 Ext. 406*

Responsible relative: Name *Betty Durall—Mother*

                            Address *Same*

Address for appointment *Same*

What seems to be the problem? (Remarks) *Stuttering*

Any previous evaluations or therapy at ESHC?   Yes _____   No ✔

                            Recorded by *Gretchen Redlands*

- -

Correspondence record (Please initial each entry.)

	Date sent	Date returned
		Rec'd 9-15-74
Acknowledgment, client history, release forms	_____	*with referral*
Follow-up acknowledgment letter	_____	_____
Letters to other sources (name and address)		
_____	_____	_____
_____	_____	_____
_____	_____	_____
_____	_____	_____

Scheduled for diagnosis: Date *9-20-74* Time *9:00* Diagnostician *D. Cook*

Appointment letter sent: Date *Telephone appointment 9-18-74*

REFERRAL LETTER: Michael Durall

September 9, 1974

Eastern Speech and Hearing Center
2661 Coventry Road
Cleveland, Ohio 44106

Dear Sirs:

We have accepted Michael T. Durall as a client for vocational rehabilitation services. As part of those services, we are requesting a speech evaluation for his stuttering disability.

Michael has previously worked in a cemetery as a groundskeeper for 3 years and for 3 years as a truck driver for his mother's catering service. We have no other reports available nor has Michael had any special training for any particular job skills.

We would like a speech evaluation and a request for therapy and amount of therapy if applicable. Enclosed is the history questionnaire completed by Mr. Durall.

Sincerely,

Al Butts
Vocational Counselor
Bureau of Vocational Rehabilitation
Room 104
Eastern Speech and Hearing Clinic

AB:jen
Encl.: (1)

HISTORY QUESTIONNAIRE: Michael Durall

Eastern Speech and Hearing Clinic
2661 Coventry Road
Cleveland, Ohio 44106

1. Name of client *Michael T. Durall*	Sex *Male*	Date of birth *July 17, 1951*

2. Your address *432 East 96th Street*	Phone no. *822-1933*

3. Where are you employed and for how long?

   Unemployed

4. What is your occupation? (Briefly describe what you do.)

   Driver and maintenance

5. Name and address of person who recommended this center to you

   Mr. Al Butts, Bureau of Vocational Rehabilitation

FAMILY HISTORY

6. Name of wife/husband *None*	His/her occupation

7. Names of children	Age	Sex	Speech problem	Remarks
a.				
b.				
c.				

8. What other relatives have a speech problem? Is it similar to yours?

   None

Continued.

HISTORY QUESTIONNAIRE: Michael Durall—cont'd

MEDICAL

9. List any serious illnesses, injuries, childhood diseases, and operations. Give dates and length of disabilities. Include any physical handicaps, prolonged fevers, convulsions, after effects, etc.

   Tonsils—5 years old
   Appendix—11 years old

10. Describe any past or present hearing problems. This to include any history of hearing loss, ear infections, ear surgery, etc.

    None

11. Do you have a medical problem now that may be related to your speech problem? State whether or not you are presently under the care of a physician, and whether you are taking any medication.

    None

12. What hand do you use for skills such as writing?	Have you ever changed hands? If so, when and why?
Right	*No*

EDUCATION

13. Schools attended	Where	What grade
a. *Garfield Heights*	*Garfield Heights*	*11*
b.		
c.		
d.		

14. Describe your speech problem.

    I have been stuttering for as long as I can remember

HISTORY QUESTIONNAIRE: Michael Durall—cont'd

15. What do you think caused your speech problem?

    I don't know.

16. How do you feel your speech problem has affected your social life?

    It is difficult to really have meaningful relationships with people when you have a hard time expressing yourself.

17. How do you feel your speech problem has affected your occupation?

    I can't get employment that involves talking to other people.

18. If you didn't have a speech problem, how would your life be different?

    I know I would be able to lead a fuller life than what I am now.

19. Describe the reaction of people, including your immediate family, to your speech problem.

    They try and act like they don't notice it.

20. If you have received previous help with your speech problem, give details such as from whom, when, where, how long, etc.

    None

21. What have you tried to do to correct your speech problem?

    I have tried to talk slower.

22. Write down any additional information you feel will help us in understanding your speech problem.

    It's a bad habit that I have had for as long as I can remember.

Signature: _____

Kankakee General Hospital
Kankakee, Illinois 30603

Name: Marie Abadie

Admitted: 4/28/70

Discharged: 5/22/70

Neurology-Neurosurgery
6 West

Diagnosis: Left internal carotid artery aneurysm

Procedures: 1. Clamp application left internal carotid artery
2. Ligation left internal carotid artery
3. Right brachial arteriogram
4. Left carotid arteriogram

Reason for admission: Severe headache and nuchal rigidity

Present illness: This 57-year-old white female tried to change her position to rest her head while watching television but on twisting her body felt a sudden severe pain in her head. The pain radiated down the spine to her back and right thigh. She was grasping and wringing her arms and trying to hold onto something. She was awake until the following morning but remembers nothing. She was seen by her private physician who referred her to this hospital.

Past medical history: Reveals no history of headache, dizziness, hypertension, or trauma. Operations include bilateral exploration for chocolate cyst of the ovaries and subtotal hysterectomy at St. Alexis Hospital in 1951; underwent thyroidectomy for adenoma of thyroid in 1961; allergy to codeine; smoking—history of a package of cigarettes a day for many years.

Physical examination: Reveals an alert, conscious, coherent female who is in no acute distress. She is cooperative and complaining of mild to moderate headache. Her general physical examination including cardiovascular system is entirely normal. Pulses are 2+ and equal with bruits. Neurologically, the patient is alert to time and place. Her cranial nerve examination was entirely normal as was the remainder of the general neurologic examination including her reflexes. The patient does have moderate stiffness in neck flexion and rotation.

Laboratory and x-ray data: Includes hematocrit of 40% and white blood cell count of 12,600 with a normal differential count. Urinalysis and SMA-12 were entirely normal. Chest and skull x-ray films and brain scan were entirely normal.

Hospital course: The patient was placed on bed rest and underwent initial lumbar puncture that revealed grossly bloody fluid. Protein cerebrospinal fluid was 26 mg/100 ml, and sugar was 91 mg/100 ml. The patient underwent a right brachial arteriogram that was entirely normal. (Lumbar puncture opening pressure was 140 mm H_2O.) The patient underwent a right retrobrachial arteriogram that was entirely normal followed in 4 days by left carotid arteriogram that revealed a long, lobulated left internal carotid artery aneurysm. The patient at this time exhibited dilation of her left pupil with slight ptosis on the left, which improved over the next several days. She remained afebrile and had gradual diminution of her headache over the next several days. Her repeat lumbar puncture revealed 13,000 red blood cells and normal pressure. The patient remained perfectly alert with minimum symptoms. On May 11, 1970, she underwent application of a Ferguson clamp to her left internal carotid artery. Some difficulty was encountered in maintaining the clamp's pressure, but the patient evidenced no neurologic difficulty throughout this time. Following the application of the clamp, she states that her diplopia, which had been present for several days, had been resolved. She underwent removal of the clamp and ligation of her left internal carotid artery on May 13, 1970, and postoperatively remained entirely normal, afebrile, and asymptomatic. She was finally discharged on the ninth day postligation, ambulating with no neurologic deficit. She was discharged on no medication. Follow-up through Dr. White's office.

Discharge diagnoses: As noted above.

Denise Aronson, M.D.

DISCHARGE SUMMARY II: Marie Abadie

Kankakee General Hospital
Kankakee, Illinois 30603

Name: Marie Abadie

Admitted: 5/23/70

Discharged: 6/13/70

Neurology-Neurosurgery
6 West

Diagnosis: 1. Left cerebrovascular accident
2. Left internal carotid artery aneurysm, status postligation of left internal carotid artery May 13, 1970

Procedures: Lumbar puncture

Reason for admission: Sudden onset of aphasia at home.

Present illness: This 57-year-old white female, discharged on May 22, 1970, following successful left internal carotid artery ligation for treatment of left internal carotid artery aneurysm, had experienced a benign postoperative course and was fully ambulatory when discharged. She did well at home on only moderate activity. Having spent a quiet evening asleep, she was noted on the morning of admission to be entirely well but was found that afternoon by her friend lying on the floor unable to speak with a right hemiparesis. She was brought to the hospital immediately.

Past medical history: Please see old chart.

Physical examination: Revealed an alert patient who was trying to sit up. She was very calm; she was gazing to all fields, left more than right; she was not moving her right side, and she seemed to recognize people by smiling. Pulse was 80 and regular. Blood pressure was 160/80 mm Hg; respirations were 60; temperature was 36.5° C. The general physical examination revealed carotids that were 2+ and full. General physical examination was entirely normal and her neurologic examination revealed her mental status to be as stated previously. She was unable to follow commands or to verbalize. Cranial nerves all revealed no response to threat on the right side. The discs were both sharp. Her doll's eye movements were full without nystagmus. There was no ptosis, and her pupils were equal and rapidly reactive to light. She had a decreased corneal reflex on the right. There was normal sensation to pin prick on the face. She had inability to test lower cranial nerves. Motor examination revealed hemiparesis on the right with increased tone, lower extremity greater than upper extremity. Reflexes were 3+ on the right with an 8+ and upgoing toe, normal on the left. Sensory examination revealed bilateral response to pin prick with no motor response on the right side. The patient was gazing 2 to left and disregarding the right. Cerebellar function not tested.

Laboratory and x-ray data: Included hematocrit of 35% and white blood cell count 17,000/cu mm. Normal urinalysis. Chest and skull x-rays and brain scan normal. Electrolytes were generally normal.

Hospital course: The patient was placed on bed rest. Lumbar puncture was done with an opening pressure of 110 mm H_2O. Cells revealed 3 to 6 white blood cells, 0 to 1 red blood cells, sugar, protein and culture negative. The sugar was 18 mg/100 ml and protein 15 mg/100 ml. The patient was essentially placed on bed rest over the next several days. It was felt that she had experienced a left cerebrovascular accident related in some way to a stressful social situation. It was later discovered that the patient had been presented with multiple bills and announcement of foreclosure because of her past due mortgage payments. Over the next several days she exhibited normal reflexes with downgoing toes and no ankle clonus and gradual and persistent return of strength on her right side. However, her speech remained with marked deficits in that she had a marked and mixed receptive aphasia and for a full 2 weeks could only respond by saying, "Ah, you." She was able to write her name. She could at times demonstrate full sentences and solve simple problems. She could count by mimicry and she said reasonable sentences; she says "Hello" and "Goodbye" and "Thank you." She remained very anxious and was desirous to return home throughout all of her course. She is being transferred to the rehabilitation unit where Dr. Sandy Mayfield will follow her for speech and language services.

Discharge diagnoses: As noted above.

Denise Aronson, M.D.

SPEECH PATHOLOGY FINDINGS: Marie Abadie

Kankakee General Hospital
Kankakee, Illinois 30603

Name: Marie Abadie

Admitted: 6/13/70

Tested: 6/14/70

Rehabilitation Unit
3 West

This information will be presented as a sequence of tasks used for testing Marie Abadie, pointing out certain features for analysis consideration. This is not to be considered as all the testing and information that was obtained on Ms. Abadie.

A. Test samples used to measure
   1. Fluency in
   2. Comprehension of
   3. Formulation of
   4. Repetition of

   } Semantics, syntactics, and phonemics

B. The emphasis of the tasks is on verbal output as related to the above processes. The attempt is to discover processing deficits for planning therapy around language processing rather than on specific language products that are deviant.

C. On all tasks given observations should be made about all processes and behaviors elicited by the task.

D. Tasks
   1. Fluency measures elicited by two tasks from the *Boston Diagnostic Aphasia Examination*
      a. Spontaneous speech sample requiring
         (1) General biographical information
         (2) Yes/no responses
         (3) Descriptive answers
      b. More confrontation situations in which Marie has to describe or tell a story about a picture that involves a cookie theft. This task should be more difficult since it is tied to a specific stimulus that is unfamiliar information.
      c. Responses to this task
         (1) Rate: slow; generally under 50 words/minute
         (2) Prosody was abnormal—slow and halting
         (3) Pronunciation was abnormal
            (a) Sounds or syllables have slipped out of sequence, have been deleted, or are entirely extraneous to desired response; but more than half of the response corresponds to more than half of the required word. Use of one phoneme for another or a breakdown in the word structure but the meaning of the word is preserved.
         (4) Phrase length was short, which relates to the slow and halting speech.
         (5) Effort in initiation is noted, and this can be seen in the abnormal prosody and short phrase lengths. Facial grimacing and body movements used as attempts to facilitate speech production.
         (6) Pauses are frequent.
            (a) According to *Boston Diagnostic Aphasia Examination,* pauses are more for articulation difficulties
            (b) Pauses are attempts to correct error or to decide to continue despite errors

SPEECH PATHOLOGY FINDINGS: Marie Abadie—cont'd

D. Tasks—cont'd

    (c) Pauses result because the patient cannot continue because of difficulty producing the words

    (d) Patient who demonstrates effort to produce words will pause preceding and following phonation

    (e) May be pauses for word finding but mostly for difficulty in initiating proper phoneme

  (7) Word choice was mostly substantive words with grammatical errors noted. More concentration and effort noted when Marie is attempting to use pronouns, tenses, and functor words.

  (8) Up to this point comprehension skills appear intact.

2. Comprehension task from the *Minnesota Test for Differential Diagnosis of Aphasia*
   a. Semantic: patient points to appropriate letter named
   b. Syntactic
      (1) Identifying three items named serially
      (2) Following directions
   c. Responses to the comprehension tasks
      (1) No errors made

3. Formulation tasks: a variety of tasks for naming, producing sentences, cloze procedures, describing pictures, etc.
   a. Primary problems seem to center more on the pronunciation of words rather than word-finding problems. Phrase length was short, effort present, syntactical errors seen in tense, pluralization, and use of functor words. Phonemic substitutions present, difficulties with distinctive features and careful use of the articulators noted during speech production. Throughout, her rate is slow; effort and pauses are seen between syllables as she strives to produce the correct sounds. Her naming abilities are good and she does recall the words needed whether they and of, although all the substantive words were preserved.

4. Repetition tasks: words, phrases, and sentences with complex phonemic sequences
   a. Most errors produced were in pronunciation and not in remembering what the stimulus was. In the longer sentences she tended to omit syntactic words such as they and of, although all the substantive words were preserved.
   b. Many phonemic errors seen, occurring more frequently on the more complex phonemic sequences such as "Methodist Episcopal" and "My favorite vegetable." More effort and pauses occurred in these instances.

Sandy Mayfield, Ph.D.

Tests and tools available for designing the diagnosis: a tool-retrieval source

Appendix III is a presentation of tests and tools available for measuring various dimensions of speech and language disorders, causal factors, and associated problems that frequently accompany speech and language disorders.

The appendix is designed as an extension of Chapters 13 and 14 covering the design of the diagnosis and collection of the clinical data. As discussed in those chapters, selection of appropriate tools for data collection is critical to diagnosis.

We have developed this appendix of testing tools to assist the student with his diagnostic design. We have attempted to be rather comprehensive in our listing, providing tools for speech, language, and hearing disorders; tools that may be used for causal testing and tools for associated problems. However, the inclusion of a tool in this appendix does not reflect a quality judgment or an endorsement on our part. Rather, we see all tools and procedures as being potentially useful with some client at some time. We feel the student in training needs to explore many different tools of varying quality, rather than being given a set of tools to use for the different speech and language disorders. This selection and organization should serve as a starting point for the student in training—as the beginning of a tool-retrieval source. As he develops in his diagnostic skill, he can add and delete tools from this ever-changing list.

On the tool-retrieval table the tests and tools are listed alphabetically, irrespective of their purpose. We have listed the tool by its name, followed by one or more references to help in the location and evaluation of the tool.

The tools that measure some dimension of speech, language, and hearing are coded within the SLPM framework—speech and language product, behavioral correlates, and internal speech and language processes. These tools are used to measure or infer information about the cause-effect relationship expressed in the clinical hypothesis. A P will be used to code primary uses of the tool and at times an S will be used to code important secondary uses. The student should keep in mind, however, that these tools might be useful for purposes other than those coded here.

Tools that are viewed as measuring other causal factors and associated problems are simply listed; no coding is done.

In order to retrieve tools for use in diagnostic design the student can go down the appropriate columns on the form and find those tools that may be potentially appropriate for measuring aspects of his cause-effect relationship. He can then view the references for the tool to explore its specific relevance to the client he will be seeing for diagnosis.

TOOL-RETRIEVAL TABLE

Name of tool	Internal processing segments								Behavioral correlates							Speech product				Language product			
	Reception segment	Central segment	Production segment	Breathing	Phonation	Resonation	Articulation	Prosodation	Sensation	Perception	Comprehension	Formulation	Repetition	Sequencing	Motor control	Voice	Resonance	Phonetic structure	Prosody	Pragmatic	Semantic	Syntactic	Phonologic
Anton Brenner Developmental Gestalt Test of School Readiness Brenner, A., *Anton Brenner Developmental Gestalt Test of School Readiness*. Los Angeles: Western Psychological Services (1964).		P																					
Appraisal of Language Disturbances Emerick, L. L., *Manual for Appraisal of Language Disturbances*. Marquette, Mich.: Northern Michigan University (1971).			P								P	P								P	P	P	P
Arizona Articulation Proficiency Scale Fudala, J. B., *Arizona Articulation Proficiency Scale*. Los Angeles: Western Psychological Services (1970).		S	P				P					S		S	P			P					P
Arthur Adaptation of the Leiter International Performance Scale Arthur, G., *Arthur Adaptation of the Leiter International Performance Scale*. Washington, D.C.: The Psychological Service Center Press (1952).																							
Leiter, R. G., *Leiter International Performance Scale*. Washington, D.C.: The Psychological Service Center Press (1948).																							
Articulation Testing for use with Children with Cerebral Palsy Irwin, O. C., A manual of articulation testing with children with cerebral palsy. *Cerebral Palsy Rev.,* **22**, 1-24 (1961).		S	P				P					S		S	S			P	S				S

Continued.

TOOL-RETRIEVAL TABLE—cont'd

Name of tool	Reception segment	Central segment	Production segment	Breathing	Phonation	Resonation	Articulation	Prosodation	Sensation	Perception	Comprehension	Formulation	Repetition	Sequencing	Motor control	Voice	Resonance	Phonetic structure	Prosody	Pragmatic	Semantic	Syntactic	Phonologic
Assessment of Children's Language Comprehension — Foster, R., Giddan, J. J., and Stark, J., *Manual for the Assessment of Children's Language Comprehension*. Palo Alto, Calif.: Consulting Psychologists Press (1972).		P									P												
Assessment in Infancy: Ordinal Scales of Psychological Development — Uzgiris, J. C., and Hunt, J., *Assessment in Infancy: Ordinal Scales of Psychological Development*. Urbana, Ill.: University of Illinois Press (1975).																							
Audiometric Procedures — Pure Tone Audiometry — Speech Audiometry — Special Testing Procedures — Katz, J. (Ed.), *Handbook of Clinical Audiology*. Baltimore: The Williams & Wilkins Co. (1972). — Rose, D. (Ed.), *Audiological Assessment*. Englewood Cliffs, N.J.: Prentice-Hall, Inc. (1971).	P								P	P													
Auditory Analysis Test — Rosner, J., and Simon, D., *Auditory Analysis Test*. Pittsburgh: Learning Research and Development Center, University of Pittsburgh (1970).	P	S	S							P	S	S	S					S					S

Reference								
Auditory Behavior Observation Guides McConnell, F., and Ward, P., *Deafness in Childhood.* Nashville: Vanderbilt University Press (1967).	P	S			P	P	S	
Myklebust, H. R., *Auditory Disorders in Children.* New York: Grune & Stratton, Inc. (1954).								
Rose, D. E. (Ed.), *Audiological Assessment.* Englewoods Cliffs, N.J.: Prentice-Hall, Inc. (1971).								
Auditory Discrimination Test Wepman, J., *Auditory Discrimination Test.* Chicago: Language Research Associates (1958).	P	S			P	P	S	
Auditory Memory for Speech Sounds Metraux, R. W., Auditory memory span for speech sounds of speech defective children compared with normal children. *J. Speech Dis.*, **6**, 33-36 (1942).	P	S	S		P	S		S
Metraux, R. W., Auditory memory span for speech sounds: Norms for children. *J. Speech Dis.*, **9**, 31-38 (1944).								
Ayres Space Test Ayres, A. J., *Ayres Space Test.* Los Angeles: Western Psychological Services (1962).								
Basic Concept Inventory Engelmann, S., *The Basic Concept Inventory.* Chicago: Follett Educational Corporation (1967).								
Bayley Scales of Infant Development Bayley, N., *Bayley Scales of Infant Development.* New York: Psychological Corporation of America (1969).								
Aram, D. M., and Nation, J. E., Intelligence tests for children: A language analysis. *Ohio J. Speech Hearing,* **6**, 22-43 (1971).								

Continued.

TOOL-RETRIEVAL TABLE—cont'd

Column groups: Internal processing segments (Reception segment, Central segment, Production segment, Breathing, Phonation, Resonation, Articulation, Prosodation) · Behavioral correlates (Sensation, Perception, Comprehension, Formulation, Repetition, Sequencing, Motor control) · Speech product (Voice, Resonance, Phonetic structure, Prosody) · Language product (Pragmatic, Semantic, Syntactic, Phonologic)

Name of tool	Reception segment	Central segment	Production segment	Breathing	Phonation	Resonation	Articulation	Prosodation	Sensation	Perception	Comprehension	Formulation	Repetition	Sequencing	Motor control	Voice	Resonance	Phonetic structure	Prosody	Pragmatic	Semantic	Syntactic	Phonologic
Bender-Gestalt Test for Young Children. Bender, L., A visual motor gestalt test and its clinical use. New York: American Orthopsychiatric Association, *Research Monogr. No. 3* (1938).																							
Koppitz, E. M., *Bender-Gestalt Test for Young Children.* New York: The Psychological Corporation (1964).																							
Berry-Talbott Tests of Language: I. Comprehension of Grammar. Berry, M. *Berry-Talbott Tests of Language: I. Comprehension of Grammar.* Rockford, Ill.: 4322 Pinecrest Road (1966).		P									P	P										P	
Boston Diagnostic Aphasia Examination. Goodglass, J., and Kaplan, E., *The Assessment of Aphasia and Related Disorders.* Philadelphia: Lea & Febiger (1972).		P									P	P	P							P	P	P	P
Bryngleson-Glaspey Articulation Test. Bryngleson, B., and Glaspey, E., *Speech in the Classroom (with Speech Improvement Cards).* (3rd ed.) Chicago: Scott, Foresman & Co. (1962).		S	P				P					S			P			P					P
Bzoch Error Pattern Diagnostic Articulation Test. Bzoch, K. R., Introduction to section C: Measurement of parameters of cleft palate speech. In W. C. Grabb, S. W. Rosenstein, and K. R. Bzoch, *Cleft Lip and Palate: Surgical, Dental, and Speech Aspects.* Boston: Little, Brown & Co. (1971).		S	P			P	P					S			P		P	P					P

Test / Reference							
California Test of Personality Thorpe, L. P., Clark, W. W., and Tiegs, E. W., *California Test of Personality.* Monterey, Calif.: California Test Bureau (1953).							
Carrow Elicited Language Inventory Carrow-Woolfolk, E., *Carrow Elicited Language Inventory.* Austin, Tex.: Learning Concepts (1974).	P			P			P
Cattell Infant Intelligence Scale Cattell, P., *The Measurement of Intelligence of Infants and Young Children.* New York: The Psychological Corporation (1947).							
Aram, D. M., and Nation, J. E., Intelligence tests for children: A language analysis. *Ohio J. Speech Hearing,* **6,** 22-43 (1971).				S			
Check List of Stuttering Reactions Johnson, W., Darley, F., and Spriestersbach, D., *Diagnostic Methods in Speech Pathology.* New York: Harper & Row, Publishers (1963).		P	P P		P	P	
Chicago Non Verbal Examination Brown, A. W., and Stein, S., *Chicago Non Verbal Examination.* New York: The Psychological Corporation (1936).							
Child Behavior Rating Scale Cassell, R., *Child Behavior Rating Scale.* Los Angeles: Western Psychological Services (1962).							
Children's Apperception Test Bellak, L., and Bellak, S. S., *Children's Apperception Test.* (5th ed.) Los Angeles: Western Psychological Services (1971).							
Bellak, L., *The Thematic Apperception Test and the Children's Apperception Test in Clinical Use.* New York: Grune & Stratton, Inc. (1954).							
Haworth, M. R., *The CAT: Facts About Fantasy.* New York: Grune & Stratton, Inc. (1966).							

TOOL-RETRIEVAL TABLE—cont'd

Name of tool	Internal processing segments								Behavioral correlates							Speech product				Language product			
	Reception segment	Central segment	Production segment	Breathing	Phonation	Resonation	Articulation	Prosodation	Sensation	Perception	Comprehension	Formulation	Repetition	Sequencing	Motor control	Voice	Resonance	Phonetic structure	Prosody	Pragmatic	Semantic	Syntactic	Phonologic
Columbia Mental Maturity Scale Burgemeister, B., Blum, L., and Lorge, I., *Columbia Mental Maturity Scale*. New York: Harcourt Brace Jovanovich, Inc. (1953).																							
Communicative Evaluation Chart From Infancy to Five Years Anderson, M., Miles, M., and Matheny, P., *Communicative Evaluation Chart from Infancy to Five Years*. Cambridge, Mass.: Educators Publishing Service, Inc. (1963).	P	P	P																				
Deep Test of Articulation McDonald, E. T., *A Deep Test of Articulation*. Pittsburgh: Stanwix House, Inc. (1964). McDonald, E. T., *A Screening Deep Test of Articulation*. Pittsburgh: Stanwix House, Inc. (1968).		S	P				P					S		S	S P			P					P
Denver Articulation Screening Exam Drumwright, A. F., *Denver Articulation Screening Exam*. Denver: University of Colorado Medical Center (1971). Drumwright, A., Van Natta, P., Camp, B., Frankenburg, W., and Drexler, H., The Denver articulation screening exam. *J. Speech Hearing Dis.*, **38**, 3-14 (1973).		S	P				P					S		S	S P			P					P

Test (reference)												
Denver Developmental Screening Test — Frankenburg, W. K., and Dodd, J. B., *Denver Developmental Screening Test.* Denver: University of Colorado Medical Center (1967).												
Frankenburg, W., Dodds, J., and Fandal, A., *Denver Developmental Screening Test.* Denver: University of Colorado Medical Center (1970).												
Detroit Tests of Learning Aptitude — Baker, H. J., and Leland, B., *Detroit Tests of Learning Aptitude.* Indianapolis: The Bobbs-Merrill Co., Inc. (1959).												
Developmental Articulation Test — Hejna, R., *Developmental Articulation Test:* Ann Arbor, Mich.: Speech Materials (1959).	S	P			S		P		S	P		P
Developmental Potential of Preschool Children — Haeussermann, E., *Developmental Potential of Preschool Children.* New York: Grune & Stratton, Inc. (1958).												
Developmental Sentence Types / Developmental Sentence Scoring / Developmental Sentence Analysis — Lee, L., *Developmental Sentence Analysis.* Evanston, Ill.: Northwestern University Press (1974).	P	S			P				P		P P P	P P P
Longhurst, T. M., Review of Lee's developmental sentence analysis. *Asha,* **17,** 429-430 (1975).												
Developmental Test of Visual Perception — Frostig, M., Lefever, D., Maslow, P., and Whittlesley, R., *Marianne Frostig Developmental Test of Visual Perception.* Palo Alto, Calif.: Consulting Psychologists Press (1964).	S	P					P		S			P
Diagnostic Sentences — Schoolfield, L., *Better Speech and Better Reading.* Magnolia, Mass.: Expression Co. (1951).	S	P					S		P			P

Continued.

TOOL-RETRIEVAL TABLE—cont'd

Name of tool	Internal processing segments								Behavioral correlates							Speech product				Language product			
	Reception segment	Central segment	Production segment	Breathing	Phonation	Resonation	Articulation	Prosodation	Sensation	Perception	Comprehension	Formulation	Repetition	Sequencing	Motor control	Voice	Resonance	Phonetic structure	Prosody	Pragmatic	Semantic	Syntactic	Phonologic
Durrell Analysis of Reading Difficulty. Durrell, D. D., *Manual of Directions for Durrell Analysis of Reading Difficulty.* New York: Harcourt Brace Jovanovich, Inc. (1937).		P																					
Environmental Language Inventory. MacDonald, J. D., and Nickols, *Environmental Language Inventory.* Columbus, Ohio: The Nisonger Center, Ohio State University (1974).												P									P	P	
Examining for Aphasia. Eisenson, J., *Examining for Aphasia.* New York: The Psychological Corporation (1954).		P									P	P								P	P	P	P
Examining for Harshness. Fairbanks, G., *Voice and Articulation Drill Book* (2nd ed.) New York: Harper & Row, Publishers (1960).			P		P										P	P							
Fer-Will Object Kit. Ferger, and Williams, *Fer-Will Object Kit.* West Sacramento, Calif.: King Company Educational Publishers.		S	P				P					S			P			P			S		P
Fisher-Logemann Test of Articulation Competence. Fisher, H. B., and Logemann, J. A., *Fisher-Logemann Test of Articulation Competence.* Boston: Houghton Mifflin Co. (1971).		S	P				P					S			P			P					P

Test								
Flowers-Costello Tests of Central Auditory Abilities Flowers, A., Costello, M., and Small, V., *Flowers-Costello Test of Central Auditory Abilities*. Dearborn, Mich.: Perceptual Learning Systems (1970).	P		P	P		S			P
Full-Range Picture Vocabulary Test Ammons, R. B., and Ammons, H. S., *Full-Range Picture Vocabulary Test*. Missoula, Mont.: Psychological Test Specialists (1958).	P					P			
Functional Communication Profile Sarno, M. T., *Functional Communication Profile*. New York: New York University Medical Center, Institute of Rehabilitation Medicine (1963).	P	P	P			P	P	P	P
Goldman-Fristoe Test of Articulation Goldman, R., and Fristoe, M., *Goldman-Fristoe Test of Articulation*. Circle Pines, Minn.: American Guidance Service, Inc. (1969).	S	P			S	P			P
Goldman-Fristoe-Woodcock Test of Auditory Discrimination Goldman, R., Fristoe, M., and Woodcock, R., *Goldman-Fristoe-Woodcock Test of Auditory Discrimination*. Circle Pines, Minn.: American Guidance Service, Inc. (1970).	P	P	P	S					
Goodenough-Harris Drawing Test Goodenough, R. L., and Harris, D. B., *Goodenough-Harris Drawing Test*. New York: Harcourt Brace Jovanovich, Inc. (1963). Harris, D., *Children's Drawings as Measures of Intellectual Maturity*. New York: Harcourt Brace Jovanovich, Inc. (1963).									
Hannah-Gardner Preschool Language Screening Test Hannah, E., and Gardner, J., *Hannah-Gardner Preschool Language Screening Test*. Northridge, Calif.: Joyce Publications (1974).	P		P		P	P	P	P	P

Continued.

TOOL-RETRIEVAL TABLE—cont'd

Name of tool	Internal processing segments								Behavioral correlates							Speech product				Language product			
	Reception segment	Central segment	Production segment	Breathing	Phonation	Resonation	Articulation	Prosodation	Sensation	Perception	Comprehension	Formulation	Repetition	Sequencing	Motor control	Voice	Resonance	Phonetic structure	Prosody	Pragmatic	Semantic	Syntactic	Phonologic
Harris Tests of Lateral Dominance Harris, A. J. *Harris Tests of Lateral Dominance.* New York: The Psychological Corporation (1955).																							
Hiskey-Nebraska Test of Learning Aptitude Hiskey, M., *Hiskey-Nebraska Test of Learning Aptitude.* Lincoln, Neb.: University of Nebraska Press (1966).																							
Hiskey, M. S., *Nebraska Test of Learning Aptitude for Young Deaf Children.* New York: The Psychological Corporation (1941).																							
Houston Test for Language Development Crabtree, M., *Houston Test for Language Development.* Houston: Houston Test Co. (1963).		P									P	P								P	P	P	P
Illinois Test of Psycholinguistic Abilities Kirk, S. A., McCarthy, J., and Kirk, W. D., *Illinois Test of Psycholinguistic Abilities.* (Rev. ed.) Urbana, Ill.: University of Illinois Press (1968).		P									P	P								P	P	P	P
Iowa Pressure Articulation Test See: Templin-Darley Tests of Articulation Morris, H. L., Spriestersbach, D. C., and Darley, F. L. An articulation test for assessing competency of velopharyngeal closure. *J. Speech Hearing Res.*, **4**, 48-55 (1961).			P			P	P								P		P	P					

Test									
Iowa Scale for Rating Severity of Stuttering — Sherman D., *Iowa Scale for Rating Severity of Stuttering.* Danville, Ill.: The Interstate Printers & Publishers, Inc. (1961).	P			P		P	P		P
Kindergarten Auditory Screening Test — Katz, J., *Kindergarten Auditory Screening Test.* Chicago: Follett Educational Corporation (1971).	P	P			P P S				P P P
Language Modalities Test for Aphasia — Wepman, J., and Jones, L., *Studies in Aphasia: An Approach to Testing; Manual of Administration and Scoring for the Language Modalities Test for Aphasia.* Chicago: Education-Industry Service (1961).	P			P P					P
Laradon Articulation Scale — Edmonston, W., *Laradon Articulation Scale.* Los Angeles: Western Psychological Services (1963).	S	P		P	S	P	P		P
Lindamood Auditory Conceptualization Test — Lindamood, C. H., and Lindamood, P. C., *Lindamood Auditory Conceptualization Test.* Boston: Teaching Resources Corp. (1969).	P			P	P P S				
Measure of Adaptation of Stuttering — Johnson, W., Darley, F., and Spriestersbach, D., *Diagnostic Methods in Speech Pathology.* New York: Harper & Row, Publishers (1963).				P		P P	P		
Measure of Consistency of Stuttering — Johnson, W., Darley, F., and Spriestersbach, D., *Diagnostic Methods in Speech Pathology.* New York: Harper & Row, Publishers (1963).				P		P P	P		
Merrill-Palmer Scale of Mental Tests — Stutsman, R., *Mental Measurement of Preschool Children.* Yonkers-on-Hudson, New York: World Book Co. (1931). Aram, D. M., and Nation, J. E., Intelligence tests for children: A language analysis. *Ohio J. Speech Hearing,* **6,** 22-43 (1971).									

Continued.

TOOL-RETRIEVAL TABLE—cont'd

Name of tool	Internal processing segments								Behavioral correlates							Speech product				Language product			
	Reception segment	Central segment	Production segment	Breathing	Phonation	Resonation	Articulation	Prosodation	Sensation	Perception	Comprehension	Formulation	Repetition	Sequencing	Motor control	Voice	Resonance	Phonetic structure	Prosody	Pragmatic	Semantic	Syntactic	Phonologic
Memory-for-Designs Test. Graham, R., and Kendall, B., *Memory-for-Designs Test*. Missoula, Mont.: Psychological Test Specialists.																							
Graham, F. K., and Kendall, B. S., Memory-for-Designs Test: Revised general manual. *Percept. Motor Skills*, **11**, 147-190 (1960).																							
Miami Imitative Ability Test. Jacobs, R. J., Phillips, B. J., and Harrison, R. J., A stimulability test for cleft-palate children. *J. Speech Hearing Dis.*, **35**, 354-360 (1970).			P			P	P						P		P		P	P					
Michigan Picture Language Inventory. Lerea, L., *Michigan Picture Language Inventory*. Ann Arbor, Mich.: University of Michigan Press (1958).		P									P	P								P	P	P	
Wolski, W., *The Michigan Picture Language Inventory*. Ann Arbor, Mich.: University of Michigan Press (1962).											P	P								P	P	P	P
Miller-Yoder Test of Grammatical Comprehension. Miller, J. F., and Yoder, D. E., *The Miller-Yoder Test of Grammatical Comprehension: Experimental Edition*. Madison, Wisc.: Department of Communicative Disorders, University of Wisconsin (1972).		P									P												

Minnesota Test For Differential Diagnosis of Aphasia
Schuell, H.. *Administrative Manual for the Minnesota Test for Differential Diagnosis of Aphasia.* Minneapolis: University of Minnesota Press (1965).

Schuell, H., *Differential Diagnosis of Aphasia with the Minnesota Test.* Minneapolis: University of Minnesota Press (1965).

Mother-Child Relationship Evaluation
Roth, R. M., *Mother-Child Relationship Evaluation.* Beverly Hills, Calif.: Western Psychological Services (1961).

"Neuropsychological" Tests
Spreen, O., and Gaddes, W. H., Developmental norms for 15 neuropsychological tests age 6 to 15. *Cortex*, **5**, 170-191 (1969).
Many of these tools are perceptual-motor tests.

Neurosensory Center Comprehensive Examination for Aphasia
Spreen, O., and Benton, A. L., *Neurosensory Center Comprehensive Examination for Aphasia.* Victoria, B. C.: University of Victoria, Department of Psychology (1969).

Northwestern Syntax Screening Test
Lee, L., *Northwestern Syntax Screening Test.* Evanston, Ill.: Northwestern University Press (1969).

Oral Reading Sentences for Breathy Quality
Fairbanks, G., *Voice and Articulation Drill Book.* (2nd ed.) New York: Harper & Row, Publishers (1960).

Orzeck Aphasia Evaluation
Orzeck, A., *Orzeck Aphasia Evaluation Manual.* Beverly Hills, Calif.: Western Psychological Services (1964).

Continued.

TOOL-RETRIEVAL TABLE—cont'd

Name of tool	Internal processing segments								Behavioral correlates							Speech product				Language product			
	Reception segment	Central segment	Production segment	Breathing	Phonation	Resonation	Articulation	Prosodation	Sensation	Perception	Comprehension	Formulation	Repetition	Sequencing	Motor control	Voice	Resonance	Phonetic structure	Prosody	Pragmatic	Semantic	Syntactic	Phonologic
Oseretsky Test of Motor Proficiency Doll, E. A. (Ed.), *Oseretsky Test of Motor Proficiency*. Circle Pines, Minn.: American Guidance Service, Inc. (1964).																							
Parent Attitudes Scale Wiley, J. H., A scale to measure parental attitudes. *J. Speech Hearing Dis.*, **20**, 284-290 (1955).																							
Parsons Language Sample Spradlin, J. E., Assessment of speech and language of retarded children: The Parsons language sample. *J. Speech Hearing Dis., Monogr. Suppl.* **10**, 8-31 (1963).		P									P	P	P							P	P	P	P
Peabody Picture Vocabulary Test Dunn, L. M., *Expanded Manual for the Peabody Picture Vocabulary Test*. Circle Pines, Minn.: American Guidance Service, Inc. (1965).		P									P										P		
Photo Articulation Test Pendergast, K., Dickey, S., Selman, J. and Soder, A., *Photo Articulation Test*. Danville, Ill.: The Interstate Printers & Publishers, Inc. (1969).			P				P								P			P					P
Pictorial Test of Intelligence French, J. L., *Pictorial Test of Intelligence*. Boston: Houghton-Mifflin Co. (1960).																							
Aram, D. M., and Nation, J. E., Intelligence tests for children: A language analysis. *Ohio J. Speech Hearing*, **6**, 22-43 (1971).																							

Test / Reference											
Picture Story Language Test Myklebust, H., *Development and Disorders of Written Language: Picture Story Language Test.* (Vol. 1) New York: Grune & Stratton, Inc. (1965).											
Pitch Analysis Test Van Riper, C., *Speech Correction: Principles and Methods.* (4th ed.) Englewood Cliffs, N. J.: Prentice-Hall, Inc. (1963).				P	P						
Porch Index of Communicative Ability Porch, B. E., *Porch Index of Communicative Ability.* Palo Alto, Calif.: Consulting Psychologists Press (1967).	P	P	P					P			
Porch, B. E., *Porch Index of Communicative Ability: Theory and Development.* (Vol. 1) Palo Alto, Calif.: Consulting Psychologists Press (1967).											
Porch, B. E., *Porch Index of Communicative Ability: Administration, Scoring, and Interpretation.* (Vol. 2, Rev. ed.) Palo Alto, Calif.: Consulting Psychologists Press (1971).											
Porch Index of Communicative Ability in Children Porch, B. E., *Porch Index of Communicative Ability in Children.* Palo Alto, Calif.: Consulting Psychologists Press (1974).	P	P	P				P				
Predictive Screening Test of Articulation Van Riper, C., and Erickson, R., *Predictive Screening Test of Articulation.* Kalamazoo, Mich.: Western Michigan University Press (1968).	P			P			S		P		S
Preschool Attainment Record Doll, E. A., *Preschool Attainment Record.* Circle Pines, Minn.: American Guidance Service, Inc. (1966).											

Continued.

TOOL-RETRIEVAL TABLE—cont'd

Name of tool	Internal processing segments								Behavioral correlates							Speech product				Language product			
	Reception segment	Central segment	Production segment	Breathing	Phonation	Resonation	Articulation	Prosodation	Sensation	Perception	Comprehension	Formulation	Repetition	Sequencing	Motor control	Voice	Resonance	Phonetic structure	Prosody	Pragmatic	Semantic	Syntactic	Phonologic
Preschool Language Manual Zimmerman, I., Steiner, V., and Evatt, R., *Preschool Language Manual*. Columbus, Ohio: Charles E. Merrill Publishing Co. (1969).	P		S								P	P						S		P	P	P	P
Primary Visual Motor Test Haworth, M., *The Primary Visual Motor Test*. New York: Grune & Stratton, Inc. (1970).																							
Pupil Rating Scale: Screening for Learning Disabilities Myklebust, H. R., *Pupil Rating Scale: Screening for Learning Disabilities*. New York: Grune & Stratton, Inc. (1971).																							
Purdue Pegboard Tiffin, J., *Examiner Manual for the Purdue Pegboard*. Chicago: Science Research Associates (1948).																							
Purdue Perceptual-Motor Survey Roach, E., and Kephart, N., *The Purdue Perceptual-Motor Survey*. Columbus, Ohio: Charles E. Merrill Publishing Co. (1966).																							
Quick Test Ammons, R. B., and Ammons, C. H., *Quick Test*. Missoula, Mont.: Psychological Test Specialists (1962).																							

Test / Reference													
Rainbow Passage Fairbanks, G., *Voice and Articulation Drillbook.* (2nd ed.) New York: Harper & Row, Publishers (1960).	P	P	P				P	P	P		P			P
Receptive-Expressive Emergent Language Scale (REEL) Bzoch, K., and League, R., *Assessing Language Skills in Infancy.* Gainesville, Fla.: Tree of Life Press (1971).	S				P					S			P	P
Reynell Developmental Language Scales Reynell, J., *Reynell Developmental Language Scales: Manual (Experimental Edition).* Buckinghamshire, England: National Foundation for Educational Research in England and Wales (1969).	P		P						P		P		P	P
Riley Articulation and Language Test Riley, G., *Riley Articulation and Language Test.* Beverly Hills, Calif.: Western Psychological Services (1966).	P		P			P	S		P		P		P	P
Screening Speech Articulation Test Mecham, M., Jex, J. L., and Jones, J. D., *Screening Speech Articulation Test.* Salt Lake City: Communication Research Associates (1970).	P				S		S		P		S			P
Screening Test for Auditory Comprehension of Language Carrow-Woolfolk, E., *Screening Test for Auditory Comprehension of Language.* Austin, Tex.: Learning Concepts (1973).					P						P			
Screening Tests for Identifying Children with Specific Language Disability Slingerland, B. H., *Screening Tests for Identifying Children with Specific Language Disability.* Cambridge, Mass.: Educators Publishing Service, Inc. (1967).														
Short Examination for Aphasia Schuell, H., A short examination for aphasia. *Neurology,* **7,** 625–634 (1957).	P				P						P	P	P	P

Continued.

TOOL-RETRIEVAL TABLE—cont'd

Name of tool	Internal processing segments								Behavioral correlates							Speech product				Language product			
	Reception segment	Central segment	Production segment	Breathing	Phonation	Resonation	Articulation	Prosodation	Sensation	Perception	Comprehension	Formulation	Repetition	Sequencing	Motor control	Voice	Resonance	Phonetic structure	Prosody	Pragmatic	Semantic	Syntactic	Phonologic
Sklar Aphasia Scale — Sklar, M., *Sklar Aphasia Scale Manual.* Beverly Hills, Calif.: Western Psychological Services (1966).		P									P	P								P	P	P	P
Southern California Figure-Ground Visual Perception Test — Ayres, A. J., *Southern California Figure-Ground Visual Perception Test.* Los Angeles: Western Psychological Services (1966).																							
Southern California Kinesthesia and Tactile Perception Tests — Ayres, A. J., *Southern California Kinesthesia and Tactile Perception Tests.* Los Angeles: Western Psychological Services (1966).																							
Southern California Motor Accuracy Test — Ayres, A. J., *Southern California Motor Accuracy Test.* Los Angeles: Western Psychological Services (1964).																							
Southern California Perceptual-Motor Test — Ayres, A. J., *Southern California Perceptual-Motor Test.* Los Angeles: Western Psychological Services (1968).																							
Southern Illinois University Behavior Check List — Brutten, G. J., and Shoemaker, D. J., *Southern Illinois University Behavior Check List.* Carbondale, Ill.: Southern Illinois University (1974).																							

Test / Reference															
Southern Illinois University Speech Situations Check List Brutten, G. J., and Shoemaker, D. J., *Southern Illinois University Speech Situations Check List*. Carbondale, Ill.: Southern Illinois University (1974).												P	P		
Spontaneous Speech and Language Sample Analyses Lee, L., *Developmental Sentence Analysis*. Evanston, Ill.: Northwestern University Press (1974).	P	P				P	P	P	P	P	P			P	
See: References (Chapters 13 through 16)															
Stanford-Binet Intelligence Scale Terman, L. M., and Merrill, M. A., *Stanford-Binet Intelligence Scale: Manual for the Third Revision, Form L-M*. Boston: Houghton Mifflin Co. (1960).															
Aram, D. M., and Nation, J. E., Intelligence tests for children: A language analysis. *Ohio J. Speech Hearing*, **6**, 22–43 (1971).															
Supplementary Examination for Breathiness Johnson, W., Darley, F., and Spriestersbach, D., *Diagnostic Methods in Speech Pathology*. New York: Harper & Row, Publishers (1963).	P	P			P	P									
Supplementary Examination for Nasality Johnson, W., Darley, F., and Spriestersbach, D., *Diagnostic Methods in Speech Pathology*. New York: Harper & Row, Publishers (1963).	P	P			P	P									
Templin-Darley Tests of Articulation Templin, M. C., and Darley, F. L., *Templin-Darley Tests of Articulation*. (2nd ed.) Iowa City, Iowa: Bureau of Educational Research and Service, University of Iowa (1969).	S	P			S	P								P	

Continued.

TOOL-RETRIEVAL TABLE—cont'd

Name of tool	Reception segment	Central segment	Production segment	Breathing	Phonation	Resonation	Articulation	Prosodation	Sensation	Perception	Comprehension	Formulation	Repetition	Sequencing	Motor control	Voice	Resonance	Phonetic structure	Prosody	Pragmatic	Semantic	Syntactic	Phonologic
	Internal processing segments								Behavioral correlates							Speech product				Language product			
Templin Picture Sound Discrimination Test. Templin, M., *Certain Language Skills in Children.* Minneapolis: University of Minnesota Press (1957).	P	P							P	P	S												
Test of Listening Accuracy in Children. Mecham, M. J., Jex, J. L., and Jones, J. D., *Test of Listening Accuracy in Children.* Provo, Utah: Brigham Young University Press (1969).	P	P							P	P	S												
Test for Auditory Comprehension of Language. Carrow-Woolfolk, E., *Test for Auditory Comprehension of Language.* Austin, Tex.: Learning Concepts (1970).		P									P												
Thematic Apperception Test. Murray, H. A., *Thematic Apperception Test.* Cambridge, Mass.: Harvard University Press (1943).																							
Bellak, L., *The Thematic Apperception Test and the Children's Apperception Test in Clinical Use.* New York: Grune & Stratton, Inc. (1954).																							
Tina Bangs Language Scale. Bangs, T. E., Evaluating children with language delay. *J. Speech Hearing Dis.*, **26**, 6-18 (1961).		P									P	P								P	P	P	
Bangs, T. E., *Language and Learning Disorders of the Pre-academic Child.* New York: Appleton-Century-Crofts (1968).											P	P									P	P	

Token Test
DeRenzi, E., and Vignolo, L. A., The Token Test: A sensitive test to detect receptive disturbances in aphasia. *Brain*, **85**, 665-678 (1962).

Spellacy, F., and Spreen, O., A short form of the Token Test. *Cortex*, **5**, 390-397 (1969).

Total Dysfluency Index
Johnson, W., Darley, F., and Spriestersbach, D., *Diagnostic Methods in Speech Pathology*. New York: Harper & Row, Publishers (1963).

Travis-Rasmus Test of Auditory Discrimination Ability
Travis, L. E., and Rasmus, B. J., The speech sound discrimination ability of cases with functional disorders of articulation. *Quart. J. Speech Educ.*, **17**, 217-226 (1931).

Utah Test of Language Development
Mecham, M., Jex, J., and Jones, J., *Utah Test of Language Development*. Salt Lake City: Communication Research Associates (1967).

Verbal Language Development Scale
Mecham, M., *Verbal Language Development Scale*. Circle Pines, Minn.: American Guidance Service, Inc. (1958).

Vineland Social Maturity Scale
Doll, E. A., *Vineland Social Maturity Scale: Condensed Manual of Directions*. Circle Pines, Minn.: American Guidance Service, Inc. (1965).

Vocabulary Usage Test
Nation, J. E., A vocabulary usage test. *J. Psycholing. Res.*, **1**, 221-231 (1972).

Weschler Adult Intelligence Scale
Weschler, D., *Manual for the Weschler Adult Intelligence Scale*. New York: The Psychological Corporation (1955).

Continued.

TOOL-RETRIEVAL TABLE—cont'd

Name of tool	Reception segment	Central segment	Production segment	Breathing	Phonation	Resonation	Articulation	Prosodation	Sensation	Perception	Comprehension	Formulation	Repetition	Sequencing	Motor control	Voice	Resonance	Phonetic structure	Prosody	Pragmatic	Semantic	Syntactic	Phonologic
	Internal processing segments								**Behavioral correlates**							**Speech product**				**Language product**			
Weschler Intelligence Scale for Children — Weschler, D., *Manual for the Weschler Intelligence Scale for Children.* New York: The Psychological Corporation (1949).																							
Aram, D. M., and Nation, J. E., Intelligence tests for children: A language analysis. *Ohio J. Speech Hearing,* **6,** 22-43 (1971).																							
Weschler Preschool and Primary Scale of Intelligence — Weschler, D., *Weschler Preschool and Primary Scale of Intelligence.* New York: The Psychological Corporation (1963).																							
Aram, D. M., and Nation, J. E., Intelligence tests for children: A language analysis. *Ohio J. Speech Hearing,* **6,** 22-43 (1971).																							
Wide Range Achievement Test — Jastak, J., *Wide Range Achievement Test.* Wilmington, Del.: Charles L. Story Co. (1946).																							
Word Intelligibility by Picture Identification — Ross, M., and Lerman, J., *Word Intelligibility by Picture Identification.* Pittsburgh: Stanwix House, Inc. (1971).	P	P							P	P	S												

Speech mechanism examination form

SPEECH MECHANISM EXAMINATION

Name _____ Birth date _____ Age ____ Center No. ____

Examiner _____ Date _____

Adequacy for speech ratings

1 = Normal

2 = Slight deviation—probably no adverse effect on speech

3 = Moderate deviation—possible adverse effect on speech; remedial services may be required particularly if other structures of the speech mechanism are also deviant

4 = Extreme deviation—sufficient to prevent normal production of speech; modification of structure required if possible, either with or without clinical speech services, or speech services needed to compensate for the structural deviation

General physical appearance _____

_____

_____

General appearance of head and face

Symmetry, size and shape of head and face _____

_____

Scars _____

_____

Facial grimaces noted during speech _____

_____

Muscles of facial expression—ability to: Smile _____ Wink _____ Wrinkle forehead _____

Eyes

  Intraocular distance: Normal _____ Other _____

  Ptosis: None _____ Right _____ Left _____ Bilateral _____

Nose

Structure

  Deviated septum: No _____ To right _____ To left _____

  Deviated columella: No _____ To right _____ To left _____

Continued.

SPEECH MECHANISM EXAMINATION—cont'd

Nose—cont'd

Function

History of upper respiratory infections: No _____ Yes _____ Explain _____

_____

Nasal obstruction: No _____ Right _____ Left _____ Bilateral _____ Describe _____

_____

Mouth breathing: No _____ Yes _____ Chronic _____ Acute _____ Describe _____

_____

Adequacy for speech: 1 _____ 2 _____ 3 _____ 4 _____

Lips

Structure

Upper lip length: Normal _____ Short _____ Markedly short _____

Symmetric: Yes _____ No _____

Do lips touch when teeth are in occlusion? Yes _____ No _____

Other abnormalities _____

_____

Function

Describe instructions necessary to obtain performance (e.g., imitation, tactile stimulation, etc.) _____

_____

Protrude: Yes _____ No _____   Tense and press: Yes _____ No _____   Eversion:
Yes _____ No _____

Retraction: Right _____ Left _____   Bilateral symmetry: Yes _____ No _____

	Trials			Rating		
	1	*2*	*3*	*Above av.*	*Av.*	*Below av.*
Rounding and retraction of lips (o-ee o-ee) in 10 sec. (5 times in 15 sec)[1]						
Number of times can say /pʌ/ in 5 sec (range 3.0-5.5 per sec)[2,3]						

Description of function _____

Adequacy for speech: 1 _____ 2 _____ 3 _____ 4 _____

Mandible

Structure

Size _____

_____

Shape _____

_____

SPEECH MECHANISM EXAMINATION—cont'd

Mandible—cont'd

Function

Ability to chew _____

Diadochokinesis (rate and rhythm) _____ /ja/

Adequacy for speech: 1 _____ 2 _____ 3 _____ 4 _____

Teeth

Occlusion: Normal _____ Neutroclusion _____ Distoclusion _____ Mesioclusion _____

Vertical relationship of anterior teeth: Normal _____ Open bite _____ Closed bite _____
Crossbite _____

Maxillary collapse: No _____ Yes _____ Right _____ Left _____ Bilateral _____

Anterior-posterior relation of incisors: Normal _____ Linguoversion _____ Labiover-
sion _____ Mixed _____

Diastema: No _____ Yes _____ Mild _____ Moderate _____ Severe _____ Which teeth _____

Missing teeth:

8 7	6 5 4 3 2 1	1 2 3 4 5 6	7 8
8 7	6 5 4 3 2 1	1 2 3 4 5 6	7 8

(Circle)

Condition of dental hygiene: Excellent _____ Good _____ Poor _____

Dental prosthesis: No _____ Yes _____ Partial _____ Complete _____

Adequacy for speech: 1 _____ 2 _____ 3 _____ 4 _____

Tongue

Structure

Size in relation to dental arches: Normal _____ Large _____ Small _____

Atrophy: No _____ Yes _____ Fissures: No _____ Yes _____ Frenum: Normal _____
Short _____

Function

Tremors or fasciculations at rest: Yes _____ No _____

Extension-retraction pattern present: Yes _____ No _____

Describe instructions needed to obtain performance (e.g., imitation, tactile stimulation,
etc.) _____

_____

_____

_____

Protrude: Yes _____ No _____ Deviation: To right _____ To left _____

Lateralize: Right _____ Left _____

Elevate

Tip: Yes _____ No _____ Back: Yes _____ No _____ Relationship of elevation to
lingual frenum and extent of mouth opening _____

_____

Continued.

SPEECH MECHANISM EXAMINATION—cont'd

Tongue—cont'd

	Trials			Rating		
	1	*2*	*3*	*Above av.*	*Av.*	*Below av.*
Number of times can say /tʌ/ in 5 sec (range 3.0-5.5 per sec)[3]						
Number of times tongue can touch alveolar ridge without speech (range 3.5-6.0 per sec)[4]						
Number of times can move tongue tip from one corner of mouth to the other in 5 sec (can use above ranges for average)						
Number of times can say /kʌ/ in 5 sec (range 3.5-5.5 per sec)[2,3]						
Number of times can say /pʌ tʌ kʌ/ in 5 sec (range 1.0-1.75 per sec)[3]						

Description for possible tongue thrust pattern (swallowing)

Extreme tension in muscles of mastication and orbicularis oris: Yes _____ No _____

Lack of contraction of masseter muscle when swallowing: Yes _____ No _____

Tongue protrusion when labial seal is broken: Yes _____ No _____

Adequacy for speech: 1 _____ 2 _____ 3 _____ 4 _____

Hard palate

Width: Normal _____ Narrow _____ Wide _____   Height: Normal _____ Vaulted _____
Low _____

Symmetric: Yes _____ No _____ Explain _____

_____

Color of tissue: Pink _____ Whitish _____ Mottled _____

Cleft: Repaired _____ Unrepaired _____ Submucous _____ Describe degree and condition

_____

_____

Adequacy for speech: 1 _____ 2 _____ 3 _____ 4 _____

Velopharyngeal port mechanism

Structure

Soft palate and uvula

At rest: Deviation _____ Right _____ Left _____

Length of soft palate in relation to depth of oropharynx: Adequate _____ Inadequate _____ Describe _____

_____

SPEECH MECHANISM EXAMINATION—cont'd

Velopharyngeal port mechanism—cont'd

Cleft: Absent uvula _____ Bifid uvula _____ Repaired _____ Unrepaired _____ Describe degree and condition _____

Fauces

Palatoglossus: Present _____ Absent _____ Scarred _____

Palatopharyngeus: Present _____ Absent _____ Scarred _____

Faucial isthmus: Average _____ Large _____ Restricted _____

Tonsils: Normal _____ Atrophied _____ Enlarged _____ Inflamed _____ Absent _____

Function

Velopharyngeal closure: Blow out match _____ Drink from straw _____

Soft palate movement

Prolonged /a/: Elevation pronounced and maintained _____ Elevation pronounced and erratic _____ Moderate movement _____ Slight movement _____ No movement _____ Other _____

Levator dimples: Prominent _____ Slight _____ Absent _____

Short rapid productions of /a/: Elevation pronounced and maintained _____ Elevation pronounced and erratic _____ Moderate movement _____ Slight movement _____ No movement _____ Other _____

Panting: Elevation pronounced and maintained _____ Elevation pronounced and erratic _____ Moderate movement _____ Slight movement _____ No movement _____ Other _____

Gag reflex

Could not be elicited _____

Movement of palate and pharyngeal walls: Vigorous _____ Moderate _____ Slight _____

Symmetric movement: Yes _____ No _____ Other observations _____

Movement of posterior pharyngeal walls (noted under the above activities): Mesially _____ Superiorly _____ Both _____

Pressure ratio: Instrument used_____

	Trials			
	1	*2*	*3*	*Notes*
Nostrils open				
Nostrils occluded				
Obtained ratio				

Continued.

SPEECH MECHANISM EXAMINATION—cont'd

Velopharyngeal port mechanism—cont'd

Comments regarding velopharyngeal closure for speech production _____
_____
_____

Adequacy for speech: 1 _____ 2 _____ 3 _____ 4 _____

Breathing

"Clavicular breathing" noted: Yes _____ No _____

Voluntary control of breathing: Rhythm _____ Inhalation

_____ Exhalation _____ Panting _____

	Trials			Rating		
	1	*2*	*3*	*Above av.*	*Av.*	*Below av.*
Ability to sustain steady exhalation (10 sec)[1]						
Length of time can sustain steady phonation of /ɑ/ or /m/ (10 sec)[1]						

References

1. Westlake, H., Suggested minimum physiological essentials for speech. In *A system for developing speech with cerebral palsied children.* Available from the National Society for Crippled Children and Adults.
2. Bloomquist, B. L., Diadochokinetic movements of nine-, ten-, and eleven-year-old children. *J. Speech Hearing Dis.,* **15,** 159-164 (1950).
3. Sprague, A. L., The relationship between selected measures of expressive language and motor skill in eight-year-old boys. Doctoral dissertation, University of Iowa (1961).
4. Fairbanks, G., and Spriestersbach, D. C., A study of minor organic deviations in "functional" disorders of articulation: 1. Rate of movement of oral structures. *J. Speech Hearing Dis.,* **15,** 60-69 (1950).

Report writing: articles reproduced from Asha

Pathological writing[*]

Mary Virginia Moore[**]

Auburn University

Report writing is defective when it is (1) unintelligible, (2) conspicuous, or (3) causes the reader to be confused. Every professional worker in speech pathology and audiology occasionally reads a clinic report that is built on a rickety skeleton, loosely hung with rambling sentences, and embellished with fancy, empty words. Let us be honest! Every professional worker occasionally writes such a report!

The penalties for pathological writing are much the same as those for pathological speech, with one important addition. The written word remains after the oral word is spent. The case for cleanliness, accuracy, and brevity in the use of English is seldom greater than in clinical writing. Yet, the profession which gives primacy to oral communication sometimes fails miserably in written communication.

Few guidebooks are more helpful in the diagnosis and correction of defective writing than Strunk and White's pithy collection of "Thou shalts" and "Thou shalt nots," *The Elements of Style* (1959). The theme of this small book is a 63-word quotation from the master teacher, William Strunk, Jr., quoted by his master pupil, E. B. White:

Vigorous writing is concise. A sentence should contain no unnecessary words, a paragraph no unnecessary sentences, for the same reason that a drawing should have no unnecessary lines and a machine no unnecessary parts. This requires not that the writer make all his sentences short, or that he avoid all detail and treat his subjects only in outline, but that every word tell.

The authors boldly dictate a series of rules that may serve the hesitant and the timid among us by allowing no leeway for ambivalence. With each rule go "before and after" excerpts of offensive writing and how it may be purged. These examples of unintelligible, conspicuous, or confusing writing might well have been drawn from clinical reports, had Strunk and White been privy to that information.

The Strunk and White dicta may be applied in heavy doses to the ills of report writing. I will discuss the three symptoms of defective writing with Strunk and White prescriptions (italicized), and give illustrations of the before and after treatment.

SYMPTOM: WRITING IS UNINTELLIGIBLE

The first requirement of clinic reporting is that information be accurately transmitted. The goal of "clarity, clarity, clarity" is a moral as well as a literary obligation. (Read *The Moral Obligation to be Intelligible,* Stevens, 1950.) To fall short of intelligibility is of grave concern when

---

[*]From *Asha,* **11,** 535-538 (1969).
[**]Mary Virginia Moore M.S., formerly Coordinator, Speech and Hearing Clinic, Auburn University, Auburn, Alabama.

the welfare of living persons rather than storybook heroes is at stake. Consider the following rules:

Strunk and White Rule: *Use definite, specific, concrete language. Prefer the specific to the general, the definite to the vague, the concrete to the abstract.* The discipline of this rule forces the clinician to report particulars (right column) instead of generalizations (left column):

The child appeared to be mentally retarded.	The child, 10 years, did not match colors, did not hand the examiner three blocks, did not draw a recognizable man.
The mother had little understanding of her child's problem.	The child's mother said that his stuttering was caused by his missing teeth.
The child's speech was characterized by numerous articulation defects especially involving the sibilant sounds.	The child made these errors: s/z, sh/s, and th/sh.

Strunk and White Rule: *Do not take shortcuts at the cost of clarity.* Avoid the use of initials unless they will be easily and accurately translated by all readers. Even the sophisticated reader appreciates having test names written out in full until he gets his bearings.

The PPVT, VSSM, WISC, MLDS and SBIS-LM were administered.	These tests were administered: Peabody Picture Vocabulary Test Vineland Scale of Social Maturity Wechsler Intelligence Scale for Children Stanford-Binet Intelligence Scale, Form L-M

Strunk and White Rule: *A participial phrase at the beginning of a sentence must refer to the grammatical subject.* The sentence in the left column is puzzling. Who administered the Vineland Scale? Who was enuretic?

Administering the Vineland Scale of Social Maturity, the mother admitted that enuresis was still a problem.	Replying to questions on the Vineland Scale of Social Maturity, the mother said that the child was enuretic.

SYMPTOM: WRITING IS CONSPICUOUS

Unintelligibility may strike the mortal blow to good writing, but conspicuousness, like a sub-clinical infection, saps writing of its vitality. Report writing is conspicuous when a reader pays more attention to how the report is written than to what it says. Conspicuousness must be excised without leaving the report dull and stereotyped.

Strunk and White Rule: *Avoid fancy words.* The line between the fancy and the plain, between the atrocious and the felicitous, is sometimes alarmingly fine, Strunk and White warn. It is a question of "ear." Cultivating ear, as every Van Riper student appreciates, is not quick and is not simple. During the ear-training process, the report writer is wise to deliberately avoid an elaborate word when a simple one will suffice. The clinic report must not become a two-page exhibition of the writer's professional vocabulary. The speech pathologist or audiologist comes of age when he declares independence from the mimeographed glossary distributed in Speech Pathology 608. He writes best when he uses vocabulary true to his own experience. How does the ear respond to the following?

The patient exhibited apparent partial paralysis of motor units of the superior sinistral fibres of the genioglossus resulting in insufficient lingual approximation of the palato-alveolar region. A condition of insufficient frenulum development was noted, producing not only sigmatic distortion but also obvious ankyloglossia.	The patient was tongue-tied.

Strunk and White Rule: *Omit needless words. Make every word tell.* Overweight in clinic reports is as undesirable as overweight in women. Strunk and White give the first five reducing hints. The next should also be added to the clinician's writing diet.

the question as to whether	whether
he is a man who	he
call your attention to the fact that	remind you (notify you)
his brother, who is a member of the same firm	his brother, a member of the same firm

due to the fact that	because
the patient, a forty-eight year old male, according to the history given by the mother	Mr. John Jones, age 48, the mother reported
Although it cannot be definitely established, it is quite probable that the patient, in all likelihood, is suffering some degree of aphasia.	The patient is probably aphasic.

Strunk and White Rule: *Express co-ordinate ideas in similar form.* The content, not the style, should protect the clinic report from monotony.

The patient sat alone at six months. At eight months crawling began. Walking was noted at twelve months.	The patient sat alone at 6 months, crawled at 8 months, and walked at 12 months.

Strunk and White Rule: *Do not affect a breezy manner.* "Be professional, serious, sincere in tone" (Johnson, Darley, and Spriesterbach, 1963). Avoid pet ideas and phrases (Huber, 1961). Cultivate a natural rather than a flippant style of writing. To write as one speaks is as artificial as to speak as one writes. But consider Jerger's powerfully presented philosophy, "Write it the way you would say it" (1962).

Would you believe, Ma and Pa had a fuss right in the middle of the interview over when the child began to walk.	The patient's parents disagreed on the date of walking.
The evaluation got off with a bang with the child yelling his head off.	The patient cried when separated from his mother.

SYMPTOM: THE READER IS CONFUSED

The etiology of a confused reader is probably a confused writer. Two possibilities exist when a report is ambiguous. The writer may have a muddy report because his thinking is muddy. This paper does not attempt to deal with the muddy thinker. However, the writer may be thinking clearly. Clear thinking (even, "I don't know") should not be dissipated by fuzzy writing. The Strunk and White rules do speak to this problem:

Strunk and White Rule: *Do not overstate. When you overstate, the reader will be instantly on guard, and everything that had preceded your overstatement, as well as everything that follows it, will be suspect in his mind because he has lost confidence in your judgment or your poise.* The inexperienced clinician is vulnerable to this mistake and is poorly equipped to place superlatives into a frame of reference.

There is no tension in the home.	The father reported no tension in the home.
The patient is absolutely brilliant.	The patient scored 141 on Stanford-Binet Intelligence Scale, presented an all A report card, and was voted "most intelligent" by the high school faculty.

Strunk and White Rule: *Avoid the use of qualifiers. Rather, very, little, pretty—these are the leeches that infest the pond of prose, sucking the blood of words.* The clinician knows other leeches: *somewhat, probably, seems to be, appears, quite, sort of, kind of.* It may give the clinician courage to omit these if he remembers that the clinic report is not and does not purport to be a divine revelation of wisdom. It is not the "pure" truth. It is the truth according to a particular writer. Certainly it must not be overstated but neither should it be a timid collection of "maybes" authored by a Milquetoast.

The patient was very attentive.	The patient was attentive.
She was a pretty good student.	She was a good student.
	or
	She was a mediocre student.
	or
	She had a grade point average of 1.4.
The mother was somewhat reluctant.	The mother was reluctant.
a pretty important rule	an important rule

Strunk and White Rule: *Work from a suitable design.* The blueprint for a clinic report may be supplied by a more experienced architect: Van Riper (1963), Johnson, Spriesterbach, and Darley (1963), Huber (1961), or others. Hopefully it will be adapted for the information that must be transmitted, for the audience who will read the report, and for the peculiarities of the writer. The structure of the report should be flexible, complete, and logical. The design must serve the writer—it is the means to an end rather than the end itself.

> . . . planning must be a deliberate prelude to writing. The first principle of composition, therefore, is to foresee or determine the shape of what is to come and pursue that shape . . . the more clearly he perceives the shape, the better his chances of success. (Strunk and White, 1959)

Strunk and White Rule: *Put statements in positive form. Make definite assertions. Avoid tame, colorless, hesitating, noncomittal language. Consciously or unconsciously, the reader is dissatisfied with being told only what is not; he wishes to be told what is.* Let's go over that last sentence again: Tell what is as well as what is not. If the clinician can delineate the threshold between what a patient can and cannot do, and if he can accurately report this threshold to another person, the danger of a confused or confusing report is negligible.

The child did not know his colors.	The child did not name the colors of the red and blue blocks. He did separate the blocks by color and matched them to other red and blue objects in the room.
The patient did not have good motor control.	The patient stacked two blocks. He did not stack three blocks.
The patient was uncooperative.	The patient did not point to the pictures in the Peabody test. He did point to his nose, mouth, and eyes.

Strunk and White Rule: *Do not inject opinion.* The clinician must amend this law: Do not inject opinion unless it is labeled. Opinion is the reason for the existence of a clinic report. It is not the accumulation but the interpretation of the data that makes the report valuable. The two must be differentiated, however. The reader must know when the reporter is acting as newscaster and when he is a commentator.

John was a late walker.	Mrs. Smith said, "John was a late walker."
	or
	John was reported to walk at 16 months.
	or
	impressions: John was a late walker.

The umbrella, "impressions," is useful equipment for the report writer. Statements that are labeled as impressions can be clearly separated from the data itself.

CONCLUSION

The plague of unintelligible, conspicuous, and confusing writing is attacked by Strunk and White. The recommendations which are illustrated in this paper are only a few of the suggestions made in *The Elements of Style*.

Linguist John Nist, in his chapter "The Future of the English Language" criticizes the puritanical approach of scholars who, "by duty and by conscience," proscribe laws of decent English usage. Nist challenges students of language:

> . . . to encourage creative imagination and inventive language rather than merely to discourage lapses in the logic and violations of the rules.
> . . . to eradicate both the fear of error and the mania for correctness in speaking and writing English.
> . . . to respect function rather than rule in the study and use of English (1966).

Do Strunk and White offer "prejudiced prescriptions" rather than "positive prescriptions?" Do they denounce, forbid, interdict? Are they shackling us with prohibitions and chaining us with the fear of error? Are their rules picayunish and petty?

I don't think so. The power for abandoned writing is rooted in the precision for controlled writing. The "mania for correctness" is most often found in the self-consciousness of the unsure. It is from discipline that freedom grows and from rules that discipline grows.

Strunk and White do not guarantee that adherence to a regime of correct usage will produce writing that is distinguished and distinguishing. They seem to agree that "it is easier to say what cannot be done than what is desirable" (Mukarovsky, 1964). They promise no sugar-coated pill, no wonder drugs. "Writing is, for most, laborious and slow," they warn. "Writing good standard English is no cinch, and before you have managed it you will have encountered enough rough country to satisfy even the most adventurous spirit."

The author is indebted to her colleagues in the Auburn University Speech and Hearing Clinic for isolating the examples of poor writing from her clinic reports and diligently calling them to her attention.

REFERENCES

Huber, J. T., *Report Writing in Psychology and Psychiatry*. N.Y.: Harper (1961).

Jerger, J., Scientific writing can be readable. *Asha,* **4,** 101-104 (1962).

Johnson, W., Darley, F., and Spriesterbach, D. C., *Diagnostic Methods in Speech Pathology.* N.Y.: Harper & Row (1963).

Mukarovsky, J., The esthetics of language. *A Prague School Reader on Esthetics, Literary Structure, and Style,* Paul L. Garvin, Translator, Washington, D.C.: Georgetown Univ. Press (1964).

Nist, J., *A Structural History of English.* N.Y.: St. Martin's Press (1966).

Stevens, N. E., The moral obligation to be intelligible. *Sci. Mon.,* **70,** 111-115 (1950).

Strunk, W., Jr., and White, E. B., *The Elements of Style.* N.Y.: Macmillan (1959).

Van Riper, C., *Speech Correction: Principles and Methods,* 4th ed., Englewoods Cliffs, N.J.: Prentice-Hall (1963).

Scientific writing can be readable*

James Jerger**

Veterans Administration and Gallaudet College

Nowadays scientists have to write in three different styles; one for research proposals, one for progress reports, and one for the serious reporting of research in books and journals.

"Proposalese" is a fairly stereotyped language system in which you must stress, by any means at your disposal, how it is that no one ever thought of this clever idea before in view of its far-reaching theoretical import, as well as its significant implications for imminent clinical practice and rehabilitation. The secret is long words, complicated subordinate clause structures, and good old-fashioned evasion.

In progress reports the problem is how to make it look like you've been doing much more than you really have all these months. The secret is long sentences, the longer and more complicated the better. This gives the reader the impression that at least you have been thinking about these things pretty hard, while at the same time you are tiring him out so rapidly that he doesn't have the energy to go back over it carefully and see exactly what you did.

Both proposalese and progress-report writing are specialized journalistic forms. They have evolved as the best methods for doing a particular job; that is, concealing the actual circumstances in a protective cloud cover of expensive language. The only criteria on which these two styles can be judged are whether you get the grant and whether it is renewed.

There is absolutely no reason why this writing style needs to carry over into the serious reporting of research findings. Here the criterion is whether or not you are getting your message across to the reader. The requirements for success are quite different from the first two areas. In scientific reporting the object is to convey to the reader what you did, why you did it, and what you found. This objective is not always achieved in our Association Journals. I believe that four major problems can be identified. First, sentences are frequently much too long and complicated. Second, language is often painfully artificial. Third, we use the passive voice to excess in verb construction. And, finally, authors are most emphatically discouraged from using the sparkling gems of our language, personal pronouns.

Here is an example of what I mean by long, complicated sentences. This appeared in a recent issue of the *Journal of Speech and Hearing Research:*

> Concerning the motivational component it seems noteworthy to report that several teachers in three different schools for the deaf mentioned to the experimenter that their pupils, when they reach the age of starting in intermediate grades, show a lessing of interest and lack of progress in scholastic achievement.

*From *Asha,* **4,** 101-104 (1962).

**James Jerger, Ph.D., formerly Director of the Auditory Research Laboratory, Veterans Administration, and Research Professor of Audiology, Gallaudet College, Washington, D.C.

Since the sole purpose of this paper is to offer some suggestions for improving the readability of Journal articles, references to many direct quotations are purposely not cited. The editors have assured themselves, however, that each excerpt not cited has, in fact, been published in an Association Journal.

Now this is really three different sentences all wrapped up in one. We can unravel it as follows:

(1) Motivation could be a factor.
(2) Several teachers in three different schools for the deaf mentioned this.
(3) They said that their pupils showed less interest and lack of progress in scholastic achievement when they started the intermediate grades.

This example illustrates an important principle in how to make scientific writing readable. *Write short sentences. Use a new sentence for each new thought.* This sounds vaguely familiar doesn't it; something they told us in the ninth grade or thereabouts? Apparently it was not reinforced on the right schedule.

Here is another example from *JSHD:*

Assessment of the child by the speech pathologist with his training and experience in the physiological and psychological aspects of speech often provides important leads indicating a more refined analysis of psychological variables is needed for a thorough understanding of the speech problems.

If you had trouble with this the first few times through it is because, again, there are three different ideas in the same sentence:

(1) The speech pathologist has training and experience in the physiological and psychological aspects of speech.
(2) By virtue of this training his assessment of the child often provides important leads.
(3) These leads may indicate that thorough understanding of the speech problem requires a more refined analysis of psychological variables.

Long complicated sentences, however, are not nearly as serious a problem as artificiality. A second useful principle in making scientific writing readable is to *write it the way you would say it.* Consider, for example, this sentence from a recent issue of the *JSHR:*

Because of the smallness of the group and the close proximity of its members, the distance variance among the subjects was not considered to be an important factor with respect to the test results.

This style of writing is difficult to read because it is not the kind of English we hear everyday. People just don't talk that way. If the author were telling you about this in person he would probably say something like this:

All subjects were not exactly the same distance away. But the group was small and they were sitting fairly close together; so we didn't think that the slight differences would affect the results.

Here is another example from *JSHD:*

Limitations imposed by the strata from which this sample was drawn preclude the use of the data as normative.

Now can you imagine anyone actually talking this way? Picture two fellows in the locker room. One says to the other, "Limitations imposed by my wife's attitude, preclude my participation in tonight's poker game." The lesson is this. Language that is patently artificial is difficult to read. If you want to make it easier, write the kind of language that people actually use when they talk to each other. Just to prove that no one is immune to this sort of thing, here is a sentence I wrote a few years ago.

Recognizing the constraints necessarily imposed by the small sample sizes, the small number of frequencies, and the particular automatic audiometric instrumentation employed in this study, the following conclusions are offered with respect to automatic audiometric methods in which the subject traces his threshold for a fixed frequency over time by controlling the direction of rotation of a motor-driven attenuator.

That is almost bad enough to build a proposal around. It translates as follows:

We realize that we haven't run very many subjects, and we haven't done too many frequencies, but here is what we found out about automatic audiometry. It only applies to fixed-frequency, Békésy-type tracings.

A third factor that tends to make scientific writing difficult to read is an almost religious dedication to the use of the passive-verb construction. Consider the following example from a recent issue of *JSHR:*

However, if it can be demonstrated that children with articulation problems can learn a newly taught sound task as well as children considered to have normal articulation then it would appear justifiable to assume that present differences in articulation are not a result of the present operation of certain physical and psychological factors.

This sentence is a bit too long and involved to begin with, but notice how much we can improve it by just changing the verb structure:

However, if children with articulation problems can learn a newly taught sound task as well as children considered to have normal articulation, then we can justifiably assume that present differences in articulation do not result from the present operation of certain physical and psychological variables.

I had the good fortune to uncover a monumental string of passive constructions in a recent monograph supplement to *JSHD*.

> With the subject seated in full view of the recording equipment, a tape-recorded speech sample was obtained. First, the tape recorder was turned on and the subject was asked for identifying information such as name, age, level of education and marital status. He was then asked why he had come to college and what previous experience he had had in having his speech recorded. The main purpose of this interview was to accustom the subject to the experimental situation. After two or three minutes of conversation the recorder was turned off and instructions were given for the first speaking performance, the job task. The subject was instructed to perform this task by talking for three minutes or so about his future job or vocation. It was suggested that he tell about the vocation, why he chose it, and anything else about it that he wished to discuss. If the subject had not yet chosen a vocation he was asked to tell about jobs he had held in the past. He was allowed one minute to think about what to say. The recorder was then turned on and the subject was asked to begin speaking.

There is nothing seriously wrong with a passage like this except that it makes insufferably dull reading. As an exercise, try your hand at brightening it up by changing passive constructions (e.g., "was obtained, was asked, was turned off, were given, etc.") to active constructions wherever possible. You might begin something like this:

> The tester seated the subject in full view of the recording equipment, then obtained a speech sample in the following way. First he turned on the tape recorder and asked the subject for identifying information such as . . . etc.

Finally, and perhaps most importantly, nothing livens up dull material like *personal references*. Use them often. Especially, use personal pronouns like I, me, we, you, she, they, etc. Don't use them to excess—the excessive repetition of anything makes dull reading—but don't be afraid to use them when they are clearly necessary in order to say a thing naturally. Here is an example from the same *JSHD* monograph:

> For the reason just mentioned, the regression equation based on 100 samples of speech . . . is not recommended for predicting a single speaker's median rating of severity of stuttering.

Now scientists make a big thing of precision in language, but here is a case where the circumlocution required to avoid the use of a personal pronoun actually degrades precision. The use of this regression equation is "not recommended." Not recommended by whom? By ASHA? By a majority of experts in stuttering? By the author's major professor? No, I think that what the author wanted to say was:

> For the reason just mentioned, *I* do not recommend the use of this regression equation for predicting a single speaker's median rating.

By using the personal pronoun the author makes this sentence not only more readable but more precise.

I will never understand how this compulsion to avoid personal pronouns at all costs in scientific writing ever got started. Scattering them about is one of the easiest ways to make dull prose come alive. Notice how the following sentence—impossibly long and involved by any standards—still sparkles with a personal touch. It is from Galileo's description of the discovery of Jupiter's satellites (3, p. 59):

> On the 7th day of January in the present year, 1610, in the first hour of the following night, when I was viewing the constellations of the heavens through a telescope, the planet Jupiter presented itself to my view, and as I had prepared for myself a very excellent instrument, I noticed a circumstance which I had never been able to notice before, owing to want of power in my other telescope, namely that three little stars, small but very bright, were near the planet.

At this point many of you are undoubtedly feeling that perhaps there is some point to what I have been saying for certain kinds of articles, but the reporting of really intricate, subtle, and significant research findings just has to be written in a dull way. Consider, then, this model of simplicity and clarity in scientific writing by Nobel Laureate Georg v. Békésy (1, p. 371):

> When we compare research with animals to research carried out on man, we see that we are dealing with two quite different situations. With animals we can always start from the normal condition, whereas with man we must first make a diagnosis in order to determine the starting point. Most diseases have more than one symptom, and since the disease may have progressed in any one of several different ways, two cases will rarely have similar starting points. This simple fact indicates that, for effective investigation, interaction must take place between clinical and animal experimentation.

Let's see if we can't take what we've learned so far and rewrite this in a manner suitable for an Association Journal. We can begin by eliminating the offensive personal pronouns, then make the sentences much longer, and finally change the phraseology so that it will impress rather than inform:

> Previous attempts to equate research endeavors concerned with physiological experimentation carried on in the laboratory on animal preparations with psychophysical and psychological behavior of the human organism inevitably suggest the existence of a fundamental multi-dimensionality which cannot be easily resolved or effectively reconciled under present circumstances.
>
> In the case of animal preparations it is preeminently feasible to take as a point of departure the fact that the basic frame of reference encompasses an organism that is initially intact, whereas, in the case of human behavioral investigative techniques, factors intrinsic to the determination of the pre-experimental status of the organism manifestly dictate the necessity for assessment and evaluation of that organism's status with respect to diagnostic categorization. . . . etc., etc.

Well, we could go on and on like that. If you think this is stretching the point at all, consider the following excerpt from a recent issue of *JSHD:*

> Articulatory patterns of speech develop as one aspect of the psychophysical systems encompassing total growth and development of an individual in conjunction with maturation and learning. Articulation is dependent upon a continuous process of development from a simple and homogeneous medium to a highly complex, modified and differentiated level of growth. As a child matures, he must endeavor to make a fundamental adjustment to his intrinsic and extrinsic environments, regardless of what prospects they hold in store for him. Whether or not the child develops acceptable patterns of articulation depends upon numerous complex and multidimensional elements. In the final analysis, it is not practicable to relegate articulatory maturation to any one single variate of growth and development. Actually, competency in articulation

seems to focus upon the extent to which all developmental propensities contribute to the eventuation of speech out of the psychophysical inherent in the human organism. . . .

I would try to translate this for you, but I honestly do not understand what it means.

In summary we can all do four concrete things to improve our writing.

(1) Write short sentences. Use a new sentence for each new thought.

(2) Avoid artificiality and pompous embellishment. Write it the way you would say it.

(3) Use active verb construction whenever possible. Avoid the passive voice.

(4) Use personal pronouns when it is natural to do so.

There are many reasons why it would be to our advantage as a profession to improve the readability of our publications. One of the more important is the fact that you cannot communicate your research findings to other people unless you write about them in a way that allows other people to understand what you are talking about. And communication with other people is, after all, the reason for scientific publications.

Let us bring our unique professional talents to bear on our own communicative disorder.

ACKNOWLEDGMENT

I am indebted to my colleagues, Stanley Zerlin and Laszlo Stein. They contributed their own unique obfuscatory talents to the rewriting of the Békésy passage.

REFERENCES

1. Békésy, G. v., Are surgical experiments on human subjects necessary? *Laryngoscope,* **71,** 367-376, 1961.
2. Flesch, R., *The Art of Plain Talk.* New York: Harper and Bros., 1946.
3. Galilei, Galileo, *The Sidereal Messenger,* 1610. (quoted in Shapley, H., Rapport, S. and Wright, H., *A Treasury of Science.* New York: Harper and Bros., 1943).

Examples for writing clinical reports and parental (client) report letters

THE CLINICAL REPORT

The following are *example* excerpts from reports demonstrating how the various sections of reports may be written. We have provided different types of information within each section. Following the excerpts is an entire example clinical report. The student should return to Chapter 17 for a discussion of what is included within each section, potential ways of ordering the information, and variations that might exist depending on the nature of the client and his problem.

I. Identification

As previously mentioned, this section is generally dictated by the work setting.

II. Statement of the problem

- Mrs. Sam Whaley, age 48 years, was referred to this clinic by Dr. Paul Keller after being diagnosed as having vocal nodules and periodic hoarseness during the 3 months prior to April 1, 1975. Mrs. Whaley reported that she seems to have a mild case of laryngitis and often loses her voice completely.
- James "Michael" Lund, 5 years, 0 months of age, was brought to the speech and hearing clinic by his mother for an evaluation of "unclear" speech. Miss Martha Moore, Director of Services for Exceptional Children in Cobb County, suggested that Mrs. Lund contact the speech and hearing clinic concerning the problem.

During the interview, Mrs. Lund stated that Michael seemed to understand everything said to him but talked infrequently. She further reported that his speech is very hard to understand and he frequently "points" without using speech.
- Rodney McCoy, 7 years, 7 months old, was referred to the University Speech and Hearing Clinic by Mrs. Frances T. Horseman, Public Health Nurse of Clarke County. Since Rodney is not yet in school and has not been provided with a special educational program, Mrs. Horseman wanted further evaluation of speech, hearing, psychological, and educational needs.

III. Background history

- According to Mr. and Mrs. Jen, Herman babbled and cooed during his first 6 months and spoke his first word at 10 months. During the first year, he was not indifferent to sound and responded when he was spoken to. He had acquired some meaningful speech. At 13 months of age Herman contracted bacterial meningitis (see medical history). Following this, Herman's vocalizations consisted of yelling and screeching to attract attention or express annoyance. He became markedly alert to gesture, facial expression, and movement.

Presently, Herman has little meaningful speech, but he does use the words "stop," "mama," and "daddy." He points to things he wants and babbles for objects. He is alert to gestures but does not respond to speech.
- Mrs. Lund stated that Michael babbled and cooed within the first 6 months. The date of Michael's first intelligible word could not be determined. Jargon was used in place of meaningful speech until the age of 2 years. Between the ages of 2 and 3 years single distorted words such as "mama," "boy," and

"girl" were first spoken. Two-word sentences and short phrases have increased in frequency up to the present time.

Mrs. Lund first became concerned about Michael's speech in the summer of 1964. At that time Michael appeared to comprehend the speech of others but spoke very little. Gestures were used in situations where speech was more applicable. Speech was highly distorted and almost unintelligible when attempted. Hesitations and repetitions of single words and sounds were also noted by Mrs. Lund.

• According to a medical report received from Dr. Paul Keller, Mrs. Whaley was seen by him in April, 1975, at which time she complained of periodic hoarseness. On examination she was found to have "very small vocal nodules on the anterior third of her vocal cords bilaterally." She was therefore advised to use her voice as little as possible, and if the nodules persisted, voice retraining was recommended. Mrs. Whaley reported that she took a short vacation at the doctor's suggestion but had to return home sooner than planned because of a family problem. After returning to work, she found it difficult to follow the doctor's orders of vocal rest since she felt that her customers would not understand.

• When Herman was 10 months old, he had severe bronchial pneumonia with fevers up to 104° F. At 13 months of age, December, 1962, he had acute bacterial meningitis accompanied by high fevers (104° F) and convulsions. Herman had 3-day measles at 1 year and a head injury at 14 months of age; both of these conditions were reported to be mild.

• Mrs. Nat had a normal pregnancy with Steve. The length of labor was 23 hours, and instruments were used in delivery. There was no supplementary oxygen required and no evidence of jaundice at birth. Birth weight was 7 pounds, 9½ ounces. No health or feeding problems occurred during the first 2 weeks of life.

• Mrs. Lund reported that labor was induced by drugs because she was 3 weeks overdue. It was feared that serious complications might result if the child was carried for a longer period. Labor lasted 3 hours. No instruments were used, but anesthesia was administered. Birth weight was 9 pounds, 2 ounces, and was regained during the first week. No postnatal problems were reported for the first 2 weeks of life.

Mrs. Lund stated that Michael held his head erect while lying on his stomach at an age comparable to his siblings. Michael sat alone unsupported at 6 months, crawled at 9 months, walked unaided at 16 months, was fed with a spoon at 2 weeks, and was toilet trained while awake at 2 years and while sleeping at 3 years.

• Jeffrey entered Mrs. Richards' kindergarten class in Lapham School on November 12, 1973. Mrs. Richards indicated the following: "Our readiness activities do not spark his interest, and he has shown he needs help with many primary concepts such as color recognition, counting and number recognition, knowledge of shapes, etc."

• During the interview with Mrs. Lund, she reported that Michael is rejected by playmates his age due to "his speech problem." As a result, he tends to play with children younger than himself or alone.

According to Mrs. Lund, Michael is easily frustrated when others fail to understand his speech. It appears to irritate Michael that he cannot talk as well as his 2-year-old brother Billy. Michael becomes very "stubborn" and hard to discipline when such frustrations occur. During these periods Michael chews his fingernails and toenails.

• Mrs. Ober described Jeffrey as a happy child "who likes school and his teacher but is very conscious of talking." Mrs. Richards indicated that Jeffrey has shown "immaturity in social and emotional growth." According to her, "Jeffrey needs firm control because he is impulsive in his actions. He becomes very restless and disturbs other children." She also mentioned that he fidgets, daydreams, and is irresponsible.

• Larry has been seen at the Psycho-Educational Clinic in regard to his learning and behavior difficulties. A report dated January 2, 1974, from Robert Birch stated that Larry obtained an intelligence score of 94 on the *Stanford-Binet Intelligence Scale* (Form L-M). His performance on the *Bender-Gestalt Test for Young Children* and the Graham-Kendall *Memory-for-Designs Test* shows "immature, but adequate, perceptual abilities." The report also states that Larry is an anxious child whose anxiety is "manifest in rapid speech, motor hyperactivity, short attention span, and inability to concentrate for extended periods of time." It is felt that this excessive anxiety underlies Larry's learning difficulties. Larry has been referred to the Dane County Guidance Center for further evaluation and therapy.

IV. Testing and observation

- Rodney went willingly with the examiners. He was responsive to visual stimuli and movement. He attended visually to people moving about the room as well as objects that were new to him. He also responded readily to touch by turning in the appropriate direction and smiling. It was evident throughout this examination that Rodney responded very favorably to human contact, concern, and approval.
- Eleanor separated easily from her parents. Testing was begun with a spontaneous speech sample talking about toys to be unwrapped. The majority of her language consisted of one-word responses, consonant-vowel syllables, or vowel sounds. Approximately 10% of her spontaneous speech consisted of nine two-word phrases: no more, more toy, no toy, big ball, big baby, bye bunny, my book, two eye, and more pow, in descending order of frequency. Total vocabulary output was less than 25 words. Intonation was appropriate and used to indicate a question or a statement.

  The *Peabody Picture Vocabulary Test* (PPVT), Form B, was administered. Without a basal being established, Eleanor received a vocabulary comprehension age of 2 years, 1 month (chronological age of 3 years, 0 months). The reliability of this test is questionable for Eleanor's responses were erratic.

  The *Utah Test of Language Development* yielded a language-age equivalent of 2 years, 2 months. She could follow simple instructions, recognize body parts, recognize the names of common objects, and identify common pictures when named. Expressively, she named two common pictures and used some two-word combinations spontaneously. She did not respond to simple commands, name colors, or identify action in pictures.
- Mrs. Smith was very cooperative and said that she understood the purpose of testing and was willing to do her best. The *Language Modalities Test for Aphasia* designed by Wepman and Jones was administered and the entire test completed. The only errors on the screening section were spelling and articulation; the response for "cat" was "C-A . . . oh, oh, C-A-C," with no response ("I don't know")

to spelling and writing "give." The repetition of words on the screening test was characterized by the production of incorrect phonemes with the exception of the correct production of "seven." Matching of both visual and auditory stimuli to pictures presented few problems for Mrs. Smith; one error was pointing to a picture of two tops instead of one (visual sentence); the second error was pointing to one plant growing rather than to several (visual sentence); the third error was pointing to "these bells ring" for "three bells ring" (auditory sentence). Oral responses showed mainly errors consisting of using an incorrect phoneme usually, but not exclusively, in the initial syllable of a word. Once she got past the first syllable, a sequence of syllables could usually be produced without the pauses that characterized the initiation of the sequence. Graphic responses were either correctly done, not attempted, or not completed after a correct attempt was begun. When Mrs. Smith wrote, she did it slowly, had to use her nonpreferred left hand, and often paused after writing one or more letters. The tell-a-story items evoked responses that were mainly content words containing incorrect phonemes, some phrases that were ended by hesitation, and a few sentences. In general, the stories told by Mrs. Smith were short, did not describe all aspects of the picture, contained many pauses and interjections, and were usually ended by "I don't know" after being urged by the examiner to tell more. According to Wepman and Jones' scoring, the patient exhibited syntactic and some semantic language problems on the tell-a-story items, phonemic and semantic errors on oral responses to visual and auditory stimuli, and correct or "no response" errors on graphic responses to visual and auditory stimuli. In cycles 1 and 2 of the *Language Modalities Test for Aphasia,* about 50% of the oral and graphic responses were correct and only 3 out of 60 matching items were missed.

- Tim went willingly with the examiner and adjusted quickly to the testing situation. He understood all the tasks and worked steadily for over 1½ hours. The following testing procedures were used:
  1. *Peabody Picture Vocabulary Test* (PPVT), Form B
  2. *Vocabulary Usage Test* (VUT)
  3. Wepman's *Auditory Discrimination Test*

4. *Templin-Darley Screening Articulation Test*
5. Hejna's *Developmental Articulation Test*
6. Speech mechanism examination
7. Pure tone air conduction audiometric screening
8. Stimulability testing as well as informal measures for auditory comprehension and retention span, cognitive behavior, and sentence structure

The primary finding was inadequate phonologic development. On the *Templin-Darley Articulation Screening Test* he had one correct response out of 50. Children his age and sex should have approximately 35 correct responses. An analysis of his errors on the sounds tested on both the Templin-Darley and Hejna tests revealed a rather consistent use of the /t/ and /d/ phonemes or these phonemes in combination with another distorted phoneme for most all of the consonant singles and blends. Other phonemes he used correctly with some consistency were /p, b, m, n, k, g/ and occasionally /f and v/. The vowels used were almost always distorted. Another phoneme problem that revealed itself was a pattern of unvoicing a final voiced consonant as in the word "bed." This phoneme pattern resulted in speech that was unintelligible unless the examiner knew the subject matter. (See articulation tests for detailed articulation results.)

- The 50-item screening test and the 43-item *Iowa Pressure Test* from the *Templin-Darley Tests of Articulation* were administered. Donna produced nine correct responses on the screening test. By 12 years of age a perfect score should be obtained. On the *Iowa Pressure Test* Donna produced three correct responses. The *Iowa Pressure Test* includes items selected to assess the adequacy of intraoral pressure for speech production and thus, inferentially, the adequacy of velopharyngeal closure.

  Donna generally produced bilabial plosives in all positions. A velar or pharyngeal fricative was substituted for the linguoalveolar and linguovelar plosives in most positions, while a glottal stop was substituted for medial / k and g/; /t/ was transcribed as correct in the medial position by two examiners, but apparently it was an acoustic approximation. Most fricatives were either omitted or substituted by the velar fricative. /z/ was transcribed in the word 'crayons' by both examiners. /f/ was never produced, although Donna sometimes put her lower lip in contact with the upper central incisors but no sound was produced. Affricates always had the velar substitution. All nasals were produced as were the glides /r/ and /l/ as singles. In the final position the r-colored vowel occasionally had no coloring. Glides were generally produced in two- and three-item consonant clusters; two-item clusters involving any fricative or plosive were always substituted by the velar fricative.

  Varying amounts of nasal emission and nasality accompanied the phonemes that were produced.

  Modifiability was attempted on all plosives, fricatives, and affricates. Even with intensive stimulation involving manipulation of the articulators, /t, d, k, g, / were always substituted by the velar fricative; there was no anterior approximation at all. A fairly good /s and z/ could be produced in isolation; in syllables the tendency was toward a more posterior production. An anterior approximation was achieved on /ʃ, θ, ð, ʒ, tʃ/; /dʒ/ was still produced with a velar substitution.

- Observations of Mrs. Whaley's voice quality were made for different types of vocalizations such as production of isolated vowels /a, i/, reading of words and sentences, and conversational speech. Speaking situations differed in the following ways: the voice was high, then low; the muscles were tensed, then relaxed; the head was bent forward, then backwards. In general her voice quality was hoarse; however, it was much clearer when producing isolated sounds and reading than in conversational speech. Mrs. Whaley was unable to increase the loudness of her voice to any noticeable degree, and when attempts were made, pitch breaks were evident. When speaking softly, she used a "loud whisper," and her voice was as strained as in habitual use.

- A speech mechanism examination revealed a postoperative left unilateral complete cleft of the primary and secondary palates. Some asymmetry of the vermilion border of the lip and depression of the left nares are evident. Asymmetry of the palate is also evident; the left half of the soft palate is more elongated than the right. Two potential fistulas were noted; one in the medial portion of the hard palate, and the second in the posterior aspect of the soft palate. It is not known if these fistulas are complete. The premaxilla is partially collapsed, resulting in a mesiocclusion. The low attachment of the superior labial frenulum is restricting the mobility of the upper lip. The tonsils are present and do not appear inflamed. On phonation of "ah" only slight movement of the soft palate on the left was noted and no lateral wall movement was noted. The oral manometer readings, indicating Maury's ability to build intraoral breath pressure, revealed an average of 3.6 ounces with the nostrils unoccluded and 4.5 ounces with the nostrils occluded. The measure was not considered reliable because of a weak labial closure that allowed air to escape out of the mouth. It does indicate, however, that velopharyngeal closure is probably not complete. Tongue protrusion, lateralization, and elevation were adequate.

V. Clinical evaluation

• From all indications, Mrs. Whaley's voice problem is a manifestation of her difficulties in coping with day-to-day problems. The vocal nodules have apparently resulted from excessive strain and tension brought on by increased responsibilities and greater use of a voice that even in its normal function was not a good speaking voice.

Throughout the interview she displayed signs of general tension, particularly in speech musculature, which probably has some relationship to her voice disorder. Although Mrs. Whaley is aware that she has tensions, she evidently does not understand the possibility of casual relationships between these tensions, her voice abuse, and resulting vocal nodules.

• A review of the case history and evaluation of present speech and language abilities suggests the possibility of brain injury, resulting in both an aphasic disorder and retarded mental development.

The case history gives evidence of the possible occurrence of brain injury. The umbilical rupture and necessity for induced labor serve as possible causal factors. Michael's expressive language problems, reduced attention span, retarded language development, distractibility, difficulties in visual discrimination and relationships, and intense preoccupation with very fine detail are behavioral characteristics indicative of possible central nervous system dysfunction.

Mental retardation was also indicated by many of Michael's behaviors. The *Leiter International Performance Scale* and *Peabody Picture Vocabulary Test* results indicated slow mental development. However, due to the language problems, these test results should be interpreted with caution.

It is therefore believed that Michael should presently be considered as having aphasic problems with an accompanying delay in mental development.

• Donna has a severe articulation-resonation disorder, the main component being production of a velar fricative as a substitution for most plosives, fricatives, and affricates. Her articulation scores on both tests were extremely low and were commensurate with the performance of a normal child 3 years of age and below. Although both parents stated that Donna was easy to understand, this examiner does not concur. Even when the subject was known, intelligibility was below 50%.

The nature and severity of Donna's disorder are the product of many variables. It is generally believed that children cannot improve phonemic production unless they are able to practice and experiment with their articulators. Donna was confined to bed because of her heart problem for the first 4 years. She had major illnesses and surgery throughout her life, significantly the laryngeal operations at 8, 9, and 10 years of age with varying lengths of forced vocal rest. When Donna did learn to speak, she did so with an incompetent mechanism, that is, inadequate velopharyngeal closure. The paralysis of the palate was not discovered until she was 10 years old, and corrective surgery was not performed until the following year. Therefore the patterns of speech that were first developed were perpetuated; that is, the sounds that require a buildup of intraoral pressure could not be produced, so Donna compensated by producing a velar fricative or glottal stop as substitutions. At the present time it seems possible that Donna has *potential* velopharyngeal closure as evidenced by the pressure ratios, her ability to modify some of the speech sounds, and the *Iowa Pressure Test*, which showed that an increase in the number of items in consonant clusters did not affect production.

VI. Diagnosis

• Mrs. Janes has a severe aphasia resulting from a cerebrovascular accident.
• Gary's speech and language problem is very

complex. The case history, previous speech therapy, and the present speech and language evaluation suggest the possibility of an aphasic language disorder and slow mental development stemming from brain injury.

- Grady has a mild articulation disorder associated with tongue thrust.
- Karyn has a severe speech production problem affecting all speech production subprocesses resulting in disordered voice, resonance, prosody, and phonetic structure. This major disorder is associated with the neurologic damage sustained in an automobile accident.
- Jess is delayed in all language abilities; this is apparently related to both intellectual and emotional factors.
- It is felt that Robert's major problem is one of general retardation. However, language comprehension and formulation appear to be poorer than would be expected from the retardation.
- Mr. Natjen has an extremely hoarse voice quality due to ventricular phonation.

VII. Recommendations

- Intensive language stimulation and articulation therapy should be initiated in an effort to prepare Ramon for entrance into school. A group situation with children his age might be especially helpful in preparing him to interact socially in kindergarten.

    Referral for psychological testing is recommended and would best be presented to the parent as an aid in determining Ramon's readiness for school.

    Referral for a dental evaluation would be helpful in planning articulation therapy and in helping the child to have a better facial appearance.

    Parent counseling with Mrs. Jablonski should be continued to help in parental attitudes toward the speech problem and reduce tendencies toward overprotection.

- Voice therapy to begin in the Fall of 1965 and designed to relax muscular tension in the laryngeal area, establish adequate breathing patterns, and alter vocal usage.

    Counseling in regard to the many pressures present in her life that may be affecting vocal use.

    Periodic examinations by an otolaryngologist.

    Periodic audiometric examinations.

    The following recommendations were given to Mrs. Whaley in regard to use of the speech mechanism until therapy can be arranged:

    1. Reduce the amount of coughing and clearing of the throat
    2. Vocal rest
    3. Use soft vocal attacks and breathy voice
    4. Eliminate speaking on residual air

- Because Larry's behavior at this time limits any improvement that could result from speech therapy, a program of speech therapy is not recommended at the present time. It is recommended that Larry be seen by the Dane County Guidance Center for an evaluation of his behavioral problems and recommendations for treatment.

    Following this evaluation and the recommendations made by the Center, further plans for speech therapy can be made. In accordance with their advice a choice can be made between the following possibilities.

    1. If it is felt that treatment of Larry's underlying difficulties will allow him to modify his behavior, speech therapy can be delayed until such modifications have taken place.
    2. If Larry's behavior problems are not felt to be symptomatic of underlying emotional difficulties but are felt to exist independently from such difficulties, speech therapy can begin immediately. If this is the case, attempts will be made during therapy to deal with Larry's behavior as it exists.
    3. Speech therapy for Larry must be directed to correction of articulation errors, elimination of word and sound omissions, and establishment of an appropriate rate of speech. Control must then be developed so that these techniques can be carried over into conversational speech.

CLINICAL REPORT EXAMPLE

November 22, 1975

I. IDENTIFICATION

Name: James Richards
Birth date: October 19, 1965
Parents' name: Mr. and Mrs. James W. Richards
                      1322 Glen Street
                      Belton, Wisconsin
Examined at: United Speech and Hearing Services
                      Belton General Hospital
                      Belton, Wisconsin
Date of examination: October 22, 1975
From: Dr. James Edwards

II. STATEMENT OF THE PROBLEM

James Richards (Ricky) was seen at the United Speech and Hearing Services Clinic (USHS) for speech evaluations and therapy. The present consultation was to determine how much speech progress might be expected with the existing speech mechanism. At this time, Ricky is 10 years of age.

III. HISTORY

A. Medical and surgical history

Ricky was born on October 19, 1965, following a normal pregnancy. The length of labor was approximately 6 hours and no instruments were used in delivery. Birth weight was 6 pounds, 8 ounces. Apparent at birth was an extensive cleft lip and palate. At 1 month of age Ricky was referred to the Cleft Lip and Palate Clinic and has been followed by them since. The original diagnosis of the cleft condition at that time by Dr. Jackson, pediatrician, stated: "Bears a severe cleft on the left side that involves a large portion of the palate. There is some rotation of the dental ridge on the right side of the cleft. The lip and nose are involved in the process."

Ricky's surgical history reveals a cleft lip repair on December 2, 1965, and a cleft palate repair on August 2, 1967. A clinic visit on January 13, 1968 revealed that the palate and lip were closed. Dr. Thompson suggested that "in a few years he will need narrowing of the left nares."

From 1968 to the present, Ricky has been followed by the Cleft Lip and Palate Clinic. Dental treatment has been carried out, but no orthodontic work has been recommended by Dr. Wells. No further surgical procedures have been done although the possibility of narrowing the left nares (Dr. Thompson, 1968), an Abbe Estlander flap (Dr. Thompson, 1971), and work on the upper lip and narrowed "arphis" (Dr. Grimball, 1973) were considered.

In October, 1974, Mr. Poolwall, speech pathologist, indicated limited improvement in speech apparently related to inadequate velopharyngeal closure. (See speech history.) He felt that pharyngeal flap surgery should be considered. In October, 1975, Dr. Grimball concurred. The possibility of pharyngeal flap surgery will be discussed by Dr. Thompson with Dr. Nelson in Madison, Wisconsin.

B. History of speech development and hearing

According to Mr. and Mrs. Richards, Ricky began to say single words at 20 months of age and began using simple sentences at age 22 months. The parents talked baby talk to

Continued.

CLINICAL REPORT EXAMPLE—cont'd

III. HISTORY—cont'd

B. History of speech development and hearing—cont'd

the child but felt that he received much speech stimulation. At times they would anticipate his wants before he could communicate his need. They believe that Ricky's present vocabulary is average but his speech is inferior. They do not feel that Ricky's cleft palate condition interferes with his amount of communication.

On March 14, 1970, Ricky was first seen by a speech pathologist (Mr. Obers, United Speech and Hearing Services). He was unable to get an adequate speech sample, but from the sounds that were heard and the parent's report of speech, he felt that a marked nasality and articulatory involvement were present. Speech therapy was recommended but was not initiated. A reevaluation (Mr. Obers) on May 5, 1971 revealed adequate vowel production but severe sibilant distortions. Speech therapy was again recommended.

Ricky has received periodic speech therapy from June, 1971, to the present time. Therapy has been concentrated around improving articulatory skills by increasing Ricky's ability to direct and control the breath stream. Some nasality and nasal emission have been decreased as a result of this therapy. On June 28, 1975, Mr. Poolwall, speech pathologist (USHS), believed that with Ricky's present inadequate velopharyngeal closure as much speech compensation as possible had taken place. He suggested the possibility of pharyngeal flap surgery. (See medical history.)

Mr. and Mrs. Richards do not believe that Ricky has heard adequately during his development. Previous otologic and audiometric examinations bear this out. A series of air conduction audiograms taken from 1971 to 1973 reveal a mild bilateral hearing loss. An otologic report to the speech clinic in 1972 indicated "fluid in the ears," scarring of the tympanic membrane, and inflammation of the tonsils and adenoids, which were removed at age 5 according to the parents.

C. Educational history

Ricky's parents report that he makes average grades in the fourth grade at Central Grammar School where Mrs. Wicker is his teacher. He attended Marshall School during the first three grades, failing the first grade. He likes school.

D. Personality adjustment

Ricky has many playmates with whom he usually gets along well. He prefers outdoor activities and likes to participate in activities involving others. He belongs to the Cub Scouts. He is taken care of by his grandmother when his mother is away. His parents stated that Ricky is concerned about the "bump on his mouth and he wants to have lips." He doesn't seem shy about it and will talk to other children about this problem when they ask him what is wrong. However, children tease him sometimes and he does mind this.

The other children in the family don't say anything to him about his problem, and they all understand his speech.

E. Family history

Ricky is the oldest of five children. He has three sisters, ages 7, 5, and 3, and a brother who is 20 months old. No speech, hearing, or physical problem is reported for any of the other children. Ricky's mother, who is 27 years old, completed the ninth grade and is a textile worker. His father, who is 30 years of age, also completed the ninth grade. They are both employed at the Belton Yarn Plant where Mr. Richards is a textile supervisor. They own their six and a half room home, which is located within the city limits.

CLINICAL REPORT EXAMPLE—cont'd

IV. TESTING AND OBSERVATION

Selected parts of the *Templin-Darley Test of Articulation* were administered to assess adequacy of articulation.

One of Ricky's primary substitution errors in the initial position was using the nasal /m or n/ sound in place of a sound requiring buildup of oral breath pressure, for example, /m/b, m/s, m/st, m/sm, s̃m/sp, mp̃/spl, mp̃/spr, n/sn, and nl/sl/. This nasal sound substitution error was used primarily in words containing an /s/ sound.

Other errors of substitution in blends in the initial position included: /w/sw, w/kw, w/tw, l/sl, l/kl, r/dr, r/pr, r/kr, r/fr, r/tr, and r/ʃr/. The common error here generally is one of omitting the aspect of the blend that required buildup of oral breath pressure. The /l, r, and w/ are produced correctly according to articulatory position but at times are nasal.

Errors of omission occurred on /p, k, t, d, s, and ʃ / in the initial position, /k, t, s, and ʃ / in the medial position, and /t and s/ in final position. Many of the sounds tested were distorted by nasality and nasal emission.

The errors of omission and distortion reveal that certain sounds are inconsistently produced. The plosives, fricatives, and affricates are at times omitted but when produced are almost always characterized by nasality (∼) or nasal emission (>). All vowels were at times produced nasally. Ricky's best consonant production requiring oral breath pressure was the production of /g/. Whenever Ricky was instructed to try very hard when producing consonant sounds, greater nasality and nasal emission were noted.

In spontaneous speech the above errors tended to make Ricky's speech highly unintelligible unless the context was known. His sentences contained many nasalized vowels, glottals, and some weak consonants.

Integral stimulation revealed that Ricky had only limited ability to modify his production of speech sounds in isolation. Most modifications still resulted in the sound being nasally emitted.

A. Oral examination

Examination of the peripheral speech mechanism revealed a repaired cleft lip and palate with the upper lip being extremely tight. This seems to interfere with protrusion and eversion of the upper lip as Ricky was observed to speak primarily out of the left side of the mouth. Scar tissue is present on both the hard and soft palate. The nasality and nasal emission noted in his speech indicated that he is not attaining proper velopharyngeal closure. Very little movement of the palate was noted on phonation of "ah." The oral manometer was used to obtain an indication of intraoral breath pressure. The average breath pressure with the nostrils open was 10 ounces. The average with the nostrils occluded was 15. This indicates that velopharyngeal closure is not adequate.

B. Hearing examination

An audiometric pure tone air conduction test was administered bilaterally for the frequencies from 250 to 8,000 Hz. The results indicated acuity within the normal range (approximately 10 to 15 dB over the speech frequencies).

V. CLINICAL EVALUATION

Ricky has a severe articulation-resonation problem including errors of substitution, distortion, and omission accompanied by excess nasality and nasal emission. The examination indicates that the problem is primarily related to his inability to obtain the adequate velopharyngeal closure needed to produce speech sounds requiring intraoral breath pressure.

Continued.

CLINICAL REPORT EXAMPLE—cont'd

V. CLINICAL EVALUATION—cont'd

The history of limited success in speech therapy, the present oral manometer readings, the limited palatal movement seen, and his inability to reduce the nasality and nasal emission on sounds under stimulation indicate that his present mechanism is not adequate. It is therefore not expected that much improvement is to be gained with a speech therapy program alone.

Richard was cooperative throughout the testing, and it would seem that his motivation for speech would be high. During the examination, he not only answered questions readily, but conversed easily.

VI. DIAGNOSIS

Ricky has a severe articulation-resonation problem accompanied by excessive nasality and nasal emission resulting from inadequate velopharyngeal closure.

VII. RECOMMENDATIONS

1. Consideration for further surgical or prosthetic procedures to obtain better velopharyngeal closure.
2. Consideration for further surgical procedures to gain better flexibility of the upper lip.
3. Continued audiometric and otologic examinations. Any further hearing loss must be prevented.
4. Speech therapy after the completion of any procedure utilized for obtaining better closure. (NOTE: Ricky should be evaluated carefully after the procedures for closure have been completed. His ability to produce each sound must be noted as well as his ability to modify any incorrect sounds. Speech therapy must proceed with direction if it is to be successful.)

James Edwards, Ph.D.
Speech Pathologist

THE PARENTAL (CLIENT) REPORT LETTER

This report is generally a brief letter to the parents or the client and should be worded so that they understand most of the terms used. Remember, however, that these reports follow your discussions with the parents or client during the interpretive conference. They should not include information that has not been previously discussed, unless you indicated during the interpretive conference. They should would be provided.

These reports in some way should incorporate the following:

1. Identification of the client
2. When and where the client was examined
3. The results of the examination
4. The diagnosis
5. Possible causal and related factors
6. The recommendations
7. The action being taken

Dear Mr. and Mrs. Rostar:

As you know, Leon was seen in our clinic on November 19, 1975. At this time we tried to find out what Leon's problem might be. At present we feel that it may be related to a hearing loss; however, we are not certain. We need to see Leon for regular observations and testing. We would like to start this as soon as possible beginning in December. Before that time you can help us a great deal by finding out as much as you can about his hearing. We would like for you to tell us such things as what he does when you tell him to do something such as "Look for your shirt," or whether or not you have to point to things you want him to get, and how much attention he pays to your face when you talk, etc. Thank you very much for your help, which will aid us in helping Leon.

We will let you know when we can begin seeing Leon on a regular basis.

If you have any questions or need help with Leon, please call Miss Josephine.

Dear Mrs. Whaley:

As you know, our voice examination results revealed that your voice has a hoarse quality that is a result of the vocal nodules and related to the increased amount of tension present in your life.

We feel that voice therapy beginning in 2 months when you return from vacation will be helpful in teaching you a better voice quality and reducing the amount of vocal misuse resulting from the increased muscular tension. Until then, however, we would like to remind you of the following recommendations in regard to the use of your voice:

1. Reduce the amount of coughing and clearing of the throat.
2. Talk as little as possible, especially under strained conditions.
3. Begin your words with a breathy voice and continue talking with this breathy quality.
4. Remember to take another breath of air rather than to talk when you are out of breath.

We will notify you in September to schedule voice therapy.

If we fail to contact you or if you have any questions concerning your problem, please feel free to call us.

Dear Mr. and Mrs. Whitney:

As you know, Scott was seen in our clinic on February 11, 1975. At that time we found that he has a problem of delayed use of sounds characterized by sound substitutions, omissions, and distortions. We found that his vocabulary comprehension is adequate for a child of his age. As you had pointed out, he is using his tongue inappropriately during conversation.

We also noted that Scott had some negative reactions to speech as evidenced by his responding with "I don't know" and "I don't want to." He also asked the examiner to name a number of objects that probably were familiar to him rather than having to name them himself. We believe that he may feel that his speech is inadequate or not understandable to the listener; thus the negative reactions on his part.

We recommend speech therapy and are placing Scott's name on the waiting list. In the meantime, we would suggest that you reinforce his speech with correct words rather than repeating his errors; for example, if he says, "Where's my 'woo' (for shoe)?" respond with the word in a sentence such as "Let's look for your shoe, Scott," etc. It is recommended that he never be forced to say a word correctly. At his age he probably is not ready to produce some of the more difficult sounds such as (ch) and (sh). Also, he should not be given directions as to tongue placement for certain sounds with which he is having difficulty.

Attention to Scott's speech can be given indirectly through certain activities such as looking at pictures and books together and letting him make responses when he wishes. Spontaneous responses, without pressure, should be acceptable in every situation.

We feel that maturation, along with reducing any pressures regarding speech, and a therapy program would indicate a favorable prognosis for Scott.

We will contact you concerning a therapy schedule for him.

If you have any questions, please do not hesitate to call or write.

Dear Mr. Herber:

As you know, your daughter Donna Kay was brought to the Speech and Hearing Clinic on November 5, 1975, by her grandmother Mrs. Hart for a speech evaluation. Results of our examination indicated that Kay has a severe articulation problem accompanied by excessive nasality. A test of hearing also indicated a moderate hearing loss in both ears. Kay was found to be below average for her age in vocabulary comprehension; she does not understand as many words as she should for a child her age.

Our main concern at the time of the evaluation was to try to find a reason for Kay's excessive nasality. An examination of her speech mechanism indicated that Kay has a very immobile soft palate. This makes it difficult, if not impossible, for Kay to get enough closure in the back part of her mouth to keep sounds from coming out of her nose. It is our belief that this lack of movement of the palate may be caused by a physical abnormality in that area. We want Dr. George Erwin to see Kay again to help us determine any physical problems she may have. Dr. Erwin will advise you concerning further medical examinations for Kay. In the meantime, we will arrange for Kay to be seen in our clinic for more extensive hearing tests and for tests to determine any special educational needs.

We will advise you as to a time that Kay can be scheduled for the two examinations in our clinic. We do feel that Kay's speech can be improved and that we will be better able to help her after the other examinations have been made.

Dear Mr. and Mrs. Bobkoff:

As you know, Juan was seen in our clinic on July 20, 1973, for a speech evaluation. At that time, a test was administered to assess Juan's use of speech sounds. Certain sounds were found to be in error; however, we are not overly concerned about the errors at this time because Juan is just about 3 years old, and his sound system will still be developing for several more years. With maturation the sounds should be correctly incorporated into his sound system.

Since you were most concerned about Juan's "stuttering" behavior, the major portion of the evaluation time was spent in evaluating Juan's spontaneous speech. Before discussing the results obtained from this speech sample, we would like to review in a general way, the development of speech in children. Rather than using the term "stuttering," we will refer to the behavior of hesitating on words or repeating words or sounds as "disfluent" speech. All normal children in the process of acquiring speech and language hesitate and repeat on words. Young children must, within the space of several years, acquire a complex language system. From the one-word level of a 1-year-old, they progress through several stages until they are speaking in complex sentences. During their second year, children learn simple and compound sentences. Their speech rhythm is often broken. Many children use gestures and other substitutive behavior while they are developing a growing vocabulary. During the third and fourth years, the length of sentences increases, and parts of speech such as pronouns, prepositions, and conjunctions are added. Many children of 3 and 4 years of age do not have the vocabulary, the articulation skills, or the facility with grammar to keep their fluency or speech rhythm up to adult standards. Children may try to master the adult patterns of speech too quickly and their attempts may be marked with disfluencies. It is similar to children tripping themselves when they try to run when they are just learning to walk.

Juan is still at the age of acquiring a language system. If one compared him to an adult speaker, his disfluent behavior might seem excessive. However, it is important to remember that he is not an adult speaker. Children lack both the fine muscular ability and the knowledge of a complete language system that adults have. It is also important to remember that all children acquire this ability at different rates, while still being within normal limits.

There are some conditions that have been thought to increase the amount of disfluent speech. Examples are a lowered physical vitality or sickness, lack of sufficient sleep and rest, competition with another child, a feeling of not being loved or wanted by one or both parents or a teacher, overprotection by a parent or another person, an aggressive or domineering person in the home or school, and the expectation of too much from a child either at home or at school. It is known, too, that disfluent speech varies with situations of emotional stress. It may increase at times when the speaker feels fear, insecurity, or excitement.

When Juan was playing with the examiner, his spontaneous speech had very few disfluencies. Later, he seemed excited to be with you again, and when he talked to you, we did hear the repetitions that you had described to us. Your telling us that Juan is most disfluent when he is tired, excited, or talking at the same time as his brother was also helpful to our assessment of Juan's speech. Because of his young age and because so much of Juan's speech does run smoothly, his disfluencies cannot be classified as excessive at the present time. We feel, however, that you were very wise to bring him in for an evaluation because at a later time, should this behavior continue, it might be significant. Although Juan's disfluencies are not a serious problem, we do have several suggestions for you that may help his speech develop normally without excessive repetitions.

It has been found that disfluent speakers are often very fluent when they feel secure and relaxed. You have already noted this, for Juan speaks smoothly when playing quietly. By your appearing calm and relaxed about Juan's speech, you can set an atmosphere that will help him to also feel calm and relaxed about his own speech. It is important to avoid giving undue attention to any periods of disfluent speech. Therefore it would be helpful to avoid discussing his speech with anyone in Juan's presence and also to avoid saying directly to him such statements as, "Stop and begin again" or "don't talk so fast." (Many 3- and 4-year-old children speak very fast because they want to say so much at one time.) Similarly, do not try to speak for him or supply him with a word or phrase. Just wait until he finishes what he is saying. Honest, sincere praise for tasks well accomplished will help a disfluent child feel more competent and important and help bolster his feelings of security and accomplishment.

The most important thing is that Juan continue to enjoy talking and to have the opportunity to share his feelings and experiences with those who are important to him. Always listen to Juan and allow him to talk when he wants to without pressuring him to talk by asking excessive questions. Your practice of preventing competition between your two sons by giving each a turn to speak when they begin talking together is a good one, so keep it up.

Because disfluencies are less frequent when Juan is relaxed and calm, it would be a good idea to set aside a short period of time during the day when Juan could be alone with you just to talk together. Early in the morning, after lunch, or perhaps right before bedtime might be suitable for this "quiet talking time." You can just chat, or talk about pictures, or play a quiet game together. You did this very naturally at the center when we asked you to play with Juan. It will give Juan a chance to talk when calm and relaxed, a break from the normal excitement of a little boy's day. Both of you could spend this time with Juan if you have time or perhaps you could take turns.

We hope that these suggestions will assist you in working with Juan. The center will contact you in 6 months to schedule a reevaluation time so that we can see how Juan is progressing. If, before then, you notice that Juan's disfluencies are becoming much more frequent, you can call the center and the appointment can be set up at an earlier time. Should you have any questions, please do not hesitate to get in touch with us.

Author index

Index